AANN's Neuroscience Nursing

Phenomena and Practice
Human Responses to Neurologic Health Problems

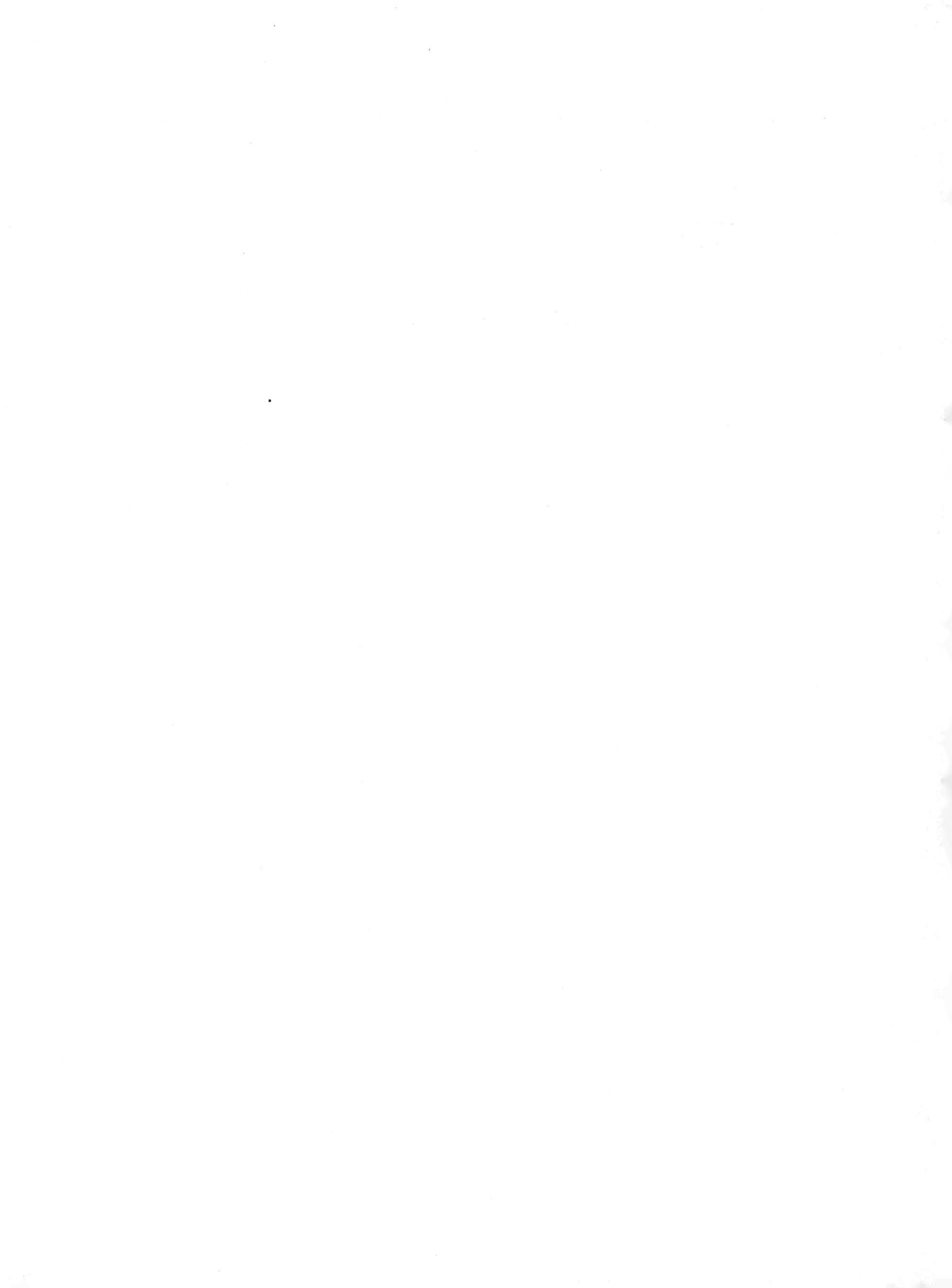

AANN's Neuroscience Nursing

Phenomena and Practice
Human Responses to Neurologic Health Problems

EDITED BY

Pamela Holsclaw Mitchell, R.N., M.S., CNRN, FAAN
Professor, Department of Physiological Nursing
University of Washington
Seattle, Washington

Linda C. Hodges, R.N., Ed.D.
Associate Dean for Academic Programs
University of North Carolina at Greensboro
Greensboro, North Carolina

Marylou Muwaswes, R.N., M.S., CNRN
Assistant Clinical Professor, Department of Physiological Nursing
University of California, San Francisco
San Francisco, California

Connie A. Walleck R.N., M.S., CNRN
Associate Director of Clinical Nursing
The Maryland Institute for Emergency Medical Services Systems
Baltimore, Maryland

APPLETON & LANGE
Norwalk, Connecticut/San Mateo, California

0-8385-0038-2

Notice: Our knowledge in clinical sciences is constantly changing. As new information becomes available, changes in treatment and in the use of drugs become necessary. The author(s) and the publisher of this volume have taken care to make certain that the doses of drugs and schedules of treatment are correct and compatible with the standards generally accepted at the time of publication. The reader is advised to consult carefully the instruction and information material included in the package insert of each drug or therapeutic agent before administration. This advice is especially important when using new or infrequently used drugs.

Copyright © 1988 by Appleton & Lange
A Publishing Division of Prentice Hall

All rights reserved. This book, or any parts thereof, may not be used or reproduced in any manner without written permission. For information, address Appleton & Lange, 25 Van Zant Street, East Norwalk, Connecticut 06855.

88 89 90 91 92 / 10 9 8 7 6 5 4 3 2 1

Prentice-Hall International (UK) Limited, *London*
Prentice-Hall of Australia Pty. Limited, *Sydney*
Prentice-Hall Canada, Inc., *Toronto*
Prentice-Hall Hispanoamericana, S.A., *Mexico*
Prentice-Hall of India Private Limited, *New Delhi*
Prentice-Hall of Japan, Inc., *Tokyo*
Simon & Schuster Asia Pte. Ltd., *Singapore*
Editora Prentice-Hall do Brasil Ltda., *Rio de Janeiro*
Prentice-Hall, *Englewood Cliffs, New Jersey*

Library of Congress Cataloging-in-Publication Data

AANN's neuroscience nursing.

  1. Neurological nursing.   I. Mitchell, Pamela Holsclaw, 1940– .   II. American Association of Neuroscience Nurses.   III. Title: Neuroscience nursing.   [DNLM: 1. Nervous System Disease—nursing. 2. Nursing Assessment.   WY 160 A111]
RC350.5.A22   1988   610.73'68   88-16706
ISBN 0-8385-0038-2

Design: M. Chandler Martylewski
Production Editor: Monica L. Messina

PRINTED IN THE UNITED STATES OF AMERICA

Contents

Contributors ix
Preface xiii

PART I. NEUROSCIENCE NURSING IN MODERN HEALTH CARE

1. The Scope of Neuroscience Nursing
   Connie A. Walleck 3

2. Human Responses: The Phenomena of Neuroscience Nursing
   Pamela H. Mitchell and Linda C. Hodges .9

3. Common Neurologic Health Problems: The Phenomena of Neuroscience Medicine
   Pamela H. Mitchell and Glenna A. Dowling 19

4. Nursing Management Strategies: An Overview
   Mariah Snyder 41

PART II. PHENOMENA CENTRAL TO NEUROSCIENCE NURSING

Section 1. Consciousness Phenomena

5. Consciousness: An Overview
   Pamela H. Mitchell 57

6. Decreased Behavioral Arousal
   Pamela H. Mitchell 67

7. Abnormally Increased Behavioral Arousal
   Mariah Snyder 85

8. Intermittent Loss of Arousal
   Judith Ozuna 99

9. Rhythmic Alterations in Consciousness: Sleep
   Mary A. Chuman 115

Section 2. Cognition Phenomena

10. Cognition: An Overview
Barbara Boss 137

11. Assessment of Cognition
Margarethe Cammermeyer 155

12. Alterations in Memory
Rebecca Sisson 171

13. Alterations in Cognitive Processing
Sister Callista Roy 185

Section 3. Communication Phenomena

14. Communication Disorders: An Overview
Roberta Schwartz-Cowley and William R. Roth 213

15. Management of Neurogenic Communication Disorders
Roberta Schwartz-Cowley and Andrew K. Gruen 231

Section 4. Affiliative Relationships Phenomena

16. Affiliative Relationships: An Overview
Catherine Ecock Connelly 247

17. Alterations in Affiliative Relationships
Susan A. Sutcliffe 259

Section 5. Mobility Phenomena

18. Human Mobility: An Overview
Linda C. Hodges and Christine Callihan 269

19. Assessment of Human Mobility
Ann D. Hollerbach 283

20. Abrupt Alterations in Mobility
Jeanette C. Hartshorn and Mary Gokey 303

21. Chronic Alterations in Mobility
Katharine M. Donohoe, Charlyne Miller, and Brenda Craig 319

22. Swallowing Dysfunction in Patients with Altered Mobility
Roberta Schwartz-Cowley and Andrew K. Gruen 345

Section 6. Sensation Phenomena

23. Sensation: An Overview
Judith A. Metcalf 359

24. Alterations in the Special Senses
Sharon A. Bray 373

25. Alterations in Peripheral Senses
Carol Gohrke Blainey 385

26. Pain: Acute and Chronic
    Nancy Wells 397

Section 7. Elimination Phenomena

27. Elimination: An Overview
    E. Elaine Lloyd, Janet Giroux, and Linda Toth 419

28. Alterations in Bladder Elimination
    Janet Giroux 431

29. Alterations in Bowel Elimination
    Linda L. Toth 441

Section 8. Human Sexuality Phenomena

30. Human Sexuality: An Overview
    Nancy F. Woods 459

31. Alterations in Human Sexuality
    Nancy F. Woods 471

Section 9. Self-Care Phenomena

32. Self-Care: An Overview
    Margaret Auld Bruya 483

33. Alterations in Self-Care
    Christina Mumma 489

Appendix: Neuroscience Nursing Practice

Process and Outcome Standards for Selected Diagnoses
*American Nurses Association Council on Medical-Surgical Nursing Practice and
American Association of Neuroscience Nurses* 501

Index 519

Contributors

EDITORS

Pamela Holsclaw Mitchell, R.N., M.S., CNRN, FAAN
Professor, Department of Physiological Nursing
University of Washington
Seattle, Washington

Linda C. Hodges, R.N., Ed.D.
Associate Dean for Academic Programs
University of North Carolina at Greensboro
Greensboro, North Carolina

Marylou Muwaswes, R.N., M.S., CNRN
Assistant Clinical Professor, Department of Physiological Nursing
University of California, San Francisco
San Francisco, California

Connie A. Walleck R.N., M.S., CNRN
Associate Director of Clinical Nursing
The Maryland Institute for Emergency Medical Services Systems
Baltimore, Maryland

CONTRIBUTORS

Carol Gohrke Blainey, R.N., M.N.
Associate Professor, Department of Physiological Nursing
University of Washington
Seattle, Washington

Barbara Boss, R.N., Ph.D.
Professor, School of Nursing
University of Mississippi Medical Center
Jackson, Mississippi

Sharon A. Bray, R.N., M.S.
Clinical Nurse Educator
Critical Care and Heart, Lung, and Blood Nursing Service
National Institutes of Health
Bethesda, Maryland

Margaret Auld Bruya, R.N., D.N.Sc.
Associate Professor, Intercollegiate Center for Nursing Education
Spokane, Washington

Christine Callihan, R.N., Ph.D.
Assistant Professor, College of Nursing
Medical University of South Carolina
Charleston, South Carolina

CONTRIBUTORS

Margarethe Cammermeyer, R.N., M.A., CNRN
Neuroscience Clinical Nurse Specialist
American Lake Veteran's Administration Hospital
Tacoma, Washington

Mary A. Chuman, R.N., D.N.Sc., Ph.D.
Department of Physiology and Department of Psychiatric Nursing
Multiple Sclerosis Research Center
Rush–Presbyterian–St. Luke's Medical Center
Chicago, Illinois

Catherine Ecock Connelly, R.N., D.N.Sc.
Associate Professor and Associate Dean for Graduate Programs
School of Nursing
George Mason University
Fairfax, Virginia

Brenda Craig, R.N., M.S.
Assistant Professor, College of Nursing
Medical University of South Carolina
Charleston, South Carolina

Katharine M. Donohoe, R.N., M.S.
Doctoral Student, School of Nursing
Clinician, Department of Neurology
University of Rochester
Rochester, New York

Glenna A. Dowling, R.N., M.N., Ph.C.
Doctoral Student, School of Nursing
University of Washington
Seattle, Washington

Janet Giroux, R.N., M.S.
Research Staff Nurse, Spinal Cord Injury Center
Veteran's Administration Medical Center
Palo Alto, California

Mary Jordheim Gokey, R.N., M.S.N., CCRN, CNRN
Adjunct Professor of Nursing
Tri College University Nursing Program
Concordia College
Moorhead, Minnesota

Andrew K. Gruen, M.S., CCC-SLP
Clinical Speech–Language Pathologist, Speech–Communications Disorders Program
The Maryland Institute for Emergency Medical Services Systems
University of Maryland Medical System
Baltimore, Maryland

Jeannette C. Hartshorn, R.N., Ph.D., CCRN
Assistant Professor, College of Nursing
Medical University of South Carolina
Charleston, South Carolina

Ann D. Hollerbach, R.N., M.N.
Associate Professor, College of Nursing
Medical University of South Carolina
Charleston, South Carolina

E. Elaine Lloyd, R.N., M.S., C.S.
Clinical Nurse Specialist, Spinal Cord Injury Center
Veteran's Administration Medical Center
Palo Alto, California

Judith A. Metcalf, R.N., M.S.N.
Formerly, Clinical Specialist, Intermediate Neuro Care Unit
Thomas Jefferson University Hospital
Philadelphia, Pennsylvania

Charlyne Miller, R.N., M.S.
Instructor of Nursing and Neurology
Clinician, Department of Neurology
Schools of Nursing, Medicine, and Dentistry
University of Rochester
Rochester, New York

Christina M. Mumma, R.N., Ph.D., CCRN
Clinical Nurse Specialist, Neurology and Rehabilitation
Providence Medical Center
Seattle, Washington

Judith Ozuna, R.N., M.N., CNRN
Clinical Nurse Specialist, Neurology
Seattle Veteran's Administration Hospital and Medical Center
Seattle, Washington

William R. Roth, M.S., CCC-SLP
Clinical Speech–Language Pathologist, Speech–Communication Disorders Program
The Maryland Institute for Emergency Medical Services Systems
University of Maryland Medical System
Baltimore, Maryland

Sister Callista Roy, R.N., Ph.D.
Professor, School of Nursing
Boston College
Chestnut Hill, Massachusetts

Roberta Schwartz-Cowley, M.Ed., CCC–SLP
Director, Speech–Communication Disorders Program
The Maryland Institute for Emergency Medical Services Systems
University of Maryland Medical System and Montebello Rehabilitation Hospital
Baltimore, Maryland

Rebecca Sisson, R.N., Ph.D.
Assistant Professor, Department of Physiological Nursing
University of California of San Francisco
San Francisco, California

Mariah Snyder, R.N., Ph.D.
Professor, School of Nursing
University of Minnesota
Minneapolis, Minnesota

Susan A. Sutcliffe, R.N., M.S.N.
Vice President, Nursing
Roanoke-Chowan Hospital
Ahoski, North Carolina

Linda Toth, R.N., M.S., CCRN
SCI Nurse Practitioner, Rehabilitation Clinical Nurse Specialist, Spinal Cord Injury Center
Veteran's Administration Medical Center
Palo Alto, California

Nancy Wells, R.N., M.N., Ph.C.
Doctoral Student, School of Nursing
Boston University
Boston, Massachusetts

Nancy Fugate Woods, R.N., Ph.D., FAAN
Professor and Chair, Department of Parent Child Nursing
University of Washington
Seattle, Washington

Preface

Neuroscience nursing is simultaneously a highly specialized and a highly generalized field. It is specialized in the knowledge that one must possess to nurse skillfully persons with nervous system disorders. At the same time, nervous system disorders affect the totality of human experience, so that the neuroscience nurse must understand the integrated generalized experience of ill human beings. Although the specialized care of people with disorders and dysfunctions of the nervous system is often viewed as difficult and esoteric, it is really the most fundamental of all nursing care. The phenomena most relevant to neuroscience nursing concern such human responses as consciousness, thinking, mobility, breathing, eating, and emotion. These are categories of human functioning that organize our understanding of human responses to any set of life events, developmental stages, or illness categories. The purpose of this book is to help nurses make that link between the specialized aspects of caring for persons with neurologic disorders and the generalized nursing model of assisting persons in adapting their biologic and psychosocial responses to actual or potential illness.

This is a book in evolution. It began when the Board of Directors of the American Association of Neuroscience Nurses recognized a need for a comprehensive text to aid nurses caring for persons with neurologic illness. They commissioned the editors to develop such a book, under the auspices of the specialty organization. At the same time a number of textbooks addressing care of persons with specific neurologic disorders were published and it became evident that what was now needed was a book to bridge the gap between medical and nursing models for understanding the phenomena of clinical neuroscience.

The phenomena of neuroscience nursing articulate with, but are different from, those of neuroscience medicine. Neuroscience medicine (neurology, neurosurgery, neuroradiology, neuropathology, etc.) is primarily concerned with the phenomena of diseases and disorders of the nervous system. In contrast, neuroscience nursing is primarily concerned with *human responses* to such actual or potential disorders and dysfunctions. The editors and the American Association of Neuroscience Nurses believe that the nursing literature is adequately supplied with clinical reference texts that demonstrate the articulation of nursing care with the diseases that provide the distinguishing phenomena for neuromedical care. There is a need, however, for a comprehensive text that is organized around major concepts comprising nursing phenomena and relating nursing phenomena and diagnoses with the associated medical phenomena and diagnoses. This book intends to demonstrate that articulation between neuroscience nursing and neuroscience medicine.

This text is organized around nine phenomena considered central to the practice of neuroscience nursing by the America Association of Neuroscience Nursing and expressed in its conceptual framework. Standards of practice have been formulated by the American Nurses' Association and the American Association of Neuroscience Nurses for seven of those phenomena. We make several assumptions in organizing the book around human response phenomena rather than around the more common disease entities that occur in people whom we nurse. First, we believe that nursing practitioners have access to many texts which describe relevant nursing care for people with a variety of nervous system diseases and disorders. On the other hand, many practitioners do not have ready access to text materials organized by the human response, or nursing model. The dilemma for nurses practicing in modern health care systems is that entry to these systems is predicated on receiving a medical diagnosis. One of the first pieces of information we have about a person is the name of the disease or disorder, that is, the health problem. Yet, if our nursing task is to assist that person with the human responses to that health problem, the name of the disease may not be the best way to organize our knowledge. The purpose of this book is to help nurses make that blend between organizing knowledge necessary for clinical care around the client's medical diagnosis (or affected body system) and organizing it around the human responses people have to health problems—specifically, responses to health problems that affect the nervous system.

Consequently, because of its purpose, this book is organized around nine phenomena: consciousness, mentation, communication, affiliative relationships, mobility, sensation, elimination, sexuality, and self-care. Each phenomenon constitutes a section of the book, with each section broken into chapters that discuss the characteristics of the overall concept or phenomenon, the assessment or measurement of relevant clinical aspects of the phenomenon, specific alterations in functioning (nursing diagnoses) that stem from neurologic disorders, and the management of those human responses. Case studies are used in each section to illustrate specific nursing diagnoses that are part of the larger phenomena. Medical diagnoses that commonly activate or coexist with the nursing diagnoses are listed illustratively in each chapter. In addition, Chapter 3 summarizes these diagnoses as common health problems that elicit human responses of interest to nursing. This chapter serves as a cross-referencing device to allow the reader to locate nursing diagnoses relevant to a specific medical diagnosis.

We believe that neuroscience nursing is not limited to acute care hospitals, but exists wherever persons with neurologic dysfunction are found—in hospitals, rehabilitation centers, nursing homes, clinics, and in their own homes and communities. Therefore, the phenomena of interest, the related human responses (nursing diagnoses) and management, are discussed with respect to the focus of care (individual, family, community) and the spectrum of care delivery. Further, nursing management is discussed both from the perspective of the nurse generalist (the nurse who works with general populations and sometimes cares for persons with neurologic problems) and the nurse in specialized neuroscience settings.

The book is directed primarily to nurses with experience in neuroscience nursing. It will also be of interest to nurses who occasionally encounter individuals with nervous system problems. We hope it will be of more than passing interest to scholars of nursing who seek to understand the phenomena addressed by nurses in the clinical arena. As the profession and its specialized branches interact more clearly with the nature of nursing phenomena, this text will evolve to an increasingly precise record of the nature of neuroscience nursing practice. We regard this book as a pioneering effort in the initial articulation of the core of that practice.

Pamela H. Mitchell
Linda Hodges
Marylou Muwaswes
Connie Walleck

for the
American Association of Neuroscience Nurses
Chicago, Illinois, 1988

PART I
Neuroscience Nursing in Modern Health Care

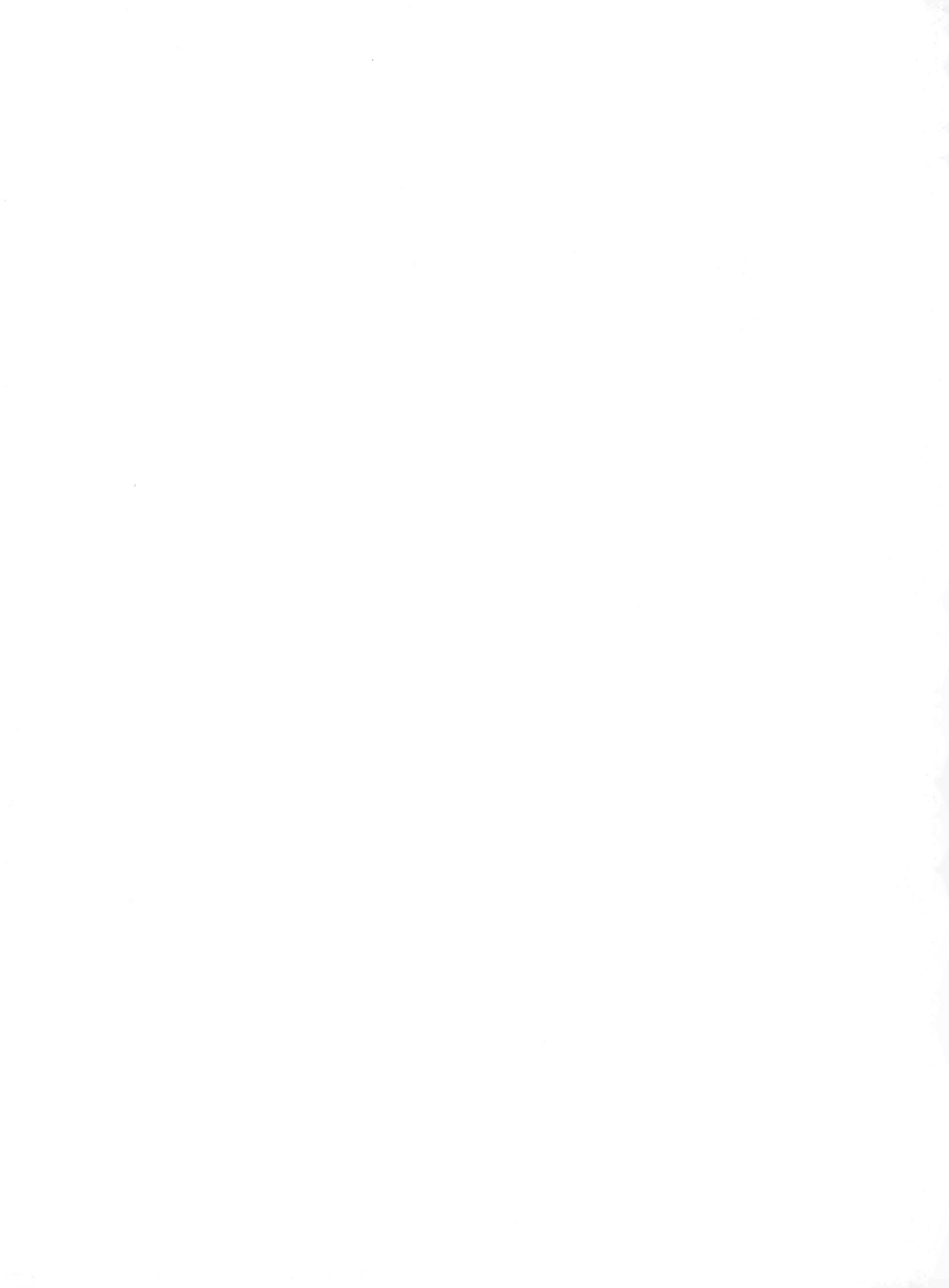

1

The Scope of Neuroscience Nursing

Connie A. Walleck

NEUROSCIENCE NURSING PRACTICE IN RELATIONSHIP TO THE PROFESSION

Nursing has been striving to be recognized as a profession since its beginnings. Questions such as "What is nursing?" "What do nurses do?" "What is nursing practice?" are being asked today as they were a century ago. Nursing is at last beginning to explore and answer these and other questions. In 1980, the American Nurses' Association (ANA) published a document entitled, *Nursing: A Social Policy Statement*, in which the nature and scope of nursing practice and the characteristics of specialization in nursing were delineated. This document is intended as a fundamental and undergirding delineation, providing a foundation that promotes unity in nursing by a basic and common approach to practice. It provides enabling definitions and descriptions, seeking to clarify the direction in which nursing has evolved and to provide a means for distinguishing between desirable and undesirable directions for future development (ANA, p. 1).

Historically, the focus of nursing has been on the individual's optimal functioning in the environment. In Florence Nightingale's *Notes on Nursing: What It Is and What It Is Not*, published in 1859, nursing was defined as having "charge of the personal health of somebody . . . and what nursing has to do . . . is to put the patient in the best condition for nature to act upon him" (Nightingale, 1946). Almost 100 years later, Virginia Henderson defined nursing as an action:

> to assist the individual, sick or well, in the performance of those activities contributing to health or its recovery (or to a peaceful death) that he would perform unaided if he had the necessary strength, will or knowledge. And to do this in such a way as to help him gain independence as rapidly as possible. (Henderson, 1961, p. 42)

The American Nurses' Association's definition of nursing contained in the *Social Policy Statement* maintains this historical orientation of Nightingale and Henderson and at the same time reflects the influence of nursing theory that is a part of nursing's evolution. "Nursing is the diagnosis and treatment of human responses to actual or potential health problems" (ANA, 1980, p. 9). This definition points to four defining characteristics of nursing: phenomena, theory application, nursing action, and evaluation of effects of action in relation to phenomena (ANA, 1980, p. 9).

The ANA definition of nursing and the characteristics of nursing derived from the definition describe the practice of nursing in the 1980s. The approach to this practice is reflected in the use of the nursing process, which serves as an organizing framework for practice. The nursing process encompasses all significant steps taken in the care of the patients: systematic assessment, diagnosing, planning, implementing the plan, and continual evaluation of the plan. This process is used by all of nursing and reflects both independent and interdependent care provided for the patient.

In the last two decades, nursing has moved from the realm of rote behavior to the era of nursing diagnoses and the application of theory. Nursing practice demands professional intention and commitment. Although all nurses are responsible for practice in accordance with the Standards of Nursing Practice, the level and sophistication of application vary with the education and skills of the individual nurse. Nursing is practiced by nurses who are generalists and by nurses who are specialists. Each nurse remains accountable for the quality of his or her practice within the full scope of nursing practice (ANA, 1980, p. 19).

The ANA describes the nurse generalist as one who has a comprehensive approach to health care and can meet the diversified health care concerns of individuals, families, and communities. Nurse generalists provide most of the nursing care for most of the people served by nursing (ANA, 1980, p. 19). Basic educational programs in nursing prepare nurse generalists.

SPECIALIZATION

Just as the field of medicine developed subspecialties to allow for quality delivery of care for all types of people, so nursing had a need for specialization. Specialization arises in five main ways:

> The amount and complexity of knowledge and technology create a demand for a few professionals to give special attention to applications in delineated practice areas.
>
> A few professional pioneers seek to obtain greater depth of understanding of phenomena related to a segment of nursing and to test new practices intended to correct or ameliorate recognized conditions.
>
> Public attention and available funds become focused on an area of practice in which heretofore there has been a lack of interest, knowledge, and skilled practitioners.
>
> The complexity of services exceeds the prevailing knowledge and skills of general practitioners, and this problem is approached by intense personal studies or post-basic study by a few interested professionals.
>
> A part of a professional field expands and simultaneously some of its members seek ways for expanded use of their intellectual and other capacities. (ANA, 1980, p. 21)

Specialists in nursing are experts in providing care focused on specific clusters of phenomena drawn from the area of general practice. The phenomena of concerns selected by specialists in a nursing practice may relate either to a specialized field or to the interaction among specialized fields (ANA, 1980, p. 19). Specialization in nursing marks its growth as a profession.

The specialty practice of neuroscience nursing can be traced back to the latter part of the nineteenth century in England and France (Hartshorn, 1986, p. 45). From that time until the 1960s, nurses learned the special knowledge and skills needed to care for the neurologic patient through informal courses taught by physicians and nurses and on-the-job training. As the subspecialties of neurosurgery and neurology continued to grow, formal courses to educate nurses caring for these patients were developed, and in 1967 the University of California at San Francisco initiated a master's degree program in neurologic and neurosurgical nursing (Hartshorn, p. 46).

To recognize the common needs of nurses caring for neurologic patients and to provide a forum for these nurses to share concerns, the American Association of Neurosurgical Nurses (AANN) was founded in 1968 in affiliation with the American Association of Neurological Surgeons. The AANN was renamed the American Association of Neuroscience Nurses in 1983. The purpose of the AANN is to foster and promote interest, education, and high standards of practice in the specialized field of neuroscience nursing. Over the years since its establishment, the AANN has developed a number of documents to assist the nurse caring for the neurologic patient.

DEFINING NEUROSCIENCE NURSING PRACTICE

The first document, published in 1977 in conjunction with the ANA, was *Standards of Neurological and Neurosurgical Nursing Practice*. These standards reflected the generic standards as established by the ANA in 1973 as they were applied to the neurologic patient.

Conceptual Framework

In preparation for the revision of these Standards, a Conceptual Framework for Neuroscience Nursing was developed. The conceptual framework identifies and links the concepts inherent in the art and science of neuroscience nursing practice. The six essential components of the conceptual framework are (1) recipients of care, (2) settings for practice, (3) definition of nursing, (4) human responses, (5) responsibilities of nurses, and (6) characteristics of nurses (AANN Standards Committee, 1984, p. 119).

The framework identifies the recipient of neuroscience nursing care as the individual with nervous system dysfunction, the individual's family or significant other, and the community and society in which the individual lives. By identifying these three groups of recipients, the framework can be applied to the various settings in which the neuroscience nurse practices, including primary care, secondary care, and tertiary care facilities.

The AANN adopted the ANA definition of nursing found in *Nursing: A Social Policy Statement* (ANA, 1980). This broad definition allows for the specialty association to specify the health problems, human responses, nursing diagnoses, and interventions unique to the neurologic patient, as well as the other recipients of neuroscience nursing care.

The framework helped to clarify the focus of nursing intervention as the human response rather than the health problem. The phenomena of concern to neuroscience nurses include communication, consciousness and cognition, mobility, protective reflexes, rest and sleep, sensation, and sexuality. From these phenomena, the neuroscience nurse derives the specific human responses to the identified phenomena, determines the appropriate nursing diagnoses, and states the nursing interventions that are needed to treat the response. The nursing focus is on the biopsychosocial response of the recipient of care rather than on the medical diagnosis. Following is the heart of the conceptual framework:

> The essence of neuroscience nursing practice is its theory developed upon sound principles of nursing science and research as well as those derived from the fields of neuroanatomy, neurophysiology, pharmacology, nutrition, rehabilitation, biological science, behavioral and social sciences and learning theories. Nursing is an applied science, so neuroscience nurses apply knowledge and theory from other fields to care for their clients in various roles and settings. Their practice may encompass clinical teaching, administrative, consultative and research roles. Nursing responsibilities, in any of the roles identified, may include the following: to care for, to support, and to teach.

Advocacy and accountability are characteristics inherent in professional behavior and, therefore, are salient characteristics of neuroscience nurses. Advocacy is demonstrated by collaborating with, or acting for, the recipient of nursing care to: 1) establish goals; 2) identify options and resources; 3) choose treatments; 4) make decisions and implement plans; and 5) formulate opinions and evaluations. Accountability requires that each neuroscience nurse insures the quality of his/her own practice by identifying and applying requisite knowledge and utilizing evaluation criteria. Individual responsibility and commitment are essential for the development of advocacy and accountability and are demonstrated by involvement in continuing education activities, academic education, certification, professional nursing organizations, standards and quality assurance, or nursing research.

The nursing process is the vehicle utilized to operationalize neuroscience nursing practice. Initial and ongoing assessment includes: physical assessment, especially of the nervous system aspects; emotional and behavioral responses to illness; and socio-cultural parameters. The nursing diagnoses, with associated etiologies and defining characteristics, are based on such assessment data and reflect current nursing knowledge. Goals are established which demonstrate patient and family involvement as well as a projected time frame for attainment. The intervention process and patient outcome criteria are developed mutually with and reflect the participation of the patient and family. Outcome criteria, which describe a measurable change in either the biological or psychosocial state of the recipient of nursing care, are utilized by the professional nurse in evaluating the quality of his/her nursing care.

In summary, the following statements are identified as essential to neuroscience nursing practice and serve as the basis for the AANN conceptual framework:

1. Neuroscience nurses diagnose and treat human responses to actual or potential health problems.
2. The phenomena of concern to neuroscience nurses include: consciousness/cognition, mobility, protective reflexes, rest and sleep, sensation, and sexuality.
3. The potential recipients of neuroscience nursing care include the individual with nervous system dysfunction, the individual's family or significant other, and society.
4. Responsibilities of neuroscience nurses include: to care for, to support, and to teach.
5. The setting for neuroscience nursing practice encompasses primary, secondary, and tertiary care.
6. Advocacy and accountability are characteristics inherent in professional behavior and are salient characteristics of neuroscience nurses.
7. Professional responsibility is demonstrated by involvement in continuing education activities, academic education, certification, professional nursing organizations, standards and quality assurance, or nursing research.
8. The nursing process is the framework under which nursing care is provided.
9. Standards of practice, which incorporate patient outcomes and the nursing process, direct and guide neuroscience nursing care. (AANN Standards Committee, 1984, pp. 118–119)

Scope of Neuroscience Nursing Practice

The development of the Conceptual Framework for Neuroscience Nursing Practice was a landmark activity for a specialty nursing association. The framework moved neuroscience nursing practice into the realm of scientific care delivery based on a conceptual approach to the care provided. From this conceptual framework, the AANN, through the Nursing Practice Committee, developed in 1985 the Scope of Practice Statement:

Neuroscience nursing is a unique area within the nursing discipline in that it encompasses all levels of human existence, from the basic bodily functions to the advanced processes of the human mind. Neuroscience patients/clients encounter extraordinary problems because dysfunction in these human processes affects the quality of life for themselves, their families, and the society in which they live. Neuroscience nurses act for, support, and teach such specialized patients/clients and families and, therefore, must be educationally and experientially prepared to assume these significant responsibilities. The scope of practice for this area of nursing includes the recognition of the area's uniqueness, a description of the recipients of this type of nursing care, a determination of the qualifications of the nurse who renders the care, and the establishment of the parameters of neuroscience nursing practice.

Neuroscience nursing practice is the specialized care of individuals who have biopsychosocial alterations due to nervous system dysfunction. Potential recipients of neuroscience nursing care are individuals with nervous system dysfunction, the individual's families or significant others, and the society in which they live.

Neuroscience nurses practice in various roles and settings, i.e., as teachers, administrators, researchers, consultants, clinical practitioners, but in any of the identified roles or settings, their primary intent is to act for, support, and teach the recipients of their care. Neuroscience nurses diagnose and treat human responses to actual or potential health problems concerned with phenomena affected by nervous system dysfunction, such as cognition, communication, consciousness, mobility, protective mechanisms, rest and sleep, sensation, and sexuality.

The nature of the patient's/client's dysfunction mandates that the neuroscience nurse have requisite knowledge and advanced clinical competency. The neuroscience practitioner is a registered professional nurse who gains such knowledge and competency by formal and informal continuing education endeavors, research activities, and participation in the specialty's certification process. Professionalism is demonstrated by assuming accountability for maintaining excellence in practice through self-motivated ventures as well as collaborative efforts with other professional nursing colleagues, organizations, and intra-professional associates. The parameters of nursing practice for the neuroscience nurse are dependent upon basic academic preparation, advanced formal/informal educational pursuits, and clinical experiences entered into and mastered while rendering care to the patient/client and family. The nurse may assume this specialized care as a neuro nurse generalist, a neuro nurse clinician, a neuro nurse clinical specialist, or a neuro nurse practitioner. Each advancing practice role requires additional knowledge of nursing theory, the applied sciences and the social and behavioral sciences. Each advancing nursing role is based upon increased clinical expertise through nursing clinical research and promotion of creative therapeutic nursing interventions for improved patient/client care.

The practice of neuroscience nursing is guided by the standards of practice developed for this discipline. The neuroscience nurse uses the nursing process to implement such standards, thus planning, giving and evaluating the quality of nursing care on a continuous basis. The ultimate goal of this practitioner is consistent with and flows from that of the entire nursing profession, to provide the highest quality of care to patients/clients to attain and maintain wellness, a type of wellness that is consistent with the quality of life desired by the patient/client and family. (AANN Nursing Practice Committee, 1985, pp. 1–3)

The current Scope of Practice Statement reflects neuroscience nursing in the 1980s. The future may hold new, expanded roles for the neuroscience nurse. The fields of neurosurgery and neurology are expanding and changing. New diagnostic methodologies, new treatment techniques, and the rapidly expanding research base in the neurosciences have already had an impact on the role of the nurse. The move from the era of needing only to provide good physical, hygienic care to the patients with severe neurologic dysfunction to the explicit incorporation of rehabilitation techniques in the intensive care unit is one mark of the change in the nurse's role. Another difference is the number of patients surviving the devastating effects of many neurologic diseases. These survivors will possibly create new phenomena of concern for the neuroscience nurse of the future.

Another major impact on the scope of practice in neuroscience nursing is the changing health care delivery system. Prospective payment plans have forced the entire health care system to examine itself and develop more cost-effective means to meet the health care needs of the public. One strategy for containing costs is to use specialists to deliver care. Theoretically, the nurse specialist, with the expanded knowledge base and expertise in the speciality, can provide high quality care to patients in a more cost-effective manner. The specialist also can function as a consultant to nurse generalists caring for the neurologic patient and other health care team members involved in providing the care needed. This consulting function can be used to determine appropriate care and will be expanded in the new health care delivery system.

The changing health care market will have an impact on the practice of the neuroscience nurse. New opportunities for roles in prevention, health maintenance, and home and community care are developing (Lipe & Doolittle, 1983, p. 317). Even in these roles, the major responsibility of the neuroscience nurse remains the diagnosis of human responses to actual or potential health problems.

Nursing has defined its practice, and the AANN has defined the practice of neuroscience nursing using a conceptual framework to link the concepts inherent in the art and science of neuroscience nursing. The boundaries of practice are changing and expanding in response to the needs and demands of the times. This chapter has presented the current conceptualization of the scope of practice in neuroscience nursing.

REFERENCES

American Association of Neuroscience Nurses Nursing Practice Committee. (1985). Scope of practice statement. *Synapse, 13,* 1.

American Association of Neuroscience Nurses Standards Committee. (1984). The AANN conceptual framework. *Journal of Neurosurgical Nursing, 16,* 117.

American Nurses' Association. (1980). *Nursing: A social policy statement.* Kansas City, MO: American Nurses' Association.

Hartshorn, J.C. (1986). Aspects of the historical development of neuroscience nursing. *Journal of Neuroscience Nursing, 18,* 45.

Henderson, V. (1961). *Basic principles of nursing care.* London: International Council of Nurses.

Lipe, H., & Doolittle, N. (1983). The neuro nurse specialist—Present and future considerations. *Journal of Neurosurgical Nursing, 15,* 317.

Nightingale, F. (1946). *Notes on nursing: What it is and what it is not.* London: Harrison & Sons, 1859. (Facsimile edition: Philadelphia: Lippincott.)

2

Human Responses: The Phenomena of Neuroscience Nursing

Pamela H. Mitchell and Linda C. Hodges

Neuroscience nursing is simultaneously among the most generalized and the most specialized groups in nursing. Because the nervous system is the central controller and integrator of all that we do, full knowledge of neuroscience nursing in relation to human responses implies knowledge and skill in the full range of human responses in both health and illness. At the same time, understanding the human response to health problems (disorders) of the nervous system is a highly specialized set of knowledge.

Because of the central role of the nervous system in human functioning, the phenomena of concern to neuroscience nursing are those most fundamental to human existence: consciousness, cognition, communication, sensation, sexuality, and relationships ([AANN] Standards Committee, 1984). All of these are part of an integrative phenomenon central to nursing—the phenomenon of self-care.

This book is based on the premise that it is necessary to understand those phenomena that underlie and stem from responses to disorders of the nervous system in order to deliver the highest quality nursing care to people with neurologic problems. *Phenomena* are observable events or facts, able to be explained or predicted through systematic observation (American Nurses' Association [ANA], 1980). Thus, phenomena relevant to people with nervous system dysfunction are:

- The events or facts that allow one to understand, explain, or predict the course of the disease or disorder
- The events or facts that allow one to understand, explain, or predict the responses of human beings to that disease or disorder

The first set of phenomena (related to the neurologic disease) are those studied and formulated by medicine. The set of phenomena related to understanding and predicting human responses to neurologic disease are the phenomena of nursing.

In this book, we seek:

- To present these phenomena from the perspective of neuroscience nursing in particular
- To distinguish the phenomena of neuroscience nursing from those of neuroscience medicine

- To show explicitly the relationship between the phenomena of medicine (disease) and of nursing (human response)
- To relate the phenomena to their larger concepts and to the subsequent nursing therapy of the phenomena

In order to accomplish these aims, it is helpful to define some terms. The terms frequently used in this chapter and throughout this book include concept, phenomenon, and sources of knowledge.

DEFINITIONS

A *concept* is a mental idea; it is not an observable or tangible entity but is known only through indicators that can be observed. Further, concept implies that there is a complex organization of multiple, related entities. Meleis (1985) describes concepts as "organized perceptions." For example, consciousness is a concept—an idea that exists in our minds and is composed of perceptions about arousability, awareness of self, awareness of others, and shared views of reality. One can only infer, however, that consciousness exists by observing behaviors that most people agree are present in the state of consciousness. Much of the difficulty that we have in developing adequate clinical indicators of level of consciousness stems from the fact that consciousness is a concept, and one that is not easily measured.

The difference between concept and phenomenon is subtle, and the two terms are often used interchangeably in the nursing literature. There is a difference, however. A phenomenon is an *observable* event or fact, susceptible to scientific explanation or prediction. Thus phenomena become the *indicators of concepts*, with the scientific meaning or concept indicators capable of verification by others. In other words, one's private observations or concept definitions can be made public and confirmed or disconfirmed by the observations of others. As an example, the Glasgow Coma Scale was an attempt to define a phenomenon, *coma*, that is part of the concept of consciousness. The developers of the scale created repeatable and observable indicators of the state of arousal or responsiveness to stimuli and assigned a precise, observable definition to the phenomenon coma: absence of eye opening, absence of intelligible verbalization, plus abnormal or no motor response to painful stimuli. Further, concepts are generally organized ideas that are composed of many phenomena. Concepts usually emerge from multiple phenomena rather than being synonymous with any one phenomenon.

Nursing and medicine share many concepts, such as health, illness, disease, and helping. Yet, the phenomena considered most salient to each discipline vary according to the primary focus and the applied practice of each discipline. The primary phenomena of medicine are diseases, expressed in terms of signs, symptoms, and pathology. In contrast, the phenomena of nursing are human responses to actual or potential health problems, including states of disease. At present there is no consensus regarding the level of abstraction or specificity at which these phenomena are described. Some are labeled the same as concepts (e.g., pain), some are behavioral responses (e.g., incontinence), some are experiential responses (e.g., dyspnea), and some might be considered physiologic or pathophysiologic responses (e.g., ischemia, immune activation). The movement to identify and label nursing diagnoses might be considered one approach to developing the observable indicators (defining characteristics) of the phenomena that are central to our discipline's practice. The attempt of nurse theorists to organize those diagnoses into a taxonomic framework can be seen as one attempt to organize and relate phenomena (e.g., diagnoses) into the larger concepts of which they are a part.

FROM CONCEPT TO PHENOMENON: A HISTORICAL OVERVIEW

Every specialty group in a profession is a part of the philosophy and history of the parent profession. The developing conceptualization of neuroscience nursing as distinct from and complementary to the specialty fields of neurosurgery and neurology parallels the growth of the profession of nursing in understanding itself to be concerned with related but different phenomena from those of interest to medicine.

Throughout its history, the practice of nursing has been closely allied with and viewed as dependent on the authority of medicine. Yet it is clear that, even in our earliest days, our leaders and academicians were describing an interest in phenomena that were not the same as those focused on by physicians. Throughout Florence Nightingale's writings, the recurrent themes are the concepts of health and the environment (not disease and assisting the physician). These conceptual themes became submerged in the early twentieth century as training schools gave increasing emphasis to the techniques and procedures of nursing's implementation of medical therapy. Nonetheless, these themes remained an unarticulated but viable component of nursing care and reemerged in formal descriptions and theories of the central nature of nursing.

Meleis (1985) categorizes these changes in articulation of nursing's concepts into four stages of development of the profession: (1) practice, (2) education and administration, (3) research, and (4) nursing theory. Nightingale's time was the beginning of the formalization of practice and its attendant goal of providing for hygiene and environmental manipulation. Formalization of the key concepts and phenomena of nursing began in the 1950s as the profession moved from emphasis on defining curricula and roles for practice to developing the research-based knowledge that underlies the unique discipline of nursing. The development of research skills and the attempt to define the concepts and phenomena that are the appropriate focus of nursing research are a major intellectual thrust of the current era in nursing development.

Fawcett (1984) has identified four major themes that are evident in the works of all the nursing theorists. Each of the theories addresses assumptions and generalizations related to the person, the environment, health, and the nature of nursing. In the 1960s, there seemed to be a sense that nursing as a discipline must *choose* one theory to guide the whole of nursing practice and research. We have come to agree in the 1980s that existing conceptualizations of nursing describe different aspects of the discipline and its practice. We are moving from developing grand theories about the whole of nursing to describing better the phenomena that must be related in order to develop larger concepts and theories.

This book is an attempt to bring together the thoughts of experts in one specialized area of nursing practice, neuroscience nursing. The phenomena and concepts described herein have been derived from the thinking of these experts, working with the ANA social policy statement (ANA, 1980), the AANN conceptual framework (Standards Committee, 1984), and the process and outcome criteria for selected diagnoses in neuroscience nursing (ANA Council on Medical–Surgical Nursing Practice and AANN, 1985).

Phenomena Identified in the American Nurses' Association Social Policy Statement

In 1980, the ANA published an important document delineating the nature and scope of nursing practice, described in the context of the implied social contract between society and the profession. Nursing is defined as the diagnosis and treatment of human responses to actual or potential health problems; the phenomena of central concern to nurses are the human responses, not the health problem (ANA, 1980). This does not imply that nurses are ignorant of or uninterested in the health problems of their clients. It indicates that such knowledge about health problems occurs at the intersection of the profession of nursing with the profession of medicine rather than at the core of nursing itself. The practice of nursing requires that we become knowledgeable about the phenomena of both nursing and medicine.

The social policy statement illustrates human response phenomena with a list of 10 categories of physical, attitudinal, behavioral, cognitive, and affective responses relevant to nursing intervention: self-care limitations; impaired functioning in such areas as rest, sleep, ventilation, circulation, activity, nutrition, elimination, skin, and sexuality; pain and discomfort; emotional problems related to illness and treatment, life-threatening events, or daily experiences; distortion of symbolic function, reflected in interpersonal and intellectual processes; deficiencies in decision making and ability to make personal choices; self-image changes required by health status; dysfunctional perceptual orientation to health; strains related to life processes, such as birth, growth and development, and death; and problematic affiliative relationships.

Phenomena Identified by the American Association of Neuroscience Nurses

The AANN built on the framework of the ANA and identified 17 phenomena. These phenomena are regularly encountered in the care of people with dysfunction of the nervous system and their families or significant others and in the interactions of these groups with society:

Affiliative relationships	Mobility
Circulation	Nutrition
Communication	Orientation to health
Consciousness–cognition	Protective reflexes
	Rest and sleep
Coping	Self-care
Elimination	Self-perception
Emotional–behavioral responses	Sensation
	Sexuality
	Ventilation

Six of these phenomena, consciousness–cognition, communication, mobility, sensation, rest and sleep, and sexuality, were identified as core phenomena for neuroscience nursing by a joint committee of the ANA Council on Medical–Surgical Nursing and the AANN. Process and outcome criteria were developed for selected nursing diagnoses in each of these categories of phenomena and provide a model for development of standards for the profession (ANA & AANN, 1985).

Nursing practice knowledge in most reference books in the specialized area of neuroscience nursing is organized by neurologic diseases or classes of neurologic disease; in other words, by the phenomena of medicine. This book is organized by the phenomena of nursing: human response categories commonly forming the basis for nursing intervention in people with actual or potential nervous system dysfunction. The categories of phenomena have been selected from those identified by the ANA and AANN, plus those additional categories that the editors believe are central to the care of most adults with neurologic health problems. These categories are:

Consciousness	Sensation
Cognition	Elimination
Communication	Sexuality
Affiliative relationships	Self-care
Mobility	

This book is our attempt to gather the most current knowledge about (1) the general categories of phenomena, (2) specific phenomena, stated as classes of nursing diagnoses, and (3) relevant interventions. This knowledge is gathered from accumulated clinical wisdom, from nursing and related research, and from our emerging nursing science. In order to avoid complacency in accepting this or any other reference book as the final authority for clinical practice, however, it is useful to reflect for a moment on the origins and development of the knowledge that we apply to practice.

SOURCES AND DEVELOPMENT OF CLINICAL KNOWLEDGE

A clear view of the phenomena of concern to nursing as an applied discipline with its own unique body of knowledge has emerged as a result of the work of nurse theorists, the ANA, and nursing specialty organizations. In recent years, a consensus on a metaparadigm of nursing has appeared in the literature with the central concepts—person, environment, health, and nursing—identified as the foundation on which to build the structure of the discipline (Fawcett, 1984). This metaparadigm provides boundaries for research efforts that will describe, promote understanding of, and predict the nature of phenomena that lie within the major concepts. To identify an approach to the methods of research that will assist in the development of a science of nursing, it is important to examine the ways of knowing that currently direct practice.

Ways of Knowing

In clinical practice, decisions may be made based on knowledge gained from experience, tradition, authority, and science. In the past and to a large extent today, most nurses rely primarily on ways of knowing other than science when confronted with situations that require a decision. Although each type of knowledge has something to offer, the goal of the profession is to move decision making into the realm of science as practice becomes more grounded in significant research findings.

Experience

Knowledge resulting from experience is knowledge that Benner defines as practical or know-how (Benner, 1983, 1984). This type of knowledge is developed before theory. It is gained through actual practice situations during which preconceived notions and expectations are challenged, revised, or disconfirmed according to events that unfold within the experience.

Accumulated knowledge is characteristic of knowledge developed by the practicing expert. Not all of practical knowledge, according to Benner, can be contained within theoretical propositions or within logical elements that map out strategies for decision making. Knowledge that results from the experience of experts can, however, be described through theory-based scientific studies. These concrete experiences affirmed by experts can serve as a beginning point for theory generation.

Because the knowledge of experts results in sound clinical decision making, it is important that this knowledge be uncovered and expanded. Practical knowledge can be viewed as the raw material for the making of a scientific body of nursing knowledge. One method for expanding practical knowledge is the interpretive approach. In this approach, the goal is synthesis rather than analysis. The descriptions of practice are examined holistically for their meanings in an attempt to understand the world shared by experts in a particular area of nursing practice (Benner, 1983).

Tradition

Knowledge that stems from tradition is knowledge that can be termed as common sense. This form of knowledge, generally accepted within a given culture, may have endured for centuries. It is usually characterized by beliefs and practices that are seldom scrutinized, having a singular point of view that focuses on practical matters of interest (Hurley, 1979).

Traditional knowledge lacks supporting scientific evidence. Some examples that many nurses learned and practiced without question include avoiding iced beverages and the use of rectal thermometers in cardiac patients for fear of stimulating the vagal response. In recent years, many traditional practices in nursing, such as these, have been questioned through scientific study.

Current nursing practice in many areas is still grounded in traditional knowledge. It is important that research projects be designed to validate continued practice based on this way of knowing.

Authority

Knowledge derived from authority stems from a source accepted as authoritative in a particular field. Children, to a large degree, rely on knowledge based on the authority of such adult figures as parents and teachers when making decisions (Kerlinger, 1973).

In the past, nurses made many clinical decisions in their practice based on knowledge derived from authorities in their work world.

Among those who provided this form of knowledge were physicians who instructed nurses in "how" or "what to do," supervisors, and other nurses in positions of authority. As nursing moves to a more autonomous model of professional practice and as significant scientific studies become available to direct practice, reliance on knowledge developed from authority will diminish.

Science
The primary aim of knowledge derived from scientific inquiry is the generation of theory that can explain natural phenomena. The acceptable method of scientific inquiry is characterized by an approach that is systematic, controlled, critical, and empirical in nature. Hypotheses about relationships among elements within and among natural phenomena are investigated to determine validity. Scientific knowledge offers the practitioner of nursing explanations about phenomena of practice that are grounded in factual evidence.

Scientific inquiry seeks to discover, organize, and classify knowledge according to explanatory principles, thus providing a factual basis for beliefs that stem from experience, tradition, and authority. Unlike other forms of knowing, scientific knowledge has a brief life span, since new evidence through scientific discovery often invalidates what is known currently.

Most disciplines use the scientific method as a means for describing, explaining, and predicting phenomena. There are at least three basic approaches within the method that can be used to construct and test theory. One approach is inductive and is based on the idea of *research, then theory*. It is employed primarily for studies that describe or explain the nature of phenomena. A second approach is deductive and is based on the idea *theory, then research*. In this approach, the aim is to predict the nature of phenomena within given situations. The third approach combines both inductive and deductive methods. This type of scientific inquiry was used by Freud and Piaget and requires clinical observations of phenomena to be used for devising theory. Theories are then tested for predictability in subsequent clinical situations. In this method of inquiry, the process of scientific discovery takes on a cyclical life as theory becomes more refined (King, 1985).

Current Status of Nursing Knowledge
At present, the majority of nursing knowledge comes from experience and tradition. Continued reliance on these ways of knowing as a basis for practice can be traced to dependence on other disciplines for knowledge, the slow growth of nursing research, and the tendency to embrace quantitative methodology as the primary method of research.

Perhaps one of the major factors in nursing's dependence on other disciplines for knowledge lies in a lack of a clear identity of the discipline. For years, untold hours were spent trying to define nursing or the nature of professional practice. Up until the 1950s, it was viewed as a myriad of borrowed knowledge. The primary model for education and practice was eclectic, with a huge component of watered-down medical knowledge at its center. Based on the work of nursing theorists and nursing organizations, the knowledge required for practice is now thought to be a synthesis of what is known about person, health, environment, and nursing, rather than a mere combination of these. The phenomena of concern that emerge from this metaparadigm are conceptualized as holistic in nature, requiring a humanistic approach as opposed to rational positivism. This approach assumes that nursing knowledge exists to be discovered not as a collection of separate parts but as a unified whole—a social reality.

The slowness of discovery within the discipline of nursing can be attributed to the current infantile stage of nursing research. Before 1960, the primary focus of study within nursing was the nurse (Gortner, 1983). Twenty-five years ago, studies of nurses outnumbered those on patient care 10 to 1. Lack of a well-defined knowledge base for nursing practice prompted both the ANA and the United States Public Health Service to issue statements calling for priority to be given to problems encountered in patient care.

The emphasis on practice-related research, therefore, has been concentrated in the past 25 years. This work has been primarily experiential and lacking in solid conceptual or theoretical frameworks. In a study of types of research published in *Nursing Research* in the two 5-year periods of the 1970s, Downs argued that the use of experimental designs has not necessarily produced better research. She cited the extremely low correlations among variables as evidence of inadequate descriptive research and the resulting lack of testable theories as a major contributing factor (Downs, 1980).

The inability of many experimental research studies to contribute significantly to the development of a science in nursing has spurred an interest in qualitative methods of research. Many nurse researchers now argue that there is a need to verify preconceived notions of reality through descriptive studies. They posit that the use of qualitative methods can assist in the identification of variables and their relationship, thus building a theory of the phenomena of concern before beginning experimental studies (Swanson & Chenitz, 1982; Field & Morse, 1985).

Scientific Methods: Developing a Science in Nursing

If nursing as a profession is to advance, there is a desperate need to identify research methods that will address the questions needed to delineate the phenomena of concern to nursing, especially those in neuroscience nursing. Perhaps a way to consider the approach is to think about how learning occurs and relate this process to the three approaches to scientific inquiry previously identified.

Kolb has developed an experiential learning model that provides a framework for categorizing the various research methods (Kolb, 1986). Kolb argues that knowledge is developed through experiencing the world (concrete experience), reflecting on that experience, forming abstract concepts of the experience (theory building), and testing the abstraction for validity in the real world again (experimental research).

A consideration of the fit of inductive, deductive approaches and descriptive, predictive methods reveals that the research process is not linear. It is, instead, part of a larger, cyclical process identified earlier as the third approach, which incorporates both basic types of methodology. Descriptive research and the inductive method begin with concrete experience and end with theory generation. In this phase, both qualitative and quantitative methods may be used as dictated by the problem statement. Predictive research or the deductive approach begins with theory and ends with concrete experience growing out of an experimental design (Fig. 2–1).

The Descriptive Phase

The primary purpose of the descriptive phase of research is to explicate the elements within a given phenomenon and describe the relationship among the elements. This method is used primarily when there is little known about a phenomenon, when what is known is suspected to be biased, or when the purpose is to develop an understanding from the emic perspective (the subject's point of view). Methods of research commonly associated with the descriptive phase are phenomenology, grounded theory, and rational empiric work.

Phenomenology. Phenomenology represents an attempt to describe the human experience as it is lived (Oiler, 1982). As a method, it grew out of the phenomenological school of philosophic thought initially developed by Edmund Hesserl. Some view its genesis as a reaction to the denigration of philosophic knowledge and the objectification of human beings spawned by an age of rational positivism. The goal of the method is to describe the entire systematic structure of the lived experience, or what Hesserl called the "essence," including the meanings that the experience had for those living them.

Phenomenology as a method does not propose to generate theories or models or gen-

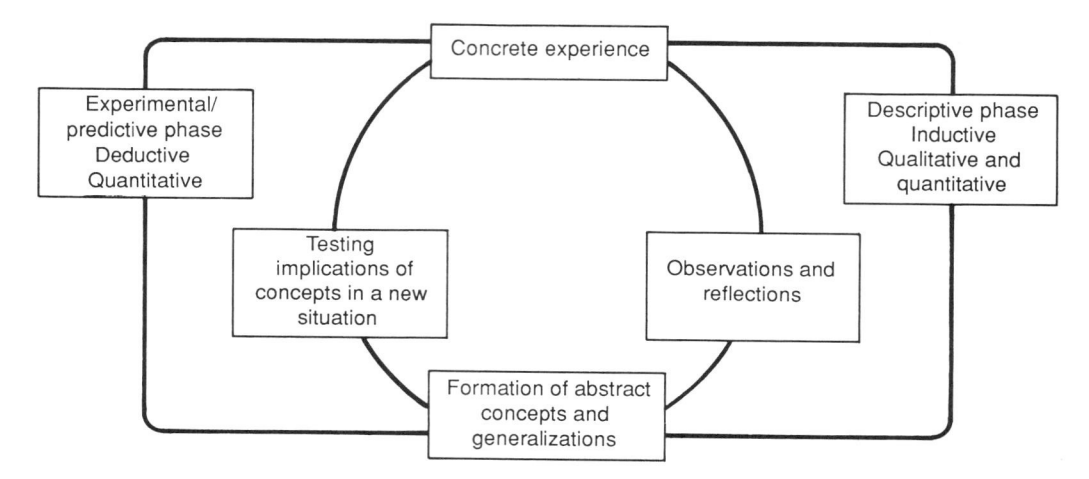

Figure 2–1. Research methods as related to learning. *(Adapted from Kolb.* Learning style inventory: A self-study booklet, *1986. Courtesy of McBer & Company.)*

eralize to other subjects the same understanding of experience. To use the method, the researcher must lay aside preconceived ideas, theories, and frameworks. Data are collected in the natural setting using a variety of methods, including participant observation, interviews, videotaping, and journals. All data generated in the experience are accepted as given, including the subjective meanings of the participants. When analyzing the data, an attempt is made to identify patterns of recurrent elements that constitute the phenomenon, determining the structure of the elements as they prove necessary to the essence of the experience (Oiler, 1982). The test of validity is the ability of the reader of the description of the phenomenon to experience the same meaning in a lived experience.

Grounded Theory. Grounded theory as a method can be considered a form of ethnographic data analysis in that the purpose of ethnography is to develop concepts helpful in understanding human behavior from the emic perspective. Unlike phenomenology, grounded theory assumes that a process is inherent in a phenomenon. Both inductive and deductive approaches to the generation of theory are used as concepts and constructs emerge from the data and are tested (Field & Morse, 1985).

Rational Empiric Studies. The purpose of rational empiric studies is to develop inferences or conclusions based on observations of phenomena. The empiric method relies on evidence obtained in a systematic and controlled manner. In this approach, questions are raised about the nature of a given phenomenon and observations are recorded to answer the questions. Data are studied and subjected to statistical analysis to determine significance. The researcher then interprets the findings, draws inferences based on the data, and discusses their implications for nursing practice.

This method of descriptive research may be either qualitative or quantitative in design. Currently, rational empiric studies make up a large part of the approach being used in descriptive studies because few nurse researchers are prepared to use such methods as ethnography, grounded theory, and phenomenology. As greater emphasis is placed on the use of a variety of qualitative research methods as legitimate for answering questions of concern to nursing and as more nurses are prepared at the doctoral level to use these methods, an increase in qualitative research studies can be expected.

Experimental or Predictive Studies

Experimental or predictive research designs probably are most appropriate for testing nursing theory derived from understanding of the phenomenon. These studies are usually quantitative in nature and are designed to generate data that explicate the interrelationships among variables posed in hypotheses derived from theories. The aim of experimental research is to preduct outcomes that will result as specific variables are manipulated. As predictability increases, the theory from which hypotheses are drawn becomes more reliable as a framework for nursing practice.

SUMMARY

The phenomena of concern to the neuroscience nurse are central to the development of a science of nursing, since they represent the core elements of self-care. Through the work of nurse theorists, beginning with Nightingale, and through the contributions of such organizations as the ANA and the AANN, there is now a better understanding of the metaparadigm of nursing and the nursing phenomena inherent within the central concepts. The profession must now move to ask the questions that will describe, explain, and predict phenomena essential to professional nursing practice.

Nursing research must include a combination of different types of inquiry, since no one method is, of itself, the avenue to scientific discovery and theoretic breakthrough. The tendency to dichotomize research into mutually exclusive categories of qualitative and quantitative designs espousing that one and not the other will lead to truth must be laid aside. The road to development of scientific knowledge is not linear but circular. The nature of the question dictates the point at which to enter the cycle.

REFERENCES

American Association of Neuroscience Nurses Standards Committee. (1984). The AANN conceptual framework. *Journal of Neurosurgical Nursing, 16*, 117.

American Nurses' Association. (1980). *Nursing: A social policy statement.* Kansas City, MO: American Nurses' Association.

American Nurses' Association Council on Medical–Surgical Nursing Practice & American Association of Neuroscience Nurses. (1985). *Neuroscience nursing practice: Process and outcome for selected diagnoses.* Kansas City, MO: American Nurses' Association.

Benner, P. (1983). Uncovering the knowledge embedded in clinical practice. *Image, 11*(2), 36.

Benner, P. (1984). *From novice to expert.* Menlo Park, NJ: Addison-Wesley.

Downs, F. (1980). Relationship of findings of clinical research and development of criteria: A researcher's perspective. *Nursing Research, 29*, 94.

Fawcett, J. (1984). *Analysis and evaluation of conceptual models of nursing.* Philadelphia: Davis.

Field, P.A., & Morse, J.M. (1985). *Nursing research: The application of qualitative approaches.* Rockville, MD: Aspen.

Gortner, S.R. (1983). The history and philosophy of nursing science and research. *Advances in Nursing Science, 5*(2), 1.

Hurley, B. (1979). Why a theoretical framework in nursing research? *Western Journal of Nursing Research, 1*, 29.

Kerlinger, F.N. (1973). *Foundation of behavioral research.* New York: Holt, Rhinehart & Winston.

King, I.M. (1985). Theory and research in nursing. *Search, 8*(2). Charleston, SC: College of Nursing, Medical University of South Carolina.

Kolb, D. (1986). *Learning style inventory–A self-study booklet.* Boston, MA: McBer & Company.

Meleis, A.I. (1985). *Theoretical nursing: Development and progress.* Philadelphia: Lippincott.

Oiler, C. (1982). The phenomenological approach in nursing research. *Nursing Research, 31*, 178.

Swanson, J.M., & Chenitz, W.C. (1982). Why qualitative research in nursing? *Nursing Outlook, 30*, 241.

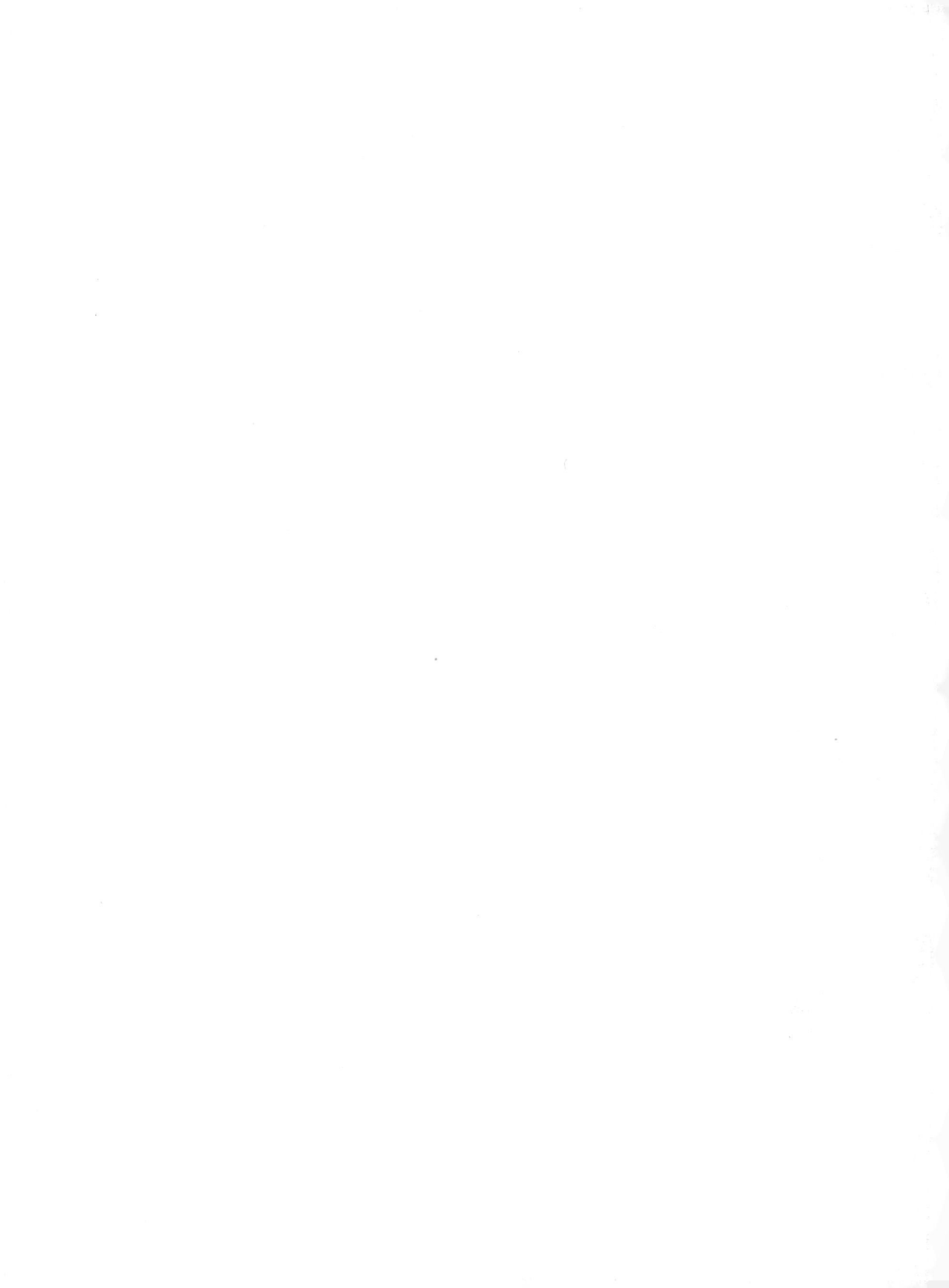

3

Common Neurologic Health Problems: The Phenomena of Neuroscience Medicine

Pamela H. Mitchell and Glenna A. Dowling*

Nurses diagnose and treat human responses to actual and potential health problems (American Nurses' Association [ANA], 1980). Examples of human responses to neurologic health problems include pain related to changes in pain signal processing, potential for falling related to loss of proprioceptive input, and social isolation related to fear of seizures.

Nursing practice occurs, for the most part, in settings at which people arrive because of their health problem—the disease, disorder, or condition that is diagnosed and treated by physicians. Neurologic disorders include such diseases as multiple sclerosis and myasthenia gravis, and such conditions as closed head injury and central nervous system tumors.

The majority of nursing practice therefore requires considerable knowledge of both the health problem and the human responses to those problems. Neuroscience nurses care for people with disorders of the nervous system. Diagnosis and treatment of the neurologic disease are directed by the physician specialist—the neurologist, neuroradiologist, or neurosurgeon—or in some cases by the physician generalist—the internist, family practitioner, or general surgeon. Diagnosis and treatment of the human responses to actual or potential neurologic disease are directed by the nurse who specializes in neuroscience nursing or, in many cases, by nurse generalists who sometimes encounter patients with neurologic disorders.

The purpose of this chapter is to present an overview of common neurologic and neurosurgical health problems and medical treatments with reference to the categories of human responses (nursing diagnoses) often associated with those health problems. Part II of this book concentrates on the phenomena of human functioning in which those nursing diagnoses cluster. Textbooks of neurology and neurosurgery should be consulted for details of the pathophysiology and medical diagnostics and therapeutics for specific medical diagnoses.

The chapter is organized into a classification of neurologic disorders with reference to

---

*Portions of this chapter on motor disorders were contributed by Katherine Donahue, Charlyne Miller, and Brenda Craig.

the parts of the neuraxis affected. The neuraxis refers to subsets of the nervous system:

Axis I	Cerebral hemispheres and diencephalon
Axis II	Brainstem and cerebellum
Axis III	Spinal cord
Axis IV	Peripheral nerves and junctions with innervated organs

Because the human functions served differ with each of the segments of the neuraxis, the nursing diagnoses tend to cluster with respect to the part of the neuraxis affected rather than by the disease classification. The purpose of including both disease and neuraxis classification is to assist nurses to correlate medical and nursing diagnoses.

CEREBROVASCULAR DISORDERS

Cerebrovascular accidents, or stroke, and vascular headache are the primary categories of cerebrovascular disorders resulting in human responses of concern to neuroscience nurses.

Cerebrovascular Accident

Cerebrovascular accident (CVA), or stroke, is the third largest cause of death in the United States (American Heart Association, 1987). In 1984, 155,000 Americans died from stroke of all types, and 1,960,000 survived a stroke. Stroke is a major cause of disability, accounting for one half of all patients hospitalized for acute neurologic disease. The American Heart Association estimated that the cost of stroke-related health care would be $12.8 billion dollars in 1987.

Stroke is defined as a sudden and focal neurologic deficit that results from cardiovascular disease (Adams & Victor, 1985, p. 570). There are three main types of stroke: thrombotic, embolic, and hemorrhagic. Thrombotic and embolic strokes are the most common, although hemorrhagic stroke has the highest mortality.

Cerebral thrombosis usually occurs in cerebral vessels damaged by atherosclerosis. Onset is usually at night or early in the morning, when systemic blood pressure is low. Thrombotic strokes often are preceded by transient ischemic attacks (TIA) (focal neurologic deficits that resolve within minutes to hours) and occur in people at high risk for other forms of cardiovascular disease (e.g., myocardial infarction, peripheral vascular insufficiency). Cerebral embolism accounts for 5% to 14% of all strokes, with cardiac valvular emboli and atrial fibrillation being the most common sources of the embolus.

Subarachnoid and cerebral hemorrhage account for 7% and 10%, respectively, of all strokes. Spontaneous subarachnoid hemorrhage is associated with ruptured cerebral aneurysm or arteriovenous malformation in younger people and with systemic hypertension in older people. Intracerebral hemorrhage may result from rupture of aneurysms, less commonly from arteriovenous malformations, and from hypertension. Head injury also is a common source of traumatic subarachnoid and intracerebral hemorrhage.

The amount and location of the hemorrhage determine the severity of symptoms in hemorrhagic stroke. In subarachnoid hemorrhage, vasospasm of cerebral vessels 4 to 7 days posthemorrhage can worsen symptoms by producing cerebral ischemia.

Altered Human Responses with Cerebrovascular Accident in Axis I

Strokes of all types that affect Axis I (cerebral hemispheres and diencephalon) will produce symptoms referable to the portions of the cerebral hemispheres and diencephalon supplied by the vascular distribution of the affected extracerebral or intracerebral vessels. The majority of CVAs are in the distribution of the anterior circulation to the brain, supplied by the common and internal carotid arteries: middle cerebral, anterior cerebral, and penetrating arteries. These arteries and their branches supply circulation to the frontal and parietal lobes, lateral temporal lobe, basal ganglia, and internal capsule. The posterior circulation, supplied from the vertebral arteries, provides blood to the caudal portion of the brain: occipital lobes, thalamus, and inferior temporal lobes, as well as to Axis II (brainstem and cerebellum).

The internal carotid artery supplies the ophthalmic artery and the vessels of the ipsilateral hemisphere. Sudden occlusion of the artery will thus produce severe contralateral hemiplegia and hemianesthesia, profound aphasia if on the dominant hemisphere, and often unilateral blindness. We would expect, therefore, to see alterations in communication, mobility, sensation, perhaps cognition, and vision (see Chapters 13, 15, 20, and 24).

The middle cerebral artery is the major branch of the internal carotid and supplies most of the lateral cortex of the brain: lateral frontal and parietal lobes, temporal pole and insula of the temporal lobe, and the caudate and putamen via penetrating branches. These structures serve the majority of our higher cerebral processes of communication, interpretation of language, perception and interpretation of space, form and sensation, and voluntary movement. Depending on the hemisphere involved, one could expect stroke of the middle cerebral artery distribution to alter communication, cognition, mobility, and sensation.

The anterior cerebral artery supplies the medial surfaces and the upper convexities of the frontal and parietal lobes and the cingulate gyrus (medial surface of the hemisphere), which includes the motor and somesthetic cortex serving the legs. Stroke of this distribution therefore affects mobility and sensation of the lower extremities more than the upper, may produce urinary incontinence secondary to loss of inhibition of the micturition reflex, and may produce emotional lability and confusion. Altered human responses will thus be possible in the categories of cognition, mobility, and elimination.

The posterior cerebral artery supplies the medial and inferior temporal lobe and the medial occipital lobe, including the visual receptive area, the thalamus, and the posterior portion of the hypothalamus. Occlusion of portions or all of this artery can result in hemianesthesia (due to involvement of the sensory portions of the thalamus), hemiplegia (as fibers pass through the cerebral peduncle), homonymous hemianopsia (visual radiations as they pass through the temporal lobe), receptive aphasia, particularly with written language, and cortical blindness (inability to interpret visual events). Thus, altered responses may occur in the areas of mobility, sensation, and language.

Altered Human Responses with Cerebrovascular Accident in Axis II

The posterior circulation derives from the vertebral arteries, which give rise to the basilar artery, supplying Axis II (brainstem and cerebellum) and the posterior cerebral artery (described under Axis I). The posterior and anterior circulations are joined by the posterior communicating arteries to form the circle of Willis at the base of the brain.

Disruption of circulation to the brainstem has the potential to alter all primary human functions except cognition. The nerve fibers carrying motor and autonomic information to and sensory information from the periphery must all pass through the compact tracts of the brainstem. In addition, the nuclei and peripheral branches of all the cranial nerves except I and II are in the brainstem.

A variety of vascular syndromes of the brainstem are described, depending on the particular vascular distribution involved. Partial occlusion of the vertebral or basilar arteries can produce transient ischemic attacks characterized by unilateral or bilateral weakness of limbs or even total loss of tone, diplopia, nausea, vertigo, tinnitus, dysphagia or dysarthria, and sometimes confusion or drowsiness. These symptoms all reflect transient ischemia to corticospinal tracts in the brainstem, brainstem consciousness system, and cranial nerve dysfunction.

Basilar artery occlusion or hemorrhage affects all functions of the brainstem and, if complete, results in coma, miotic pupils, decerebrate rigidity, and respiratory and circulatory abnormalities, and ultimately death. Partial basilar artery thrombosis can produce the *locked-in syndrome,* in which anterior portions of the pons are affected, thus precluding all movement except that of the eyelids. Sensation and consciousness are preserved.

There are a number of medullary syndromes produced by vascular disorders of the cerebellar arteries. Cerebellar arteries are branches of the vertebral artery. The most common is the lateral medullary, or Wallenberg syndrome, produced by thrombosis of the posterior inferior cerebellar artery (PICA). The circulation to the lateral and posterior portion of the medulla is disrupted, resulting in dysfunction of the nucleus ambiguus, fibers and tracts of cranial nerves V, IX, and X, descending sympathetic pathways, afferent spinocerebellar tracts, and lateral spinothalamic tract. The person thus exhibits dysphagia and dysphonia related to ipsilateral paralysis of the soft palate, larnyx, and pharynx, ipsilateral anesthesia of the face and cornea for pain and temperature but not touch, ipsilateral Horner's syndrome (miosis, ptosis, and anhydrosis), ipsilateral cerebellar dyssynergy (decomposition of movement), and contralateral loss of pain and temperature sensation in the trunk and limbs. The primary alteration in human response is in communication and swallowing (see Chapters 14 and 15) and unilateral lack of coordination, with potential safety problems related to the loss of pain and temperature sensation. Cognition and most aspects of mobility are intact.

Hemorrhage into or ischemia of the cerebellum can occur from thrombosis or aneurysms of the posterior inferior, anterior inferior, or superior cerebellar arteries, all branches of the vertebral arteries. Problems in motor coordination, synergy, tone, station, and gait can occur with cerebellar vascular lesions. These may be manifest in difficulties in articulation (due to dyssynergies of speech), swallowing, eye movement (nystagmus), or gross motor movements of the limbs.

Altered Human Responses with Cerebrovascular Accident in Axis III

The spinal cord (Axis III) circulation is supplied by the anterior and posterior spinal arteries. The anterior spinal artery branches from the vertebral arteries and travels the length of the anterior spinal cord, reinforced by branches of lateral spinal arteries. The anterior spinal cord controls voluntary and reflex movement via the anterior horn motor neurons and carries descending motor and ascending touch, pain, and temperature sensations. Thrombosis of the anterior spinal artery results in a transverse myelitis with flaccid paralysis at the level of the lesion, spastic paralysis below the lesion, and loss of pain, touch, and temperature but sparing of proprioception (posterior columns). Dissecting aortic aneurysm, complications of arteriography, or disseminated atherosclerosis are the most common causes. Human responses are altered in a pattern similar to that in acute spinal cord injury (see Chapter 20) but with preservation of proprioceptive sensation.

The posterior spinal arteries are really a series of plexiform channels, rather than single vessels, and arise from the vertebral arteries. Isolated ischemia or thrombosis of posterior vessels in disseminated vascular disease would produce sensory loss, particularly of proprioception, vibration, touch, and pressure, with preservation of movement.

Vascular Headache

A vascular etiology for migraine and cluster headaches has come to be accepted. Vasodilation and pulsation of the external carotid artery during an attack have been documented in about one third of patients. Decreased pulsation results in disappearance of the headache. Migraine headache is prevalent and found in 3% to 5% of the general population, and in 15% of women in their reproductive years (Adams & Victor, 1985). The incidence in women is about twice that in men, although cluster headaches (severe vascular headaches that occur in seasonal clusters) occur most commonly in men.

Although numerous symptom constellations are described in the literature, migraine is usually characterized by periodic, commonly unilateral, throbbing or pounding head pain. Symptom onset is typically early in life (childhood, adolescence, or early adulthood), with attacks diminishing with advancing age. Often a family history of similar headaches exists. The classic syndrome begins with an alteration in neurologic function (flashing lights, zigzag lights, less commonly speech arrest or unilateral weakness), followed in 15 to 20 minutes by hemicranial pain and often nausea and vomiting. The neurologic symptoms abate with the onset of the headache. Common migraine is typified by the onset of throbbing headache without prodromal neurologic symptoms.

Medical therapy includes ergot derivatives (ergotamine tartrate), taken at the onset of headache to promote constriction of extracranial vessels, or beta blockers (propranolol hydrochloride) or calcium channel blockers (verapamil) taken prophylactically to prevent wide swings in vascular reactivity thought to cause vascular headache. Nonpharmacologic therapy includes biofeedback and progressive muscle relaxation to reduce sympathetic reactivity. These may be more effective in reducing the muscle contraction components of the headache than in any direct effect on the vascular headache itself.

Human responses to the condition, vascular headaches, are all referable to Axis I, the cerebral hemispheres and diencephalon, since both the pain and its interpretation are a function of these structures. Responses can be classified into two categories: (1) concerns about the meaning of the pain and (2) behaviors in response to or anticipation of head pain. Vascular reactivity is the source of chronic but intermittent head pain, often accompanied by transient neurologic dysfunction and gastrointestinal symptoms. Before definitive medical diagnosis of the cause of the vascular headache, many people fear that it is a sign of a brain tumor or some other fatal brain disease. If the source is indeed an arteriovenous malformation or an aneurysm, definitive neurosurgical intervention may be lifesaving. In the vast majority of cases, however, the pain is a symptom of a nonlife-threatening condition that can be managed reasonably well with either vasoactive drugs or nonpharmacologic techniques. Chronic pain and its nursing management are discussed in Chapter 26.

DEGENERATIVE DISORDERS

The degenerative disorders are those characterized by loss of neurons or neuronal processes. They usually exhibit progressive loss of both structure and associated human function. The demyelinating diseases and peripheral neuropathies might be considered special cases of degenerative disorders in that portions of the nerve processes (axons and dendrites) or their coverings (myelin) undergo degenerative changes. In many of these disorders, the process is reversible and cellular repair occurs.

Degenerative Disorders of Axis I

Parkinson's Disease
Parkinson's disease is a common disorder, with an incidence of 20.5 cases per 100,000, prevalent in approximately 500,000 persons in the United States at any one time (Rajput et al., 1984; Adams & Victor, 1985). Onset is usually between 40 and 70 years of age, with the peak onset in the sixth decade. The disease affects men and women of all socioeconomic groups and varied occupations equally.

A loss of pigmented, dopamine-producing cells in the substantia nigra and other pigmented nuclei in the basal ganglia is believed responsible for the clinical symptoms. Although some cases are directly attributable to conditions known to destroy the substantia nigra (carbon monoxide poisoning, manganese poisoning, and certain illicit so-called designer drugs, such as 1-methyl-4-phenyl-1, 2, 3, 6-tetrahydropine [MPTP]) or to block the action of dopamine (phenothiazine-type antipsychotic agents), the cause is unknown in the majority of cases.

The early symptoms of aching, fatigue, and slowness are often overlooked and attributed to arthritis or other effects of aging. Eventually, stiffness and slowness progress into the classic triad of tremor, rigidity, and bradykinesia. Loss of automatic movement and righting reflexes is prominent as well. Symptoms frequently are unilateral in the beginning and then progress to bilateral involvement. It is not uncommon for the classic pill-rolling tremor to be absent or a very minor manifestation. Bradykinesia is the most disabling symptom for most people. Although the course of the disease does not shorten the life span appreciably, as the disorder progresses, all spheres of function mediated by the brain may be affected: mood, cognition, social and work ability, sleep, and sexual function. Medical treatment is most commonly pharmacologic, with dopamine precursors (L-dopa, L-dopa/carbidopa combination) and anticholinergics (trihexyphenidyl, benztropine mesylate) used to control the motor problems. Occasionally, thalamotomy is still used for severe unilateral tremor, and transplantation of catecholamine-producing adrenal medullary tissue into the brain is being explored. With the exception of experimental tissue transplantation, medical and surgical therapies do not alter the basic degenerative process but merely supplement the body's waning ability to produce neurotransmitters that control movement. These therapies maintain functioning for a longer period of time than was the case before their advent, but the disease process continues to progress slowly, resulting in severe disability.

Human responses are potential in all areas directly and indirectly mediated by the cerebral dopamine and acetylcholine neurotransmitter systems: movement, cognition, mood, sleep, and hypothalamically integrated autonomic functions (e.g., blood pressure control, appetite, sexual function), with mobility problems being the most prominent. Chapter 21 illustrates some of these problems.

Dementias

Collectively, many of the degenerative disorders of Axis I comprise the dementias or produce generalized cognitive and intellectual deterioration (Reisberg, 1983). Clinically, the term "dementia" denotes a syndrome involving intellectual deterioration, changes in personality, and a variety of behavioral abnormalities. Examples of dementing diseases include Alzheimer's disease, multiinfarct dementia, alcoholism, intracranial tumors, normal pressure hydrocephalus, and Huntington's disease. The annual incidence of the dementias collectively is estimated to be 50 per 100,000 population, with a prevalence of 250 per 100,000 population. The prevalence increases with age.

Dementias of the Alzheimer's type are the most common, estimated to account for between 33% and 50% of all cases (Schoenberg, 1986; Adams & Victor, 1985). Alzheimer's disease is estimated to affect 4% of the population over age 65 and reach 20% by age 80 (Kwentus et al., 1986). Terry and Katzman (1983) report that Alzheimer's disease accounts for 90,000 to 100,000 deaths per year.

Huntington's disease is a disorder of movement, mentation, and behavior and is inherited in an autosomal dominant pattern, with the genetic defect now localized to chromosome 4. The defect causes atrophy of cells in the caudate nucleus and putamen. Huntington's disease occurs worldwide, with a prevalence of 5 to 10 per 100,000 population (Hayden, 1981). In the United States, approximately 25,000 people have clinical features of Huntington's disease, and another 125,000 are immediately at risk (i.e., have parents with the disorder) (Conneally, 1984). Age of onset is estimated at 38 years, with the duration of illness ranging from 10 to 25 years. The life span is estimated to be shortened to approximately 57 years (Shoulson, 1984).

Motor signs of the disease consist of involuntary hyperkinesias (chorea and dystonia) and, in the later stages, bradykinesia and rigidity. These movements interfere with safety, speech, swallowing, nutrition, and self-care skills. Dementia may not be evident for several years but eventually becomes manifest with the same signs as the other dementias. Behavioral outbursts and dyscontrol syndromes are common.

The clinical course of the dementias is variable and may occur rapidly over a few years or slowly over 15 or more years. The earliest symptoms include gradual development of forgetfulness, lack of initiative, and neglect of routine tasks and are so subtle as to be noticed only in retrospect. As the disorder progresses, the person experiences increased deficits with recent memory, decreased ability to concentrate, and inability to manage personal and work or financial affairs. It is in this phase that family members often experience the strain of coping with the changing person and seek professional help. Eventually, the person becomes unable to function independently, experiences difficulties in simple activities of daily living (such as dressing), and may experience hallucinations or delusions and exhibit socially problematic behaviors, such as wandering or combativeness. In the final phases, the person even loses self-orientation, and becomes bedridden and incontinent.

The symptoms of the various dementias are related to structural degeneration of neurons in the cerebrum and diencephalon, with the specific structures varying with the particular disease. For example, Huntington's chorea is characterized by degeneration of neurons in the caudate nucleus and has both cognitive and motor symptoms (involuntary choreiform movements). In contrast, Alzheimer's disease involves loss of neurons and accumulation of argyophylic plaques and neurofibrillary tangles, primarily in the hippocampus (Kwentus et al., 1986).

Although the dementing diseases have varying pathologic and structural markers that differentiate them at autopsy, the human responses are much the same. They all affect cognition and mood because of their effects on the cerebral hemispheres, diencephalon, and limbic system. Some, such as Parkinson's disease with dementia and Huntington's disease, also affect movement because of the involvement of the basal ganglia in the pathologic process. All dementing diseases create a variety of problems for family and community in terms of safety and supplementation of self-care activities, which can no longer be performed by the afflicted person. Chapters 10 through 13 and 33 discuss cognition responses and self-care alterations relevant to this group of disorders.

Degenerative Disorders of Axes II, III, and IV

Axes II, III, and IV are the brainstem and cerebellum, spinal cord, and peripheral nerves and junctions with innervated organs, respectively. They all serve various components of the integration of motor and sensory function in the peripheral and central nervous system.

Multiple Sclerosis

Multiple sclerosis (MS) is the most prominent of the diseases that destroy the myelin covering of axons and dendrites in the central nervous system. It is the third most common cause (after trauma and stroke) of severe disability between the ages of 15 and 60. Given the early age of onset (in the second and third decades), chronicity (approximately 30 years duration), and cost per individual (50% greater than stroke on a per-person per-year basis), MS has been estimated to cost a person nearly 40% of his or her lifetime earnings (Weinfeld & Baum, 1984).

The risk of developing MS is related to place of residence. Prevalence studies in many countries have demonstrated that there is a high risk (prevalence of 40 per 100,000 or more) above 40 degrees latitude and the Tropics of Capricorn and Cancer and a low risk (less than 19 per 100,000 cases) between the Tropics (McDonald, 1984). Migration studies have shown that moving to a lower prevalence region before age 15 results in a decreased incidence of the disease. These results suggest a mixture of genetic susceptibility and environmental factors in the etiology of the disease. The occurrence of clusters of the disease suggests that the environmental factor may be infectious (McDonald, 1984).

The etiology is postulated to be late activation of a slow virus or, more likely, an autoimmune response triggered by a virus. Multiple sclerosis is a disease of the white matter (myelinated tissue), associated with multifocal inflammatory demyelinating lesions or diffuse axonal demyelinating lesions that leave the nerve cell process itself intact. It is not strictly a disorder of Axes II and III, since there may be lesions in the white matter of the cerebrum as well. Manifestations, however, most commonly are related to formation of plaques (areas of demyelination) in the spinal cord, brainstem, cerebellum, and visual pathways.

The earliest clinical signs are often vague, such as weakness or numbness and tingling in one or more limbs, visual blurring, difficulty walking, or urinary frequency and urgency. The diagnosis has been considerably aided by the use of magnetic resonance imaging (MRI)—which often demonstrates plaques—visual evoked responses, and special techniques of spinal fluid examination. Diagnostic criteria include visualization of plaques that are consistent with clinical signs, episodes of neurologic deficit separate in space and time, and symptoms in more than one neurologic system that cannot be explained on the basis of a single lesion. Clinical syndromes can be classified into the following types: mixed or generalized (50% of cases, with involvement of the optic nerve, brainstem, cerebellum, and spinal cord), spinal (30% to 40% of cases, characterized by spastic ataxia and deep sensory changes), cerebellar or pontobulbar–cerebellar (5% of cases, characterized by problems with coordination, equilibrium, speech, and swallowing), and amaurotic (5% unilateral visual deficits). Seventy percent of patients experience the typical acute-onset exacerbating and remitting type. Fewer than 10% suffer from the malignant form with early cerebellar signs and rapid progression to severe disability (Smith & Sheinberg, 1985).

A large number of treatments of MS have been attempted, all of which are difficult to evaluate because of the exacerbating–remitting natural course of the disease. Adrenocorticotropic hormone (ACTH) and corticosteroids are often administered to shorten the course of an exacerbation. Immunosuppressive therapy and plasmapheresis have been evaluated, based on the theory of autoimmune response. Cyclophosphamide has been reported helpful in chronic progressive MS, with 70% to 80% of patients stable after 1 year in one study, compared to 50% of those treated with plasma exchange and 20% of those treated with ACTH alone (Sibley, 1985).

As is evident from the large portion of the central nervous system that can be affected by MS, human responses vary widely. There may be alterations in vision, cognition, mobility (related to weakness or coordination), somatic sensation, communication (related to coordination of speaking mechanisms), nutrition (related to swallowing difficulties), elimination, and self-care. Alterations in human responses discussed in Chapters 11, 14, 15, 21, 24, 26, 28, 31, and 33 are relevant to people with MS.

Motor Neuron Diseases

The motor neuron (or motor system) diseases are characterized by progressive degeneration of motor neurons in the anterior horns of the spinal cord and brainstem. Since the 1950s, the motor neuron diseases have replaced poliomyelitis as the most frequent cause of anterior horn cell dysfunction. *Amyotrophic lateral sclerosis* (ALS, or Lou Gehrig's disease) is the most common form of adult motor neuron disease, accounting for 1.5 of the 2 cases per 100,000 of all motor neuron disorders. The prevalence is estimated at 5 of the 6 cases per 100,000 population for all motor neuron disorders (Kurtzke, 1982). The mean duration of survival with ALS is about 3 years, although some patients live as long as 10 to 15 years and some die as soon as 1 year after diagnosis.

Pathologically, motor neurons in the brainstem or spinal cord atrophy and die, with subsequent loss of their peripheral axons. Sensory neurons are not affected. Muscles atrophy due to loss of trophic influences from the nerve fiber, and progressive muscular weakness ensues. Symptoms may begin in the periphery (usually the arms), with difficulty performing fine finger movements and wasting of the hands. Cramping and fasciculations of the muscles of the limb or trunk are evident. Reflexes may be absent in the affected limb and hyperactive in the limbs more distal. The atrophic weakness progresses to involve the neck, tongue, pharyngeal and laryngeal muscles, trunk, and lower extremities. Ultimately, the patient is unable to move, speak, swallow, and, eventually, breathe. Mentation and sensation and usually bowel and bladder control are intact throughout the course of the disease. Respiratory insufficiency frequently is the cause of death, although long-term ventilatory support can be offered if the patient wishes to extend life.

The *spinal muscular atrophies* are several types of more slowly progressive motor neuron diseases. These are inherited, usually in an autosomal dominant pattern. Symptoms are evident in early infancy or in adolescence. The childhood form, called Werdnig-Hoffmann disease, can be associated also with respiratory failure. Patients will have significant deficits in mobility and self-care. Chapters 15, 21, and 33 are most relevant to human responses common in persons with motor neuron diseases.

Degenerative Disorders of Axis IV

Neuropathy indicates damage to the peripheral nerves, regardless of cause. Infectious disorders are referred to as neuritis (as in trigeminal neuritis, a sequela of varicella infection). The neuropathies may be caused by entrapment of the nerve, with subsequent degeneration of either the myelin covering or the axons themselves, by trauma and pressure or severing of the nerve, or by metabolic processes that cause degeneration of myelin or axonal tissue. Many are reversible.

Polyneuropathies

Polyneuropathies (involvement of multiple peripheral nerves) have an annual incidence rate of 40 cases per 100,000 (Kurtzke, 1982). Most polyneuropathies exhibit a characteristic distribution of weakness, paralysis, and often sensory changes. The pathologic process begins at the most distal parts of the largest and longest nerves and advances headward along the affected fiber to the cell body. Regeneration and functional reconnections are possible unless the cell body itself dies.

Guillain-Barré syndrome, also called acute infectious polyradiculoneuritis, serves as a prototype for the problems patients face with acute polyneuropathies. The incidence of Guillain-Barré syndrome worldwide is approximately 1.5 cases per 100,000, and approximately 2 per 100,000 in the United States (Adams & Victor, 1985; Kurtzke, 1982).

The major clinical manifestation is symmetrical weakness that ascends and becomes more severe over days to 1 to 2 weeks. Distal muscles of the lower extremities usually are affected first, with progression to the lower proximal muscles and then to the trunk, intercostal, upper extremity, neck, and cranial muscles. Peak severity, which can be complete flaccid paralysis, is reached in 90% of patients within 10 to 14 days. Weakness can progress more rapidly, however, leading to total motor paralysis and respiratory muscle failure within days. The disorder affects primarily motor and autonomic peripheral nerves, leaving sensation intact. Autonomic disturbances (tachycardia, fluctuating blood pressure control, elimination disturbances) are common.

Most evidence suggests that the disorder results from a cell-mediated immunologic reaction to peripheral nerve myelin. The majority of cases remit spontaneously, with full recovery. The disorder has the potential to alter responses in all areas of human function except consciousness, cognition, and sensation.

Mononeuropathies

Mononeuropathies are disorders of single peripheral nerves secondary to trauma, entrapment, and some metabolic processes, such as diabetes or postinfectious syndromes. The symptoms depend on the specific motor, sensory, or mixed function of the involved nerve. Most commonly, mononeuropathies occur in cranial nerves (particularly V and VI) and the brachial and lumbosacral plexes. Such disorders produce problems in movement and, in some cases, pain or anesthesia. The incidence of mononeuropathies is estimated at 40 per 100,000 (Kurtzke, 1982).

TUMORS

Tumors are abnormal growths of neural or nonneural tissues in the cranial cavity or on the spinal cord or peripheral nerves. Although many central nervous system tumors are not malignant in the sense that they spread to other parts of the body, their local growth and extension may threaten function and life because of compression and destruction of tissues around them by the tumor itself and by the vasogenic brain swelling surrounding the tumor. Metastatic tumors from other parts of the body may spread to the central nervous system, producing multiple tumors within it.

Kurtzke (1982) provides the following general estimates of incidence of tumors in the central nervous system:

Type	Incidence per 100,000
Metastatic brain tumor	15
Benign brain tumor	10
Malignant brain tumor	5
Metastatic spinal cord tumor	5
Benign spinal cord tumor	1
Malignant spinal cord tumor	0.5

Tumors of the central nervous system occur in great pathologic variety, but their symptoms are based on their size, location, and invasiveness. Common symptoms of tumors in Axis I are changes in cognition, motor function, headaches, vomiting, and seizures. Increased intracranial pressure, with papilledema, is often a concomitant sign of slowly growing tumors of the cerebral hemispheres. If tumors continue to grow, they may alter consciousness and ultimately produce brain herniation and death (see Chapter 7).

Central nervous system neoplasms are classified in many ways. This discussion classifies them, first, by type of neural or supporting tissue involved and, second, by area of the nervous system affected. The classification of tumors by type of tissue is helpful to neuroscience physicians in anticipating the relative responsiveness of specific tumors to adjuvent therapies (chemotherapy, radiotherapy). Classification by area of the nervous system involved is useful to the neuroscience nurse in anticipating specific alterations in human responses related to location of specific kinds of neoplasms.

Neoplasms Classified by Type of Tissue Involved

Tumors of the nervous system may derive from neuronal tissue, supportive brain tissue, the reticuloendothelial system, brain and spinal cord coverings, residual developmental tissues, glandular structures, or nerve sheaths. In addition, tumors of either the brain or spinal cord may be metastatic from systemic carcinomas.

Tumors of Neurons or Primitive Neuronal Elements

Medulloblastomas and neuroastrocytomas are tumors derived from primitive neuronal blast cells or from neurons. Medulloblastomas account for about 7% of all central nervous system tumors and occur primarily in children. Generally arising in the fourth ventricle, medulloblastomas thus cause symptoms referable to the posterior fossa: ataxia, nystagmus, and impairment of cerebrospinal fluid flow. These tumors may metastasize throughout the neuroaxis and are treated with resection and radiation or chemotherapy. Neuroastrocytomas (or gangliogliomas) are extremely rare and occur primarily in children. They are generally located in the frontal and temporal lobes and hypothalamus. Excision may or may not be possible, depending upon accessibility. Radiation may increase length of survival.

Tumors of Central Nervous System Supportive Tissue

The most frequent central nervous system tumors are those of the supportive tissues: gliomas and tumors of the choroid plexus. Gliomas are tumors of the glial tissues and are subdivided into astrocytomas (grades I and II), glioblastoma multiforme (grades III and IV, or malignant astrocytoma), oligodendrogliomas, and ependymal tumors. Together, the gliomas account for about 46% of all central nervous system tumors.

Astrocytomas grades I and II account for 10% to 15% of central nervous system tumors and are found most commonly in children and young adults. Astrocytomas are the most common type of posterior fossa tumor in children (33%). About 1% of astrocytomas are optic gliomas, also found in children. Grades III and IV astrocytomas (glioblastoma multiforme) are seen almost entirely in adults and account for 25% of central nervous system tumors. Although grades I and II astrocytomas are often resectable and sensitive to radiation, glioblastomas are much more invasive and virtually never eradicated. Excision and subsequent chemotherapy or irradiation are used to prolong life.

Oligodendrogliomas are slowly growing lesions, usually found in the cerebral hemispheres in young adults. About 3% of tumors are this type. Excision and irradiation are used to prolong life but are rarely curative. Likewise, ependymomas are relatively uncommon (3% of all tumors) and derive from the ependymal cells lining the ventricles. Ventricular obstruction is common, and the tumor often can be completely resected, although metastasis is possible during excision. Irradiation may be used if complete resection is not possible.

Colloid cysts and choroid plexus papillomas are rare tumors of supportive tissues that occur in childhood and adolescence. Colloid cysts occur in the third ventricle, and choroid plexus papillomas occur most commonly in the lateral or fourth ventricle. Both are apt to produce hydrocephalus and may be cured if surgical excision is complete.

Tumors of the Reticuloendothelial System

Systemic diseases, such as leukemia, lymphoma, and myeloma, rarely may involve the nervous system, infiltrating either the brain or the meninges. Such involvement is more likely to occur when there is a generalized immunosuppression, such as with therapeutic immunosuppressive therapy or with acquired immune deficiency syndrome (AIDS). Irradiation, chemotherapy, and shunting to reduce intracranial pressure are all used as adjuvant therapy.

Tumors of Central Nervous System Coverings

Tumors of skull elements, such as osteomas and chondrosarcomas, are relatively rare central nervous system tumors, whereas meningiomas (tumors of the leptomeninges) account for about 15% of central nervous system tumors. Most of the bony tumors are found in children and young adults, and meningiomas are found only in adults. Meningiomas are rarely malignant, and cure is the rule when excision is complete. Meningiomas of the areas around the brainstem and base of the skull may not be accessible to complete excision, however.

Tumors of Developmental Remnants

Congenital tumors include craniopharyngiomas (about 3% of all tumors) and the more rare cholesteatomas (epidermoid cysts), teratomas, and chordomas. All are present from birth but may not be detected until later in life because of their slow growth. Craniopharyngiomas are believed to be remnants of Rathke's pouch and thus develop in the suprasellar region. Pituitary dysfunction, bitemporal visual deficits, and hydrocephalus from obstruction of the third ventricle may all occur. Complete excision is often possible.

Cholesteatomas and teratomas derive from remnants of epidermoid cells of germinal cells and are found in the cerebellopontine angle and pineal or suprasellar regions, respectively. Teratomas are usually malignant but are radiosensitive. Cholesteatomas are benign and often can be completely excised.

Tumors of Glandular Structures

Pituitary adenomas account for 5% to 15% of cranial tumors and are found in adults. Pinealomas are rare and are seen in children. Pituitary dysfunction (Cushing's syndrome, acromegaly, amenorrhea) and visual defects are indications for transphenoidal resection. Hormonal replacement is necessary postoperatively.

Tumors of Nerve Sheaths

Tumors of nerve sheaths include acoustic neuromas and fifth nerve tumors. Acoustic neuroma is the most common tumor of the cerebellopontine angle in adults and accounts for 5% to 8% of all central nervous system tumors. It usually originates on the vestibular portion of the eighth cranial nerve (CN VIII) within the auditory canal. It grows into the posterior fossa to occupy the cerebellopontine angle and may grow to impinge on CN V and CN VII (and occasionally CN IX and CN X). If not resected, it eventually will displace the pons and medulla and obstruct cerebrospinal fluid circulation. Unilateral loss of hearing, disturbed balance, ipsilateral loss of coordination, and ipsilateral facial weakness are common symptoms.

Fifth nerve tumors are rare and are usually associated with severe facial pain. Surgical resection is possible but may be limited by access at the junction of the middle and posterior fossa.

Metastatic Tumors

Tumors metastasize to the brain most commonly from the lung, followed by breast, skin, kidney, gastrointestinal tract, prostate, and thyroid. Metastatic tumors constitute about 10% of intracranial neoplasms that come to surgery. Single lesions may be excised surgically to extend life or to reduce symptoms. The edema surrounding such lesions is responsive to corticosteroid therapy.

Neoplasms Classified by Neural Structures

Axis I (Cerebral Hemispheres and Diencephalon)

Tumors of the cerebral hemispheres may occur in any of the lobes of the brain or in the diencephalon, with the symptoms referable to the particular brain area involved. Gliomas and meningiomas are the most common tumors of the hemispheres. Tumors of the sella or parasella are the most likely to produce hypothalamic, optic, and pituitary dysfunction. Craniopharyngiomas and pituitary adenomas are the most common of these. Ventricular tumors, such as choroid plexus papillomas of the lateral ventricles, may also affect the hemispheres and diencephalon.

Axis II (Brainstem and Cerebellum)

Tumors of the posterior fossa and cerebellopontine angle will all produce dysfunction of cerebellar coordination, cranial nerves, and brainstem tracts. Ventricular tumors of this area can produce obstructive hydrocephalus. Medulloblastoma, cerebellar astrocytoma, ependymona, brainstem gliomas, and acoustic neurinomas are common tumors of Axis II.

Axis III (Spinal Cord)

Spinal cord tumors are less common than intracranial tumors, constituting only about 15% of central nervous system tumors (Adams & Victor, 1985). The majority are benign and exert their effects by compression of the spinal cord. Spinal tumors can be divided into extramedullary and intramedullary. Extramedullary tumors arise outside the spinal cord, in the vertebral bodies and epidural tissues (extradural) or in the leptomeninges or roots (intradural). Intramedullary tumors arise within the substance of the spinal cord and destroy tracts and central gray structures. People with spinal cord tumors manifest one of three clinical syndromes; sensorimotor loss referable to dysfunction of spinal cord motor and sensory tracts, radicular–spinal cord syndrome referable to involvement of peripheral nerve roots as well as spinal cord tracts, and syringomyelic syndrome referable to loss of central cord function.

Human responses to tumors of Axes I and II are of three types: (1) specific symptomatic alterations referable to the portion of the brain or brainstem affected, (2) responses to the surgical, chemotherapeutic, or radiotherapeutic modality used, and (3) responses related to uncertainty about the future and residual neurologic deficits. The category of altered human response (e.g., altered communication and cognition) can be inferred from the discussion of the more common locations of brain and spinal cord tumors. All tumor-destructive medical and surgical interventions carry the potential for inflammatory response and local brain swelling. These, in turn, carry the potential for increased intracranial pressure and brain herniation. Corticosteroids reduce cerebral edema related to brain tumors and often are used to minimize the swelling associated with radiotherapy and chemotherapy as well.

Responses to the uncertainty of future function and life may create a variety of coping responses for the individual and family. Often a need arises for community support systems for people with terminal central nervous system neoplasms. Chapter 17 illustrates some of these responses.

NEUROMUSCULAR DISORDERS

The neuromuscular disorders are all disorders of Axis IV, specifically, the neuromuscular junction or the muscles themselves.

Myasthenia Gravis

Myasthenia gravis (MG) is characterized by muscular weakness and easy fatigability. The weakness increases with use and is relieved by rest (Grob et al., 1981). Facial, extraocular, masticatory, deglutitional, and lingual muscles are particularly involved, but respiratory and limb muscles also are affected. The most common symptom experienced by people with MG is double vision (41%), followed by drooping eyelid (24%), difficulty with voice (16%), weak legs (13%), general weakness (11%), difficulty swallowing (10%), difficulty chewing (7%), and weak arms and hands (7%).

The fatigability of muscles is traced to a defect at the juncture between nerve and muscle. Specifically, acetylcholine receptors on the muscle fiber are decreased in number, presumably through an autoimmune response to the receptors.

Epidemiologic studies demonstrate the incidence and prevalence of MG to be much higher in women than in men. A Norwegian study reports an incidence of 5.3 per million population for women, compared with 2.6 per million for men, as well as a prevalence of 127 per million for women and 52 per million for men (Storm-Mathisen, 1984). Two thirds of women develop symptoms before age 40, whereas two thirds of men develop them after age 40 (Kurtzke, 1984). Mortality is related to respiratory insufficiency and is higher than that of the age-matched population (1.5 times of that in women under 60, nearly 5 times that of women older than 60, and 1.4 times that of all men) (Storm-Mathisen, 1984). The outlook for a normal life span has improved considerably over the past 25 years, however. Formerly, nearly one third of patients died from respiratory complications of the disease; currently, this figure is less than 5% as a result of improvements in intensive care management, respiratory nursing care, and new treatment modalities. Spontaneous remission is said to occur in 10% to 20% of cases, and can be induced in 60% to 87% of selected cases by thymectomy (Johns, 1982).

Early in the course of the disease, patients may be managed with anticholinesterase medications: pyridostigmine bromide, prostigmine, or ambenonium chloride four to six times daily. Most patients require further medical or surgical therapy, including corticosteroids, thymectomy, immunosuppressive drugs, or plasma exchange.

Corticosteroid therapy is associated with improvement in a large proportion of patients (Johns, 1982) but carries all the numerous side effects of long-term steroid administration. Immunosuppressive drugs, particularly azathioprine, have been successful in treating symptoms of MG. Compared with prednisone, the side effects are mild, consisting of occasional gastrointestinal upset, leukopenia, liver enzyme elevation, and interstitial cystitis. The potential for teratogenesis in women of childbearing age is a concern for many MG patients, and the risk of acquired malignancy is unknown (Hertel, 1981). Plasma exchange temporarily removes antibodies to the acetylcholine receptors and may be effective in myasthenic crisis, but it does not offer long-term remission (Howard, 1982). Thymectomy is particularly effective in young women and often induces remission or marked improvement.

Botulism

Botulism is an uncommon but frequently fatal disorder caused by a bacterial toxin (*Clostridium botulinum* toxin) that acts at the myoneural junction. Botulinum toxin is produced from the spores of *C. botulinum* and prevents the release of acetylcholine from the presynaptic nerve terminal, thus preventing function of all smooth and skeletal muscle fibers. The organism is ubiquitous in the soil, but its spores normally are destroyed by acidic foods or with pressure cooking in commercial preparation. Improper home canning techniques may not kill the spores, which will then produce the toxin when the sealed container remains at room temperature. Less frequently, toxin-producing spores may enter the body through wounds contaminated with dirt. Very few cases are reported each year in the United States (e.g., 21 during 1979 and 1980), and most occur in the western United States, particularly Colorado, California, Oregon, Washington, and Alaska (Rubenstein, 1985).

Death may be rapid, depending on the amount of toxin circulating. Improvements in intensive care, particularly respiratory support, have reduced the death rate from 60% to 20% in recent years (Rubenstein, 1985). Symptoms appear within 6 hours to a few days and initially consist of dry mouth, diplopia, difficulty focusing, dysphagia, and dysarthria. Nausea, vomiting, diarrhea, and abdominal cramping are common. Descending motor weakness or paralysis and respiratory muscle insufficiency are common, and sensory involvement is rare.

Treatment is entirely symptomatic, with respiratory support and nursing prevention of immobility complications essential. Antitoxin may be of help if given early. In many cases the disease may mimic Guillain-Barré syndrome, tick paralysis, and a variety of chemical intoxications. The diagnosis is confirmed by demonstrating that the patient's serum is toxic to mice.

Recovery is slow as the patient's body gradually metabolizes the toxin. The prognosis for full recovery is good provided the intercurrent complications of immobility and respiratory insufficiency are prevented. Human responses to this disorder can be expected to be similar to those of patients with other acute immobilizing disorders, such as Guillain-Barré syndrome and acute spinal cord injury.

Myopathies

Chronic myopathies are disorders of the muscle fibers that produce weakness and progressive loss of functional mobility. The two major categories are the muscular dystrophies and the inflammatory diseases, such as polymyositis. Both categories are characterized by progressive weakness, as well as myopathic changes apparent on electromyography, high serum enzymes that reflect muscle damage (creatine kinase [CK]), and abnormal muscle biopsy findings.

Muscular Dystrophies

The muscular dystrophies are genetic diseases characterized by progressive deterioration of skeletal muscle function without associated pathologic changes in the peripheral nerves or central nervous system (Donahoe, 1979). At least nine types of muscular dystrophy are identified. The incidence of all types combined is 1.2 cases per 100,000, with a prevalence of 20 cases per 100,000 population.

The most common is Duchenne type muscular dystrophy, a sex-linked recessive disorder, with the locus of the defect on the X (female) chromosome. The disease is thus carried by the mother on one X chromosome but manifested only in her male children, who do not have a healthy X chromosome to prevent expression of the disorder. Symptoms begin when the child begins to walk. The family will notice frequent falls, a lordotic toe-walking gait, and difficulty climbing stairs and running. By age 10, the child is usually wheelchair bound. Other complications include obesity, severe contractures, scoliosis, and occasional learning disabilities. Pulmonary function abnormalities begin in the late teens and early 20s. Without respiratory intervention, these people rarely survive through their 30s.

Myotonic muscular dystrophy is an autosomal dominant disorder characterized by an abnormality in muscle relaxation, as well as defects in a variety of specialized and smooth muscle functions, such as cardiac conduction abnormalities, gastrointestinal slowing, and cataracts. The age of onset varies from childhood to early adulthood.

No medical therapies slow the progressive muscle deterioration seen in all types of muscular dystrophy. Symptomatic therapy, such as bracing of extremities, appropriate exercise, and prescription of functional wheelchairs, remains the primary therapeutic intervention. Genetic counseling is an important component of care for these families.

Inflammatory Myopathies

The inflammatory myopathies, such as polymyositis and dermatomyositis, have an incidence of 0.5 per 100,000 and a prevalence of 6 per 100,000. The symptoms include symmetric proximal muscle weakness, muscle tenderness, reduced mobility, and, in dermatomyositis, a distinctive rash. The disease can be found in all age groups but is most common in childhood and middle age. Treatment with immunosuppressive agents, such as prednisone and azathioprine, has been successful in many cases, suggesting that an autoimmune response to muscle fiber is the source of the disorder. The illness can be lifelong, being controlled rather than cured by medication.

NEUROTRAUMA

Trauma to the central nervous system is a major source of disability and death in the United States. The primary types of neurotrauma are head injury and spinal cord injury. The Department of Human and Health Services estimates that one million cases of head and spinal cord injury occur each year. The cost of these injuries totals $4.68 billion. An estimated $37.8 billion was spent on research of these disorders in fiscal year 1987. Both head and spinal cord injuries are largely preventable, since they are caused mainly by motor vehicle accidents and falls.

Head Injury

Head injury is a term for a cluster of diagnostic entities that result from trauma to the cranial cavity. Head injuries affect both Axes I (cerebral hemispheres and diencephalon) and II (brainstem and cerebellum), and the human responses reflect a combination of problems in these axes.

Frankowski (1986) estimates the incidence of fatal and nonfatal head injuries at 200 to 300 cases per 100,000 in the United States. The peak incidence of head trauma occurs in the late teens (567 cases per 100,000), with a second, smaller peak in the sixth decade (Minter-Convery, 1985). Males are more than twice as likely as females to sustain such injuries. The most common cause of head injury is transportation accidents (31% to 49%), followed by falls (20% to 32%), assault (7% to 40%), recreational accidents (3% to 14%), and miscellaneous causes (4% to 23%) (Frankowski, 1986).

The mechanism of injury largely determines the areas of the brain affected. Concussion, a transient alteration in neural function and consciousness, is an example of a minor injury in which recovery is the rule. A postconcussive syndrome may occur, however, characterized by headache, dizziness, and difficulty concentrating.

More severe injuries may result in brain contusion, bleeding at the site of impact and at distant sites secondary to movement of the brain in the cranial cavity. Tearing of extradural and subdural vessels in the brain coverings may result in hematomas, which compress underlying brain tissue and may lead to brain herniation. Hyperemic responses to injury, coupled with intracranial or extracranial bleeding, may lead to intracranial hypertension, decreased brain perfusion, and transtentorial herniation.

Hematomas often can be removed surgically, providing relief from brain compression. The majority of severe head injuries, however, are characterized by widespread disruption in neuronal function and are not treatable by surgical means. Because the cerebral hemispheres and brainstem integrate all human functions, the range of human responses to head injury potentially encompasses all aspects of living. Patients with head injuries are likely to exhibit many of the alterations in human responses discussed in the sections on consciousness (Chapters 5 through 8), cognition (Chapters 10 through 13), communication (Chapters 14 and 15), affiliative relationships (Chapter 17), and self-care (Chapters 32 and 33).

Spinal Cord Injury

Spinal cord injury reflects neurotrauma in Axis III. The annual incidence rate is 3 cases per 100,000, about 1% of that of head injury. The prevalence of permanent spinal cord injury is about 50 per 100,000, with an average duration of 18 years (Kurtzke, 1982). As with head injury, males are affected far more than females, with 72% of injuries occurring in males (Griffin et al., 1985). Sixty percent of spinal cord injuries are incurred on the highway, with another 13% at other outdoor sites, 12% in the home, and 7% at work.

Adams and Victor (1985) divide spinal cord injuries into three groups: fracture–dislocations, fractures, and dislocations. Fracture–dislocations are three times as common as the others. Fractures and dislocations of the vertebral column can cause injury to the cord itself by compression or laceration of the cord. Shearing or compression of the cord results in destruction of white and gray matter by hemorrhage and ischemia. Pathologic processes that result in the death of neurons appear to start at the time of impact and do not seem to be prevented by early decompressive laminectomy if signs of spinal cord trauma are already present. Immobilization, reduction, and stabilization of the fracture or dislocation are important to prevent further trauma to the cord. Characteristics of acute spinal cord injury and associated human responses are discussed in Chapter 20.

SEIZURES

Epilepsy

Epilepsy (recurrent seizures) is among the most common neurologic disorders. An estimated 2 million people in the United States are affected by this disorder, with an annual incidence of 50 per 100,000 persons and a prevalence rate of 650 per 100,000 or nearly 1 in 25 (Kurtzke, 1982). Epilepsy is a sudden, intermittent alteration in consciousness or function resulting from excessive discharge of cerebral neurons. It is entirely a disorder of Axis I (cerebral hemisphere and diencephalon). The etiologies of seizures include systemic disease (fever, neoplasm, vascular disease), sequelae of head trauma, stroke, or such disorders as multiple sclerosis and hypoxic syndromes. The largest number of cases are idiopathic, that is, they have no identifiable cause.

Seizures currently are classified on the basis of their clinical form and electroencephalographic (EEG) features as partial, generalized, unilateral, or unclassified (because of incomplete data) (Gastaut, 1970). *Partial seizures* are of three forms: elementary, complex, or secondarily generalized. Those that begin locally with elementary symptoms usually take a simple form (motor, sensory, autonomic, or a mixture of the three) and cause no impairment of consciousness. Complex partial seizures generally cause some impairment of consciousness in that the patient cannot recall events that happened during the seizure but is able to carry on automatic activities that require consciousness. The automatisms of psychomotor seizures are in this classification. Partial seizures may spread secondarily to become generalized seizures. The so-called aura for many people with epilepsy is actually a partial sensory, motor, or complex partial seizure that precedes a secondary generalization.

Generalized seizures are characterized by bilaterally symmetric EEG changes and no local onset. Consciousness is impaired for very brief (absence) or longer periods (major motor seizures). Generalized seizures may take many forms: absence (formerly *petit mal*), clonic motor, tonic motor, tonic–clonic (formerly *grand mal*), atonic, and akinetic, myoclonic, and infantile spasms.

Various anticonvulsant drugs specific to the seizure type are used to alter membrane properties and raise the seizure threshold. Therapeutic levels can be monitored in the serum or saliva to help titrate therapy for adequate seizure control. Surgical removal of epileptic foci is sometimes possible in severe cases that are uncontrolled by medication and in which a focus can be found.

Human responses to seizures are discussed in Chapter 8.

INFECTIOUS DISORDERS

Bacterial and viral organisms may gain access to the central nervous system either through the blood (as septic emboli or thrombi or in overwhelming bacteremia) or through direct extension from extracranial sources (traumatic penetrating injuries, from the nose via dural leakage, or direct extension from infections of facial, skull, or spinal bones). Neural tissue appears relatively resistant to direct bacterial and viral infection but is less resistant if there is intercurrent systemic disease and in malnourished, aged, and immunosuppressed patients.

Infectious Disorders of Axes I and II

Meningitis
Infections of the brain and spinal cord and their coverings may be caused by bacteria, viruses, or fungi. Meningitis is the most common of these infections and is characterized by inflammation of the leptomeninges of the brain and spinal cord.

Bacterial meningitis is reported to have an annual incidence varying from 3 to 10 cases per 100,000 population. *Hemophilus influenzae* is the most common causative agent, accounting for 48% of reported cases. *Neisseria meningitidis* and *Streptococcus pneumoniae* account for 20% and 13% of cases, respectively. The attack rate is highest in children aged under 1 year (7.6 per 100,000) and greater in males than females of all ages (3.3 versus 2.6 cases per 100,000 in one series) (Schlech et al., 1985).

Bacterial meningitis accounts for approximately one third of all meningitis cases (Skoch & Waling, 1985), with the remainder being termed aseptic meningitis. A virus can be demonstrated conclusively in approximately 12% of cases of aseptic meningitis (Beghi et al., 1984). Aseptic meningitis has a seasonal pattern, with the majority of cases in the summer months, whereas bacterial meningitis is more common in the winter.

Aseptic meningitis is characterized by flu-like symptoms, with fever, drowsiness, stiff neck, and often headache and paresthesias. There is no specific therapy, but recovery is usually complete and hospitalization is not commonly required.

In contrast, bacterial meningitis produces purulent exudate that can interfere with both the function of cranial nerves as they exit the meninges and with the flow of cerebrospinal fluid. Medical therapy consists of large doses of intravenous antibiotics specific to the organism. Penicillin G remains the drug of choice for most organisms, with chloramphenicol as a second choice. Gram-negative organisms respond to chloramphenicol or aminoglycosides.

Potential *human responses* include brain herniation secondary to swelling or communicating hydrocephalus, airway and visual disturbances due to cranial nerve dysfunction, and pain (headache).

Encephalitis
Encephalitis is inflammation and infection of the brain parenchyma (cortex and white matter) as well as the meninges and most com-

monly has a viral etiology. Herpes simplex type I is the most common causative virus, with arboviruses (eastern and western equine), enteroviruses (polio, coxsackie), and viruses that cause systemic illness (measles, mumps) also accounting for some cases. The attack rate for all causes is estimated at 7.4 per 100,000 persons, greater in females than in males (8.6 versus 6.3 per 100,000) and in children under 10 years old (Beghi et al., 1984). Encephalitis is seasonal, with nearly half the cases occurring in July, August, and September. Viruses gain access to the central nervous system via the blood or peripheral nerves, causing a nonexudative inflammation. Because viruses replicate inside cells, there is often neuronal degeneration, demyelination of axons and dendrites, and subsequent necrosis, hemorrhage, and cavitation. The amount of tissue destruction varies with the organism, but the potential for significant neurologic sequelae is greater for encephalitis than for meningitis.

Medical therapy is supportive, since there are few antiviral agents available. Acyclovir is effective in herpes encephalitis, but mortality remains high even with the drug (28% compared with 54% before introduction of the drug).

Human responses include the potential for brain herniation secondary to swelling, alterations in arousal that range from coma to hyperarousal, and a variety of cognitive problems, particularly memory loss.

Brain Abscess

Brain abscess is a localized area of infection usually caused by direct extension of bacteria from an infected wound or sinus. Bacteria also may enter via the bloodstream and create a localized, walled-off infection. The abscess acts as a space-occupying lesion and thus may mimic a tumor or hematoma. Medical therapy consists of systemic antibiotics or craniotomy for removal of encapsulated abscesses.

Infectious Disorders of Axis III

Poliomyelitis and tetanus are two infectious disorders that attack the spinal cord.

Poliomyelitis

Poliomyelitis is rare in developed countries because of widespread preventive immunization but remains common in developing countries. The poliovirus is an enterovirus. In the vast majority of cases, symptoms are nonspecific and flu-like, or may produce a mild aseptic meningitis. In a small percentage of cases, however, the virus gains entry to the central nervous system and is believed to travel along nerve fibers, being particularly attracted to the motor neurons of the brainstem (bulbar polio) or spinal cord. In paralytic cases, the motor neuron is destroyed, producing a flaccid paralysis of the muscles served by the portion of the brainstem or spinal cord affected. In mild cases, there may be only localized motor weakness, but in severe cases, the muscles of the limbs, trunk, head, and neck are involved. There is no specific medical therapy once the disease is established, and nursing management is identical to that of the patient with severe Guillain-Barré syndrome (see the section "Degenerative Disorders of Axis IV" in this chapter).

Tetanus

Tetanus is a rare but life-threatening disease caused by the neurotoxin tetanospasmin that is produced by the bacillus *Clostridium tetani*. The disorder is rare in the industrialized world as a result of widespread use of active immunization. Fewer than 200 cases are reported annually in the United States, and these are in nonimmunized or insufficiently immunized people. The incidence in developing countries, however, is high, with an estimate of over 1 million deaths annually (Simon & Schwartz, 1984).

The organism commonly is introduced through puncture wounds contaminated with dirt. The spores germinate and produce toxin, which then spreads along axons to the spinal cord and may spread also via the general circulation. Tetanus toxin acts on the spinal cord to suppress the reflex inhibition mediated by internuncial neurons. Thus, when a muscle contracts, the contraction of its antagonist is no longer suppressed, and muscle spasm occurs. The disease is characterized by initial spasm at the wound site, with subsequent difficulty opening the mouth (lockjaw), dysphagia related to pharyngeal spasm, and generalized muscular spasm that is both painful and metabolically costly. The sympathetic nervous system also is affected by the toxin, producing labile hypertension, tachycardia, arrhythmias, sweating, and tachypnea.

There is no specific therapy once the toxin has bound to spinal neurons, although antitoxin can neutralize circulating toxin. The primary therapy is supportive: ventilatory support, muscle-relaxing drugs, such as diazepam, paralyzing drugs, such as curare, or pancuronium to reduce the metabolic demand of uncontrolled spasms. Sensation and cognition are not affected by the toxin, so care of these patients requires continual attention to relief of pain and fear as well as respiratory support, autonomic stability, and control of muscle spasm.

Mortality varies with rapidity of onset. It has been reported at 100% when symptoms appear within 1 to 2 days of injury and 35% to 40% when incubation exceeds 10 days (Simon & Schwartz, 1984).

NEUROSURGICAL PROCEDURES

A number of disorders of the nervous system lend themselves to surgical therapy, either to remove the source of the problem, as in tumors, or to provide decompression of the brain for temporary palliation and relief of symptoms, as in intracranial hypertension or invasive tumors. It is beyond the scope of this chapter to discuss the variety of neurosurgical procedures that one may encounter in the care of patients with nervous system disorders. There are some general principles related to care of patients after neurosurgical intervention that suggest common categories of human responses that neuroscience nurses should consider. Classic textbooks of neurosurgery and basic textbooks of neurosurgical nursing should be consulted for information about specific surgical procedures and standard nursing care plans after the procedures (Hickey, 1986; Rudy, 1984; Youmans, 1982).

Surgical procedures subject tissues to controlled trauma, and the response of neural tissues to trauma is some degree of swelling. Some potential for tissue swelling always occurs, therefore, after any neurosurgical procedure that involves handling or invading the brain, spinal cord, or peripheral nerve tissues. In the case of craniotomy (removal of a part of the cranium to enter the cranial cavity), this potential for tissue swelling creates the potential for brain swelling and subsequent brain herniation. An example of such a situation is described in Chapter 7. Infratentorial craniotomy (below the tentorium, usually to gain access to the brainstem or posterior fossa) carries the additional risk of swelling that will compromise the brainstem nuclei or cranial nerves that serve swallowing and breathing. Particular attention is therefore required for monitoring respiration and airway protection. Laminectomy (removal of part of the vertebrae to gain access to the spinal canal) always carries some risk of swelling that can compromise spinal cord function. Careful monitoring for signs of worsening spinal cord function is therefore necessary.

The basic complications of immobility that attend any surgical procedure, for example, thrombophlebitis and atelectasis, are just as likely after neurosurgical procedures. In addition, the lengthy procedures carry additional risk of skin breakdown and peripheral pressure palsies related to prolong positioning on the operative table. Leg exercises, elastic stockings, and early ambulation are just as important after neurosurgery as after any other type of surgical procedure. In the case of infratentorial craniotomy and laminectomy, however, special support must be given to the operative site during dangling and ambulation to compensate for the lack of integrity of normal bony or muscle support. In the unresponsive patient, frequent repositioning and stimuli to breathe deeply must be used to compensate for the lack of voluntary movement.

SUMMARY

Human responses to any given neurologic disorder will manifest in a combination of dysfunctions that are related to the area of the nervous system involved and of the coping responses of the individual and family to the prognosis and social meaning of the specific disease. This chapter has described briefly a number of the more common nervous system disorders and human responses that often accompany them. Chapters in Part II are organized around the functional human responses, such as arousal and cognition, that may be seen in many different disorders.

REFERENCES

Adams, R.D., & Victor, M. (1985). *Principles of neurology* (3rd ed.). New York: McGraw-Hill.
American Heart Association. (1987). *1987 Stroke facts.* Dallas: American Heart Association.
American Nurses' Association. (1980). *Nursing: A social policy statement.* Kansas City, MO: American Nurses' Association.
Beghi, E., Nicolosi, A., Kurland, L.T., Mulder, D.W., Hauser, W.A., & Shuster, L. (1984). Encephalitis and aseptic meningitis, Olmsted County, Minnesota, 1950–1981: 1. Epidemiology. *Annals of Neurology, 16,* 283.
Conneally, P.M. (1984). Huntington's disease: Genetics and epidemiology. *American Journal of Human Genetics, 36,* 506.
Donohoe, K. (1979). Overview of neuromuscular disease. *Nursing Clinics of North America, 14,* 96.
Frankowski, R.F. (1986). Descriptive epidemiologic studies of head injury in the United States: 1974–1984. *Advances in Psychosomatic Medicine, 16,* 153.
Gastaut, H. (1970). Clinical and electroencephalographical classification of epileptic seizures. *Epilepsia, 11,* 102.
Griffin, M.R., Opitz, J.L., Kurland, L.T., Ebersold, M.J., & O'Fallon, W.M. (1985). Traumatic spinal cord injury in Olmsted County, Minnesota, 1935–1981. *American Journal of Epidemiology, 121,* 884.
Grob, D., Brunner, N.G., & Namba, T. (1981). The natural course of myasthenia gravis and effect of therapeutic measures. *Annals of the New York Academy of Sciences, 377,* 652.
Hayden, M.R. (1981). *Huntington's chorea.* New York: Springer-Verlag.
Hertel, G., Mertens, H.G., Reuther, P., & Picker, K. (1979). The treatment of myasthenia gravis with azathioprine. In P. Dau (Ed.), *Plasma pharesis and the immunobiology of myasthenia gravis* (p. 315), Boston: Houghton-Mifflin.
Hickey, J. (1986). *The clinical practice of neurological–neurosurgical nursing* (2nd ed.). Philadelphia: Lippincott.
Howard, J.F. (1982) Nonsteroidal immunosuppressive therapy for myasthenia gravis. *Seminars in Neurology, 2*(3), 265.
Johns, T.R. (1982). Treatment of myasthenia gravis by thymectomy. *Seminars in Neurology, 2*(3), 271.
Kurtzke, J.F. (1984). Neuroepidemiology. *Annals of Neurology, 16,* 265.
Kurtzke, J.F. (1982). The current neurologic burden of illness and injury in the United States. *Neurology, 32,* 1207.
Kwentus, J.A., Hart, R., Lingpon, N., Taylor, J., & Silverman, J.L. (1986). Alzheimer's disease. *The American Journal of Medicine, 81,* 91.
McDonald, W.I. (1984). Multiple sclerosis: Epidemiology and HLA associations. *Annals of the New York Academy of Science, 436,* 109.
Minteer-Convery, M.A. (1985). Head injury. *Annual Review of Rehabilitation, 4,* 215.
Rajput, A.H., Offord, K.P., Beard, C.M., & Kurland, L.T. (1984). Epidemiology of Parkinsonism: Incidence, classification, and mortality. *Annals of Neurology, 16,* 276.
Reisberg, B. (1983). An overview of current concepts of Alzheimer's disease, senile dementia, and age-associated cognitive decline. In B. Reisberg (Ed.), *Alzheimer's disease: The standard reference.* New York: Free Press.
Rubenstein, E. (1985). Botulism. In E. Rubenstein & D.D. Federman (Eds.), *Scientific American Medicine: Sec. 8, II* (p. 1). New York: Scientific American.
Rudy, E. (1984). *Advanced neurological and neurosurgical nursing.* St. Louis: Mosby.
Schlech, W.F., Ward, J.I., Band, J.D., Hightower, A., Fraser, D.W., & Broome, C.V. (1985). Bacterial meningitis in the United States, 1978 through 1981. *Journal of the American Medical Association, 253,* 1749.
Schoenberg, B.S. (1986). Epidemiology of dementia. *Neurologic Clinics, 4*(2), 447.
Shoulson, I. (1984). Huntington's disease: A decade of progress. *Neurologic Clinics, 2*(3), 515.

Sibley, W. (1985). Management of the patient with multiple sclereosis. *Seminars in Neurology, 5*(2), 134.

Simon, H.B., & Swartz, M.N. (1984). Tetanus. In E. Rubenstein & D.D. Federman (Eds.), *Scientific American Medicine: Sec. 7, V* (p. 9). New York: Scientific American.

Skoch, M.G., & Waling, A.D. (1985). Meningitis: Describing the community health problem. *American Journal of Public Health, 75*, 550.

Smith, C., & Sheinberg, L. (1985). Clinical features of multiple sclerosis. *Seminars in Neurology, 5*(2), 122.

Storm-Mathisen, A. (1984). Epidemiology of myasthenia gravis in Norway. *Acta Neurologica Scandinavica, 70*, 274.

Terry, R., & Katzman, R. (1983). Senile dementia of the Alzheimer type: Defining a disease. In R. Katzman & R. Terry (Eds.), *The neurology of aging* (p. 51). Philadelphia: F.A. Davis.

Youmans, J.R. (1982). *Neurological Surgery* (2nd ed.). Philadelphia: Saunders, 6 vols.

Weinfeld, F.D., & Baum, H.M. (1984). The national multiple sclerosis survey: Background and economic impact. *Annals of the New York Academy of Science, 436*, 469.

4

Nursing Management Strategies: An Overview

Mariah Snyder*

Nursing actions play a key role in the outcomes of care for people with neurologic disorders. This is true for people who have either acute or chronic problems. Assessing and monitoring patients are two important care activities that nurses perform. This chapter, however, focuses on the intervention phase of the nursing process, particularly on interventions that nurses can initiate independently. The revised Nursing Practice Acts in most states specifically provide for nurses to function in an independent manner. Patients with neurologic conditions provide unique opportunities for nurses to assess, plan, and intervene autonomously.

Only recently has nursing given attention to specific interventions that are within its realm. *Nursing Interventions*, edited by Bulechek and McCloskey and published by Saunders in 1985, and *Independent Nursing Interventions*, edited by Snyder and published by Wiley in 1985, are the first textbooks devoted entirely to this phase of care. Both provide the scientific basis for the intervention and both identify populations for whom the intervention can be used. Considerable research is needed to verify the effectiveness of these interventions. Expanding the scope of interventions that are within the purview of nursing is also necessary.

This chapter is divided into three sections—interventions that can be used with the patient, with the family, and with the community. Although an intervention is placed in only one section, many would be appropriate for use with other groups.

INTERVENTIONS FOR THE PATIENT

Movement and Proprioceptive Interventions

Promoting mobility and preventing problems associated with immobility are frequent goals for patients with neurologic problems. Cerebrovascular accidents, spinal cord injuries, head trauma, Parkinson's disease, and multiple sclerosis are among the conditions causing mobility problems and for which a number of these interventions would be appropriate.

---

*The author wishes to acknowledge Michaelene Mirr, doctoral student at the University of Minnesota, who reviewed the chapter.

Movement and proprioceptive interventions also are useful in promoting wholeness, improving self-concept, and decreasing stress. These are outcomes that are frequently seen on nursing care plans for neuropatients.

Progressive Muscle Relaxation

Progressive muscle relaxation is one of a number of interventions that are labeled as stress management techniques or relaxation techniques. The technique involves the tensing and then relaxing of successive muscle groups, with the person learning to discriminate between the feelings experienced when the muscle group is tensed and when it is relaxed. Eventually, the person is able to bring about relaxation merely by recalling the image of the muscles being relaxed. Jacobson first publicized the technique in 1938; since that time many variations of his technique have evolved and have been used in clinical settings.

Stress is pervasive in our society. People faced with new situations, such as surgery, diagnostic tests, or crisis, frequently exhibit high levels of stress. Those with a chronic condition likewise have to make many adaptations, and anxiety often occurs at such times. If a patient can use an intervention, such as progressive relaxation, some of the ill effects resulting from sustained high levels of stress can be reduced or avoided.

Brown (1977) noted that a circuitous feedback loop between the muscles and the mind operates in the stress process. The person perceives a situation as threatening; the brain sends a message to the muscles alerting them to prepare for the stressful event. The muscles tense; the proprioceptive status of the muscles is sent to the brain, which interprets this as an impending threat and sends messages to the muscles alerting them to the threat. The muscle tension thus increases. According to Brown, the scientific basis for the use of progressive relaxation in reducing tension results from fewer impulses from the relaxed muscles being sent to the brain, so there are fewer stimuli to have an impact on the cerebral cortex and keep it alerted. This, in turn, decreases the cortical action on the lower brain areas that have been maintaining muscle tension.

Physiologic findings resulting from the relaxed state include decreased oxygen consumption, metabolism, respiratory rate, heart rate, muscle tension, premature ventricular contractions, systolic and diastolic blood pressure, and increased alpha waves (Jacobson, 1964). Others have found that progressive relaxation reduces overall anxiety (Borkovec et al., 1978; Woolfolk et al., 1982).

The progressive relaxation technique is simple to teach patients. General directions for teaching progressive relaxation are given below. Modifications may be necessary for particular patient populations; some patients are unable to sit in a comfortable chair, and thus adaptations are needed.

The nurse creates a quiet environment for teaching the technique. A comfortable chair, such as a recliner, is ideal. Tight or binding clothing is loosened, and shoes and glasses are removed. The nurse is seated so that the patient can be viewed while directions are given. Before beginning the instructions, the nurse provides the patient with the rationale for use of the technique and goes through the methods used for tensing the various muscle groups. A typical session lasts 20 to 30 minutes.

In Bernstein and Borkovec's technique (1973), 16 muscle groups are alternately tensed and relaxed. These are identified in Figure 4–1, along with the combinations of muscles that are used as the person masters the technique. The patient is asked to tense (for approximately 7 seconds) and then relax each of the 16 groups. Encouragement and directions that assist the patient to concentrate on the muscle groups are provided by the nurse. The nurse notes if the patient is becoming more relaxed, as indicated by slowed breathing, decreased body movement, and feedback from the patient. Electromyography also may be used to measure the degree of relaxation of specific muscle groups. Termination of the relaxed state is brought about gradually, with the nurse instructing the pa-

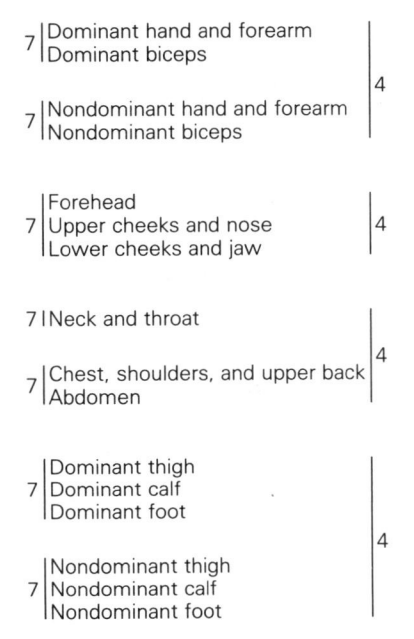

```
 ┌Dominant hand and forearm
7│Dominant biceps
                                    │
                                    │4
 ┌Nondominant hand and forearm      │
7│Nondominant biceps

 ┌Forehead
7│Upper cheeks and nose              │4
 └Lower cheeks and jaw

7│Neck and throat
                                    │4
 ┌Chest, shoulders, and upper back
7│Abdomen

 ┌Dominant thigh
7│Dominant calf
 └Dominant foot
                                    │4
 ┌Nondominant thigh
7│Nondominant calf
 └Nondominant foot
```

Figure 4–1. Combination of 16 muscle groups in sets of seven (7) and four (4). The muscle groups can be combined into seven large sets, designated by the number 7 at the left of each group, or four larger groups, designated by the number 4 at the right of each group.

tient to begin to move hands and feet, then arms and legs, and finally to open the eyes.

Four to six teaching sessions are usually needed for the patient to master the technique (Borkovec & Sides, 1979). Daily practice is a vital component of the learning process. Some people prefer practicing in the morning because it helps them relax during the day; whereas others prefer doing it in the evening because it calms them and helps promote sleep.

Although progressive relaxation seems to be a benign intervention, certain precautions are necessary. Combining several larger muscle groups (e.g., those designated seven and four in Fig. 4–1) should never be done by people with hypertension. Relaxing the large muscle groups after they have been tensed often forces a large volume of blood to be re-turned at one time to the heart, a situation which can tax the vascular system. Some patients with chronic pain find that the technique heightens the experience of pain. Hypotension may occur after total body relaxation is attained; movement in place before rising will help alleviate this problem.

Progressive relaxation has been used with many patient populations. Of particular interest to neuroscience nurses is its use in reduction of seizures (Cabral & Scott, 1976; Ince, 1976), reduction of hypertension (Pender, 1984), postoperative pain reduction (Flaherty & Fitzpatrick, 1978; Wells, 1982), reduction of headaches (Cox et al., 1978), reduction of chronic pain (Greziak, 1977), and lessening of nausea and vomiting (Cotanch, 1983).

Exercise
Exercise is an intervention used often by neuroscience nurses. Active and passive range of motion exercises, ambulation, exercises to increase muscle strength, and general exercise to promote well-being are modes that nurses prescribe routinely. Basmajian (1978) defined therapeutic exercise as the movement of the body or its parts to relieve symptoms of pathology or improve its function. Many believe that exercise promotes the optimum psychophysiologic development of humans.

Exercise can be classified in several ways: isotonic, isometric, or isokinetic or as aerobic and anaerobic. Isotonic exercise involves changing the length of muscles; range of motion exercises are an example of isotonic exercise. In isometric exercise, the length of the muscle does not change, but contraction of fibers occurs with increase in tension of the muscle; this form is used when a person has a limb immobilized, such as in a cast. Isokinetic contraction involves trying to contract the muscle group against graded resistance; it is used in rehabilitation to increase strength in a muscle group. Minimal oxygen is consumed in anaerobic exercise, whereas considerable oxygen is consumed in aerobic exercise. Efficient functioning of the heart, lungs, and circulatory systems is promoted through aerobic exercise.

For many neuropatients, exercise must be continued for extended periods of time or for a lifetime. Finding ways to make exercise sessions fun so that the person will continue to practice is a challenge. Many patients find group exercises enjoyable; socialization is an added benefit from such sessions. The family can be involved in the exercise program. Doing exercises to music, much like aerobic exercise classes, reduces boredom. Altering routines or the sequence, if possible, provides a newness to the sessions. Although other disciplines, such as physical therapy, often are involved in the exercise program, nurses play a key role in the success of this intervention. Consistency of doing transfers, range of motion exercises, and mobilization is critical to the patient's recovery. Many of these patients have cognitive problems and are unable to deal with diverse ways of doing things.

Movement Therapy
Movement therapy is closely aligned with exercise. One of the most commonly used forms of movement therapy is dance. Dance places emphasis on the holism of the human being. The person, through the body, externalizes concepts created in the mind. Movements allow people to express themselves nonverbally and release emotions in this manner. This promotes physical relaxation and increases an awareness of self. Laben (1975) described dance as:

> movement, by which I mean the interaction of effort and space through the medium of the body. Our bodily movements make shapes in space and they are charged with effort, that is energy coming from within, springing from a whole range of impulses, intentions, and desires. (p. 108)

Schoop (1974) identified four goals of dance therapy:

1. Develop functional patterns for parts of the body that have been inactive or have been misused
2. Establish unifying relationships between mind and body
3. Bring conflicting emotions into an objective physical form that allows the person to deal with them in a constructive manner
4. Assist the person to adapt to the environment

All of these purposes have relevance for patients with neurologic deficits.

Dance has been used with several neuropatient populations. Hecox et al. (1976) used dance with patients who had mild to moderately severe physical disabilities. Patients increased awareness of themselves and explored and used abilities that had been dormant. Adaptation of movement therapy has been used with quadriplegic patients to increase physical and mental well-being (Gerhart, 1979). Group dance sessions have been used to facilitate social interaction (Feder & Feder, 1982). Application of the intervention of dance with other patient populations is feasible.

Cognitive Interventions
Many interventions can be placed in this category. Sensory information, imagery, decisional control, and reminiscence are examples of cognitive interventions that neuroscience nurses can implement. Although cognitive interventions can be used to attain a variety of outcomes, one common goal is to provide the patient with a sense of control over a situation. Patients with neurologic disorders often feel overwhelmed by their condition and think that there is nothing they can do to change the situation. Cognitive interventions may help to decrease these concerns and may improve the person's functional capacities.

Sensory Information
Sensory information (sensation information) is providing the person with an objective description of what the person will see, feel, hear, smell, and taste in a specific situation. It is important that objective sensations and not subjective feelings be presented. Findings from research studies have verified that providing the patient with sensory information before a procedure or surgery will, in many

instances, decrease anxiety (Schacter & Singer, 1962; Johnson & Rice, 1974; Johnson et al., 1975; Johnson et al., 1978; Sime, 1976; Sime & Libera, 1985). According to Johnson, the basis for this is that the congruency between the expected and experienced sensations reduces the emotional responses associated with the threat situation.

Many patients with neurologic conditions experience heightened anxiety before and during diagnostic and surgical procedures. Sime (1976) reported that preoperative patients with high anxiety were particularly helped by having sensory information given to them before surgery. Findings in a recent study by Sime & Libera (1985), however, revealed that providing sensory information to patients with low anxiety may interfere with their ability to cope. Adequate assessment of the patient is needed before giving sensory information.

To develop scripts of objective sensory information relating to specific procedures, the nurse interviews patients who have undergone the procedure. Open-ended questions are best for obtaining data about experienced sensations. Only responses reported by over 50% of the patients should be incorporated into the script to be used (Leventhal & Johnson, 1981). Preparing an audiotape of the script helps to ensure completeness and accuracy. Few scripts have been developed for neurologic diagnostic procedures and tests. Sharing of scripts when they are complete will assist other neuroscience nurses.

Imagery

Imagery has been used extensively as an intervention in nursing for pain control. Imagery is defined as the formation of a mental representation of an object that is usually perceived only through the senses (Sodergren, 1985). Imagery can be of two types—free or guided. In the former, the person formulates his or her own images. The instructor provides specific images to the patient during guided imagery.

Imagery can be used to achieve several types of goals. It is sometimes used to help the patient gain insight into the nature of a problem being experienced. Imagery also may be used to help the patient work out a solution to a problem in a symbolic manner; the nurse then helps the patient apply this to real life situations. Adjustment to adaptations required by a neurologic condition would be one instance when imagery could be used. The patient with decreased mobility is asked to visualize getting around at home; barriers and problems can be identified and solutions found before the patient goes home. Imaging or fantasizing has been used to lessen anxiety; providing images of quiet meadows or seashores is often used to promote relaxation.

Visualization, or imagery, can be used as part of a multimodal treatment program for people with chronic pain. According to Korn (1983), its success may be that imagery interferes with the processing of pain information or that imagery enhances the secretion of endorphins and thereby relieves pain. He suggested using visual or auditory images because pain is a kinesthetic experience, and images of a kinesthetic nature may be blocked by the pain. McCaffery (1979) proposed using imagery to help patients remove themselves from the pain by taking imagery vacations or enjoying other pleasant experiences.

Imagery has been used to help people relearn lost functions or skills. Korn (1983) related using imagery with a girl who had a closed head injury to relearn swallowing mechanisms and motor skills. He also used it with a person who had suffered a stroke to learn balance and speech and to improve memory. The hypothesis for use in these situations is that through imagery the person reexperiences the psychomotor task, activating sensory and neuromuscular mechanisms similar to those involved when doing the task before the accident. This is similar to an athlete mentally rehearsing skills before the event. One nurse used imagery during exercises with a girl who had severe weakness from Guillain-Barré syndrome. The girl was asked to visualize herself dancing while the movements were performed. Other creative uses of imagery can be formulated.

Decisional Control

Most people like to be in control of their lives and surrounding activities, and many illnesses interfere with that control. A person who has had a cerebrovascular accident often is unable to communicate requests, to dress, to feed himself or herself, or to control when things will be done. Other neuroconditions likewise alter the person's life and control over the surrounding environment. Decisional control is one of the three types of control described by Averill (1973). This intervention provides the patient with the opportunity to choose among various courses of action.

Kallio (1979) compared intensive care unit patients who had been given control over certain activities with those who had not. Patients were given choices regarding where cards, flowers, and other articles would be displayed, when they wished to ambulate, and when they wanted their bath. The experimental group had significantly less fatigue, anxiety, anger, and depression than did the control group. The items Kallio used may seem minor, but giving the patients control of these activities improved their mental state. Langer and Rodin (1976) reported similar findings in nursing home residents who were offered choices.

Several points must be observed when using decisional control. It has to be clear to the patients that they are allowed to make these choices but do not have to do so. The options available must be ones that the patient can control and that the nursing staff will honor. The effects of the intervention may be negated if the nurse offers options and then is unable to allow the patient to make the choice. The number of choices available to the patient should be limited in scope; large numbers of options could be overwhelming.

Reminiscence

This intervention is not restricted to use with elderly patients. It can be used to help orient people who are confused, to orient closed head injury patients with short-term memory loss, to assist younger people who are facing death to reconcile past problems, and to improve feelings of self-worth (Chubon, 1980). Reminiscence is an adaptive mechanism for helping the person compensate for losses that have been experienced and for past inadequacies (Ryden, 1981). All of these purposes are applicable to patients with neurologic conditions. Reminiscence is defined as a planned strategy to help a person recall past events, feelings, and thoughts so that the person can better adapt to the present time (Snyder, 1985).

The nurse helps the patient recall past events and experiences. Asking open-ended questions assists the patient in exploring the past. Lewis and Butler (1974) used a variety of strategies to help patients explore the past: developing written or taped autobiographies, pilgrimages through correspondence, and references to scrapbooks, photo albums, and letters. All of these can help the person to reconcile differences, establish a continuity with the past, and build for the future.

Sensory Interventions

Interventions in this category may be used for stimulation, communication, healing, relearning, and stress reduction. Therapeutic touch, music, purposeful touch, massage, and biofeedback are interventions in this category that have wide use in neuroscience nursing.

Therapeutic Touch

Krieger (1975) called touch the imprimatur of nursing because nurses use it so often. Therapeutic touch differs from the usual touching in that it is a process by which it is postulated that energy is transmitted from one person to another for the purpose of potentiating the healing process of one who is ill or injured (Egan, 1985). The intervention consists of four steps: centering, assessment, unruffling, and transferring energy. The nurse first relaxes and directs attention inward (centering). In assessment, the nurse moves her hands, held several inches away, over the patient's body to determine differences in the quality of energy flow in the patient. Unruffling is done to relieve pressure in areas where the energy is dense. The hands are moved from the area of density outward with sweeping motions. The last step, transfer of energy, requires knowledge of the types of energy available and introducing the one appropriate to the patient. Blue energy is used to calm or sedate a patient, yellow energy is used to energize, and green is used for harmonizing. To transfer energy, the nurse must intend to help the patient.

There has been a great deal of controversy surrounding the effectiveness of therapeutic touch. There is scientific evidence supporting its use in specific situations (Heidt, 1981; Krieger et al., 1979). It has been used to decrease pain, to increase energy, and to decrease anxiety. These are patient outcomes frequently stated for neuropatients, and neuroscience nurses may find therapeutic touch an appropriate intervention to use. Nurses wishing to use therapeutic touch, however, should first attend a workshop on the intervention; knowledgeable use is necessary to avoid harmful effects.

Music

Music has been used since ancient times as a treatment modality for a wide variety of conditions. It is used also as an adjunct with other interventions, such as imagery, exercise, and meditation. Music as an intervention can involve active patient participation—in playing instruments, singing, or listening to musical selections. Both methods have been used by neuroscience nurses.

Alvin (1975) delineated five elements of music: frequency (pitch), intensity, tone color, interval, and duration. The nurse must have an understanding of these in order to choose judiciously selections for specific patient populations. Pitch refers to the number of vibrations; rapid vibrations tend to act as a stimulant, whereas a slow pitch induces relaxation. Intensity relates to the amplitude of the vibrations. A person's like or dislike for a selection often is based on the intensity of the piece. Tone color is determined by the harmony of the piece. The psychologic significance of a piece is created by the tone color. The interval creates the melody and harmony.

Cultural norms greatly influence a person's perception of what is pleasant to hear. Duration and rhythm are similar; duration is the length of sounds, and rhythm is a time pattern fitted into a certain speed. The rhythm of a piece is a major determinant of when it would be most appropriate to use it.

Music has been used with a number of neuropatient populations. Since music is viewed as a unifier of the person, it has been used to help orient confused patients. Music with a strong beat helps a person gain an awareness of self; both the auditory and kinesthetic senses are activated. Musical selections with which a patient is familiar are useful in orientation, and family members can assist in the selection process. Mason (1978) used music to decrease tension in elderly people with Parkinson's disease and disseminated sclerosis, which helped the patients move more freely. Hoskyn (1982) used music to promote relaxation and decrease choreic movements in people with Huntington's chorea. She found also that speech improved in these patients. Herth (1978) played music during exercises for hemiplegic patients to make the exercises less boring.

Music can be used both to calm and to stimulate patients. Soothing music has been suggested for patients prone to increases in intracranial pressure. Some believe that music familiar to the patient is more calming than unfamiliar music. Selections for stimulation should have a strong beat and intensity. Sisson (1979) used *A Fifth of Beethoven* and *Theme from Grease* to stimulate patients who had remained comatose after head injury.

Purposeful Touch

Purposeful touch is defined as any purposeful physical body contact between the nurse and the patient; it does not include the touching that occurs in the course of treatments or procedures. Purposeful touch is one of the most commonly used interventions in nursing, but nurses rarely think about its use or when it can be used therapeutically. Findings from a study by Barnett (1972) showed that nurses touch patients twice as often as do other health care personnel.

Examples of types of purposeful touch include handholding, soothing touch, and an application of greater intensity that acts as a stimulant. Knable (1981) found that adult patients in an intensive care unit reported very positive reactions to nurses purposefully holding their hand. Nurses noted that both appropriate timing and intent to help were necessary for the handholding to be therapeutic. Touch is one of the most primitive forms of communication; its use with people who have decreased levels of responsiveness or are confused is one means of conveying care and presence.

The use of soothing touch with patients who have increased intracranial pressure has been investigated by nurses (Walleck, 1982). Walleck reported that touching the hand or face resulted in a decrease in intracranial pressure. Although it is not completely clear if these findings resulted from touch or from the accompanying rest periods, the intervention holds promise as a simple means that nurses and family members can use to bring about beneficial effects.

Touch as stimulation is used early in neurorehabilitation programs (Farber, 1982). Inhibitory techniques are used first to normalize hypersensitive areas. During the inhibitory phase, constant pressure is applied to one spot for a period of time. Pressure is applied to the perioral region, abdomen, and palms of the hand. Facilitory techniques are applied after normalization is established. A moving stimulus is used in facilitory techniques; for example, the nurse moves her forefinger caudally from under the patient's nose to the tip of the chin. This is repeated a number of times with a short rest period between each repetition. Textured materials and hot and cold frequently are used in stimulation programs for head-injured patients or others recovering from coma to increase tactile stimulation.

Massage
Massage produces effects on multiple body systems: integumentary, musculoskeletal, cardiovascular, lymphatic, and nervous systems. Manipulation of the skin causes it to become more supple, and sebaceous excretion is enhanced (Wakim, 1980). Massage increases or improves movement of the musculoskeletal system by reducing edema, loosening and stretching contracted tendons, and aiding in the reduction of soft tissue adhesions. Fatigue is lessened, since massage causes a more rapid removal of waste products. All of the outcomes benefit immobile patients or patients with reduced mobility. Backrubs, one form of massage, must be considered by nurses to reduce anxiety and promote rest. Spending a few minutes giving a good backrub can do much to promote the patient's well-being.

Biofeedback
Biofeedback has been used to manipulate functions related to the autonomic, peripheral, and central nervous systems. Katkin and Goldband (1980) defined biofeedback as:

> any technique that uses instrumentation to provide a person with immediate and continuous signals concerning body functions of which that person is not normally conscious (p. 537).

This technique has been used for treating many conditions, including strokes, epilepsy, insomnia, pain, headache, chronic lower back pain, Bell's palsy, and cerebral palsy. Much of the success of the intervention depends on the patient's commitment to practice, and thus a criterion for its use is that the patient be able to cooperate. Patients experience a strong sense of personal control by mastering the process and altering certain body functions.

Nurses can learn the techniques for biofeedback by attending classes or workshops; the Biofeedback Society of America offers numerous workshops. The nurse who wishes to use these techniques needs knowledge of the instrumentation, the basis for the technique, and an understanding of conditions for which it should be used.

Other Interventions

There are many other interventions that neuroscience nurses can prescribe and use independently that do not fall into the previous categories. Several of these that seem to have particular relevance for care of neuropatients are presented.

Humor

Norman Cousins (1979) has drawn attention to the use of humor as an intervention. He watched comedies to make him laugh and attributes the cure of his illness to the use of this therapy. Humor is individualistic and even differs for the same person over time. Mindess et al. (1984) developed a questionnaire for assessing the type of humor that a person enjoys.

Humor can be used to aid in establishing relationships, to help relieve anxiety and tension, to release anger and aggression, to avoid feelings that are too painful to face immediately, and to facilitate learning (Robinson, 1970). Kubie (1971) found that humor helped to create a relaxed atmosphere that promoted communication. Patients who have been presented with a difficult diagnosis often are unable to discuss its impact on their lives. Many times, joking about an illness is viewed as denial, and although one would not want to allow the patient to remain at this level for a long period of time, humor and laughter can be helpful in alleviating anxiety, fear, and anger.

Patient education is important in the nursing care of patients with neurologic deficits. Clabby (1979) reported that information taught in a humorous manner was retained to a greater extent than was information presented routinely. Recall how many times one remembers information presented in the context of a joke or story. Humor could be added judiciously to patient teaching to enhance learning.

Timing

Findings from the field of chronobiology are relevant for neuroscience nurses. A considerable body of research is evolving concerning the impact that the time of administration of medications has on their effectiveness. If therapeutic effects can be maximized by administration at specific times of the circadian cycle, lower dosages could be used and toxic effects and side effects could be lessened. Decreasing side effects may increase patient compliance, particularly with anticonvulsants, antihypertensives, and other drugs that have notable side effects. Since nurses often establish the times for administration of medications, findings from chronobiology could assist the nurse in selecting the times of greatest benefit from the medication.

Measurement of blood pressure, temperature, and other parameters vary during the circadian cycle. Borderline hypertension, for example, may go undetected for a period of time if pressure readings are measured during only one timeframe. Measurements at varying times are needed to obtain an accurate assessment. It is believed that intracranial pressure also varies during the circadian cycle, and this has implications for selecting when activities are performed. Astute assessments by nurses can add to the body of knowledge related to rhythms.

The perception of the passage of time is changed by alterations in a person's mobility. Patients on bedrest often complain of time dragging. According to Tompkins (1980), people with restricted mobility perceive the duration of time to be shortened. She believed that this slowing helped preserve system integrity. Performing nursing care activities at a slower pace, based on nurses' awareness of this perception, would help patients maintain their sense of integrity.

Hope

Many people with neurologic problems feel devastated; life and the future hold no meaning. Miller (1985) stated that hope nurtures the person's transition from being weak and vulnerable to functioning as fully as possible.

Caregivers have the opportunity to be inspiriting to the patient. Hope arises from different sources for each person. Miller suggested the following strategies to be used by nurses to inspire hope:

1. Emphasize sustaining relationships, such as mentioning the names of loved ones to the unresponsive patient.
2. Let the patient know if the current situation is a temporary state.
3. Radiate hope by recognizing the person's intrinsic worth and viewing the person's illness as only one facet of the individual.
4. Expand the patient's repertoire of coping mechanisms.
5. Teach reality surveillance by surveying the situation and making contingency plans.
6. Assist the patient to devise and revise goals.
7. Help the patient expand the spiritual self.
8. Help guard against despair—live the moment.

Providing hope does not mean being unrealistic or masking the truth in dealing with the patient's condition, but rather helping the person find meaning in the present situation.

Presence

Presence is closely akin to caring. Gardner (1985) defined this intervention as follows:

> Presence in the cognitive domain by verbal communication of empathy or understanding of the patient's experience; Presence in the affective domain by a generation of a positive regard, trust, and genuineness, which is evidenced by interpersonal rapport; and Presence in the physical domain by being physically available as a helper. (pp. 320–321)

Presence thus means being there for the patient and conveying this to the patient. For many patients and their families, this aspect of nursing is the one most valued. Even though it is difficult to define and evaluate, it is one that neuroscience nurses can use with all patients.

INTERVENTIONS FOR FAMILIES AND SIGNIFICANT OTHERS

Nurses have placed a major emphasis on viewing the patient as part of a family group (family is used in a broad context to include people who are significant to the patient). Although this has been emphasized, frequently the business of the hospital and clinic setting has left little time for nurses to provide care for the family. This section presents interventions that have particular relevance for use with families of patients with neurologic conditions.

Groups

Establishing and conducting support groups for families falls within the realm of nursing. Groups have been formed to assist families of patients in crisis situations, such as trauma and brain tumors (Wilson, 1982), to help families deal with adjustment problems, such as with post-head injury patients (Mauss-Clum & Ryan, 1981), and families with a member having a chronic condition, such as multiple sclerosis, Parkinson's disease, Alzheimer's disease, or epilepsy. Specific strategies for developing support groups with families are described in Chapter 17.

Counseling

Although group sessions may be extremely helpful for many family members, individual counseling is an intervention that nurses may need to use to help some families or family members. Banks (1985) defined counseling as:

> an interactive helping process between a counselor and a client characterized by the core elements of acceptance, empathy, genuineness, and congruency. This relationship consists of a series of interactions over time in which the counselor, through a variety of active and passive techniques, focuses on the needs, problems, or feelings of the client which have interfered with the client's usual adaptive behavior. (p. 105)

Counseling in this context is formalized. Many times, the counseling provided to family members is more informal and may occur over a cup of coffee or during a walk.

The counselor needs to have a genuine interest in the client and accept the intrinsic worth of the person. Because of this the client senses acceptance and trusts the counselor. Caring, a key component of nursing, is felt by families as well as by patients and is one reason that families often seek out the nurse for assistance. If the nurse feels that the time demands for the assistance needed go beyond that available, referrals to appropriate resources are necessary. Referrals to a social worker, chaplain, or other health care personnel can be made. Frequently, however, the nurse is able to provide counseling about concerns related to the patient and the impact that these may have on the family.

Journal

Use of a journal is an intervention that may help families in dealing with either the acute or the long-term phase of a family member's illness. A journal is different from a diary in that in the journal the person records not only the event but also feelings and reflections on the event. There is an interplay between the conscious and the unconscious in journal entries. Putting feelings on paper can assist in giving insights into the problem or can serve as a catharsis for the person. Progoff (1975) believed that the journal aids the person in discovering new capabilities.

The nurse can suggest a journal to a family member as a means of coping with the situation. Making daily entries is suggested during times of crises. Later, the person may make less frequent entries. It should be emphasized that what is written is private and need not be shared with anyone else. Some people find it helpful to share insights they have gained or questions that may have arisen from the entries. The nurse can offer to discuss the journal, but this should be done in such a way that the person does not feel obligated to share its contents.

INTERVENTIONS FOR THE COMMUNITY

The scope of nursing practice has expanded to include working for legislation that benefits patients, working with community organizations to improve care for people with particular illnesses or conditions, providing education about certain conditions, and being an advocate for people with particular problems. Two of these—education and advocacy—are elaborated on here.

Education

Public education is an important nursing function. The public lacks knowledge about many neurologic conditions. People with epilepsy are ostracized; people with multiple sclerosis are thought to be alcoholics; employers generally do not understand the long-term effects of head injuries. These are only examples of the many areas in which nurses can provide valuable information.

Education may consist of classes for specific groups, such as firefighters or police, working to get public service commercials on radio or television, or preparing literature for distribution. Nurses have much knowledge about specific neuroconditions and are able to put this into language that the public can understand. This ability is a key ingredient to the success of the education program. Reading specialists, people in the marketing field, and media specialists can be helpful in the development of educational materials.

Advocacy

Advocacy has existed since there have been powerless groups in need of a champion (Donahue, 1985). People within the health care system or those in need of health care often feel powerless. Nurses have acted as advocates for the patient and helped the patient know his rights. The recent upsurge of consumerism has put added emphasis on this role; the introduction of advocates, particularly advocates for certain groups of patients, has resulted.

Advocacy for patient groups can be extended to the political realm. Working to get legislation passed that will provide health care for particular groups is critical. Many patients with neurologic problems are unable to return to their former work setting, yet they are capable of doing some work. If they work, however, they lose their welfare benefits, and the jobs they are able to obtain often do not pay enough to support them. Another problem related to neuropatients that requires advocates in the political arena is support for home care. Many families are unable to receive any assistance if they elect to care for a family member at home. Knowledge of the political process and willingness to become involved are key components of the advocacy role.

REFERENCES

Alvin, J. (1975). *Music therapy*. New York: Basic Books.

Averill, J. (1973). Personal control over aversive stimuli and its relationship to stress. *Psychological Bulletin, 80*, 286.

Banks, L. (1985). Counseling. In G. Bulechek & J. McCloskey (Eds.), *Nursing interventions* (p. 99). Philadelphia: Saunders.

Barnett, K. (1972). A survey of the current utilization of touch by health team personnel with hospitalized ptients. *International Journal of Nursing Studies, 9*, 195.

Basmajian, J. (1978). *Therapeutic exercise*. Baltimore: Williams & Wilkins.

Bernstein, D., & Borkovec, T. (1973). *Progressive relaxation training*. Champaign, IL: Research Press.

Borkovec, T., Grayson, J., & Cooper, K. (1978). Treatment of general tension: Subjective and physiological effects of progressive relaxation. *Journal of Consulting and Clinical Psychology, 46*, 518.

Borkovec, T., & Sides, J. (1979). Critical procedural variables related to the physiological effects of progressive relaxation: A review. *Behavior Research and Therapy, 17*, 119.

Brown, B. (1977) *Stress and the art of biofeedback*. New York: Bantam Books.

Bulechek, G., & McCloskey, J. (Eds.). (1985). *Nursing interventions*. Philadelphia: Saunders.

Cabral, R., & Scott, D. (1976). Effect of two desensitization techniques, biofeedback and relaxation, on intractable epilepsy: A follow-up study. *Journal of Neurology, Neurosurgery, and Psychiatry, 39*, 504.

Chubon, S. (1980). A novel approach to the process of life review. *Journal of Gerontological Nursing, 6*, 543.

Clabby, J. (1979). Humor as a preferred activity of the creative and humor as a facilitator of learning. *Psychology, A Quarterly Journal of Human Behavior, 16*, 5.

Cotanch, P. (1983). Relaxation training for control of nausea and vomiting in patients receiving chemotherapy. *Cancer Nursing, 6*, 277.

Cousins, N. (1979). *Anatomy of an illness as perceived by the patient*. New York: Norton.

Cox, D., Freundlich, A., & Meyer, R. (1978). Differential effectiveness of electromyograph feedback, verbal relaxation instructions, and medication placebo with tension headaches. *Journal of Consulting and Clinical Psychology, 43*, 892.

Donahue, M. (1985). Advocacy. In G. Bulechek & J. McCloskey (Eds.), *Nursing interventions* (p. 338). Philadelphia: Saunders.

Egan, E. (1985). Therapeutic touch. In M. Snyder (Ed.), *Independent nursing interventions* (p. 199). New York: Wiley.

Farber, S. (1982). *Neurorehabilitation*. Philadelphia: Saunders.

Feder, E., & Feder, B. (1982). The therapeutic use of dance and movement. In E. Nickerson & K. O'Laughlin (Eds.), *Helping through action: Action-oriented therapies* (p. 141). Amherst, MA: Human Resources Development Press.

Flaherty, G., & Fitzpatrick, J. (1978). Relaxation technique to increase comfort level of postoperative patients: A preliminary study. *Nursing Research, 27*, 352.

Gardner, D. (1985). Presence. In G. Bulechek & J. McCloskey (Eds.), *Nursing interventions* (p. 316). Philadelphia: Saunders.

Gerhart, K. (1979). Increasing sensory and motor stimulation for patients with quadriplegia. *Physical Therapy, 59*, 1518.

Greziak, R. (1977). Relaxation techniques in treatment of chronic pain. *Archives of Physical Medicine and Rehabilitation, 58*, 270.

Hecox, B., Levine, E., & Scott, D. (1976). Dance in physical rehabilitation. *Physical Therapy, 56*, 919.

Heidt, P. (1981). Effect of therapeutic touch on anxiety level of hospitalized patients. *Nursing Research, 30*, 32.

Herth, K. (1978). The therapeutic use of music. *Supervisor Nurse, 9* (10), 22.

Hoskyns, S. (1982). Striking the right chord. *Nursing Mirror, 154,* 28.

Ince, L. (1976). The use of relaxation training and a conditional stimulus in the elimination of epileptic seizures in a child: A case study. *Behavior Research and Experimental Psychiatry, 7,* 39.

Jacobson, E. (1938). *Progressive relaxation.* Chicago: University of Chicago Press.

Jacobson, E. (1964). *Anxiety and tension control: A physiologic approach.* Philadelphia: Lippincott.

Johnson, J., Kirchoff, K., & Endress, M. (1975). Altering children's distress behavior during orthopedic cast removal. *Nursing Research, 24,* 404.

Johnson, J., & Rice, V. (1974). Sensory and distress components of pain: Implications for the study of clinical pain. *Nursing Research, 23,* 203.

Johnson, J., Rice, V., Fuller, S., & Endress, M. (1978). Sensory information, instruction in a coping strategy, and recovery from surgery. *Research in Nursing and Health, 1,* 4.

Kallio, J. (1979). The relationship among perceived control, mood state, and perception of nursing care for a control-induced and comparison group of patients in the critical care setting. Unpublished master's thesis, University of Minnesota.

Katkin, E., & Goldband, S. (1980). Biofeedback. In F. Kanfer & A. Goldstein (Eds.), *Helping people change* (p. 537). Elmsford, NY: Pergamon Press.

Knable, J. (1981). Handholding: One means of transcending barriers to communication. *Heart and Lung, 10,* 1106.

Korn, E. (1983). The use of altered states of consciousness and imagery in physical and pain rehabilitation. *Journal of Mental Imagery, 5,* 25.

Krieger, D. (1975). Therapeutic touch: The imprimatur of nursing. *American Journal of Nursing, 75,* 784.

Krieger, D., Peper, E., & Ancoli, S. (1979). Therapeutic touch: Searching for evidence of physiological change. *American Journal of Nursing, 79,* 660.

Kubie, L. (1971). The destructive potential of humor in psychotherapy. *American Journal of Psychiatry, 127,* 861.

Laban, R. (1975). *Modern educational dance.* London: MacDonald & Evans.

Langer, E., & Rodin, J. (1976). The effects of choice and enhanced personal responsibility for the aged: A field experiment in an institutional setting. *Journal of Personality and Social Psychology, 34,* 191.

Leventhal, H., & Johnson, J. (1981). Laboratory and field experimentation: Development of a theory of self-regulation. In P. Wooldridge, R. Leonard, J. Skipper, & M. Schmitt (Eds.), *Behavior science and nursing theory.* St. Louis: Mosby.

Lewis, M., & Butler, R. (1974). Life-review therapy. *Geriatrics, 29,* 165.

Mason, C. (1978). Musical activities with elderly patients. *Physiotherapy, 64* (3), 80.

Mauss-Clum, N., & Ryan, M. (1981). Brain injury and the family. *Journal of Neurosurgical Nursing, 13,* 165.

McCaffery, M. (1979). *Nursing management of the patient with pain.* Philadelphia: Lippincott.

Miller, J. (1985). Inspiring hope. *American Journal of Nursing, 85,* 22.

Mindess, H., Miller, C., Turek, J., Bender, A., & Corbin, S. (1984). The Antioch sense of humor inventory. Unpublished manuscript, Antioch University, Psychology Department, Los Angeles.

Pender, N. (1984). Physiologic responses of clients with essential hypertension to progressive muscle relaxation training. *Research in Nursing and Health, 7,* 197.

Progroff, I. (1975). *At a journal workshop.* New York: Dialogue House Library.

Robinson, V. (1970). Humor in nursing. In C. Carlson (Ed.), *Behavioral concepts and nursing intervention* (p. 129). Philadelphia: Lippincott.

Ryden, M. (1981). Nursing intervention in support of reminiscence. *Journal of Gerontological Nursing, 7,* 461.

Schacter, S., & Singer, J. (1962). Cognitive, social, and physiological determinants of emotional state. *Psychological Review, 69,* 785.

Schoop, T. (1974). *Won't you join in the dance?* Palo Alto: National Press Books.

Sime, A. (1976). Relationship of preoperative fear, type of coping and information received about surgery to recovery from surgery. *Journal of Personality and Social Psychology, 34,* 716.

Sime, A., & Libera, M. (1985). Sensation information, self-instruction and responses to dental surgery. *Research in Nursing and Health, 8,* 41.

Sisson, R. (1979). The effect of stimuli on patients with closed head injuries. Unpublished doctoral dissertation, University of Texas.

Snyder, M. (1985). Reminiscence. In M. Snyder (Ed.), *Independent nursing interventions* (p. 145). New York: Wiley.

Snyder, M. (Ed.). (1985). *Independent nursing interventions*. New York: Wiley.

Sodergren, K. (1985). Guided imagery. In M. Snyder (Ed.), *Independent nursing interventions* (p. 103). New York: Wiley.

Tompkins, E. (1980). Effect of restricted mobility and dominance on perceived duration. *Nursing Research, 29,* 333.

Wakim, K. (1980). Physiologic effects of massage. In J. Rogoff (Ed.), *Manipulation, traction, and massage* (p. 45). Baltimore: Williams & Wilkins.

Walleck, C. (1982). Effect of touch on intracranial pressure. Speech at the American Association of Neurosurgical Nurses, Honolulu, Hawaii.

Wells, N. (1982). The effect of relaxation on postoperative muscle tension and pain. *Nursing Research, 31,* 236.

Wilson, L. (1982). How to develop a support group for families of open heart surgery patients. *Dimensions of Critical Care Nursing, 1,* 108.

Woolfolk, R., Lehrer, P., McCann, B., & Rooney, A. (1982). Effects of progressive relaxation and meditation on cognitive and somatic manifestations of daily stress. *Behavior Research and Therapy, 20,* 461.

PART II
Phenomena Central to Neuroscience Nursing

SECTION 1. CONSCIOUSNESS PHENOMENA

5

Consciousness: An Overview

Pamela H. Mitchell

The classic medical definition of consciousness—awareness of self and of the environment—sounds deceptively simple and leads us to think of simple dichotomies: conscious, unconscious; alert, comatose; awake, asleep. Yet, as we shall see, the concept of consciousness is far from simple and leads us from attempts to quantitate the degree of consciousness to metaphysical ventures into the relationship of mind, soul, and brain.

Clinically, we tend to think of consciousness in terms of responsiveness to the environment and try to measure it as a reflection of the intactness of the brain as a whole. This concept includes only a few of the phenomena of consciousness. Plum and Posner (1980) distinguish two aspects of consciousness: the content of consciousness (or the sum of cognitive functions) and the arousal component of consciousness (p. 11). It is far easier to evaluate arousal, in terms of responsiveness to the environment, than it is to understand and quantitate the content of the self-awareness and responsiveness-to-self components. The following definitions indicate the range of behavior and mental phenomena that philosophers and scientists have attempted to subsume in the concept of consciousness.

Definition of consciousness: (Webster's New International Dictionary of the English Language Unabridged, 2d ed., G.C. Merriam & Co., 1943)

1. a. awareness, especially of something within oneself
   b. the state or fact of being conscious with regard to something
2. Philos. That state of being which is characterized by sensation, emotion, thought or any psychical attribute whatever; mind in the broadest possible sense: that in nature which is distinguished from the physical; that form of existence which, in its full development, is able to distinguish itself from other existence.

   1) an attribute or condition of soul, or of spiritual substance, not necessarily consciously
   2) itself a spiritual substance
   3) one aspect of the real, correlative with the physical as another aspect
   4) an epiphenomenon or dependent accompaniment of physical existence

5) that of which all phenomena, physical as well as psychical, are forms, the ultimate form of existence
3. the totality of conscious states or processes connected with any single organism, as a man, or with any group of mental factors closely interrelated, as one of the personalities in the phenomenon of multiple personality; a mind; a single mental life
4. a particular consciousness or process
5. the normal state of conscious life, as distinguished from sleep, trance, etc.
6. the upper level of mental life, as contrasted with unconscious

For the purposes of this chapter, consciousness is considered to be composed of arousal and awareness. It is the substrate of all responsive behavior and, therefore, of the cues necessary to human interaction. Because this book is directed to clinicians caring for people with health problems stemming from the nervous system, the major focus of Chapters 5 through 9 is on alterations in consciousness in relation to disorders of the nervous system. Alterations in consciousness related to normal and supranormal experiences (e.g., hallucinogens, psi experience, religious ecstasy) are beyond the scope of the book.

Cognition and awareness of self cannot be separated from one another and are considered together in Section 2: Cognition Phenomena. Therefore, this chapter focuses primarily on the arousal component of the phenomenon of consciousness. Chapters 6 and 7 deal with decreased and increased arousal, and Chapters 8 and 9 focus on two forms of intermittently altered arousal.

THE PHENOMENON: AROUSAL

Arousal is defined as being awakened from sleep, stimulated to action or to physiologic readiness for activity, or excited (Webster's Ninth, 1983). Clearly, we cannot know that someone is aroused unless that person exhibits some *behavior* that communicates arousal to us. Therefore, a more clinically useful definition is that *arousal* is the *excitation of behavior by internal or external stimuli* (Daube & Sandok, 1986). Pribram (1976) describes consciousness as the "property by which organisms achieve a special relationship with their environment" (p. 299). Arousal can be viewed as the behavior by which we can infer that such a relationship is occurring. Therefore, clinical estimates of arousal are, in reality, estimates of externally observable responsive behavior. Such behaviors may include simple responses, such as eye opening, head turning, or restless movements, or more complex responses, such as obeying commands or answering questions.

Behaviors that manifest arousal may be categorized as those indicating (1) nonspecific alerting and (2) attention to specific environmental stimuli. *Nonspecific alerting* is elicited by any novel, uncertain, or incongruous stimulus or by painful stimuli in normal humans and animals, as well as in people with pathologic depression of alertness. Nonspecific alerting is characterized by the orienting response (head turning to the source of stimulus, increased muscle tone and sympathetic nervous system responses preparatory to defense or flight), and by electroencephalogram (EEG) changes (decreased amplitude, higher frequency) (Magoun, 1963). In normal humans and animals, familiarity with a stimulus or repetition of it will diminish the nonspecific alerting response, and the person will either ignore it if it is irrelevant or attend only to its particular properties. The ability to tune out or habituate oneself to such a stimulus is believed to require some degree of higher cortical inhibition (Gulbrandsen et al., 1972).

Reactivity or attention to particular alerting stimuli has been termed *vigilance* by von Cramon (1978). He considers vigilance to have two components: behavioral arousal, or the nonspecific susceptibility to stimulation described previously, and reactivity to the specific stimulus. Reactivity to a specific stimulus is characterized behaviorally by directional movements of the body and the obeying of simple and complex commands.

Neuroanatomic Basis of Arousal

Our knowledge of the neuroanatomic basis for arousal stems from extensive study of animals with respect to brain structures associated with changes in arousal behaviors. Our knowledge of clinical states associated with altered arousal stems from observation of human injury and disease, complemented by lesion studies in animals.

It is useful to consider the phenomenon of arousal as dependent on an integrated neural system. In order for behavior to occur that allows us to infer arousal, information must be received through the sensory structures, perceived in the reticular activating system, and acted on by motor and language systems. A defect in any portion of this overall system will alter the behavioral output we call arousal. This concept becomes important when we consider the dangers in inferring lack of arousal or consciousness in the person for whom brain processing is intact but sensory input or motor output is altered. It becomes necessary to use a wide range of sensory stimuli as input and to recognize special cases in which the absence of motor output should not be accepted as evidence for absence of arousal or content of consciousness (see the section "Assessing Arousal and Awareness" in this chapter).

Input

We receive information constantly from both our external and internal environments. Visual, auditory, tactile, and thermal stimuli are examples of the kind we receive from the external world. The sensory systems for vision, hearing, touch, and temperature serve as transducers of the physical information contained in those stimuli to transmit them to the central nervous system for processing.

Internal stimuli consist of the sensations from the viscera, from the muscles and joints, from the heartbeat and respiration, for example. These physical signals also are transmitted from the peripheral to the central nervous system for processing.

Processing

Some sensory information is processed at the segment of the spinal cord at which it enters as part of the reflex arcs that regulate homeostasis or vegetative functions, muscle tension, and other functions. The information that is translated into observable arousal, however, must reach the reticular activating system in order to be processed in such a way as to produce the behaviors we term arousal.

The *reticular activating system* is a physiologic concept rather than a discrete, dissectable structure. It consists of the reticular core, a diffuse collection of neurons extending from the medulla headward to the midbrain (Fig. 5–1). The projections of this core then ascend to the structures that activate behavioral arousal. Medially, the reticular core projects fibers to the thalamus and from the thalamus to the cerebral cortex. Presumably, this set of projections serves the integration of the cognitive, or consciousness content, aspects of arousal. Laterally, the fibers from the reticular core project to the hypothalamus, and from there to the autonomic nervous system and the motor reflex systems and the more basic or vegetative responses seen in arousal.

Our understanding of the key role of the reticular activating system in the maintenance of arousal stems from a series of investigations beginning in the late 1930s. In 1937, Bremer found that a very small area or core of the midbrain was critical for the maintenance of the awake state in the cat (Bremer, 1977). This area subsequently was named the "reticular core." If a lesion was made in the cat at the midbrain (the upper portion of the core), the animal remained in persistent sleep. If, however, the lesion was made in the midpons, the animal remained persistently awake; lesions in the medulla allowed normal cycling between sleep and awake. These findings suggested to Bremer that animals (and presumably people) fell asleep unless sensory stimuli from the body could travel through the brainstem to reach the cerebral hemispheres. Moruzzi and Maguoun's later discovery (1949) that electrical stimulation of midbrain reticular formation could activate arousal

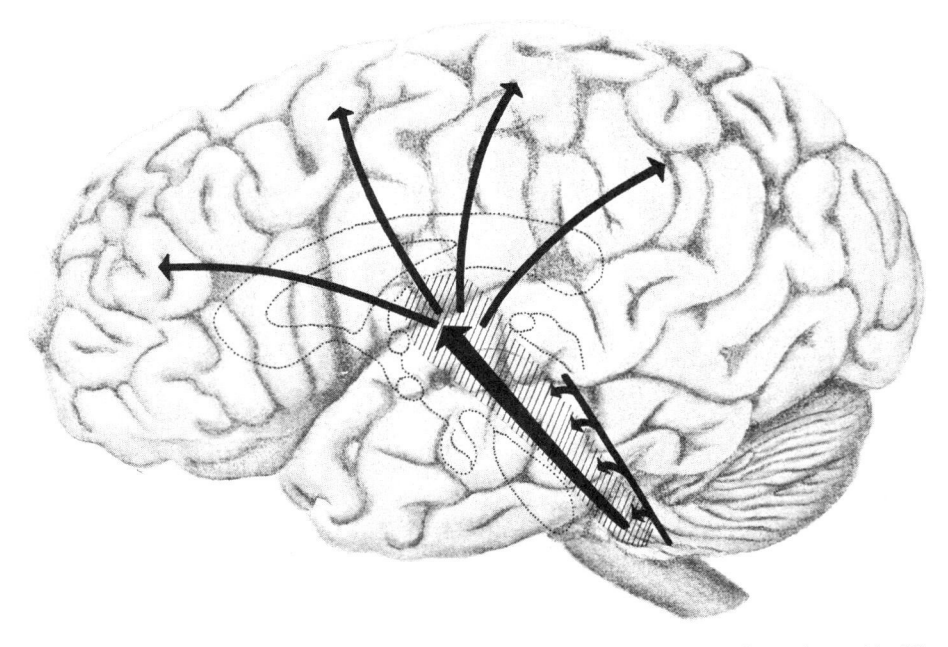

Fig. 5–1. Reticular activating system. The thick arrow represents the reticular formation, with diffuse projections to the cortex indicated by thin arrows. Sensory input to the reticular formation is indicated by connected small arrows. *(From Mitchell et al, 1984, p. 97.)*

clearly showed arousal to be a nonspecific but active process, dependent not only on the reticular core but also on the ascending projection fibers linking brainstem core to a diffuse system of fibers linking midbrain to thalamus and cortex. The term ascending reticular activating system was derived from their work.

In humans, the smallest lesions capable of causing impaired arousal occur in the brainstem central area (or paramedial tegmentum), often from hemorrhage or infarction in the pons or midbrain. Isolated lesions of the medulla have not been reported to impair arousal. Diencephalic lesions from stroke or traumatic injury also can impair arousal, particularly in bilateral paramedian areas of the hypothalamus and subthalamus. Lesions in the cerebral hemispheres generally do not impair arousal unless both hemispheres are involved. Plum and Posner, however, cite several cases of greater clouding of consciousness with massive left hemisphere infarct, compared to similar right hemisphere lesions (1980, p. 22). The various sizes of lesions that impair consciousness are shown in Figure 5–2.

Output

Fibers from the reticular core pass through the diencephalon to end diffusely at the cerebral cortex. Not only do reticular activating system fibers project to the cortex, presumably stimulating responses to arousing stimuli, but cortical fibers project to the reticular activating system. Presumably, this cortical feedback is part of the mammalian ability to modulate arousal responses depending on the psychologic qualities or interpretation of the meaning of the stimulus at the specific areas of the cerebral cortex that serve movement, language, and integrated thought. Further projections within the diencephalon pass

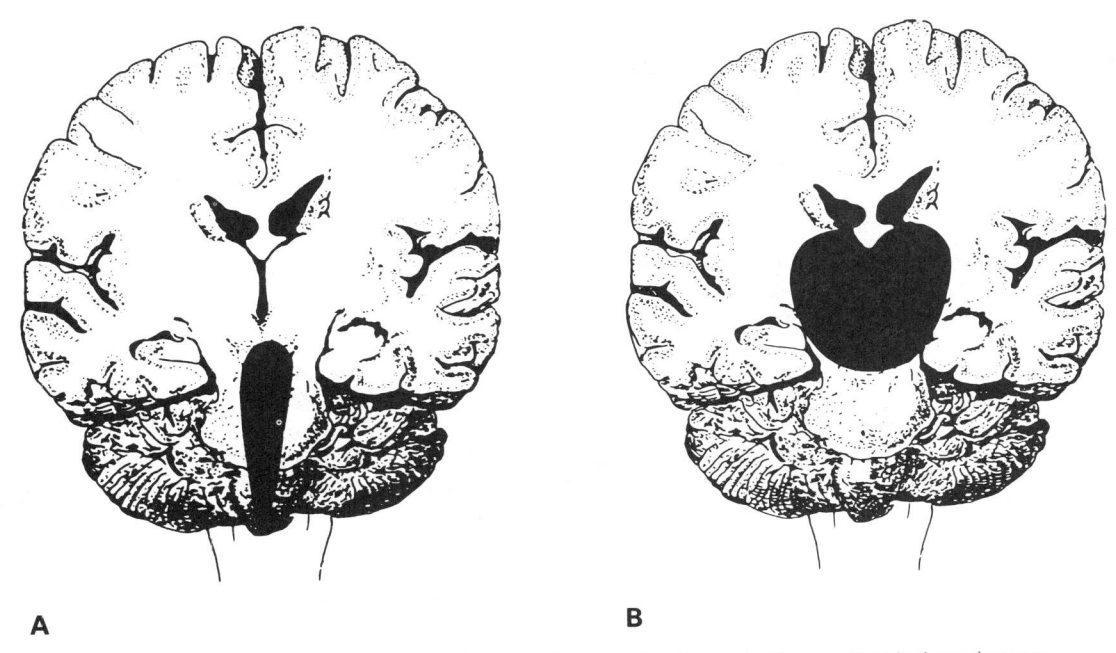

Fig. 5–2. Diencephalic and brainstem areas serving consciousness. **A.** The smallest lesions that can alter consciousness, those in the reticular core of the brainstem. **B.** Diecephalic lesions that may impair consciousness. *(From Mitchell et al., 1984, pp. 99, 100.)*

through hypothalamic structures that serve the autonomic nervous system and then project onto the basal forebrain and the limbic system, which serves primitive emotional response. Because of the diffuse innervation of the limbic cortex and neocortex, we can infer that pathways exist for behavioral output of three types: movement, language, and vegetative response. The assessment and inference of arousal from this behavior are discussed in the section "Assessing Arousal and Awareness" in this chapter.

Neurochemical Basis of Arousal

The anatomic structures described provide a framework by which information can travel from one area of the central nervous system to another. The transmission of information from the ascending reticular activating system to the cortex and back, however, requires chemical messengers to alter the membrane potential of neurons and thus stimulate or inhibit the action potentials that actually transmit information in the central nervous system. Two types of chemical substances are required to maintain consciousness and arousal. First are the basic metabolic substrates necessary for cellular function of neurons—glucose, enzymatic cofactors, and oxygen. Second are the neurotransmitters that serve the projections of the ARAS. These neurotransmitters are believed to be acetylcholine, monoamines, and possibly gamma-aminobutyric acid (GABA) (Plum & Posner, 1980).

Metabolic Substrate

Neurons, like all cells, require nutrients and enzymes to catalyze the basic chemical reactions neccessary to maintain cellular respiration and energy production. These basic processes of cellular respiration and energy consumption and production underlie the specific functions of neurons and glial cells in the central nervous system. Neurons must maintain action potentials in order to transmit information, manufacture and recover neurotransmitters, manufacture axoplasm, and repair themselves via protein and lipid synthesis. Glial cells (oligodendroglia and astrocytes) manufacture myelin, regulate the ionic environment of the brain, serve nutritional functions of the neurons, and maintain the capillary endothelial blood–brain barrier. The energy requirements for these functions exceed those of any other organ of the body and depend entirely on a constant supply of glucose and oxygen. Unlike other organs of the body, the brain cells do not store alternate energy sources, nor can alternate energy sources, such as fatty acids, pass through the capillary endothelium into the brain tissue. Enzymatic cofactors, such as the B vitamins (thiamine, pyridoxine, cyanocobalamin, and niacin), are necessary to catalyze energy production via cellular respiration. Neurons of the consciousness system seem particularly sensitive to the effects of loss of metabolic substrate. Therefore, disorders or clinical situations that result in hypoglycemia, hypoxia, or cofactor deficiency can be expected to alter arousal and self-awareness as generalized brain functions.

Central Neurotransmitters

The number of known and putative neurotransmitters in the central nervous system has grown immensely in recent years. New techniques allow the mapping of the nerve fibers served by the monoamine transmitters, detection of enzymes that serve the cholinergic transmitters, and mapping of receptors for a wide variety of central nervous system neurotransmitters (Kuhar et al, 1986).

Acetylcholine is found widely throughout the central nervous system. It is difficult to map precisely the location and fibers for this transmitter because its presence must be inferred from the activity of its enzymatic activators or inactivators or from the change in behavioral or neurophysiologic activity when cholinergic drugs or their antagonists are given systemically. A variety of indirect evidence, however, supports the existence of cholinergic neuronal fiber systems that correspond to the reticular formation–thalamic projections and to the reticular formation–basal forebrain pathways. These pathways receive fibers from the monoamine pathways in the locus ceruleus in the brainstem and project diffusely to parietal and frontal cortex (Shute & Lewis, 1967; Bartus et al., 1982; Whitehouse et al., 1982).

The monoamines found in the brain (norepinephrine, dopamine, and serotonin) are implicated in consciousness primarily in terms of their role in regulating waking and sleeping. Since a substantial number of people in long-term states of decreased arousal (persistent vegetative state) appear to recover normal sleep–wake cycles, it is clear that sleep–wake components of consciousness are at least partly independent of systems that maintain high-level vigilance behavioral arousal. Given the anatomic connections between the brainstem monoamine pathways and the forebrain cholinergic pathways, it may be possible that disorders that result in persistent vegetative states with preserved sleep–wake cycles may represent a disconnection of two components of an integrated consciousness system.

Gamma-aminobutyric acid (GABA) is an inhibitory neurotransmitter and is found widely throughout the brain. A relative decrease in GABA has been implicated in generalized seizures, which are characterized by loss of consciousness. Plum and Posner (1980) cite evidence that cortical levels of GABA are low during periods of wakefulness and higher during cortical inhibition.

Normal Alterations in Arousal

Sleep, as described more fully in Chapter 8, represents a normal alteration in arousal and consciousness. As noted previously, normal cycles of sleep and waking can exist in people with intact brainstems but with injuries that impair their ability to respond to stimuli from

TABLE 5–1. CLASSIFICATION OF DISORDERS THAT IMPAIR AROUSAL.

Damage to Structures

Destructive lesions:
- Thalamic infarcts
- Pontine (other brainstem) infarcts
- Massive hemispheric infarct

Mass lesions:
- Hemorrhage (subdural, epidural, intracerebral, pituitary, cerebellar)
- Tumors (abscesses: supratentorial, cerebellar)
- Closed head injury

Loss or Alteration in Brain Metabolites

Oxygen deprivation:
- Hypoxia (pulmonary disease, anemia, carbon monoxide poisoning, inadequate atmospheric oxygen)
- Ischemia (decreased cardiac output, low blood volume [shock], small vessel occlusion)

Hypoglycemia:
Acid–base and ion abnormalities (acidosis, alkalosis, water intoxication, hypernatremia)
Cofactor deficiency (thiamine, niacin, folic acid)
Systemic disorders (uremia, hepatic coma)

Disruption of Neurotransmitters Central to Arousal

Poisons (barbiturates, ethanol, opiates, street drugs)
Anticholinergic excess (scopolamine)
Psychotropic drugs (antihistamine excess)
Seizures

Adapted from Plum and Posner, 1980.

the environment, that is, a person in persistent vegetative state. Variants of normal sleep that represent pathologic alterations in arousal and their attendant nursing diagnoses are discussed in Chapter 8.

Abnormal Alterations in Arousal

Hypoarousal or hyperarousal can result from three main sources: (1) damage to structures of the ascending reticular activating system and its projections, (2) loss of basic metabolic substrates for brain metabolism, and (3) disruption of neurotransmitter synthesis, uptake, or release. Table 5–1 summarizes disorders that impair consciousness (arousal) in these three classifications. Nursing diagnoses that may accompany these disorders are considered in Chapters 6 through 8.

ASSESSING AROUSAL AND AWARENESS

Arousability (susceptibility to stimulus) and attention (reactivity to the stimulus) comprise the two dimensions of the assessment of *vigilance* as described by von Cramon (1977). Although a large number of tools and terminologies have been developed in an attempt to quantify level of consciousness, all implicitly contain measurement of (1) the amount and kind of stimulus required and (2) the nature of the response to the stimulus. Initially, one observes the person's response to general environmental stimuli and to specific verbal stimuli. Only if there is no response to auditory stimuli is the use of painful stimuli appropriate. The kinds of response to be observed include eye opening, movement of the head or body toward the stimulus, verbalization, and more complex responses, such as obeying commands.

At a minimum, one is attempting to distinguish the patient who is comatose (does not open the eyes) from the patient who is awake (opens the eyes) and the one who is both awake and aware (opens the eyes and follows commands) (Gamel-Bentzel, 1984). Such a minimal distinction, however, does not allow the clinician to detect subtle changes in arousal status nor to determine differences in awareness or vigilance functions of the many patients who are both awake and aware but vary in the degree to which they can sustain self-care activities. A variety of coma tools and cognitive assessment tools have been developed in an attempt to grade more accurately a patient's progress from truly comatose to fully conscious.

The Glasgow Coma Scale (GCS) is the best known of the scales that attempt to quantitate arousabilty in the acute and critical care setting (Teasdale, 1975; Teasdale & Galbraith, 1975; Teasdale & Jennett, 1974; Mitchell et al., 1983; Mitchell et al., 1984). It was developed to standardize initial observations of acutely head-injured persons in an international study of the consequences of head injury. It is the only coma scale for which test-

TABLE 5–2. GLASGOW COMA SCALE SCORING SYSTEM.

Parameter	Observation	Score[a]
Eye opening	Spontaneously	4
	To voice	3
	To pain	2
	None	1
Best verbal response	Oriented	5
	Confused	4
	Inappropriate words	3
	Incomprehensible sounds	2
	None	1
Best motor response	Obeys commands	6
	Localizes	5
	Flexion withdrawal[b]	4
	Abnormal flexion	3
	Abnormal extension	2
	None	1

[a]Maximum score 15 (awake and aware), minimum score 3 (coma).
[b]Flexion withdrawal did not appear in the early versions of the scale (Teasdale & Jennett, 1974; Teasdale, 1975). For those versions, the maximum score was 14, with only 5 points in the motor response scale.

ing of interrater reliability has been reported (Teasdale et al., 1978). As with all observational tools, specific training is required to achieve a high degree of reliability among observers.

Three parameters of behavioral response are observed in the GCS: eye opening, verbalization, and movement. The initial stimulus is the examiner's voice (asking the patient to obey a command); if no response occurs, fingertip or supraorbital pressure is applied as a painful stimulus. In each category, the patient's best response is recorded. The developer found that observers could agree much more on the best of a series of responses than on the worst. The scoring system is reproduced in Table 5–2.

The Munich Coma Scale (MCS) has been used more in research than in clinical monitoring (Brinkmann et al., 1976; von Cramon, 1977; Schuri & von Cramon, 1979, 1980, 1981). It has several attractive features for clinical use in that it grades the type of stimulus needed and is responsive to more subtle variations in motor response than is the GCS. This ability to detect more subtle change is desirable as patients with altered arousal become more stable with respect to physiologic function but are still in a state of decreased arousal. More complex behavioral indicators of arousal, however, are likely to require more training on the part of observers in order to grade responses consistently. No reports of interrater reliability are given in the literature. Some of the stimuli used may not be esthetically acceptable (electric shock and loud siren) for routine clinical use, but some groups have used more clinically acceptable stimuli, with the response monitored by the MCS reactivity scale (Smith et al., 1986). The MCS scales are shown in Table 5–3.

The Rancho Los Amigos Levels of Cognitive Functioning Scale (Malkmus et al, 1980) is another scale that has been used extensively to evaluate levels of awareness in patients who are awake but have varying levels of awareness. Dowling (1985) has shown that a reasonably high degree of interrater consistency occurs with this tool, even in untrained individuals. Levels 3 and 4 yielded the most ambiguous results, perhaps because study subjects overinterpreted behavior from the videotaped stimuli. The scale is reproduced in Table 7–2.

SUMMARY

Consciousness is a complex concept, comprised of arousal and self-awareness. The anatomic substrate for arousal consists of the brainstem reticular formation, its inputs from sensory systems, and its projections to the thalamus, hypothalamus, limbic system, and neocortex. Damage to these structures, loss of substrate necessary for brain metabolism, or interference with the function of central nervous system neurotransmitters can all act separately or together to alter arousal. Arousal can be detected only by observing behavioral indicators of the aroused awakened state: eye opening, verbalization, and simple to complex movements.

TABLE 5-3. MUNICH COMA SCALE.

MCS Stimulus	Scale of Susceptibility to Stimulation Clinical Stimuli Used by Smith et al.
Electrical (1–10 mA shock)	Olfactory (ammonia, fruit, vinegar)
Tactile (2 cm nylon hair)	Tactile (sharp, dull, varying texture)
Acoustic (90 dB siren)	Acoustic (bell, car sounds, telephone)
Optical (4000 lux flashlight)	Visual (lights, mirrors)
	Kinesthetic (range of motion)

Category of Reactivity	MCS Scale of Reactivity Response Definition
1	Any body movement; movement of head without clear-cut directional component in relation to stimulus
2	Any orofacial movements (e.g., frowning), single or repeated contraction of eyelids with closed or open eyes; any movements of perioral muscles, of tongue, or of muscles for swallowing
3	Unequivocal turning of head to or away from stimulus; opening of eyes or state of open eyes
4	Unequivocal looking at stimulus or examiner; understandable verbal utterance

Adapted from von Cramon, 1978; Smith 1986.

REFERENCES

Bartus, R.T., Dean R.L., Beer, B., & Lippa, A.S. (1982). The cholinergic hypothesis of geriatric memory dysfunction. *Science, 217.* 408.

Bremer, F. (1977). Cerebral hypnogenic centers. *Annals of Neurology, 2,* 1.

Brinkman, R., von Cramon, D., & Schulz, H. (1976). The Munich coma scale (MCS). *Journal of Neurology, Neurosurgery and Psychiatry, 39,* 788.

Daube, J.R., & Sandok, R.A. 1986. *Medical neurosciences.* (2nd ed.). Boston: Little, Brown.

Dowling, G.A. (1985). Levels of cognitive functioning: Evaluation of interrater reliability. *Journal of Neuroscience Nursing, 17,* 129.

Gamel-Bentzel, C. (1984). Nursing diagnosis: Integral to standards of practice. In M.J. Kim, G.R. McFarland, & A.M. McLean (Eds.), *Classification of nursing diagnoses: Proceedings of the fifth national conference* (p. 458). St. Louis: Mosby.

Gulbrandsen, G., Kristiansen, K., & Ursin, H. (1972). Response habituation in unconscious patients. *Neuropsycholia, 10,* 313.

Kuhar, M.J., De Souza, E.B., & Unnerstall, J.R. (1986). Neurotransmitter receptor mapping by autoradiography and other methods. *Annual Review of Neuroscience, 9,* 27.

Magoun, H.W. (1963). *The waking brain* (2nd ed.). Springfield, IL: Thomas.

Malkmus, D., Booth, B., & Kodimer, C. (1980). *Rehabilitation of the head injured adult.* Downey, CA: Professional Staff Association of the Rancho Los Amigos Hospital.

Mitchell, P.H., Cammermyer, M., Ozuna, J., & Woods, N.F. (1984). *Neurological assessment for nursing purposes.* New York: Appleton & Lange (formerly Reston).

Mitchell, P.H., Ozuna, J., & Bolles, J. (1983). *Evaluating the comatose patient.* Seattle: Health Sciences Center for Educational Resources, University of Washington (Two videotapes and observational record demonstrating use of the Glasgow Coma Scale and brainstem examination).

Moruzzi, G., & Magoun, H. (1949). Brainstem reticular formation and activation of the EEG. *Electroencephalography and Clinical Neurophysiology, 1,* 455.

Plum, F., & Posner, J. (1980). *The diagnosis of stupor and coma* (3rd ed.). Philadelphia: Davis.

Pribram, K.H. (1976). Problems concerning the structure of consciousness. In G.C. Globus, G. Maxwell, & I. Savodnick, (Eds.), *Consciousness and the brain*. New York: Plenum.

Schuri, U., & von Cramon, D. (1979). Autonomic responses to meaningful and nonmeaningful auditory stimuli in coma. *Archiv fur Psychiatrie und Nervenkrankheiten (Archives of Psychiatry and Neurological Sciences), 227*, 143.

Schuri, U., & von Cramon, D. (1980). Autonomic and behavioral responses in coma due to drug overdose. *Psychophysiology, 17*, 253.

Schuri, U., & von Cramon, D. (1981). Electrodermal responses to auditory stimuli with different significance in neurological patients. *Psychophysiology, 18*, 248.

Shute, C.C.D., & Lewis, P.R. (1967). The ascending cholinergic reticular system: Neocortical, olfactory and subcortical projections. *Brain, 90*, 497.

Smith, C., Smith, J., & Speirs, J. (1986). Coma stimulations: An interdisciplinary approach for treatment of the coma patient. Unpublished paper, Speech-Language Pathology Department, Regency Rehabilitation Center, Denver, Colorado.

Teasdale, G. (1975). Acute impairment of brain function. 1: Assessing conscious level. *Nursing Times, 71*, 914.

Teasdale, G., & Galbraith, S. (1975). Acute impairment of brain function. 2: Observation record chart. *Nursing Times, 71*, 972.

Teasdale, G., & Jennett, B. (1974). Assessment of coma and impaired consciousness: A practical scale. *Lancet, 2*, 81.

Teasdale G., Knill-Jones, R., & Van der Sande, J. (1978). Observer variability in assessing impaired consciousness and coma. *Journal of Neurology, Neurosurgery and Psychiatry, 41*, 603.

von Cramon, D. (1977). The structure of vigilance. *Archiv fur Psychiatrie und Nervenkrankheiten (Archives of Psychiatry and Neurological Sciences), 225*, 201.

Whitehouse, P.J., Price, D.L., Struble, R.G., Clark A.W., & Coyle, J.T. (1982). Alzheimer's disease and senile dementia: Loss of neurons in the basal forebrain. *Science, 215*, 1237.

6

Decreased Behavioral Arousal

Pamela H. Mitchell

Arousal is a component of consciousness. As discussed in Chapter 5, we can detect the level of arousal only through evaluation of the patient's *responsiveness*, or behavioral responses to a variety of stimuli. We therefore *infer* the degree of arousal from the nature of the behavioral response. New technologies that evaluate neurophysiologic functioning after central nervous system injury may make it possible to evaluate *internal behavior, that is, physiologic responses*, in people with decreased behavioral arousal and thus enable us to make more accurate inferences about the arousability and awareness of such people.

The focus of this chapter is the phenomenon of *decreased arousal* in people with neurologic disease and injury. Disorders that produce decreased arousal are presented briefly, categorized by their effect on input, processing, or behavioral output of the arousal system. Nursing diagnoses commonly seen in such patients are discussed in two categories: those that stem from the pathophysiologic processes that produce decreased arousal and those that stem from the diminished ability to interact with the environment.

DISORDERS PRODUCING DECREASED AROUSAL

Coma is the most profound clinical state manifested by decreased arousal and can be defined behaviorally as the absence of eye opening, absence of intelligible verbalization, and absence of following verbal commands (Jennett & Teasdale, 1981). Disorders that produce coma can be classified as *structural* and *metabolic* (Plum & Posner, 1980). Structural disorders are those, such as tumors, intracranial bleeding, and abscesses, that alter consciousness by distorting the neuroanatomic *structures* that serve consciousness. Metabolic disorders affect overall brain function by altering the supply of *nutrients* and *metabolic substrates* (oxygen, glucose, enzymatic cofactors) required by brain cells. Hypoglycemia, hypoxia, and hyperammonemia are examples of metabolic states that can produce decreased arousal and coma.

As discussed in Chapter 5, arousal requires sensory *input* into the reticular activating system, central *processing* of that input by reticular formation, limbic system, and cortex, and *behavioral output*, or the motor and

TABLE 6–1. DISORDERS THAT ALTER AROUSAL.

Diminished Input	Impaired Output	Impaired Central Nervous System Processing
Isolation Impoverished sensory environment Blindness Deafness Profound sensory neuropathy	Locked-in syndrome Paralysis	Structural lesions • Tumors (supratentorial, infratentorial) • Hemorrhage (subarachnoid, intraventricular, diencephalic, subdural, epidural) • Abscesses (large hemispheric, small infratentorial) • Meningitis (encephalitis) • Infarcts (central brainstem, diencephalic, large hemispheric) • Diffuse white matter damage (traumatic head injury) • Diffuse gray matter degeneration (Jacob-Kreutzfeld syndrome, late Alzheimer's disease, subacute combined degeneration) Metabolic disorders • Oxidative (hypoxia–anoxia, hypercarbia) • Metaboic substrate (hypoglycemia, thiamine deficiency) • Metabolic poisons (hyperammonemia [hepatic encephalopathy], hyperuremia [renal encephalopathy], drug overdose, Reye's syndrome)

verbal behaviors that indicate responsiveness. Table 6–1 shows disorders that produce decreased arousal and coma, categorized by their effect on input, processing, or behavioral output.

Diminished Input

The central nervous system must receive sensory input to maintain arousal. Sensory input can be diminished either by an impoverished sensory environment or by profound alteration in the sensory pathways that transmit information to the central nervous system. Either of these conditions produces a state of *sensory deprivation*—alteration in the pattern or meaning of sensory information. Confusion, lethargy, and diminished brain activation are well-documented effects of both experimental and clinical conditions of sensory deprivation, although coma is never the result of sensory deprivation (Wolanin & Phillips, 1981; Slade, 1984). When there is structural or metabolic injury, one might expect diminished external sensory input to compound the problem (Walsh, 1981; Le Winn & Dimanescu, 1978).

Impaired Central Nervous System Processing

The most frequent sources of decreased arousal observed by the neuroscience nurse are those diseases and conditions that impair *processing* of sensory input in the brain. As described in Chapter 5, structural lesions of the central brainstem, diencephalon, or bilateral cerebral hemispheres can impair arousal and produce coma. In addition, systemic processes that impair metabolism of the whole central nervous system can cloud consciousness and produce coma.

Disorders, such as tumors, abscesses, and hemorrhage, produce alternations in consciousness by displacing and distorting brain structures. Tumors or subdural and epidural hematomas that cause a shift of one hemisphere across the midline of the brain produce bilateral hemispheric damage and thus decreased arousal. Hemorrhage, tumor, or abscesses in the diencephalon decrease the ability of the reticular activating system to send information along the diffuse projection system from thalamus to cortex. Tumor, infarct, or compression of the brainstem produce coma by direct action on the reticular formation.

Traumatic head injury can produce coma in several ways. Diffuse white and gray matter injury at the time of impact temporarily or permanently disrupts the ability of cortical and subcortical neurons to communicate with each other. Hemorrhage from vessels damaged at the time of impact can act as a space-occupying lesion and gradually disrupt the functioning of the diffuse reticular activating system at cortical and subcortical levels. Finally, secondary injury from brain swelling and increased intracranial pressure can produce global ischemia, which disrupts the consciousness system at diencephalic and cortical levels (Jennett & Teasdale, 1981; Miller, 1985; Becker, 1987).

A smaller number of cases of coma in traumatic head injury are associated with intracerebral hemmorrhage or acute subdural or epidural hematoma. Hemorrhage produces displacement of brain tissue from the accumulating intracerebral, extradural, or subdural hematoma and thereby acts as a bilateral hemispheric or diencephalic source of coma. Hemorrhage into the ventricular system can produce rapidly increasing intracranial pressure from blockage of cerebrospinal fluid flow.

Cerebral infarct or ischemia (stroke) does not usually impair consciousness. Decreased arousal, however, can be a manifestation of stroke under three circumstances: if a whole hemisphere is infarcted, if there are old infarctions in the hemisphere opposite to the new stroke (thus producing bilateral damage), or if the infarction is of the reticular formation itself, usually at the pontine level. It is possible for certain brainstem strokes to impair the motor output necessary for behavioral evidence of arousal (see the section "Diminished Behavioral Output" in this chapter).

Disorders that impair the metabolic processes necessary for whole brain function can also alter consciousness. Exogenous poisons or drugs act to depress consciousness either by interfering with the cellular metabolic processes (e.g., carbon monoxide, cyanide) or by depressing overall brain cell functioning (e.g., barbiturates, narcotics, sedatives, tricyclic antidepressants). A variety of systemic disorders alter consciousness by depriving the brain of necessary metabolic substrate (e.g., glucose in profound diabetic hypoglycemia, oxygen in profound hypoxemia, or enzymes necessary to use glucose in thiamine deficiency). Other systemic diseases produce metabolic waste products that act as cellular poisons in the brain (e.g., urea in acute renal failure, hyperammonemia in Reye's syndrome or in acute hepatic encephalopathy).

Diminished Behavioral Output

The final category of disorders altering consciousness includes conditions that create diminished ability to produce the behavioral *output* (motor and verbal behaviors) from which we infer responsiveness. These disorders do not impair consciousness but the person's *ability to communicate consciousness* to the world.

Disorders that impair motor output so profoundly that the patient appears to be unresponsive comprise this category. For example, high cervical cord injuries leave the facial, shoulder, and neck muscles intact. Thus, no one confuses lack of verbalization by the person who is quadriplegic and on a ventilator with lack of consciousness, because the person is still capable of eye blinking and head nodding. The person who has Guillain-Barré syndrome (ascending polyneuropathy) that has affected the cranial nerves may have great difficulty communicating his or her completely intact consciousness. These patients, however, usually retain the ability to open and close the eyes.

A disorder of motor output that easily can be confused with coma is the locked-in syndrome, a relatively uncommon form of brainstem stroke in which the anterior brainstem is infarcted, usually at the base of the pons. Any anterior infarction from midbrain to lower pons can produce the syndrome. This portion of the brainstem carries all the motor fibers from the lower cranial nerves (those that serve phonation and facial expression) as well as those from the cortex to the limbs. It is anterior to the reticular formation. Consciousness is thus spared, but all motor output is disconnected between cortex and the effector cranial and spinal nerves that serve verbal and motor output. Usually, at least vertical eye movements are preserved, and the patient may be capable of communication via eye movements.

HUMAN RESPONSES ASSOCIATED WITH DECREASED CONSCIOUSNESS

People with decreased consciousness have responses, and thus nursing diagnoses, that are specifically related to the *pathophysiologic states* that produce diminished responsiveness; they have nursing diagnoses that stem directly from the *lack of volitional movement* from which we infer loss of consciousness. The nursing diagnoses related to the basic pathology commonly are clinical problems that must be managed collaboratively by nurses and other health professionals (collaborative problems), whereas the diagnoses related to lack of movement usually are managed independently by nurses (nursing diagnoses). The following case studies are used to illustrate nursing diagnoses often found in patients with coma from a variety of sources.

Case Study 1: Decreased Arousal After Neurosurgery

Mr. P is a 50-year-old man admitted to an acute care hospital for craniotomy to remove a left frontal brain mass. Over the 4 months before admission, he had been experiencing frontoparietal headaches, constant and stabbing, associated with nausea without vomiting and loss of appetite. The headaches had no apparent precipitators, nor were they relieved by aspirin, acetaminophen, or ibuprofen. His family encouraged him to seek medical attention when he began to have weakness and pain in the right shoulder, arm, and leg. In retrospect, they also noted that he seemed to have difficulty finding words and hesitancy initiating speech.

The physician's initial examination noted the following abnormalities: difficulty initiating sentences and pronouncing words with initial "n" sounds; decreased strength of the right proximal arm muscles (3/5 compared to 5/5 in the left arm and both legs), pronator drift present in the right arm, deep tendon reflexes 3+ on right compared to 2+ on left, Babinski's reflex present bilaterally. The patient was alert, oriented, and without cranial nerve deficits. A computerized tomography scan of the head revealed a probable tumor in the left frontal lobe, with left-to-right brain shift.

Mr. P underwent a left frontal craniotomy, with removal of a grade III astrocytoma. Postoperatively, he was on bedrest, with the head of the bed elevated 30 degrees. Other medical therapies included intravenous (IV) fluids to maintain normovolemia, dexamethasone 4 mg IV every 6 hours and cimetidine 300 mg every 6 hours.

Immediately postoperatively, his score on the Glasgow Coma Scale (GCS) was recorded at 14: eyes opened spontaneously; verbal response was confused ("I'm at home"); he obeyed commands. His pupils were equal at 4 mm and reactive to light, and eye movements were conjugate. The right hand grasp was weaker than the left. Respirations and cardiovascular status were unremarkable. The assessment remained much the same for about 6 hours, when the nurse's notes indicated that commands were followed slowly; the patient was "lethargic," and the right hand grasp was markedly weaker than the left. The GCS score was not reported. Vital signs and pupils remained unchanged.

The patient was judged by the night nurses to be stable, and the frequency of assessment was decreased to every 4 hours. At noon the next day, Mr. P was noted to be difficult to arouse, "sleeping at times," and the right arm was flaccid, with flexion withdrawal to painful stimuli. The ability to obey commands was inconsistent. At this point, the attending neurosurgeon was called. Intracranial pressure (ICP) monitoring, mannitol and hyperventilation were instituted. The ICP was 25 mm Hg, with rapid reduction to 8 to 10 mm Hg with therapy. The CT scan showed brain swelling on the left hemisphere but no postoperative hemorrhage, and the brain swelling was brought under control with mannitol. The patient regained his previous level of arousal within 12 hours and regained motor function on the right to his preoperative level. The remainder of his postoperative course was uneventful, and he was discharged home with plans for a course of radiation therapy.

Collaborative Problems Related to Arousal for Case 1

Mr. P's case illustrates several collaborative problems that stem from the pathophysiologic state accompanying supratentorial craniotomy. The overall category of collaborative problems is *high risk for secondary brain injury*, with specific risks including:

- Potential for brain herniation secondary to brain swelling or postoperative hemorrhage
- Potential for intracranial hypertension and cerebral ischemia secondary to brain swelling
- Potential for inadequate cerebral oxygenation related to impaired gas exchange (postoperative atelectasis)

In addition, there are several highly probable independent nursing diagnoses related to his and his family's cognitive, motor, and coping responses to the residual physical disabilities and the meaning of the diagnosis of brain tumor. These diagnoses, however, are not manifested by nor do they stem from his decreased arousal. Therefore, diagnoses related to cognitive, self-care, communication, and coping responses are more appropriately illustrated in the case studies in Chapters 12, 13, 15, 17, and 33.

Potential for intracranial hypertension and potential for brain herniation are two clinical problems that stem directly from the pathophysiologic state, *brain swelling*, that commonly follows manipulation of the brain during craniotomy.

Brain swelling is the net increase in volume of any one of the brain fluid compartments (vascular, intracellular, extracellular). *Hyperemia*, acute vasodilation of cerebral vessels, is the most immediate cause of brain swelling in acute head injury and may be caused by a combination of hypoxemia and release of vasoactive substances from injured cells. Vasodilation as a source of brain swelling is distinguished from *cerebral edema*, a more slowly developing process of accumulation of extracellular or intracellular water, resulting in a net increase in the water content of the cranial cavity 24 to 72 hours after injury (Langfitt, 1983; Miller, 1985). In Mr. P's case, the postoperative deterioration was most likely the manifestation of early brain swelling surrounding the operative site or mass effect from postoperative hemorrhage at the operative site.

Brain swelling can produce decreased arousal and coma (1) by acting as a whole brain depressant, (2) by displacing tissues onto the diencephalic and midbrain arousal structures, and (3) by producing rapidly increasing intracranial pressure.

Potential for Brain Herniation

The potential for brain herniation is a risk for all patients who undergo either supratentorial or infratentorial craniotomy. It is further compounded by the risk of postanesthesia complications that impair pulmonary gas exchange and thus the delivery of oxygen to the brain. *Defining characteristics* of brain herniation are decreasing level of consciousness, asymmetry of motor response, and signs of brainstem dysfunction (abnormal or absent extraocular movement, pupillary asymmetry, abnormal breathing patterns, and if allowed to progress, Cushing's reflex—bradycardia, increased systolic blood pressure, widening pulse pressure).

The most prominent aspect of altered arousal in Mr. P's case is the decrease in responsiveness within the first 12 hours after surgery. Although the nurses caring for him recognized the need for neurosurgical intervention relatively early in the course of probable brain herniation, there were subtle signs of decreased arousal even earlier. Had the terminology of the Glasgow Coma Scale (GCS) been used consistently throughout the early postoperative course, it is possible that the "lethargy" reported at 6 hours postoperatively would have been manifested by lack of spontaneous eye opening and confusion, thus a measurable decrease in level of arousal. Since transtentorial brain herniation progresses in a rostral–caudal fashion, one expects proximal motor function to be impaired before distal motor function. Thus, the use of hand grips to test motor function fails to detect increasing motor weakness that could indicate early progression of the motor deficit. Since this patient did obey commands, he should have been asked to hold his arms out in front of him while the nurse observed for drift and pronation of either arm.

Nursing *assessment* of this potential problem consists of *serial monitoring* for signs of brain herniation, with the *goal* of earliest possible detection of actual herniation.

At a minimum, the monitoring protocol requires assessment for level of consciousness and for brainstem functions that indicate the status of the arousal system. The GCS is a widely used assessment tool for level of consciousness but cannot be relied on as the sole indicator for brain herniation because it does not include assessment of brainstem and motor functions. One must include, therefore, serial assessment of the following:

- Symmetry of motor response to verbal or painful stimuli, including deep tendon and superficial reflexes
- Eye signs: extraocular movements, pupillary responses
- Protective reflexes: lash (corneal), gag, or swallow
- Vital signs: pulse, blood pressure, respiratory pattern

Nursing *intervention* is prompt *referral* for neurosurgical management if signs of herniation are detected. Neurosurgical intervention consists of management of intracranial hypertension, if it coexists with the impending brain herniation, and diagnosis and control of the pathophysiologic state causing the brain herniation. Brain swelling and postoperative hemorrhage are the most common causes of brain herniation after craniotomy. Many neurosurgeons, therefore, will institute measures to reduce hyperemia and brain swelling as immediate management and then obtain a CT scan for definitive diagnosis. Hyperventilation acts to constrict cerebral blood vessels and thus reduce hyperemia. Mannitol or other osmotic diuretics are used to reduce total brain water volume.

In the case of Mr. P, osmotic diuretics were adequate to reduce brain water volume sufficiently to reverse brain herniation and to prevent concomitant increase of ICP until the postoperative edema had resolved. Had this not been sufficient, more aggressive measures to control ICP might have been necessary. The CT scan did not show any signs of postoperative hematoma.

Potential for Intracranial Hypertension

Any patient with significant brain injury, including craniotomy as a controlled trauma, is at risk for intracranial hypertension. Intracranial hypertension is defined as resting ICP equal to or greater than 20 mm Hg. Although many describe a variety of clinical signs as indicators of intracranial hypertension, the only valid indicator is direct measurement of ICP. Research over the past 20 years has shown clearly that the traditional signs of increased ICP have poor correlation with the actual level of ICP. Even the level of arousal may not change in clear relationship to the measured level of ICP; that is, arousal may decrease at low levels of ICP or be unchanged until ICP is high. It is inappropriate, therefore, to define intracranial hypertension in terms of clinical signs.

In Mr. P, ICP was measured and found to be high at some point after his decrease in level of arousal. Since he also showed signs of early transtentorial brain herniation, it is impossible to determine if his decreased arousal was a manifestation of intracranial hypertension or early brain herniation or both. Medical intervention is designed to reduce ICP and to correct the underlying pathologic state if possible. Hyperventilation to control hyperemia and osmotic diuretics are used. Nursing therapies to reduce activity-related transient elevations are described in Case Study 2.

Once Mr. P's ICP was found to be elevated, it was important to monitor cerebral perfusion pressure continually to determine that brain cells were being adequately perfused. Since he had an arterial monitoring catheter in place, the monitoring was simple. Cerebral perfusion pressure (CPP) can be calculated at the bedside by subtracting mean ICP from mean arterial blood pressure. Normal CPP should be 60 to 150 mm Hg; Mr. P's CPP remained 70 to 90 mm Hg.

Mr. P's brain herniation and intracranial hypertension were detected relatively early and were reversed by neurosurgical intervention. His right-sided motor deficits were not resolved completely by removal of the tumor and probably complicated the postoperative assessment for the nurses. Those who discounted his lethargy and tested only hand grips may have assumed that the asymmetry between right and left motor function was the same as had been noted preoperatively. This case illustrates the importance of serial assessments of brainstem and motor function, as well as arousal (or level of consciousness).

Case Study 2: Sudden-Onset Coma

Alex is a 24-year-old man employed as an auto mechanic, who lived with his family in Alaska. He arrived home from a party at 3 A.M. and was noted by his father to still be resting at 6 P.M. that day. By 11 P.M. the parents had called the rescue squad to the home because Alex would not respond and seemed "stiff and strange."

In the emergency room, he was noted to have no spontaneous eye opening, although his eyes did open to painful stimuli. Pupils were fixed in midposition, and spontaneous gaze was dysconjugate. The fundi were remarkable for significant venous engorgement, although the disks were sharp and pale. He did not respond to verbal commands or verbalize intelligibly. His teeth were clenched, and there was fecal-smelling material at his mouth. Painful stimulation produced extension at both elbows, internal rotation of the shoulders, and extension at the wrists. The legs also extended. Computed tomography scanning equipment was not available, nor was there capability for ICP monitoring.

The initial impression noted by the physician was "major intracranial event." Furosemide, mannitol, intubation, and hyperventilation were instituted, and the patient was airlifted to a major medical center for further evaluation and care.

On arrival at the medical center, Alex had no spontaneous eye opening and no verbal response and exhibited flexion withdrawal to painful stimulation. Corneal reflexes were absent bilaterally, pupils were fixed in midposition, and slight conjugate movement of the eyes was present with oculovestibular testing (cold calorics). A CT scan showed intraventricular clots and dilated ventricles thought to be secondary to hemorrhage from a left posterior cerebellar artery arteriovenous malformation (AVM).

A Richmond bolt was placed to monitor ICP, and a right frontal ventriculostomy was performed to drain cerebrospinal fluid. Arterial pressure monitoring and assisted ventilation were instituted. The ICP initially was 25 mm Hg, decreasing to maintain at 8 to 10 mm Hg with intermittent ventriculostomy drainage. Dexamethasone 4 mg was given intravenously every 4 hours initially. Tube feeding was instituted, since adequate bowel tones were present, with feedings of 3,000 kilocalories daily and 100 ml free water per hour.

Over the course of the next 4 weeks, ICP stabilized as the hydrocephalus resolved. Oxygenation was adequate with spontaneous breathing. Spontaneous eye opening and eye opening to pain stimuli were present, but eye opening was not consistently present to verbal stimulation. No verbal response was present to any stimulus, and motor response remained flexion withdrawal to painful stimuli. Gaze was conjugate with spontaneous eye movements, but no orienting or tracking of objects occurred. The patient tended to gaze to the left when undisturbed. Facial grimacing was present both spontaneously and to painful stimuli; it occurred regularly when family members spoke to him. Spontaneous swallow was present, but gag was markedly diminished. Deep tendon reflexes were hyperactive in all extremities, and the plantar reflex was present on the right.

Tube feeding was necessary for nutritional intake. Although Alex was no longer hypermetabolic, the earlier hypermetabolic state had resulted in loss of weight, primarily muscle. Pressure hyperemia was evident on the hips and sacrum and did not resolve rapidly with turning from the affected areas. Elimination of urine was controlled with a condom catheter; he was incontinent of loose stool one or more times daily. Aspiration pneumonia had been present during the early hospitalization but was resolved presently.

Although the possibility of surgical embolization of the AVM had been entertained early in the course of the illness, his continued functioning at a subcortical level suggested that irreversible and massive brain damage had occurred with the initial hemorrhage. The physicians and family decided, therefore, to forego surgery and to place the patient in an extended care facility when his physical condition was stabilized. No facilities were available near the family home that offered specialized care for the brain-damaged patient, and he was transferred to a nursing home that could provide tube feedings and his basic physical care. He died 6 months later of aspiration pneumonia, never having manifested signs of arousal beyond spontaneous eye movements and facial grimacing.

Alex's case illustrates a greater variety of collaborative problems and nursing diagnoses (Table 6–2) than does that of Mr. P. Although the particular pathology in Alex's case was AVM, the clinical problems illustrated are found in a wide variety of severe brain injuries, including closed head injury.

TABLE 6–2. A SUMMARY OF NURSING DIAGNOSES FOR CASE STUDY 2: SUDDEN-ONSET COMA.

Diagnoses That Stem from the Pathophysiologic Process

For the individual
- Physiologic instability related to impaired CNS integrative functions: cardiovascular, respiratory, temperature regulation
- Intracranial hypertension: potential for decreased adaptive capacity and secondary brain injury
- Nutritional deficit related to hypermetabolism
- Potential for infection: steroids, monitoring devices

For the family
- Knowledge deficit concerning nature and prognosis of coma

For the community
- Potential knowledge deficit regarding prevention of pathology

Diagnoses That Stem from Reduced Ability to Interact with Environment

For the individual
- Self-care deficit: protective reflexes related to lack of volitional responsiveness
- Potential for skin breakdown related to nutritional deficit and self-care deficit
- Impaired mobility, level 4: potential for disuse syndrome; immobility complications
- Potential for psychologic distress related to auditory environment

For the family
- Potential for impaired family coping

For the community
- Inadequate resources for care of people with long-term decreased arousal

Diagnoses Related to the Pathophysiologic State

The sudden onset of a massive hemorrhage from the AVM precipitates a number of problems that must be managed collaboratively by nurses and physicians. These problems include multisystem physiologic instability, intracranial hypertension, and potential nutritional and infection problems that stemmed from the medical therapies.

☐ Physiologic Instability Related to Impaired CNS Integrative Functions

Cardiovascular, respiratory, temperature regulation, and fluid balance homeostatic functions are all regulated at the level of the hypothalamus. The regulatory functions of the hypothalamus can be altered in severe and generalized insult to the central nervous system (CNS) (as in head injury or massive intracranial bleeding), global ischemia from intracranial hypertension, or direct ischemia to the diencephalon (as in some strokes). Systemic problems may be evident, particularly in cardiovascular, pulmonary, temperature regulation, and fluid–electrolyte balance systems. This was the case for Alex and was manifested in cardiac arrhythmias, spontaneous hyperventilation and possible nonaspiration-related ventilation-perfusion abnormalities, and initial poikilothermia (tendency to take on the environmental temperature). There was no evidence of hyperosmolar or hypoosmolar states (fluid–electrolyte regulatory disturbance).

Defining characteristic for this class of collaborative problem is abnormal systemic function in the absence of systemic disease. Examples are cardiac arrhythmias in a young person with head injury and no history of cardiac disease, ventilation-perfusion abnormalities with no evidence of pneumonia or primary respiratory disease, fever with no evidence of infection, or hyperosmolar or hypoosmolar plasma and urinary laboratory values in the absence of diabetes, primary pituitary dysfunction, or inappropriate parenteral fluid management. Aspiration pneumonia, nosocomial infection, and inappropriate parenteral fluid management are by far the most common sources of pulmonary, temperature, and fluid balance problems in patients with central nervous system disorders and must be ruled out before assuming that they stem from disordered diencephalic regulation (Jennett & Teasdale, 1981; Mitchell, 1988).

In the case of Alex, only the cardiac arrhythmias (premature ventricular contractions [PVC] and inverted T waves) can be assumed to stem from hypothalamic regulatory dysfunction. Aspiration of gastric contents presumably occurred during the prehospitalization period, thus accounting for the pulmonary problems and fever. Some degree of shunt (ventilation-perfusion mismatch) has been shown in experimental head injury and may be present to compound the altered ventilation stemming from aspiration pneumonia.

Hyperosmolar state (diabetes insipidus [DI]) and hypoosmolar state (syndrome of inappropriate antidiuretic hormone [SIADH]) can occur in brain injury that is sufficient to cause coma and can be a direct result of hypothalamic ischemia or injury.

Hyperosmolar state results from the inability to produce antidiuretic hormone or from nonketotic hyperglycemia and results in osmotic diuresis, which is manifested by urine output in excess of fluid intake, hypotonic urine (specific gravity 1.001 to 1.005, urine osmolarity 50 to 150 mOsm/kg) and normal or increased serum sodium (and thus normal or increased serum osmolarity). *Hypoosmolar state* is caused by excess production of antidiuretic hormone and, thus, retention of excess free water. This state is manifested by low urine output compared to fluid intake, hypertonic urine (increased urinary sodium, urine osmolarity higher than serum osmolarity) and decreased serum sodium and serum osmolarity (<280 mOsm/kg) (Raimondi & Taylor, 1986; Saul, 1983).

Nursing management of these neurally induced systemic states as a class consists of (1) monitoring or surveillance to detect the problem and (2) collaborative implementation of the medical therapy for the specific systemic clinical problem. Careful monitoring of cardiac, pulmonary, temperature, and fluid balance systems is essential. Many authorities believe that the cardiac arrhythmias seen after head injury and subarachnoid hemorrhage represent microinfarcts of the myocardium and that patients who manifest them should be treated as if they had a myocardial infarction (McCarthy, 1982). Implementing a treatment plan of bedrest and graded resumption of activity is consistent with the activity capabilities of a patient with decreased level of consciousness.

Monitoring of ventilation (blood gases, respiratory response to activity) and temperature is important both in following the course of pulmonary and infectious problems and in estimating the demands of such clinical problems on the patient's metabolic capacities. Increasing activity and mobility creates demands on patients' ability to expend energy and may create a demand greater than the ability to respond in patients with compromised ventilation and the excess metabolic demands of fever. The patient with diminished consciousness cannot tell us that he or she is exhausted after sitting up 30 minutes, for example, and, therefore, changes in heart rate, respiration, and blood pressure must be used as rough estimates of the person's ability to tolerate increased activity.

Monitoring intake and output and specific gravity of the urine is warranted in any patient with severe central nervous system insult because of the potential for either neurally or iatrogenically induced fluid balance problems. Thirst is our most important signal for self-regulation of fluid intake. Although we cannot know if poeple with decreased consciousness experience thirst, we are certain that they cannot communicate it to us. We must rely on indicators of intake and output and osmolarity to detect hyperosmolar and hypoosmolar problems. Alex's fluid balance remained normal. With manifestations of hyperosmolar state, the usual medical treatment is to replace urinary losses plus insensible losses with dextrose and water rather than saline. Supplementary vasopressin (antidiuretic hormone) may be necessary to control diuresis. Hypoosmolar state is treated by fluid restriction; some physicians advocate rapid correction with hypertonic saline, titrating to urine and serum osmolarity (Saul, 1983).

☐ Intracranial Hypertension: Potential for Decreased Adaptive Capacity and Secondary Brain Injury

A clinical problem directly related to the pathophysiology of Alex's massive intracranial hemorrhage is intracranial hypertension. Intracranial pressure is normally between 0 and 10 mm Hg when the volumes of brain, blood and cerebrospinal fluid in the cranial cavity are in their normal proportions. When any of these components increases, compensatory changes occur to maintain ICP at a normal level. These compensatory changes include shifting of a larger proportion of cerebrospinal fluid to the spinal sac, a slight increase in venous outflow, and a slight compression of brain tissue. If the volume of one of the components continues to increase, ICP will eventually rise.

In the case of Mr. P, brain edema served to increase the volume of brain as the source of increased ICP. In Alex's case, the clots from the intraventricular hemorrhage blocked the flow of cerebrospinal fluid and produced noncommunicating hydrocephalus, thus increasing the volume of cerebrospinal fluid in the cranial cavity. Since the cerebrospinal fluid could not flow out of the cranial cavity by the usual route through the ventricles and basal cisterns, the normal ability to compensate by shifting cerebrospinal fluid to the spinal sac was lost. In the case of head injury, intracranial hypertension often results from a combination of reflex hyperemia (increasing intracranial blood volume), brain swelling, and cerebrospinal fluid obstruction.

A nursing diagnosis sometimes coexisting with intracranial hypertension is *decreased intracranial adaptive capacity*. The etiology of the diagnosis is failure of normal intracranial compensatory mechanisms, and its *defining characteristic* is repeated, disproportionate increases in ICP in response to noxious and nonnoxious stimuli (Mitchell, 1986, 1988). This means that a patient whose ICP increased 10 mm Hg for 3 minutes or longer with repeated episodes of turning, suctioning, and so on would be manifesting decreased adaptive capacity. Those at high risk for such repeated transient increases in ICP are patients with resting ICP >20 mm Hg, resting CPP <50 mm Hg, wide amplitude ICP tracing, or >10 mm Hg response to nursing maneuvers lasting more than 3 minutes (Mitchell, 1986).

Nursing intervention for this diagnosis consists of measures to decrease the environmental demands on the intracranial system or measures to increase the intracranial adaptive capacity. Measures designed to *reduce the demand* on the intracranial system of rapid changes in posture include turning patients with head held in midline, using turning sheets, slow turning, or mechanical turning beds. Prevention of constipation (and thus straining at stool), reduction of coughing with endotracheal tube and suctioning, and avoidance of loud noises or sudden tactile stimuli are other examples of activities that reduce demand on the cardiovascular system and thus prevent adding transient additional vascular volume to the intracranial cavity. Increase in systemic blood pressure can increase cerebral blood volume in the injured brain, and the Valsalva maneuver associated with coughing and straining acts to reduce cerebral venous outflow (and thus increase net cerebral blood volume).

Many of the medical therapies described for intracranial hypertension, for example, osmotic diuresis, act to *increase adaptive capacity*. Mechanical drainage of cerebrospinal fluid reduces the volume of cerebrospinal fluid in the cranial cavity and thus temporarily increases intracranial adaptive capacity. In Alex's case, the nurses implemented the medical protocol to drain a small amount of cerebrospinal fluid from the ventriculostomy before initiating such activities as suctioning, turning, and chest physiotherapy. This provided sufficient intracranial adaptive capacity that his resting ICP was maintained at 8 to 10 mm Hg and he never showed a peak pressure beyond 15 mm Hg in response to activities that initially produced an ICP of 30 to 40 mm Hg. Cerebral perfusion pressure remained adequate during and after all nursing care procedures. As the intraventricular clots and the blood products in the subarachnoid space were reabsorbed, the hydrocephalus resolved, and ICP remained within normal limits without ventricular drainage.

☐ Nutritional Deficit Related to Hypermetabolism

Patients who are sufficiently unresponsive to be unable to take oral food and fluids are at risk for nutritional deficits because parenteral fluids alone cannot supply enough calories to meet basal metabolic needs. Compounding this relatively simple supply problem is the fact that significant trauma, including central nervous system trauma or injury, results in a hypermetabolic state (Deutschman et al., 1986). The caloric and nitrogen needs of such patients can be approached only by hyperalimentation, enteral or parenteral (Clifton et al., 1985). Alex had bowel tones and was fed by nasogastric tube, with a high protein nutritional prescription tailored to 140% of his estimated basal metabolic needs. The nutritional problem is best managed collaboratively by nutritionist, physician, and nurse. The nutritionist's *assessment* of nutritional deficit includes serial monitoring of weight, fluid intake and output, serum sodium, albumin, glucose, lymphocyte count, and urine creatinine and urea excretion as markers of protein loss. The laboratory monitoring of markers of nutritional status is primarily a collaborative endeavor of nutritionist and physician. It is often the nursing staff, however, that recognizes the need for nutritional intervention from patterns of weight loss. The nutritional prescription and the means to deliver it require collaboration among nurses, nutritionists, and physicians. If hyperalimentation is delivered parenterally, a high risk for infection of the hyperalimentation line exists, and nursing *interventions* consist of using scrupulous aseptic technique and monitoring of aseptic technique used by others. If enteral hyperalimentation is used, the risk of aspiration of nasogastric tube feeding is present. Nursing *interventions* consist of monitoring the tube placement before each feeding, monitoring the respiratory status for signs of silent aspiration (sudden fever, atelectasis, respiratory distress), and monitoring the pulmonary secretions for signs of the dye marker that is added to the enteral formula. Since the patient cannot complain of thirst if there is insufficient free water in the feeding, the nurse should monitor serum sodium, urinary output, and specific gravity for signs of extracellular volume deficit. This is manifested by increasing serum osmolarity (estimated by doubling serum sodium) as serum water volume decreases and decreasing urine output as the body seeks to conserve free water. If long-term tube feeding is required, esophagostomy or gastrostomy decreases the risk of aspiration of tube feeding that is inherent in nasogastric feeding (Olivares et al., 1974).

☐ **Potential for Infection Related to Invasive Monitoring Devices**

Early in Alex's hospitalization, several invasive monitoring devices were used to diagnose and track the pathophysiologic problem underlying the coma. Intracranial pressure monitoring, intraarterial pressure monitoring, and parenteral delivery of medications all carry the risk of nosocomial infection, compounded by the use of corticosteroids. *Assessment* consists of monitoring for signs of infection—fever, lymphocyte count, local inflammation. *Intervention* consists of changing tubings at least every 48 hours, as recommended by the Centers for Disease Control, scrupulous handwashing, and using aseptic technique every time the monitoring system must be opened to air (e.g., calibration, removal of cerebrospinal fluid or blood specimens). The incidence of infection increases with the time that the invasive monitoring devices are in place. Some authorities recommend removal and reinsertion at a new site if ventriculostomy measurement must continue beyond 5 days (Mayhall et al., 1984).

☐ **Potential Family Knowledge Deficit for Nature and Prognosis of Coma**

At the time of Alex's transfer to the medical center hospital, his family had every hope that the cause of his coma would be removed and that he would be the same person he had been before the catastrophic illness. Although the attending neurosurgeon told them early that people with this kind of hemorrhage often do not wake up, or are left with severe deficits, they could not believe that Alex would not recover. Their hopes were particularly buoyed when he began to open his eyes and make facial grimaces when the family was in the room. As the weeks wore on, however, they began to wonder if the physician had not been correct and they reached out for the support and help with long-term placement that had been offered earlier.

Assessment and intervention in family knowledge deficit about the nature and implications of the pathophysiologic state must be a collaborative effort of physician, nurse, and often such support people as social worker and chaplain. The *goal* of increasing family knowledge is to provide an adequate information base on which to make decisions about future care.

Only in the past 15 to 20 years has sufficient evidence been accumulated to make reasonably accurate prognoses from early neurologic status for patients with traumatic and nontraumatic coma. In both head injury and nontraumatic causes of coma, the presence or absence of specific combinations of neurologic signs on admission or in the first few days of hospitalization is a more accurate prognosticator of survival and extent of recovery than is the specific disease process (Plum & Posner, 1980). Knowing that a given patient has essentially no chance of satisfactory recovery can prompt us to provide supportive rather than inappropriately heroic care, whereas knowledge that a patient has a 50% chance of meaningful recovery allows one to support honestly the family's hope and provide appropriately aggressive intensive care.

In traumatic head injury, there is less than a 5% chance of satisfactory recovery in the patient who does not open the eyes, does not make intelligible sounds, does not make localizing movements to pain, and has absent pupillary or oculocephalic responses at any point in the hospitalization. By 6 hours after the onset of coma, abnormal flexor or extensor motor responses are associated with 80% to 100% mortality if abnormal eye signs are present, and 60% mortality if eye signs are normal.

Nontraumatic coma is caused by drug overdose, cerebral vascular disease (infarct and hemorrhage), central nervous system infection, spontaneous subarachnoid hemorrhage, cardiac arrest, and such metabolic disorders as hepatoencephalopathy and renal encephalopathy. A multinational study of 500 patients in coma from medical causes showed that if coma lasted longer than 6 hours and was accompanied by abnormal neuroophthalmic signs on admission (absence of any two responses: corneal, oculocephalic, oculovestibular, or pupillary), there was less than a 1% chance of survival, regardless of the disease state. Conversely, even if coma lasted longer than 6 hours, the presence of comprehensible words, obeying commands, orienting eye movements, or localizing motor response during the first week after admission correlated with a 60% to 80% good or moderately disabled outcome (Plum & Posner, 1980). The prognosis offered to Alex's family clearly was based on the grim signs on admission: absence of pupillary response, absence of corneal response, and abnormal motor responses. Although he did regain spontaneous eye movements and eye opening, he never regained comprehensible sounds, eye movements that clearly tracked objects, or the ability to obey commands.

The intensive care team was faced with assessing the family's readiness to hear the prognostic information as well as the intervention of providing information. Nursing assessment in such situations consists of listening to the family questions for changes from "When will he wake up?" to "Do you think he will wake up?" and eliciting the family's understanding of and reaction to the information provided by the physician. In some situations, nursing intervention may be needed with the physician to encourage provision of prognostic information when the family is ready to hear it. Ways in which nursing can facilitate family support during acute hospitalization are discussed in Chapter 15.

☐ Potential Community Knowledge Deficit Regarding Prevention of Pathology

Although Alex's pathology (arteriovenous malformation) was a congenital one for which there is no known prevention, a great many of the disorders that result in prolonged states of decreased arousal are largely preventable. Examples include traumatic head injury from motor vehicle accidents, cerebral hemorrhage from hypertension, drug overdose, and alcoholic hepatic encephalopathy (McGuire, 1986). Nurses can and should be vitally involved in community organizations, such as the National Head Injury Foundation and The American Heart Association, that seek to assess community knowledge and behavior and bring about changes in health behaviors.

Diagnoses Stemming from Reduced Ability to Interact with the Environment
The diagnoses under this heading are independent nursing diagnoses that have as their etiology the patient's inability to communicate or meet voluntarily his own basic physiologic and psychosocial needs.

☐ Self-Care Deficit: Protective Reflexes Related to Lack of Volitional Responsiveness

As discussed in Chapter 33, there is a continuum of self-care deficits ranging from complete deficits, including loss of protective reflexes, to deficits in one or more aspects of daily living. In the case of Alex, the initial *assessment* demonstrated absence of corneal reflexes, pupillary responses, and presumably gag and cough reflex (based on his prior aspiration and the loss of cranial nerve reflexes located higher in the brainstem). *Intervention* consists of basic nursing care that is protective of all the vital functions usually served by those reflexes. Loss of corneal reflex implies high risk of corneal abrasion, with secondary infection and loss of eyesight should there be any functional recovery. Careful application of artificial tears and use of eyepads or eyelid taping is indicated to protect the eyes. Alex later regained the corneal reflex but still required regular eye care, since he had no ability to remove lint, dried secretions, or other material that might lodge in the eyes.

Initially, the loss of gag and cough reflex was managed medically by endotracheal tube. When spontaneous breathing and these reflexes returned and the tube was removed, nursing assessment was crucial in determining the patient's ongoing ability to swallow his secretions and avoid aspiration. Methods of assessing swallowing are described in Chapter 12.

☐ Impaired Mobility, Level 4: Potential for Disuse Syndrome, Immobility Complications

Movement and change of posture are activities that are normally automatic and serve to maintain normal ventilation via periodic full expansion of the lungs. The patient with absent volitional movement depends on the nursing staff for position change. Position change (turning) is an intervention that is useful for many disgnoses for patients with decreased arousal: prevention of inadequate gas exchange, prevention of skin breakdown, and promotion of sensory stimulation. In the early days, the nurses had to reduce ICP by ventriculostomy drainage before turning Alex, since the position change acted as an adaptive demand. Once his ICP stabilized, he could be safely turned to any position, including prone. Further assessment and intervention measures for problems induced by immobility are discussed in Chapter 20.

☐ Potential for Skin Breakdown Related to Nutritional Deficit and Self-Care Deficit

The combination of Alex's inability to respond to sensations of pressure by moving and the loss of body protein from the hypermetabolic response to injury put him at high risk for the breakdown of skin and underlying tissues and development of pressure sores.

For clinical purposes, pressure sores can be classified into two types: superficial friction lesions (sheetburn) and deep, pressure–shearing-induced tissue necrosis. If superficial redness and friction lesions do not heal, they may progress to ulcerations of the skin and underlying tissues. The costs to the patient are severe, in terms of pain and discomfort, and in monetary costs of the treatment and extra days in the acute care hospital. The costs to staff in time to treat active decubitus ulcers are far greater than the minutes needed to prevent them.

Shannon (1982) reviewed the literature and identified the major factors associated with development of pressure sores. She divided them into patient-related factors and environmental variables and postulated that the greater the number of factors present, the greater the risk of pressure sores. *Patient factors* include the degree of immobility, state of the sensorium, chronologic age, nutritional status, kind of diagnosis, presence of major surgical procedure, type of medication, presence of infection, musculoskeletal alterations, soft tissue changes, and presence of bowel or bladder incontinence. *Environmental factors* include situations that result in unrelieved external pressure (confinement to bed or chair), increased pressure at the interface of the supporting surfaces and skin, inadequate supervision of patient mobility, restriction of patient movement by external devices, increased friction, shearing forces exerted when moving the patient, lack of adequate nutritional management, and failure to maintain a dry environment. Those at highest risk are patients with paralyzing conditions (see Chapter 20), and the second highest risk group is those with decreased consciousness.

Alex had 12 of the patient and environmental risk factors identified by Shannon (1982): immobility produced by neurologic injury, unconsciousness, hypoproteinemia and cachexia, neurologic diagnosis, loss of muscle mass, steroid therapy, bowel and bladder incontinence, and sustained elevated body temperature from his pulmonary infection. Environmental risk factors included confinement to bed, shearing damage when turned, and movement without clearing body of mattress. As staff became discouraged about his prognosis, it is possible that he was repositioned less frequently than required when other patient's care assumed higher priority.

The *goal* of nursing management for the diagnosis of high risk of pressure sores is *prevention of skin breakdown*. *Assessment* has two components: assessment for risk factors and assessment for signs of beginning skin breakdown in patients ah risk. Those assessed at high risk require continual *monitoring* of skin surfaces for signs of friction or pressure lesions. One inspects the skin for redness that does not disappear with relief of pressure, excoriation or blistering of skin, or open abrasions. Simultaneously, the nursing staff uses a variety of *preventive interventions* to reposition the patient frequently (to prevent prolonged pressure on any body part), to ensure that the patient's body clears the mattress when he or she is repositioned (to prevent shearing of underlying tissues), to give enteral or parenteral hyperalimentation as ordered, and to monitor weight and serum protein (to maintain nutritional status at adequate levels), and to change bed linens promptly when they are wet (to maintain a dry environment).

☐ Potential for Psychophysiologic Alarm Response Related to Auditory Environment

One if the dilemmas faced by staff who care for unresponsive patients is the inability to gauge if the patient is influenced by events in the environment that might be distressful to people with overt awareness and responsiveness. Nearly everyone who has worked in clinical neuroscience for any length of time has had one or more experiences of patients recalling events that occurred during a time when the patient appeared unresponsive to the environment, and there are recurring anecdotal accounts in the literature of similar situations. These anecdotes suggest a potential to process complex environmental stimuli even when overt signs of awareness are not present, at least in some patients.

The dilemma posed by these observations is this: Are such observations merely of passing interest, an epiphenomenon of no particular meaning, or is it possible that the internal, not readily observable responses to environmental stimuli are potentially harmful or helpful to the recovery of patients with absent or decreased responsiveness? This question can be examined from two perspectives—the impact of environmental stimuli on physiologic stability in the acute phase of illness or injury and the impact on recovery of psychophysiologic overt responsiveness in later phases of illness.

Several investigators have documented clear and reproducible responses of the autonomic nervous system to a variety of auditory and somatic sensory stimuli in neurologic patients with varying levels of arousal. The findings may be summarized as follows:

1. Autonomic responses to new stimuli were of the alarm response nature: increased heart rate, skin conductance, in some cases electroencephalogram (EEG) activation. In patients with drug overdose, the autonomic activation did not occur without concomitant behavioral activity (e.g., grimacing, spontaneous movement [Evans, 1976; Schuri & von Cramon, 1979, 1981]). Linking of behavioral and autonomic responses has not been studied systematically in traumatic and nondrug cases of decreased arousal.
2. Stimulus intensity is more important in eliciting an alarm autonomic response than is the type or meaningfulness of the stimulus. Ability to habituate or decrease the response to repeated instances of the same stimulus was evident in patients who make eye contact or follow simple commands (Schuri & von Cramon, 1980, 1981).

In contrast to autonomic responses, EEG changes seem to vary with the type of stimulus in the few patients in whom this has been studied. Booth (1982) and Weber (1984) both used compressed spectral array to demonstrate EEG changes in response to different environmental stimuli (voice versus music;

sensorimotor therapy, respectively). A few investigators have noted decreases in ICP in patients with GCS scores less than 8 with the sensory input of stroking and talking, particularly by family members (Walleck, 1983; Pollack & Goldstein, 1981; Mitchell at al., 1986a, b; Henrickson, 1987).

The potential for an alarm autonomic response to be harmful is during the acute phase of illness or during intercurrent illness when physiologic instability is present. The nurse should, therefore, *assess* both the sources of environmental stimuli (voices, noises, alarms, abrupt contact with the patient) and the patient's physiologic response to such stimuli (heart rate, ICP, blood pressure). If all remain stable, no intervention is needed. If instability occurs, the nurse may *intervene* to reduce the intensity and frequency of the particular environmental stimulus until such time as the patient becomes more physiologically stable.

In later stages of recovery, it may be desirable to activate the patient deliberately in the hope that recovery may be enhanced. Coma stimulation programs are based on enhancing the patient's physiologic and behavioral responses to environmental stimuli (Le Winn & Dimancescu, 1978). To date there have been no adequately controlled studies to compare the efficacy of coma stimulation programs and routine care on the overall outcome in prolonged states of reduced arousal.

☐ Potential for Impaired Family Coping

Traumatic brain injury and prolonged unresponsiveness after medical sources of coma strain both financial and psychosocial family resources. Although Alex was grown, the fact that he had been living with his parents and the long period between arriving home and being found unresponsive produced strong feelings of guilt and responsibility in his parents. Because there are many similarities in family responses to a variety of devastating neurologic disease, the discussion in Chapter 17 is applicable to Alex's case as well.

☐ Inadequate Resources for Care of People with Long-Term Decreased Arousal

The final diagnosis related to Alex's state of decreased arousal is a community diagnosis—lack of adequate resources for care of patients in *persistent vegetative state* and those whose inability to initiate contact with the environment is such that they require total care of their most basic needs. Persistent vegetative state characterizes those people three or more months after neurologic insult who may open their eyes in response to verbal stimuli but do not track objects in their environment, have sleep–wake cycles with periodic spontaneous eye opening, and maintain vegetative functions (heart rate, respirations, blood pressure) but have abnormal motor responses in all four limbs, do not utter comprehensible sounds, and do not obey commands (Jennett & Plum, 1972; Jennett & Teasdale, 1981). Although these people comprise only a relatively small percentage of those surviving traumatic head injury (3% to 7%), they account for from 5% to 20% of those who survive medical coma for 1 month (Jennett & Teasdale, 1981). Subarachnoid hemorrhage accounts for the least number of survivors in the vegetative state (5%) and hypoxic-ischemic episodes the most (20%) (Plum & Posner, 1980). They, plus the unknown number of people with disability severe enough to require total custodial care, tax the resources of extended care facilities. In many cases, the inability of extended care facilities to take such patients requires many extra days of acute hospitalization until placement can be found.

The very poor prognosis for productive life gives rise to a number of ethical dilemmas for providers of care. Several nurses have identified the many sources of psychologic stress on nurses who care for these patients and some of the means they use to cope (Loen & Snyder, 1979, 1980; Flaherty, 1982). The question whether to treat intercurrent illness or even to provide nutritional support for long-term unresponsive patients has become an important ethical consideration as prognostication has become more precise (Grenvik et al., 1978; Strong, 1981). Some states have begun enacting laws allowing families to choose to withhold any form of treatment, including tube feeding, from patients in such hopelessly ill states.

The majority of patients with severe neurologic deficits who require extended care placement are not in persistent vegetative state and have a chance of recovery that is meaningful. Nurses as well as other community activists are important in monitoring and lobbying for higher standards of care in these facilities and for adequate funding to provide such care.

SUMMARY

People with decreased arousal exhibit a complex array of human responses to their neurologic insult. Because the disorders that alter arousal also alter integration of body systemic function in the cerebral hemispheres, the care of such people requires a high degree of skillful nursing monitoring of all functions, not just neurologic status. Although the basic pathology cannot be altered, a key set of nursing interventions is to manipulate the environment—initially to reduce the demands on the patient's ability to respond, and later to increase the level of stimulation to that which the patient can tolerate.

REFERENCES

Becker, D.P. (1987) Cerebral ischemia: Clinical pathophysiology. In F.B. Cerra & W.C. Shoemaker (Eds.), *Critical care: State of the art, Vol. 8*. Fullerton, CA: Society of Critical Care Medicine.

Booth, K. (1982). Responses of unconscious patients to auditory stimuli: An electroencephalographic study. Unpublished master's thesis. University of Washington, Seattle, WA.

Clifton, G.L., Robertson, C.S., & Contant, C.F. (1985). Enteral hyperalimentation in head injury. *Journal of Neurosurgery, 62*, 186.

Deutschman, C.S., Konstantinides, F.N., Raup, S., Thienprasit, P., & Cerra, F.B. (1986). Physiological and metabolic response to isolated closed-head injury. *Journal of Neurosurgery, 64*, 89.

Evans, B.M. (1976). Patterns of arousal in comatose patients. *Journal of Neurology, Neurosurgery & Psychiatry, 39*, 392.

Flaherty, M.J. (1982). Care of the comatose patient: Problems faced alone. *Nursing Management, 13*(19), 44.

Grenvik, A., Powner, D., Snyder, J., et al. (1978). Cessation of therapy in terminal illness and brain death. *Critical Care Medicine, 6*, 284.

Henrickson, S.L. (1987). Intracranial pressure changes and family presence. *Journal of Neurosurgical Nursing, 19*, 14.

Jennett, B., & Plum, F. (1972). Persistant vegetative state after brain damage. *Lancet, 1*, 734.

Jennett, B., & Teasdale, G. (1981). *Management of head injuries*. Philadelphia: Davis.

Langfitt, T.W. (1983). CT, NMR and emission tomography in the diagnosis and management of brain swelling and intracranial hypertension. In S. Ishii et al. (Eds.), *Intracranial Pressure V* (p. 54). Berlin: Springer-Verlag.

Le Winn, E.B., & Dimancescu, M.D. (1978) Environmental deprivation and enrichment in coma. *Lancet, 2*, 156.

Loen, M., & Snyder, M. (1979). Psychosocial aspects of care of the long-term comatose patient. *Journal of Neurosurgical Nursing, 11*, 235.

Loen, M., & Snyder, M. (1980). Care of the long-term comatose patient: A pilot study. *Journal of Neurosurgical Nursing, 12*, 134.

Mayhall, C.G., Archer, N.H., Lamb, V.A., et al. (1984) Ventriculostomy-related infections: A prospective study. *New England Journal of Medicine, 310*, 553.

McCarthy, E. (1982). Cardiovascular complications of intracranial disorders. In D. Nikas (Ed.), *The critically ill neurosurgical patient* (p. 53). New York: Churchill-Livingstone.

McGuire, A. (1986). Issues in the prevention of neurotrauma. *Nursing Clinics of North America, 21*, 549.

Miller, J.D. (1985). Head injury and brain ischaemia—Implications for therapy. *British Journal of Anaesthesiology, 57*, 120.

Mitchell, P.H. (1986). Intracranial hypertension: Influence of nursing care activities. *Nursing Clinics of North America, 21*, 563.

Mitchell, P.H. (1988). Neurologic disorders. In M. Kinney & S. Dunbar (Eds.), *AACN's clinical*

reference for critical care nursing (Chap. 35). New York: McGraw-Hill.
Mitchell, P.H., Johnson, F.B., & Habermann-Little, B. (1986a). Nursing and ICP: Studies of two clinical problems. In J.D. Miller et al. (Eds.), *Intracranial pressure VI* (p. 702). Berlin: Springer-Verlag.
Mitchell, P.H., Johnson, F.B., & Little, B.H. (1986b). Promoting physiologic stability: Touch and ICP (Abstr.). *Communicating Nursing Research, 18*, 93.
Olivares, L., Segovia, A., & Revuelta, R. (1974). Tube feeding and lethal aspiration in neurological patients: A review of 720 autopsy cases. *Stroke, 5*, 654.
Plum, F., & Posner, J.B. (1980). *The diagnosis of stupor and coma* (3rd ed.) (p. 325). Philadelphia: Davis.
Pollack, L.D., & Goldstein, G.W. (1981). Lowering of intracranial pressure in Reye's syndrome by sensory stimulation (Letter). *New England Journal of Medicine, 304*, 732.
Raimondi, J., & Taylor, J.W. (1986). *Neurological emergencies: Effective nursing care*. Rockville, MD: Aspen.
Saul, T. (1983). Intensive care of the brain-injured patient. *Critical Care Quarterly, 5*(4), 82.
Schuri, U., & von Cramon, D. (1979). Autonomic responses to meaningful and nonmeaningful auditory stimuli in coma. *Archiv fur Psychiatrie und Nervenkrankheiten (Archives of Psychiatry and Neurological Sciences), 227*, 143.

Schuri, U., & von Cramon, D. (1980). Autonomic and behavioral responses in coma due to drug overdose. *Psychophysiology, 17*, 253.
Schuri, U., & von Cramon, D. (1981). Electrodermal responses to auditory stimuli with different significance in neurological patients. *Psychophysiology, 18*, 248.
Shannon, M.L. (1982). Pressure sores. In C. Norris (Ed.), *Concept clarification in nursing* (p. 357). Rockville, MD: Aspen.
Slade, P.D. (1984). Sensory deprivation and clinical psychiatry. *British Journal of Hospital Medicine, 32*, 256.
Strong, C. (1981). Positive killing and the irreversibly unconscious patient. *Bioethics Quarterly, 3*, 190.
Walleck, C. (1983). The effects of purposeful touch on intracranial pressure (Abstr.). *Heart & Lung, 12*, 428.
Walsh, R. (1981). Sensory environments, brain damage, and drugs: A review of interactions and mediating mechanisms. *International Journal of Neuroscience, 14*, 129.
Weber, P.L. (1984). Sensorimotor therapy: Its effect on electroencephalograms of acute comatose patients. *Archives of Physical Medicine and Rehabilitation, 65*, 457.
Wolanin, M.O., & Phillips, L. (1981). *Confusion: Prevention and care*. St. Louis: Mosby.

7

Abnormally Increased Behavioral Arousal

Mariah Snyder*

The term altered level of consciousness makes most people immediately think of decreased levels of arousal. Abnormally increased behavioral arousal is a category that few people consider. A possible reason is that minimal attention has been given to this area in nursing research and publications. The questions proposed by Meleis (1985) for studying nursing phenomena are helpful in exploring the phenomenon of abnormally increased behavioral arousal:

1. When does the phenomenon occur?
2. Why does it occur?
3. How do we deal with it?
4. How do we prevent it?
5. What other conditions occur at the same time?

This chapter attempts to answer these questions in relation to abnormally increased behavioral arousal in patients with neurologic problems.

---

*The author wishes to thank Michaelene Mirr and Mary Wotzka, graduate students at the University of Minnesota, for their review of and comments on this chapter.

MANIFESTATIONS

Aggressive behavior, severe agitation, rage, and acting out are human responses that are difficult for the caregiver. The threat of the person's behavior both to the caregiver and to the patient increases anxiety in most caregivers. The behavior is often viewed as being "less than human." Unconsciously, we hope that the person will regain composure and behave like other human beings. Some of these feelings result from a lack of understanding about the underlying mechanisms associated with aggressive behavior. Aggressive behavior and delirium are two states that can be considered indicators of abnormally increased behavioral arousal and are discussed in this chapter.

Many definitions of *aggression* exist. Montague (1983) defined aggression in its broadest sense as "a forceful and hostile attacking action that may be expressed physically, verbally, or symbolically—real or unreal—depending on how the patient perceives and interprets the environment" (p. 140). Her definition is more applicable to patients who are hyperarousable due to neurologic conditions than are definitions that include conscious intent to harm. Inaccurate interpretation of stimuli precipitates the aggressive behavior. Often the person views the situation as a threat and uses aggressive behavior to decrease anxiety created by the threat. Accompanying autonomic nervous system findings include decreased salivation, decreased gastrointestinal activity, and increased heart rate and perspiration.

Delirium is characterized by disorientation, restlessness, hyperirritability, fear, misinterpretation of sensory stimuli, and hallucinations. People classified as delirious often have complex and protracted delusions: a dreamlike state during which the person is out of contact with the environment. Characteristic of delirium is alternation between lucid periods and times of confusion; during the lucid periods, people are terrified by their inability to control their mental functioning and actions (Montague, 1983). Delirium often lasts a relatively short time (36 to 48 hours).

Table 7–1 lists conditions in which the hyperarousal state may be found. Whether abnormally increased arousal occurs because of misperceptions from defects in the sensory system, inability to integrate new stimuli with old because of memory problems, or as a partial result of an association with the person's premorbid personality is not fully known. In this chapter particular attention is given to delirium and the aggressive state found in recovery from head trauma. The former state may be observed in neuropatients who have alcohol suddenly withdrawn from them. Delirium is also found in patients with encephalitis.

Anatomic Basis

The three anatomic areas primarily associated with hyperarousal are the limbic system, the temporal lobes, and the frontal lobes. Phylogenetically, limbic structures are among the oldest parts of the brain, whereas the frontal and temporal lobes are classified as neocortex. Ottoson (1983) stated that cortical areas exert little control over the functions of the limbic system. Figure 7–1 shows the components of the limbic system: the main components are

TABLE 7–1. POSSIBLE ETIOLOGIES OF ABNORMALLY INCREASED BEHAVIORAL AROUSAL.

Withdrawal from drugs, such as alcohol and barbiturates
Acute encephalitis
Head trauma, particularly during resolution of coma
Epilepsy (some forms of complex partial seizures)
Metabolic disorders (electrolyte imbalance)
Intracranial space-occupying lesions
Alzheimer's disease
Rabies
Cerebrovascular accidents, particularly right hemispheric lesions
Multiple sclerosis

the hypothalamus, amygdala, hippocampus, and septal area.

The hypothalamus has control over some visceral, autonomic, and endocrine functions. It has multiple connections with other parts of the brain and limbic system. Ottoson (1983) stated:

> In broad outline, the hypothalamus receives its major input from the non-specific reticular system and from the olfactory system and the hippocampus. There are also less well defined pathways connecting the hypothalamus with the limbic system, the frontal cortex, the thalamus, and the periaqueductal grey matter. The hypothalamus in turn sends projections to most of these regions. (p. 290)

Animal studies have provided some knowledge about the functions of specific regions of the hypothalamus. Stimulation of the dorsal hypothalamus results in flight behavior, whereas stimulation of the ventral hypothalamus produces defensive behavior. Electrical stimulation of the medial hypothalamus results in feelings of restlessness, anxiety, depression, and fright. Strong stimulation of the posterior hypothalamus produces a rage reaction (Byers & Guthrie, 1984).

7. ABNORMALLY INCREASED BEHAVIORAL AROUSAL 87

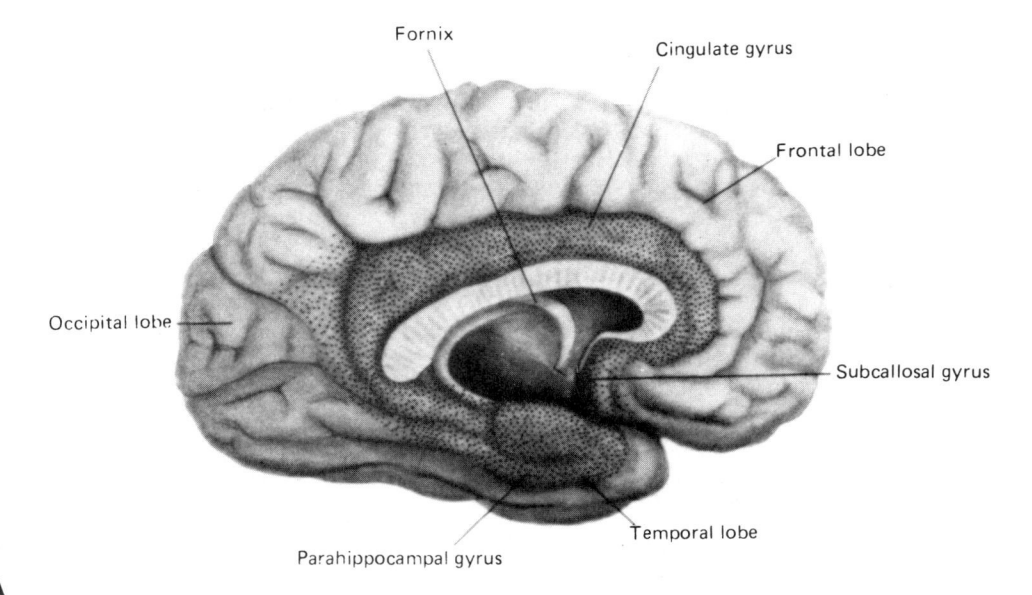

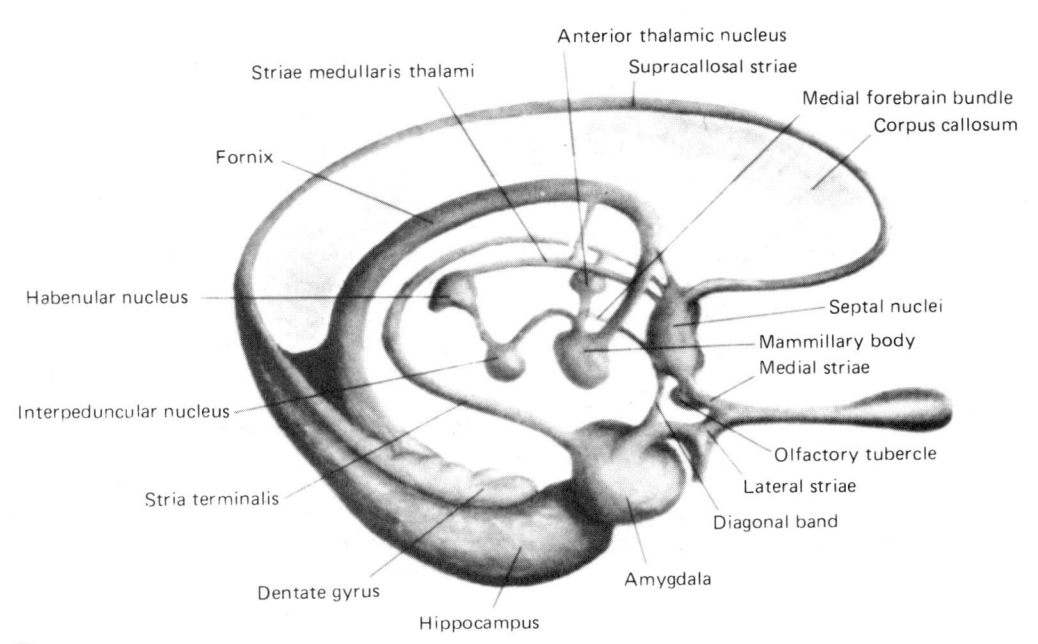

Figure 7–1. Dotted area in top figure shows the location of the limbic system in relation to other cerebral structures. The bottom figure shows the many structures of the limbic system. *(Reprinted by permission of the publisher from Kandel & Schwartz [Eds.], Principles of neural science [2nd ed.], p. 613. Copyright 1985 by Elsevier Science Publishing Co., Inc.)*

The amygdala lies under the uncus of the temporal lobe. It has connections with the hypothalmus, preoptic area, septum, and thalamus. The amygdala receives input directly and indirectly from the sensory systems, particularly from the olfactory system. Stimulation of the amygdala results in flight and defense behaviors but not in aggressive behaviors. The amygdala may be involved in integrating environmental cues with appropriate affective states that govern behavior. Kupfermann (1985) noted that lesions and stimulation of the amygdala produced effects similar to those found for the lateral or medial regions of the hypothalamus.

The hippocampus is located in proximity to the lateral ventricle. Afferent pathways connect it with sensory areas of the cortex, and a main efferent connection is the subiculum, which has numerous links with the many areas of the brain, including the neocortex (Kupfermann, 1985). Breathnach (1980) believed that the hippocampus was associated intimately with short-term memory, whereas Bennett (1971) thought that it was involved in orientation and attention.

The septal complex lies under the corpus callosum. It is believed to have both an inhibitory and a facilitory influence on the hypothalalmus. Septal lesions can reduce the rage or fear precipitated by hypothalamic lesions.

The temporal lobe is in close proximity to components of the limbic system and has many connections with the structures of this system. Injury to the temporal lobe often includes damage to these underlying structures. One function of the temporal lobe is memory. Interference with memory can cause problems with perception and integration of new stimuli. Frustration that may result from memory impairment may manifest itself in aggressive behaviors.

The prefrontal area of the frontal lobe is associated with higher intellectual functions. Personality changes, lack of initiative, poor judgment, inappropriate sexual behavior, and occasionally aggressive behaviors occur when the frontal lobes are damaged. These manifestations are rarely seen, however, when only one hemisphere is involved. The bifrontal area is readily damaged in head trauma; impact thrusts the lobes down against the orbital roof of the skull. People who have suffered frontal damage have a poor prognosis for full recovery of functions located in this area.

Case Studies

Two case studies are presented to typify the responses in people who manifest abnormally increased behavioral arousal: aggression after a head injury and delirium resulting from withdrawal from alcohol. This latter example was chosen because of the high incidence of trauma resulting from alcohol intoxication.

Case Study 1: Aggression After Head Trauma

Andy, 30 years old, suffered a closed head injury in a motorcycle accident. The computed tomography (CT) scan showed a subdural hematoma in the right temperoparietal area causing a shift of the midline structures, small areas of contusion in the right temporal lobe, and a nondepressed fracture of the left occipital bone. The subdural hematoma in the right temporal lobe area was evacuated, and part of the temporal lobe from the temporal gyrus to the tentorial notch was removed also. After surgery, Andy had a left hemiparesis, which gradually lessened.

Andy had a long hospitalization primarily because of behavioral problems. Behaviors included wandering aimlessly, spitting out pills, yelling, taking off his clothes in the hall, striking out at staff or biting them, kicking and hitting people, and incoherent speech. Many episodes of severe agitation and violence occurred. In addition, slight conductive aphasia, poor orientation, and poor short-term memory were present. Lithium, haloperidol, physostigmine, and lethicin were administered at various times during the recovery to help subdue the violent behavior. At the end of 3 months, Andy was less violent but still manifested aggressive behavior, poor short-term memory, and difficulty in interacting.

TABLE 7–2. RANCHO LOS AMIGOS LEVELS OF COGNITIVE FUNCTIONING SCALE AFTER HEAD TRAUMA.

Level	Response	Description
1	None	Completely unresponsive to any stimulus
2	Generalized	Reacts inconsistently and nonpurposefully to stimuli; may respond with physiologic changes, gross body movements, or utterances
3	Localized	Reacts specifically but inconsistently to stimuli; responds directly to a stimulus; shows vague awareness of self and body; may pull at tubes and react to discomfort
4	Confused Agitated	Heightened state of activity but unable to process information correctly; reacts to internal confusion; nonpurposeful behavior with confabulation present; cries, screams, and manifests aggressive behavior; cannot discriminate among people; performs gross motor activities but not self-care activities
5	Confused Inappropriate	Follows simple commands; may show agitated behavior from inability to cope with external demands; gross inattention to environment, easily distracted; impaired memory and inappropriate verbalization; cannot initiate tasks; often uses things incorrectly
6	Confused Appropriate	Displays goal-directed behavior but requires direction from others; follows simple commands; shows carryover of information from previously learned tasks; memory problems persist; inconsistently oriented to time and place; increased awareness of self and others
7	Automatic Appropriate	Oriented in hospital and home settings; performs tasks in robot-like manner; superficial awareness of own condition but lacks good problem-solving abilities; carryover for new learning; independent in self-care activities; needs structure but can initiate tasks of interest
8	Purposeful Appropriate	Alert and oriented; few memory problems; can begin vocational rehabilitation; carryover for new learning; social, emotional, and intellectual capacities may be decreased from pretrauma level

From Malkmus et al., 1980.

Andy falls into level 4 of the Rancho Los Amigos Levels of Cognitive Functioning Scale for head injury patients (Malkmus et al., 1980). Table 7–2 provides a description of each of the levels. Not all post-head injury patients pass through this level 4, and for those who do, the length of time spent in this state varies. A few, like Andy, never progress beyond this level.

Case Study 2: Delirium From Alcohol Withdrawal

Paul is a 40-year-old businessman who was hospitalized after being involved in a motor vehicle accident in which he sustained a fractured femur and a mild concussion. Paul was alert when he was admitted to the emergency department. In response to questioning about alcohol consumption, he stated that he was a social drinker. Two days after admission, the nurses noted that Paul was extremely restless, picking at the bed sheets, and jumping from one topic to another during conversations. He would begin to answer a question but, after a few words, would shift to other topics. Paul talked constantly. The nurses noted that he had difficulty holding eating utensils and his electric razor because of a tremor. Vital signs revealed a heart rate of 112, a temperature of 100°F, and a slightly elevated systolic blood pressure from that at admission.

When his wife came to visit in the afternoon, Paul believed that she was his mother. Paul was unable to rest or sleep and was in constant motion. He reached for objects in the air and hit staff who tried to measure vital signs or provide care. He perspired profusely. His heart rate increased to 130 and his temperature to 101°F. The severe delirium phase lasted 24 hours. After this had subsided, Paul was exhausted and slept a great deal of the time.

Medical treatment included administering chlorpromazine, paraldehyde, and phenytoin. Phenytoin was given to decrease the likelihood of seizures. Intravenous fluids were begun and vitamins were given.

HUMAN RESPONSES ASSOCIATED WITH ABNORMALLY INCREASED BEHAVIORAL AROUSAL

In this section nursing diagnoses appropriate for patients who manifest abnormally increased behavioral arousal are presented, along with assessment and interventions that nurses can use to meet outcomes for these diagnoses.

Diagnoses for the Patient
The nursing diagnoses that pertain to the patient include:

1. Injury, potential for
2. Nutrition, alteration in; less than body requirement
3. Self-care deficits
3. Sensory–perception alterations
4. Sleep pattern disturbance (particularly in delirium)
5. Thought processes, alteration
6. Violence, potential for

Other diagnoses may be appropriate in some situations, but those listed are common for hyperactive patients.

☐ Potential for Injury

This diagnosis is defined as, "The interactive conditions between individual and environment which impose a risk to the defensive and adaptive resources of the individual" (Kim & Moritz, 1982, p. 194). *Defining characteristics* of this diagnosis include sensory and integrative dysfunction, problems in orientation, cognitive impairment, and environmental variables. People in the abnormally increased behavioral arousal state are prone to injury because they are unable to make correct judgments about their own capabilities, misperceive items in the environment, or act impulsively.

Assessment includes surveying the environment for objects that could be harmful to the patient, determining the patient's cognitive state, and evaluating the staff's knowledge of the condition. The *goal* for the patient with this diagnosis is, "The patient will remain free of injury."

Although it may seem simplistic to list removal of harmful objects from the immediate environment as a nursing *intervention* for this diagnosis, many nurses who do not routinely care for the hyperarousal patient do not remember to survey the environment for such objects. All glass objects, items that have sharp edges, and substances that can be consumed must be removed from the patient's immediate territory. Rubbing alcohol, lotion, and other skin care materials are items in the last category that often are at the bedside and could be harmful to the patient.

Restraints sometimes are necessary to prevent the patient from removing tubes or from getting out of bed, but they should be used sparingly. Because these patients have a high level of activity, sites under the restraints need frequent assessment to determine the integrity of the underlying tissue and any nerve or circulatory impairment. Providing periods when restraints can be removed helps to reduce agitation.

The presence of tubes and catheters often increases agitation. Whenever possible, these stimuli should be removed (Malkmus et al., 1980). Hand mitts are useful to help prevent dislodgment of tubes and catheters if it is necessary to keep them in place. People who are delirious must be monitored frequently because of the severity of their condition and the strain of the high level of activity on the heart.

Brigman et al. (1983) suggest using a floor bed for patients who are in the confused–agitated phase of recovery after a head injury (Fig. 7–2). Such a bed eliminates the need for restraints to keep the patient in bed, and patients can move about, which helps dissipate energy and aggression. Feeding tubes and tracheostomies pose no care problems on

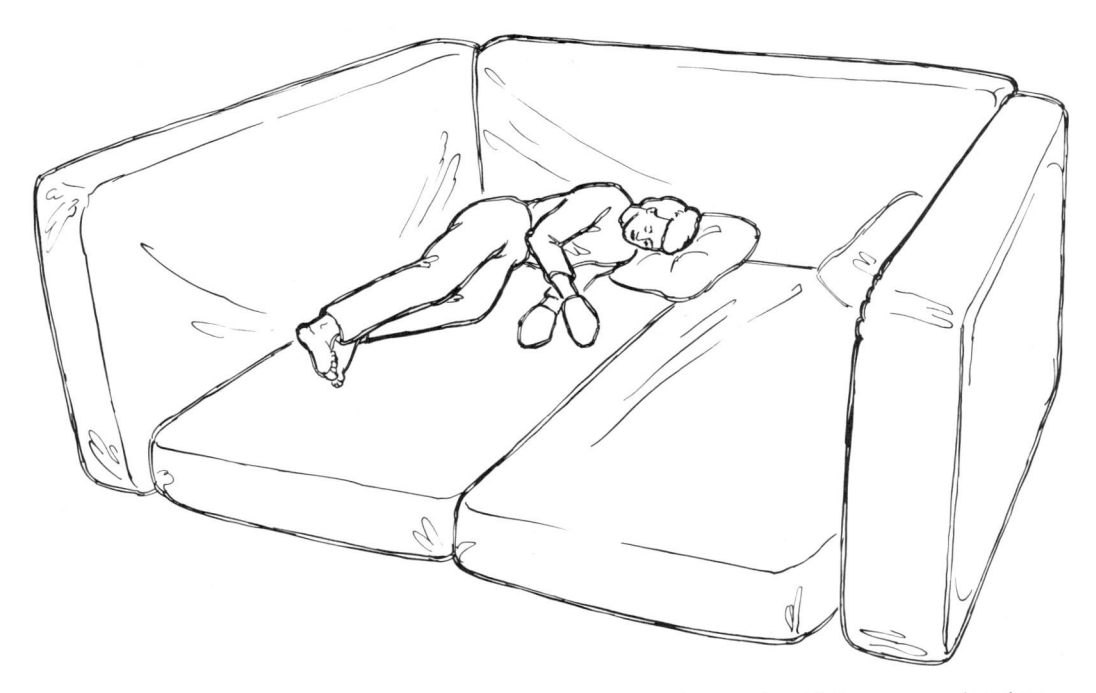

Figure 7–2. A floor bed used for head-injured patients who are hyperactive. Mattresses are placed on the floor and as padding on the sides. Patients can move about without fear of injury.

floor beds. It is not possible, however, to use an indwelling catheter, since the urine would not drain, and an external catheter is needed.

The frequent assessment of this patient population must be part of the care plan. It is easy to forget this on a busy unit, and injuries can occur very quickly unless there is adequate supervision.

☐ **Alterations in Nutrition; Less Than Body Requirements**

The nursing diagnosis as presented by Kim and Moritz (1982) does not include among the *defining characteristics* people who require additional nutrients because of their high level of activity. Many people in the hyperarousal state, however, particularly those in delirium, manifest signs of inadequate nutritional and fluid intake. They also lack the ability to concentrate and thus forget the food placed before them. Patients in delirium frequently have elevated temperature, which places an added demand on their nutritional status.

Assessment includes determining the patient's needed caloric level in relation to his or her activity level by observing the patient and using charts for energy expenditure associated with exercise. The patient's temperature is noted in determining the number of calories required. The nurse must consider the patient's past nutritional status, such as having been given intravenous fluids for protracted periods. The *goal* of this diagnosis is that the patient will have sufficient intake of nutrients to meet energy expenditure.

Safety measures must be considered in providing interventions for nutritional needs. Sturdy plastic glasses are preferred for patients who can hold them, since glass utensils are easily broken and patients may use the broken pieces to harm themselves. Styrofoam or paper cups collapse if the patient grasps them tightly. Covered, untippable cups (like the Tommy Tippy for infants) are practical (Wells, 1983). These are especially helpful for people who have a tremor, have difficulty with coordination, or are hemiparetic. Small, frequent feedings are best because of the person's short attention span. Malkmus et al. (1980) suggested promoting participation in simple, automatic self-care activities, such as eating finger foods. Nutritional items such as cheese, fruits, vegetables, hard cookies, and crackers are finger foods that can be given. If the patient has muscle wasting, protein supplements may be needed. Collaboration between the dietitian and the nurse is needed to plan and implement a nutrition program that will provide an adequate supply of nutrients for the hyperactive patient.

□ Self-care Deficits

People in the abnormally increased behavioral arousal state will manifest various levels of self-care deficits from the completely dependent state to ability to perform much of their own care. The self-care deficits may be a result of the use of restraints to prevent injury, the person's inability to concentrate, or the presence of associated problems.

Assessment includes noting the capabilities of the patient so that these can be incorporated into the plan of care. Self-care deficits in hygiene, elimination, and eating are of particular concern. The *goals* for this diagnosis are that the patient's basic needs will be met and that the patient will progress, as his condition permits, toward independence. A scale (Table 7–3) for rating the self-care deficit of a patient has been developed (Baer et al., 1984) that can be used in evaluating the progress of the patient toward the goal.

Interventions include using automatic, familiar gross motor activities to help the person regain motor coordination. Such activities place few demands on the patient (Malkmus et al., 1980). Some of these are self-care activities, such as combing the hair and washing the face. The nurse initiates the activity, since the person would most likely only look at the utensils or use them for other purposes. Emphasis is not placed on completing the task; at this stage of recovery, this would only increase agitation.

Hygiene requires close attention. For the patient with an elevated temperature, frequent bathing and skin care are required. If the person is incontinent, care is needed to prevent skin breakdown. Taking the patient to the bathroom at regular intervals often prevents incontinence. Tub baths may prove to be both relaxing and helpful in promoting the integrity of the skin.

TABLE 7–3. SELF-CARE DEFICIT SCALE.

Numerical Index	Definition
0	Independent, able to perform activity with no one present
1	Requires use of equipment or device
2	Requires help from another person for assistance, supervision, or teaching
2.2	Supervision—may include verbal reinforcement or standby assistance
2.4	Minimal assistance, patient does 75% of work
2.6	Moderate assistance, patient does 50% of work
2.8	Maximal assistance, patient does 25% of work
3	Requires help from another person and equipment or device
4	Dependent, does not participate in activity

Reproduced by permission from C. Baer, M. Delorey, & J. Firzmaurice, A study to evaluate the validity of the rating system for self-care deficit. In M. Kim, G. McFarland, & A. McLane, Classification of Nursing Diagnoses. *St. Louis, 1984, C. V. Mosby.*

☐ Sensory–perceptual Alterations

The *etiology* for this diagnosis includes altered environmental stimuli that may be either excessive or insufficient (Kim & Moritz, 1982). Steinhart (1979) concurred that delirium could originate from sensory overload or sensory deprivation. Altered sensory integration is another possible etiology of this diagnosis. *Defining characteristics* include disorientation, altered abstraction, change in problem-solving abilities, change in behavior pattern, anxiety, change in usual response to stimuli, restlessness, irritability, and possibly hallucinations. All of these may be observed in people with abnormally increased behavioral arousal.

Assessment is aimed at determining the extent of the alteration. In people in delirium, the type and extent of the hallucinations must be evaluated. Whereas the medical diagnosis seeks to determine the underlying pathology resulting in the alterations in perception, the nurse is concerned with identifying the problems that interfere with the patient's functional ability and safety. The *goal* for this diagnosis is that the patient will be able to interpret the immediate environment correctly.

Interventions vary depending on whether the etiology is excessive stimuli or inadequate stimuli. If it is excessive stimuli, interventions to decrease stimuli are indicated. Placing the patient in a quiet atmosphere, reducing activity, and avoiding loud noises and sudden changes will help the person to interpret the environment correctly. A structured environment also is helpful (Malkmus et al., 1980). A calm manner and a soothing voice and playing quiet, restful music are other interventions that can be used. Brigman et al., (1983) suggested using a quiet room for patients who seem to become agitated from too much stimulation. They call this the time-out room, where the patient can go to get away from unit activities. In most instances, the staff has to make this determination for the patient, since the person is usually unaware of his or her need for decreased stimulation.

In patients having hallucinations, the nurse does not support or encourage the patient's misperceptions. The nurse may ask the patient to describe the environment without arguing with the patient. Providing reassurance that the patient is safe decreases the patient's anxiety and lessens restlessness. Whispers and muffled conversations should be avoided, since they can be misinterpreted by the patient and serve to increase anxiety.

☐ Alterations in Sleep Patterns

This diagnosis is made frequently in people in delirium. Lack of sleep contributes to the symptoms found. Chapter 9 provides a discussion of the phenomenon sleep.

☐ Alterations in Thought Processes

This diagnosis is common to all people with abnormally increased behavioral arousal and accounts for many of the other problems found. *Defining characteristics* of this diagnosis include impaired attention span, inappropriate behavior, impaired recall ability, decreased ability to grasp ideas, decreased ability to order ideas, impaired ability to reason, impaired judgment, impaired decision making, hypervigilance, and inappropriate and nonreality-based thinking.

The *goal* for this diagnosis is to increase the person's ability to process information correctly. Malkmus et al. (1980) noted that the patients in level 4 of the Ranchos Los Amigos Levels of Cognitive Functioning Scale of recovery from head injury cannot be held accountable for their behavior because they are not yet capable of producing thought-out actions. The person experiences inner confusion originating from cognitive disruption and is unable to process information from the environment correctly. This often is manifested in agitated behaviors.

Chapters 12 and 13 provide *interventions* that are useful in caring for people with alterations in cognitive processes.

☐ Potential for Violence

Aggressive behavior is a frequent finding in people manifesting abnormally increased behavioral arousal. Some of the *defining characteristics* of this diagnosis include body language of clenched fists, facial expressions, rigid posture, and tautness; increased motor activity, such as pacing; overt aggressive acts; rage; and suspicion of others, delusions, and hallucinations. Some of the other characteristics are increased anxiety, fear of self or others, argumentative behavior, and vulnerable self-esteem.

The *goal* for this diagnosis is that the patient will not harm self or others. A number of *interventions* can be used to achieve this goal, but one of the most important considerations is the knowledge nurses have about techniques they can use to protect themselves from assaultive and aggressive behaviors. If the nurse feels secure, it is communicated to the patient, which helps in decreasing the patient's anxiety and aggressive behavior. Since many nurses may have little knowledge about techniques that are effective in dealing with potentially violent patients, staff education is indicated. A calm, quiet, but firm approach conveys to the patient that the nurse is in control. This helps alleviate the fear the patient has of losing control and striking out at those present. If a patient is aggressive or assaultive, sufficient staff are needed to provide care. If an injection is to be given, three people can do this without undue attention and scuffling. If there are too many people present, however, the patient's apprehension and aggressive behavior can increase.

Working with patients who have aggressive tendencies taxes the nursing staff. Booth et al. (1980) stated, however, that a patient's agitation is not a reason to keep the patient from therapy. They believe that all staff, not just the nursing staff, must be involved in the care of the agitated patient. A care conference is helpful, in which fears and concerns can be voiced along with suggestions for planning consistent care.

Interventions that serve to calm the patient are appropriate. These include the use of soothing music and tapes of familiar voices when the patient must be left alone. The patient should be left alone as little as possible, since human contact tends to reduce the fright of these patients (Booth et al., 1980). Activity is alternated with rest. Such activities as throwing a Nerf ball and other gross motor actions help to lessen aggressive actions. Activities should be geared to the patient's level of cognitive functioning to avoid insulting the person's intelligence, that is, using activities deemed childish. Allowing freedom of movement as much as possible is desirable, since restraints tend to increase agitation. Because the patient's cognitive abilities are extremely limited in this stage of recovery, minimal demands should be placed on the patient. The goal is to have the patient progress through this phase rather than to acquire any specific skills (Booth et al., 1980).

It is important to speak directly to the patient in a calm voice. All care activities are explained to the patient so that the element of surprise is decreased. Information is repeated as often as seems necessary to ensure understanding. If the patient appears to be coming agitated, the amount of stimulation is lessened.

Behavior modification has been used with people who manifest aggressive behavior after head injury (Brigman et al., 1983; Hollon, 1973; Muir et al., 1983; Wood, 1984). This intervention is not appropriate for aggressive behavior manifested soon after recovery from coma (Muir et al., 1983). Both family and staff must be involved in the use of behavior modification techniques for them to be effective. Rewards are given for completing tasks, and deviant or aggressive behavior is ignored. The patient's attention span and cognitive abilities are important points to assess in implementing a behavior modification program; the expectations should not exceed the patient's abilities.

It is recommended that medications to lessen agitation be used sparingly and only when all other measures have proven ineffective, because the use of medications prolongs the time spent in this stage of recovery (Brigman et al., 1983). This is not true, however, for people in delirium, for whom medications often are required because of the extreme agitation present.

Diagnoses for the Family and Significant Others

The nursing diagnoses that relate to the family include:

1. Knowledge deficit regarding the condition
2. Ineffective coping

☐ **Knowledge Deficit Regarding the Condition**

Behaviors found in the increased arousal state can be very frightening to the patient's family. A number of the *etiologies* suggested by the North American Nursing Diagnosis Association (NANDA) for lack of knowledge are applicable for families of patients who manifest abnormally increased behavioral arousal: inability to seek information, such as not knowing about resources, lack of readiness for reception of information, and lack of external support and resources. *Defining characteristics* include verbalization of the problem. *Assessment* may reveal high anxiety because of lack of understanding about the condition, undue expectations of the patient, and denial. The *goal* for families with this diagnosis is that the family will express an understanding and acceptance of the patient who is manifesting abnormally increased arousal behavior.

Support groups are one type of *intervention* for providing information to families. Both the nurse group leaders and other group participants are sources of information. Knowledge about the cause of the behavior manifested, the length of time that such behavior can be expected to exist, and ways the family can assist the patient are presented. Information provides the family with a sense of control. Knowledge can lead to a reduction in anxiety. Support can be gained from hearing others relate the process that their relative has gone through and ways that they have dealt with the condition. A more detailed discussion of support groups and networks is found in Chapter 17.

Role modeling by nurses is another intervention nurses can implement in helping families of patients acquire knowledge about the hyperarousal state. Just as nurses may at first be frightened by aggressive behavior, family members may also be afraid. Being present with the family when they visit is one method for instructing them in techniques that can be used to improve interaction with the patient. Sensitivity to family members' reaction to the condition is needed; they should never be pushed into staying alone with the patient if they feel insecure or afraid.

☐ **Ineffective Coping**

For family members, this is a very trying time. Seeing a loved one unable to control behavior or even striking out and hitting staff and family members is extremely difficult. *Behavioral indicators* of ineffective coping include crying, avoiding the patient and care setting, being critical of care and caregivers, and actions associated with high levels of anxiety. *Causes* of ineffective coping may be inadequate information or disability progression that exhausts the supportive capacity of the family members. *Defining characteristics* include the significant other's describing preoccupation with personal reactions to the patient's condition, the family member's attempting supportive behaviors that are less than adequate, and the family member's withdrawing from the situation. An *outcome* for the family for whom the diagnosis of ineffective coping has been made is that the family will exhibit minimal anxiety in dealing with the patient.

Interventions given for the preceding diagnosis, "Knowledge Deficit," are appropriate for meeting this goal. Other resources may be needed to assist the family to cope with the patient's condition. Providing time and opportunities for the family to discuss their concerns is helpful. This is especially needed if the patient has been abusive to family members or staff. Offering realistic hope is another intervention that can be used. Knowing that most patients are in this state—be it post-trauma or delirium—for a limited period of time provides the family with an end goal. Interacting with a loved one who is abusive or aggressive is very taxing. Suggesting that family members take time away—a free day or free weekend—can do much to renew their energies. If the family seems anxious about doing this, giving them a telephone number and a specific nurse to call will help to ease their fears about not being present all the time.

Diagnoses for the Community

☐ Knowledge Deficit

The nursing diagnosis related to abnormally increased behavioral arousal that is found in the community is that of knowledge deficit. Knowledge is lacking about the long-term effects of trauma and about the seriousness of the delirious state associated with withdrawal from drugs such as alcohol. Public education is needed to alert the public to means that can be used to prevent head trauma. Increased public support for seatbelt legislation, control of drunk driving, mandatory insurance for license renewal, and safety in sports can do much to alleviate the cause of the underlying problem. People who have not had close interaction with anyone who has suffered a severe head injury are often unaware of the behavioral problems present in the recovery phases. Society is now being forced to look at management for severely disabled head injury patients; in the past, these people rarely survived the trauma. Making the public more knowledgeable about the serious implications of head injury and the often permanent effects may assist in decreasing trauma in our society. A more detailed discussion of community assessment and intervention with regard to head injury prevention is found in Chapter 6.

REFERENCES

Baer, C., Delorey, M., & Fitzmaurice, J. (1984). A study to evaluate the validity of the rating system for self-care deficit. In M. Kim, G. McFarland, & A. McLane (Eds.), *Classification of nursing diagnoses* (p. 185). St. Louis: Mosby.

Bennett, T. (1971). Hippocampal theta activity and behavior—A review. *Communications in Behavioral Biology, 6,* 37.

Booth, B., Doyle, M., & Malkmus, D. (1980). Meeting the challenge of the agitated patient. In Professional Staff Association of Rancho Los Amigos Hospital (Eds.), *Rehabilitation of the head injured adult* (p. 43). Los Angeles: Rancho Los Amigos Hospital.

Breathnach, C. (1980). The limbic system. *Journal of Irish Medical Association, 73,* 331.

Brigman, C., Dickey, C., & Zegeer, L. (1983). Agitated aggressive patient. *American Journal of Nursing, 83,* 1409.

Byers, V., & Guthrie, M. (1984). The limbic system and behavior. *Journal of Neurosurgical Nursing, 16,* 80.

Hollon, T. (1973). Behavior modification in a community hospital rehabilitation unit. *Archives of Physical Medicine, 54,* 65.

Kim, M., McFarland, G. & McLane, A. (1984). *Classification of nursing diagnoses.* St. Louis: Mosby.

Kim, M., & Moritz, D. (1982). *Classification of nursing diagnoses.* New York: McGraw-Hill.

Kupfermann, I. (1985). Hypothalamus and limbic system I: Pepidergic neurons, homeostasis, and emotional behavior. In E. Kandel & J. Schwartz (Eds.), *Principles of neural science* (2nd ed.) (p. 609). New York: Elsevier/North-Holland.

Malkmus, D., Booth, B., & Kodimer, C. (1980). *Rehabilitation of the head injured adult—comprehensive cognitive management.* Downey, CA: Professional Staff Association of the Rancho Los Amigos Hospital.

Meleis, A. (1985). *Theoretical nursing: Development and progress.* Philadelphia: Lippincott.

Montague, M. (1983). Altered levels of responsiveness: Hyperactivity. In M. Snyder (Ed.), *Guide to neurological and neurosurgical nursing* (p. 139). New York: Wiley.

Muir, C., Haffey, W., Ott, K., Karaica, D., Muir, J., & Sutko, M. (1983). Treatment of behavioral deficits. In M. Rosenthal, E. Griffith, M. Bond, & J. Miller (Eds.), *Rehabilitation of the head injured adult* (p. 381). Philadelphia: Davis.

Ottoson, D. (1983). *Physiology of the nervous system.* New York: Oxford University Press.

Steinhart, M. (1979). Treatment of delirium. *International Journal of Psychiatry in Medicine, 9,* 191.

Wells, R. (1983). Impairment of mobility: Lack of voluntary control and resistance to movement. In M. Snyder (Ed.), *Guide to neurological and neurosurgical nursing* (p. 354). New York: Wiley.

Wood, R. (1984). Behavior disorders following brain injury: Their presentation and psychological management. In N. Brooks (Ed.), *Closed head injury* (p. 195). Oxford: Oxford University Press.

8

Intermittent Loss of Arousal

Judith Ozuna

SOURCES OF INTERMITTENT LOSS OF AROUSAL

There are several ways in which intermittent loss of arousal can occur. Among these are alteration of circulation to the brain, excessive electrical discharge of neurons in the brain, and psychogenic phenomena. The most common types of intermittent loss of arousal are syncope and seizures.

Syncope

Syncope, or faint, involves an episodic interruption of consciousness, usually of abrupt onset and brief duration. Recovery from syncope is usually complete. The physiologic causes of syncope fall under two categories: decreased blood flow to the brain and altered state of blood to the brain. Clinical states in the latter category include hypoxia and anemia. Conditions commonly leading to decreased blood flow to the brain (Adams & Victor, 1985) include vasovagal syncope, which results from vasodilation of peripheral resistance vessels. It can be induced by physical injury, strong emotion (these may occur together), or hot, crowded environments. A vagal response, which includes bradycardia, perspiration, nausea, salivation, and increased peristaltic activity, may accompany the faint. Postural (orthostatic) hypotension occurs in people with unstable or defective vasomotor reflexes from a variety of causes, for example, prolonged bedrest, drug side effects, peripheral nerve dysfunction, hypovolemia, and autonomic insufficiency.

Syncope of cardic origin is due to a sudden reduction in cardiac output, usually because of a dysrhythmia. Pulse rates less than 40 beats per minute impair cerebral circulation and can lead to syncope. The cardiac condition most frequently causing syncope is complete atrioventricular block. Carotid sinus syncope is due to an overly sensitive carotid sinus. In this condition, fainting can occur when slight pressure is applied to the neck area where the carotid sinus is located. A person with this condition may faint with head turning while wearing a tight collar or even by shaving over the region of the carotid sinus.

Seizures
Certain types of seizures produce intermittent loss of arousal, and some of these may closely

resemble syncope. The pathophysiology of seizures, however, arises within the brain itself rather than in the circulation to the brain. A seizure is a paroxysmal, uncontrolled excessive firing of hyperexcitable neurons within the brain. There are several causes of neuronal hyperexcitability, for example, metabolic imbalance, trauma, tumor, hemorrhage, infection, genetic predisposition, degenerative disease, and drug side effects. Epilepsy is defined as a tendency for recurring seizures, regardless of cause, and is treated with chronic use of anticonvulsant medication. Seizures owing to reversible causes, such as metabolic imbalance and drug side effects, are usually not considered epileptic because once the underlying cause is corrected the seizures do not recur.

The most common seizure resulting in loss of arousal is the generalized tonic–clonic (grand mal) seizure. It is characterized by sudden loss of consciousness that is followed by stiffening of the body for several seconds (tonic phase) and subsequent jerking of the extremities (clonic phase). Some people experience only tonic or only clonic seizures, but these are usually accompanied by loss of consciousness. Recovery of consciousness after a tonic–clonic seizure is gradual, unlike recovery from syncope, which is usually rapid once the blood supply to the brain has been restored. The time for recovery after a seizure depends on how quickly the neurons regain normal functioning from their exhausted state. This may take up to several hours.

Two other types of seizures involve an alteration in consciousness rather than complete loss of consciousness. Because of this, the likelihood of falling is not as great as it is with a tonic–clonic seizure. The more common of these two types is the complex partial (temporal lobe, psychomotor) seizure. This seizure type has a wide range of duration (seconds to minutes) and of manifestations, from simple staring and relatively few motor signs to very complex behaviors despite lack of awareness of one's surroundings. The second seizure type is the generalized (both typical and atypical) absence spell. In this seizure, there is alteration in consciousness and sometimes minor movements of the face and limbs, but there is usually a more rapid return to normal arousal than in a complex partial seizure.

HUMAN RESPONSES TO INTERMITTENT LOSS OF AROUSAL

A variety of behavioral and physical responses to intermittent loss of arousal forms the basis for nursing diagnoses related to the individual, family, and community.

Diagnoses for the Individual

Nursing diagnoses in people who experience intermittent loss of arousal include fear, potential for injury, ineffective coping—denial, social isolation, role disturbance, noncompliance, knowledge deficit, and memory deficit.

☐ Fear

Gordon (1987) separates fear from anxiety by noting that the source of the emotion is identifiable in fear and is unknown in anxiety. People prone to episodes of intermittent arousal manifest the *defining characteristic* fear more often than anxiety because they usually can identify the source of the emotion and verbalize expectation of danger. Fear of danger to oneself, in the form of injury and even death, has been mentioned by some patients with seizures (Ozuna, personal observation). *Etiologies* include fear of death, fear of rejection or prejudice, and fear of malformed offspring. It is probable that people prone to syncope also have this fear. The following episodes illustrate how and why these fears arise. A man blacked out while driving but fortunately was unhurt when his car ran into a ditch. Both he and his family feared he would not be so lucky if it happened again. He was diagnosed eventually as having carotid sinus syndrome, and after a pacemaker was inserted, he had no more blackouts. An elderly woman was known to have blackouts, spells supposedly from cardiac arrhythmia. Her fears and her family's fears of injury were realized when she blacked out, fell, and broke her hip. In retrospect, her new doctor decided that she was probably overdosed on her cardiac and antihypertensive medications.

People who have syncopal attacks or the types of seizures described also fear how others might perceive them if they have an attack in public. Our society affirms people who are normal, who conform to the expectations of society. Society rejects those who deviate from the norm, who display abnormal behavior, or who lack self-control. The person who has a syncopal attack, especially in public, however unwillingly, acts well outside the expected norms of society, and, therefore, the person with uncontrolled episodes of intermittent loss of consciousness is understandably fearful of rejection and prejudice.

A detailed review of the literature on epilepsy (Bagley, 1971) has indicated that prejudice against epilepsy exists in modern industrial society. A well-known businessman in a medium-sized community expressed strong fears of others' learning that he had epilepsy and even greater fear of their seeing him in a tonic–clonic seizure. He had had one seizure in the past several years, but because of fear, he withdrew from his social contacts and retired from his job as owner and operator of an automobile sales business.

There are other sources of fear in people with epilepsy. In women with idiopathic epilepsy, especially with a history of typical absence epilepsy, fear of bearing children who will develop epilepsy may be a valid concern. The offspring of a person (male or female) with typical absence epilepsy have a 50% chance of inheriting the gene for the disorder and about a 12% risk of actually having clinical seizures (Jennings & Bird, 1981). For others, fear of losing a job because of seizures may be justified. There are numerous accounts of people with epilepsy being fired from their jobs after having a seizure at work or after the employers discovered they had epilepsy (*National Spokesman*, 1985).

In *assessment*, one must explore the patient's fears with him comprehensively to identify the real source of the fear. Once this is determined, appropriate interventions can be implemented. Often, information about the disease can help alleviate fear when the source of the fear is lack of knowledge, the unknown (see the section "Knowledge Deficit" in this chapter).

Interventions should include assessment of the type and frequency of attacks, the conditions under which they occur, the treatment regimen if there is one, and compliance with that regimen. A person who has a seizure (regardless of type) only once in several months may be encouraged to pursue normal activities, but he or she should be sure to be accompanied in such activities as climbing in high places, swimming, or working around dangerous machinery. If seizures occur only when a person is very tired, regular rest periods can be planned so that seizures are less likely. Compliance with a medication regimen is very important to assess, since noncompliance is a significant factor in breakthrough seizures (see the section "Noncompliance" in this chapter). The fear of seizures and subsequent injury during a seizure may subside significantly with improved compliance and subsequent seizure control.

People with epilepsy who fear rejection by others present a challenge to caregivers from both patient care and community perspectives. Although public attitudes toward people with epilepsy have improved greatly over the years (Caveness & Gallup, 1980), some people still react negatively to people with epilepsy. Often this is because of lack of knowledge about the disorder. Thirty-nine percent of the general public surveyed in a poll in 1979 said they did not know the cause of epilepsy (Caveness & Gallup, 1980).

It is important to determine from whom the patient feels the potential for rejection (see section "Social Isolation" in this chapter). If it is family members, the nurse may find that teaching the family and the patient more about epilepsy is helpful (see section "Knowledge Deficit" in this chapter). If the person feared is an employer, the patient is probably best referred to a vocational counselor. If the people feared are classmates in school, it is best to have the school nurse or the teacher educate the students about epilepsy. Parents and teachers are role models for children, and if adults treat the epileptic child as any other child, the children will most likely do the same. For those who have fears about bearing children, it is important to determine exactly what is feared: Is it fear of the effects of pregnancy on seizure frequency, or is it fear of a bad outcome of pregnancy, for example, malformations or epilepsy? Most studies suggest that about 50% of women with epilepsy will have no change in their seizure frequency while pregnant, and 40% will have fewer seizures (Dalessio, 1985). Some of the increase in seizure frequency during pregnancy is the result of medication noncompliance, and some is due to changes in drug metabolism and clearance during pregnancy that cause drug levels to decline (Dalessio, 1985). Although children of epileptic mothers have approximately twice as many malformations as children of mothers without epilepsy (Janz, 1982), this risk is still small (about a 5% chance). The offspring of a person with epilepsy (with the exception of typical absence epilepsy) have approximately a 2% to 5% risk of having seizures (Jennings & Bird, 1981). If a family is especially concerned about the effect of a parent's epilepsy on their offspring, it is best to refer them to a genetic counselor.

☐ Potential for Injury

Anytime there is loss of awareness or an alteration in consciousness, the potential for injury exists. Both syncope and seizures, with the exception of simple partial seizures, present a risk for injury because of alteration in consciousness. Injuries encountered include head trauma, burns, bone fractures, aspiration, and multiple trauma. Head trauma occurs if there is sudden loss of consciousness that leads to a fall. The head may strike furniture or other objects during the fall or may hit the ground, resulting in scalp or facial lacerations or even skull fracture and hematoma. Burns may result from falling onto a heating element of a stove, a heater, or into a fire, or if the person is smoking. They may occur if the person is in the shower or bathtub with hot water running. Bone fractures usually are associated with falls but can result when the jerking limbs strike adjacent objects. Aspiration can occur if a person is not properly positioned during a generalized tonic–clonic seizure. Some people have had severe aspiration, leading to death by drowning, while in the bathtub or while swimming. Multiple trauma can result from a fall or an automobile accident precipitated by an epileptic or syncopal attack.

Assessment for potential for injury includes frequency of seizure or syncopal episodes, adequacy of seizure control, and the type of activities commonly performed.

It is important for the patient, family, and caregivers to understand the risk for injury, and the patient should be allowed to participate in as many activities as are within reason. As an *intervention*, people who experience episodes of loss of consciousness are advised not to go swimming alone, not to climb high places (this includes both recreation and work) without safety lines, and not to work around dangerous machinery (although some machines can be adapted so that they run only if the operator applies constant pressure via a footpedal or button). People should be advised of the legal restrictions for driving a motor vehicle. The specific interval for being free of seizures necessary to obtain a valid driver's license varies among states, usually between 6 months and 2 years. All those who come in contact with a person with seizures should have knowledge of first aid management of seizures to minimize the risk of injury.

Care of a person during a generalized tonic–clonic seizure is twofold: protection from injury and prevention of aspiration. Furniture and other large objects in the immediate surroundings should be removed so that the person's limbs do not strike them. The head should be cradled, either on someone's lap or on soft padding. No attempt should be made to prevent limb movement or place anything between the person's teeth once the jaws are tightly clenched. Because the jaws generate 1,000 pounds of pressure per square inch, no amount of human force can open the jaws during a seizure. Once the seizure is over, the person should be turned gently on the side so that saliva that has accumulated during the seizure can drain from the mouth. Someone should remain with the person until he or she regains consciousness. It should be emphasized to family members and to the general public that there is no need to call an ambulance when a tonic–clonic seizure occurs, since this results in unnecessary and expensive ambulance and emergency room bills.

Care of a person having a complex partial seizure is mostly close observation. The witness should remain with the person throughout the seizure and not attempt to restrain him or her, even if the person attempts to walk away. It is important to remember that the person's behavior is being driven by the seizure activity and he or she may become combative if restraint is attempted. The general *goals* for first aid management of seizures are to provide physical safety, emotional support, and privacy.

☐ Ineffective Coping: Denial

Denial can be defined as prolonged minimization or rejection of information when a situation requires active coping (Gordon, 1987). Among people with epilepsy, the ability to cope can vary greatly. Some people whose seizures are relatively minor and infrequent have a suprisingly difficult time adjusting to their condition, whereas others cope well with more severe epilepsy.

There are several aspects of epilepsy (Ozuna, 1979; Shope, 1982) that make it more difficult for an afflicted person to adjust than it is for a person with syncope. Epilepsy is a chronic condition, with the likelihood of seizures occurring throughout a lifetime. Epilepsy is incurable: although seizures can be controlled for a period of time, the condition itself is rarely cured. Epilepsy is invisible: it is not apparent to others that a person has this condition unless a seizure occurs. People tend not to understand epilepsy because they are not exposed to it. Epilepsy is unpredictable: other people are never prepared when a seizure occurs. Epilepsy requires that medications be taken regularly and for many years to control seizures, which forces a kind of dependency that some reject. Epilepsy means restrictions on driving, alcohol consumption, occupation, and recreation even though the person with epilepsy may not be ill between seizures. Epilepsy carries a stigma: this may be due to the public's continuing misconceptions about epilepsy or its fear about potential loss of control.

Among people with epilepsy, denial may occur when the diagnosis is first made and may continue for several years. Defining *characteristics* of denial of epilepsy include poor medication compliance, continuation of activities known to precipitate seizures, or continuing to drive a car despite a history of recent seizures.

Denial of epilepsy has a variety of *etiologies*—fear of being labeled epileptic, with its negative connotations, any of the fears discussed in the section "Fear" in this chapter, loss of independence. The following episode illustrates an instance of denial resulting from a possible misconception.

A passenger on an airplane stated that he was on his way to see a neurologist for another opinion about his blackouts (Ozuna, 1979). He had already seen five physicians. He said he was taking Dilantin (phenytoin), but when asked if he had epilepsy, he said, "Oh no, I just have blackouts, but I let them think I have epilepsy so I can get workman's compensation. I pop these pills just before I go to the doctor so it will show up in my blood." On further questioning, it became apparent that he had been injured in a construction accident 2 years previously, which resulted in a depressed skull fracture. The blackouts began shortly after that injury.

He said he was having these spells a few times a week. He continued to drive a car and fly an airplane. When asked why he did not think he had epilepsy, he could not really answer. He said, "I just don't think I have it."

When it was explained to him that epilepsy simply means recurring seizures and that many people develop seizures after a severe head injury because of damage to brain cells, he said, "Really? You're the first person who's ever told me that." He may have been denying his epilepsy because of misconceptions that only retarded or severely brain-damaged people have epilepsy.

Some people deny the prognosis that epilepsy is likely to continue throughout their lifetime. This is particularly true if they have not had a seizure for several months or years. Denial of epilepsy by family members is discussed in the section "Ineffective Coping" in this chapter.

As with other psychosocial problems, it is important to explore the patient's feelings and *assess* the patient's conception of epilepsy and its connotations. The preceding case illustrates that correcting misconceptions can reverse denial in some people. Ascertain how the patient perceives the treatment regimen and how it affects his or her lifestyle and determine if noncompliance is willful or due to forgetfulness, since *interventions* for these two situations differ (see section "Noncompliance" in this chapter).

☐ Social Isolation

Social isolation can be *defined* as a lack of societal fulfillment, a condition in which individuals set themselves apart from the societal whole with which they could be expected to interact and affiliate (Beniak & Beniak, 1983). It is evident from the preceding discussions that social isolation may not be an unusual consequence of having epilepsy. In some cases, fear of or actual rejection by others may lead an otherwise socially adroit person into seclusion.

In other cases, the condition of epilepsy removes a previously socially unskilled person even farther from the mainstream of social interactions.

Social isolation has as *defining characteristics* withdrawal from social contacts, activities, and responsibilities; lack of genuine interest in other people; little, if any, development of vocational or recreational pursuits; lack of social poise, poor communication skills; and general aloofness (Beniak & Beniak, 1983). The onset of epilepsy in childhood can make it doubly hard to develop social skills because the child may be denied early opportunities for socialization. The denial may come from the family, who unknowingly overprotect the child, or it may come from the child's classmates, friends, and siblings, who ridicule and ostracize the child.

Antiepilepsy medications can cause emotional and physical side effects (irritability, depression, aggression, sleepiness, dizziness, clumsiness) that are *etiologic factors* in social isolation. Legal, vocational, and activity restrictions on people with epilepsy also add to the likelihood that some will decrease their social interactions.

Beniak & Beniak (1983) propose the following *assessments* and *interventions* for epileptic people manifesting social isolation. One should first assess the person's level of cognitive and intellectual functioning, since this helps determine the form of therapy that might be most helpful. Formal personality assessment (Minnesota Multiphasic Personality Inventory [MMPI] and Washington Psychosocial Seizure Inventory [WPSI]; Dodrill et al., 1980) can provide additional data. One should note the person's routine behavior: how the person interacts with others and under what circumstances. It is helpful to establish indivualized *goals*, such as (1) a specific number of social interactions with staff or other patients, (2) participation in a novel social activity, and (3) responsibility on the part of the patient for some aspects of care. In settings where there are several people who experience seizures, formal group interactions can be arranged. Group discussions about common problems can help establish some socialization among all the members. Role playing can help members to practice social skills, such as greeting a stranger, asking a ticket agent for tickets to an event, and inviting someone to a function. Relaxation training is another intervention that has been used with some success (Snyder, 1983). This method enhances psychic comfort and, therefore, enables a person to interact more openly and spontaneously.

☐ Role Disturbance

Role disturbance is an internal conflict based on a discrepancy between what a person wants his role to be and what it actually is. Role disturbance can develop particularly in the adult years when certain roles have been established or at least planned for and a diagnosis of epilepsy or syncope requires changes in these roles. A person may manifest the *defining characteristics* of role disturbance by expressing frustration and feelings of inadequacy related to loss of job, inability to find work, loss of independence, or inability to participate in previous activities (e.g., child care, work, recreation). Thus, the role of breadwinner, parent, homemaker, or athlete may be perceived by the person with episodes of intermittent loss of arousal as being lost to him or her.

The *interventions* for role disturbance depend on *assessment* of the role involved. Vocational counseling and social work services are in order for the person who has employment difficulties. Family counseling can help the person with role disturbance regarding parenting and providing child care. For the woman who is worried about her role as procreator, genetic counseling may be helpful. Recreation therapists may have ideas for those who need to choose alternative diversional activities. Local affiliates of the Epilepsy Foundation of America (EFA) sponsor self-help groups.

☐ Noncompliance

Noncompliance with prescribed antiepilepsy medication is a common problem among people with epilepsy and is the most frequent cause of poor seizure control (Kutt & Penry, 1974). Certain features about epilepsy contribute to the likelihood of noncompliance: the need for long-term compliance to a medical regimen, the requirement that medications be taken regardless of the presence of symptoms (seizures) and often during symptom-free periods, a need for change in the patient's lifestyle, and the fact that the drug regimen may produce side effects (Green & Roter, 1977). Psychologic factors, such as denial and rebellion against dependency on medications, can contribute to noncompliance. These are all factors of willful noncompliance, a situation in which a person makes a conscious decision not to take medication as prescribed. There are, however, people who do not comply with an antiepilepsy medication regimen because of simple forgetfulness. These people need different interventions than do those who have willful noncompliance.

The *defining characteristic* of noncompliance, whatever the reason, is a lower-than-expected antiepilepsy drug serum level, that is, a level below what would be expected for a given patient on a given dose. Since most patients are taking sufficient dosages to achieve a therapeutic level, the drug level usually will be subtherapeutic if the person is noncompliant. It is important, however, to rule out other causes of a subtherapeutic level before making this assumption. These include altered drug metabolism (some people are fast or slow metabolizers), altered drug utilization (as a consequence of disease), altered physiologic state (e.g., pregnancy), age (children utilize drugs at a faster rate, elderly people at a slower rate) (Pippenger, 1979), and drug interactions.

Assessment of noncompliance should include both examination of the drug serum level and direct questioning of the patient. When questioned, up to half of noncompliers will admit it (Sackett, 1977), and this group responds most positively to compliance-improving strategies. (Sackett, 1979). Once noncompliance has been determined, the reason or reasons for noncompliance should be assessed. These include but are not limited to forgetfulness, misunderstanding of the medication schedule, drug side effects, complexity of the medication schedule, hesitation of taking medications in front of others (at school or work), attitude toward illness, family problems, financial problems, poor social support, poor patient–health care provider interaction, denial, and rebellion (Marston, 1970; Haynes, 1979; Shope, 1982).

The author has found the Health Belief Model (Rosenstock, 1966) to be a useful model on which to base a compliance counseling approach. The model suggests that people are not likely to take a health action (e.g., take medication) unless (1) they believe themselves susceptible to the disease, (2) they believe the disease would have serious effects on their lives, (3) they are aware of actions and treatments and believe they will help, and (4) they believe the risk of taking action is less serious than the illness itself. A prerequisite of each belief is the preceding belief in the hierarchy; for example, a person who does not believe his illness is serious is not likely to follow a treatment regimen for that illness. The nurse can evaluate the health beliefs of her patients and use the information to guide her compliance-improving interventions. The Health Belief Model is a useful guide also for general patient and family education (see section "Knowledge Deficit" in this chapter).

It is beyond the scope of this chapter to discuss interventions for each of the cited reasons for noncompliance. *Interventions* for a few of the major reasons are presented. For those who are forgetful, several methods are helpful (Ozuna & Cammermeyer, 1982). Provide the patient with written instructions for taking medication, have him or her record each taken on a calendar. Encourage the use of pillboxes or containers that have compartments for every day of the week. The Medi-Set (Drug Intelligence, Hamilton, IL 62341) has four compartments for each day of the week for patients who take several doses a day. Suggest that the patient associate taking medication with a routine daily activity, such as use of the bathroom, daily hygiene activities, meals, and so on.

A young adult male was referred by his private physician because of inability to control his seizures. After attempts by the referral physician to raise the patient's serum levels by increasing the medication dose were unsuccessful, the author asked him about his medication-taking habits. He said that he was somewhat irregular in taking his medication because he worked late hours some days and would forget to take it. When she asked him where he kept his medication, he said, "in the kitchen cupboard." She asked him if he always went to the kitchen after coming home from work, and he said, "No." She suggested that it would be easier for him to remember taking his medication if he associated it with a routine daily activity, but he said that he did not have any routine, especially when he worked such late hours. When she asked, "Do you use the bathroom every night before you go to bed?" he responded affirmatively, and she suggested that he keep the medication in the bathroom and put a note on the bathroom mirror to remind himself to take his medication. He accepted these suggestions readily and was able to obtain therapeutic serum phenytoin levels and seizure control.

Since many patients lack understanding of antiepilepsy drugs, the nurse can do much to improve compliance by providing information about the action of the drugs, their pharmacokinetics (e.g., why some drugs can be taken once a day), and a realistic perspective of their side effects. Through discussions with the primary caregiver (physician or nurse), the number of medications can be kept to a minimum, the frequency of the doses can be lowered, and the complexity of the medication regimen can be simplified.

Many patients respond well to increased supervision (Haynes, 1979). Regular feedback to them about their drug levels and regular discussions about their seizure control and medication-taking habits can provide positive reinforcement of compliant behavior. The increased attention also gives the patient a favorable impression of his relationship with the health care provider, a factor known to influence compliance behavior (Shope, 1982).

Contributions by nurses in specialized roles in promoting compliance have been particularly important in chronic disease, partly because of their supportive role functions and, in some situations, because of their ability to provide greater continuity in care (as opposed to physicians who rotate through outpatient clinic settings) (Hogue, 1979). Hogue suggests that nurses can employ several strategies to improve compliance: use clear, concise information when instructing patients, help the patient feel competent to manage the treatment regimen, encourage the use of natural support systems (family, friends), and facilitate teamwork with others interested in the patient's progress.

☐ Knowledge Deficit

Gordon (1987) operationally *defines* knowledge deficit as the "inability to state or explain information or demonstrate a required skill related to disease management procedures, practices, and/or self-care–health-care management" (p. 186). Knowledge deficits among people with epilepsy can occur in several areas: the disorder of epilepsy, diagnostic procedures and rationale, medications and the medication regimen, follow-up care, legal restrictions, community resources.

Because of the relatively high percentage of people who lack knowledge about epilepsy (Caveness & Gallup, 1980) and the persistence of misconceptions about what epilepsy is, basic teaching in layman's language about the pathophysiology of epilepsy should be a priority not only in newly diagnosed patients but in long-term patients as well. A useful way to *assess* patients' knowledge is to ask them to describe what epilepsy is and why they think they have it. For some, the first step is to acknowledge that they have epilepsy (see section "Ineffective Coping" in this chapter). Some physicians tell patients they have a seizure disorder, and they are shocked to learn that this term is synonymous with epilepsy. In addition to offering verbal explanations of epilepsy, one can provide the patient and family with educational pamphlets published by the EFA.

Patients must understand through nursing *intervention* that epilepsy is not a curable condition but can be controlled in most cases with regular use of antiepilepsy medication. The patient should be made aware of his or her seizure type and its manifestations. Incorrect labeling of seizure type could lead to improper treatment, since most medications used to treat partial seizures are not useful in treating generalized nonconvulsive seizures, and vice versa. Patients should know what they do during seizures so that loved ones and co-workers will know what to expect should a seizure occur. Although some people choose not to reveal their epilepsy to their employers because of a sometimes valid fear of losing their jobs, much of the frightening aspects of a seizure can be lessened by knowing what to expect.

The patient should know what kind of first aid care will be needed. Patients and their families should be reminded that unless an injury results from a seizure or the seizure is prolonged, there is no need to summon medical help. Lack of this information often leads to unnecessary and very expensive medical bills. Table 8–1 is a teaching plan based on the Health Belief Model.

When a person is undergoing a diagnostic workup for epilepsy, one should explain both the value and the limitations of the electroencephalogram (EEG) and computerized tomography (CT). It should be explained that much of the diagnosis still depends on the history and on the descriptions by those who witness the seizures.

Once the diagnosis is made and antiepilepsy medication is started, information about the prescribed drugs should be provided, including the mechanism of action of the drugs, their side effects, interactions with other drugs, and the need for routine assessment of serum drug levels. The patient should be instructed to report any side effects or changes in well-being. The patient should be reminded not to change the dosage of medication without first consulting the health care provider and should be warned that abrupt discontinuation of antiepilepsy drugs can precipitate seizures and even lead to status epilepticus.

The nurse in the inpatient setting should include information about follow-up care in dis-

TABLE 8–1. TEACHING PLAN BASED ON HEALTH BELIEF MODEL.

Outcome Criteria	Teaching Plan	Evaluation
Patient and family state that patient is likely to have another seizure (acknowledge susceptibility)	Review with patient and family: • Anatomy and physiology of nerve impulse transmission in brain • Probable cause of patient's seizures • Pathophysiology of epilepsy • Body functions governed by specific brain regions and how patient's seizures relate to these functions	Patient and family regularly indicate knowledge of susceptibility to recurring seizures
Patient and family recognize possible consequences of seizures on patient's life: • More seizures, less likely to be controlled • Risk of physical injury during seizure • Difficulty finding employment • Inability to legally drive if not seizure free	Review with patient and family: • Seizures beget more seizures • Physical danger if patient loses consciousness, falls, drives during seizure • Benefits and risks of telling employer about having epilepsy • State driving law	Evidence that patient has adjusted to his or her epilepsy • Demonstrates acceptance of epilepsy • Admits having seizures • Gainfully employed according to abilities
Patient and family demonstrate positive actions toward controlling patient's seizures • Identify names of prescribed medications, dosage, time schedule, side effects • State understanding of differences in dosage needs for individuals • List factors that precipitate seizures • States understanding of need for follow-up by health provider • States advantages and disadvantages of identification tags • Demonstrates appropriate first aid procedure for all seizure types	Review with patient and family: • All aspects of medication regimen • Use of serum level determinations • How to avoid or better handle precipitating factors • Pros and cons of identification tags • First aid procedures	Evidence that patient is taking health action for his epilepsy: • Obtains maximal seizure control with minimal side effects • Maintains therapeutic serum drug levels • Gives no history of activities or situations that precipitate seizures • Returns regularly for follow-up visits • Has made logical decision about wearing identification tag • Shows minimal, if any, physical injury after a seizure

charge planning of newly diagnosed patients. Follow-up visits are needed to ascertain drug efficacy and side effects and overall adjustment. The nurse should supply information about community resources (both educational and vocational) and the state driving laws.

Similar patient education topics should be addressed when advising people with syncope. Patients should be informed about the cause and treatment of their disorder and should be told about the legal restrictions about driving. They should be advised that activities that put them at risk for injury if they lose consciousness (e.g., climbing high places, swimming alone, working with heavy machinery) should be avoided.

Memory Deficit

The *defining characteristic* of memory deficit is the inability to recall recent or current events and activities (Gordon, 1987). The author has observed that this is a frequent complaint among patients with epilepsy. It is known that memory problems, particularly those involving short-term memory, can be a result of antiepilepsy medications (Trimble & Reynolds, 1976; Giordani et al., 1983) and, probably, the disorder itself (Mungus et al., 1985; Loiseau, et al. 1983). The degree of memory impairment can range from relatively benign forgetfulness to severe cognitive dysfunction. In addition, the memory disturbance can affect medication compliance adversely (see section "Noncompliance" in this chapter).

Many patients with a memory problem recognize it themselves. They complain of forgetting such things as conversations they had recently, what their spouse has asked them to do, what they were supposed to get at the store, or what they had intended to do at work on a given day. In other situations, a family member or the employer notes the memory deficit. In some cases, the nurse can *assess* a memory deficit by testing immediate and recent recall, although, in other cases, these tests are normal. Most often, the memory problem is brought to the nurse's attention by the patient or patient's family.

It is important to rule out overdosage of antiepilepsy medication as a cause of memory disturbance. In some cases, reduction of medication dosage can improve memory problems without adversely affecting seizure control.

The following *interventions* are designed for those who have minor verbal memory disturbance. Interventions for those more severely impaired are discussed in Chapter 12. The patient should be advised to use memory aids, such as written reminders and daily or weekly calendars. Since memory problems can influence medication compliance, the patient should be encouraged to associate medication taking with routine daily activities, keep a written log, and use pill containers (see section "Noncompliance" in this chapter).

Patients will have less difficulty if their daily routine is structured and unchanged from day to day. This kind of repetition, as well as repetition of new information, can improve memory and provide a sense of comfort and security to the person with minor memory disturbance.

Memory problems have significant implications for patient education and discharge planning. Any new information that is to be given to a person should be written down and shared with family members or significant others.

Diagnoses for the Family and Significant Others

Ineffective Family Coping

Gordon (1987) *defines* this nursing diagnosis as a condition in which the usually supportive person provides insufficient, ineffective, or compromised support, comfort, assistance, or encouragement that the client may need to manage or master adaptive tasks to a health challenge. Epilepsy and syncope, as many other health conditions, can generate ineffective coping within certain families and close friendships. Problems in coping with intermittent loss of arousal are addressed from two perspectives: the child with the disorder and the adult with the disorder.

When a child develops epilepsy, one of several alterations in coping can occur in one or both of the parents (Ozuna, 1979). The first is denial. The parents may refuse to believe that their child has epilepsy, that a product of themselves is imperfect. Some parents who are fearful about epilepsy and deny its existence are unable to assist the child with his own fears (Voeller & Rothenberg, 1973). This denial may have serious consequences if the parents refuse to give the child his antiepilepsy medication. Once epilepsy is accepted by the parents, feelings of guilt may result from unconscious rejection of the imperfect child. The parents may blame themselves for the child's disorder. They may overprotect the child and severely limit his or her activities, or they may overindulge and spoil the child to avoid causing aggravation and causing a seizure. The child then learns to manipulate the parents and get whatever he or she wants. This may lead to an alteration in the family process. If the child's demanding personality carries over into adulthood, difficulty in getting along with others and rejection may result (see section "Social Isolation" in this chapter).

In other families, the parents may blame the epileptic child for the family's difficulties. This maladaptive coping can cause the child to lose self-esteem and the ability to develop relationships with others, thereby leading to social isolation.

Siblings may have difficulty coping with an epileptic child. If the child gets most of the parental attention, siblings may become jealous and exclude him or her from their activities. They may reject their brother or sister as a source of embarrassment, or they may use the child as a scapegoat when altercations occur.

When epilepsy develops in an adult, stresses on the family occur. The spouse may be faced with getting a new job or obtaining a driver's license. If the spouse cannot face this challenge, he or she may blame the person with epilepsy for disrupting their lifestyle. Fear and denial may be evident, as may blame, overprotection, and scapegoating.

The children of a parent with epilepsy may have difficulty coping. The author is aware of several cases in which the children were afraid that their parent was going to die when he or she had a seizure. An exploratory study of children's adaptation to epilepsy in a parent revealed four major problems that occurred in families: learning about the disorder, fear of abandonment, overresponsibility of children for their parents, and fear of developing epilepsy (Lechtenberg & Akner, 1984). It was concluded that children who adjusted most poorly to epilepsy in a parent were those from whom the seizure disorder had been concealed.

Ineffective family coping may be detected during an encounter with family members in either an inpatient or an outpatient setting. Comments and behaviors of children, spouses, and friends provide valuable clues in the *assessment* of family coping. The nurse should explore feelings that are expressed. Reflective listening can bring out more detailed aspects of the coping pattern. Once the coping problem is identified, *interventions* can be planned.

If denial is present in a family member, further exploration about the reason for the denial may help determine how to intervene. For instance, if the family member exhibits lack of knowledge or misconceptions, providing accurate information about epilepsy may help (this presumes that the person is ready to learn). If parents are overprotecting the child, one may offer information that it is in the child's best interest to treat him or her like any other child. If parents or siblings are blaming the child for their problems, formal family counseling may be needed.

In view of the findings of Lechtenberg and Akner (1984), it appears that lack of information about epilepsy is an important cause of coping problems among family members. They suggest that the least disruptive approach to children of epileptic parents is a frank discussion of what epilepsy is and what is being done to control it because parental efforts to conceal the problem breed distrust in the children.

☐ Alteration in Family Process

Inability of the family system to meet the needs of members, carry out family functions, and maintain communications for mutual growth and maturation are *defining characteristics* of alteration in family process (Gordon, 1987). This problem often is an outgrowth of family coping problems. If mother and father have different perceptions of epilepsy in their child, controversy over child rearing can develop. The father may blame the mother, or vice versa, for the child's epilepsy, and as a result, the child suffers. He or she begins to lose self-esteem and withdraws. For children of epileptic parents, family process alterations may include taking on responsibilities for family functioning beyond those of other children of the same age. Some children may function successfully in these responsibilities, but for others, it may prove to be too great a burden. The child may miss normal opportunities for growth and development because of self-imposed or parent-imposed responsibilities for the epileptic parent.

As with family coping alterations, family process alterations necessitate further data gathering for *assessment*. The nurse may need to speak to family members individually in order for them to express frank, uninhibited feelings. If both parents agree that they need help, the nurse can offer simple guidelines as nursing *interventions*. Discipline of the child should be no different from that of the other children. Limitations on the child's activities can be obtained from the child's primary caregiver and should be followed by both parents in a consistent manner. Responsibility for the child's medication should be assumed by one or both parents until the child is old enough to take responsibility. In situations where disagreements between parents are too great, the nurse may refer parents to family counseling or to a parent support group. Support groups are sponsored by children's hospitals and by local chapters of the EFA.

☐ Knowledge Deficit

The previous discussions about family problems imply that lack of knowledge is an important component. Lack of knowledge and misconceptions may become apparent during interviews with family members, and some members may admit openly their lack of knowledge. Teaching approaches are guided by the type of knowledge deficit, the readiness of the learner, and the age of the learner.

Diagnoses for the Community

☐ Stigma Related to Knowledge Deficit

Misconceptions and prejudice about people with epilepsy still exist despite improvement in public attitudes toward epilepsy over the last 40 years (Bagley, 1972; Caveness & Gallup, 1980). Many patients report that well-meaning bystanders call an ambulance when a seizure occurs, regardless of its severity. Patients are then faced with expensive, and unnecessary, emergency medical care. On one occasion, a bystander who witnessed a seizure forced a plastic pen into the person's mouth. The cap broke off and was aspirated into a bronchus. The person complained of an irritating chronic cough for several weeks before the offending object was detected on an x-ray. Many witnesses of a seizure continue to force hard objects into a person's mouth, resulting in aspiration of broken teeth or parts of the object. The author is aware of one occasion on which a teacher ran out of the room in a state of fear when a child had a seizure in the classroom.

Articles about and letters from people who have difficulty with employment because of their epilepsy can be found in almost every issue of the EFA *National Spokesman* (newsletter). A national survey found that discrimination in jobs was the most serious problem facing the person with epilepsy. Employers may have misconceptions that all epileptic people are mentally deficient, have poor work attendance, and perform less well than nonepileptic people, or they may fear that an epileptic employee will disrupt the performance of coworkers if he has a seizure on the job (Ozuna, 1979). In fact, employment seems to have a beneficial effect on the physical we well as the psychologic aspects of the person with epilepsy (Risch & Rose, 1957).

It is important for any professional who cares for people with epilepsy to provide the *intervention* of education about epilepsy to people in the community, including teachers, employers, police, firefighters, airline attendants, and the general public. A resource for public education is the EFA, which sponsors nationwide programs on many aspects of epilepsy. Local chapters of EFA sponsor educational programs and support groups. EFA publishes a number of educational brochures that are available for a fee and can be used for patient and family teaching and has educational program packages for both lay and professional audiences. Information about these resources should be shared with teachers, librarians, physicians, and employers.

☐ Knowledge Deficit Regarding Health Promotion, Disease Prevention, and Community Resources

Head trauma is one of the most preventable causes of acquired epilepsy. Campaigns to make the public aware of measures to prevent head trauma should include advocating wearing of seatbelts and helmets and participating in sports safely (i.e., avoiding diving in shallow water and wearing protective helmets in such sports as football, baseball, hockey, cycling).

For many people with epilepsy, psychosocial problems far outweigh the physiologic problem of seizures. Knowledge of community resources for employment, financial assistance, housing, child care, transportation, patient advocacy, and social skills improvement should be shared with all health care providers who assist people with epilepsy.

NURSING ROLES IN MANAGEMENT OF INTERMITTENT LOSS OF AROUSAL AND AWARENESS

Ensuring patient safety is a primary responsibility of the nurse generalist. Patients with syncope or epilepsy are at great risk for injuring themselves during loss of arousal and, therefore, require preventive measures. The nurse must be knowledgeable about the frequency of the patient's seizures, their precipitating factors, and their warning signs so that appropriate safety measures can be instituted for patients with poorly controlled seizures. In the hospital, siderails should be padded, and a padded tongue blade should be taped at the head of the bed. (One should realize, however, that the nurse rarely has enough time to place a tongue blade or plastic airway between a patient's teeth before they become tightly clenched in a tonic–clonic seizure.) Patients with either uncontrolled syncopal episodes or seizures should never ambulate or transfer unassisted. The nurse generalist is responsible for ensuring that the patient knows about his or her disorder. Pamphlets from the EFA or other written resources can be given to patients to fortify retention of information.

The nurse generalist should be knowledgeable about the patient's medication regimen, including mechanisms of action, pharmacokinetics, usual adult dosages, and therapeutic ranges of the drugs. Discharge planning should include patient and family teaching of the drug regimen: dose, frequency, and side effects.

The nurse specialist is accountable for assisting in the management of complex patient problems in an inpatient setting and, in some cases, is responsible for directly managing patient care in an outpatient setting. The nurse specialist may help a multidisciplinary team treat complex behavioral or pathophysiologic responses. She may become involved in the identification and management of compliance problems. The specialist has a responsibility to educate the public about epilepsy: what it is, how it can be prevented, and why it should not carry a stigma.

REFERENCES

Adams, R., & Victor, M. (1985). *Principles of neurology* (3d ed.) (p. 273). New York: McGraw-Hill.

Bagley, C. (1971). *The social psychology of the child with epilepsy* (p. 106). Coral Gables, FL: University of Miami Press.

Bagley, C. (1972). Social prejudice and the adjustment of people with epilepsy. *Epilepsia, 13,* 33.

Beniak, J.A., & Beniak, T.E. (1983). Social isolation. In M. Snyder (Ed.), *A guide to neurological and neurosurgical nursing* (p. 268). New York: Wiley.

Caveness, W.F., & Gallup, G.H. (1980). A survey of public attitudes toward epilepsy in 1979 with an indication of trends over the past thirty years. *Epilepsia, 21,* 50.

Dalessio, D.J. (1985). Seizure disorders and pregnancy. *New England Journal of Medicine, 312*(9), 559.

Dodrill, C., Batzel, L., Queisser, H., & Temkin, N. (1980). An objective method for the assessment of psychologic and social problems in epileptics. *Epilepsia, 21*, 123.

Giordani, B., Sackellares, J.C., Miller, S., et al. (1983). Improvement in neuropsychological performance in patients with refractory seizures after intensive diagnostic and therapeutic intervention. *Neurology, 33*, 489.

Gordon, M. (1987). *Manual of nursing diagnosis: 1986–87*. New York: McGraw-Hill.

Green, L., & Roter, D. (1977). The literature on patient compliance and implications for cost-effective patient education programs in epilepsy. In Commission for the Control of Epilepsy and Its Consequences (Eds.), *I. Plan for nationwide action on epilepsy* (Vol. II, Part I, Sections I-IV). Washington, DC: Dept. of HEW.

Haynes, R.B. (1979). Determinants of compliance: The disease and the mechanics of treatment. In R.B. Haynes, D.W. Taylor, & D.L. Sackett (Eds.), *Compliance in health care* (p. 49). Baltimore: Johns Hopkins University Press.

Haynes, R.B. (1979). Strategies to improve compliance with referrals, appointments, and prescribed medical regimens. In R.B. Haynes, D.W. Taylor, & D.L. Sackett (Eds.), *Compliance in health care* (p. 121). Baltimore: Johns Hopkins University Press.

Hogue, C.C. (1979). Nursing and compliance. In R.B. Haynes, D.W. Taylor, & D.L. Sackett (Eds.), *Compliance in health care* (p. 247). Baltimore: Johns Hopkins University Press.

Janz, D. (1982). On major malformations and minor anomalies in the offspring of parents with epilepsy: Review of the literature. In D. Janz, M. Dam, A. Richens, L. Bossi, H. Helge, & D. Schmidt (Eds.), *Epilepsy, pregnancy and the child* (p. 211). New York: Raven Press.

Jennings, M.T., & Bird, T.D. (1981). Genetic influences in the epilepsies. *American Journal of Diseases of Children, 135*, 450.

Kutt, H., & Penry, J.K. (1974). Usefulness of blood levels of antiepileptic drugs. *Archives of Neurology, 31*, 283.

Lechtenberg, R., & Akner, L. (1984). Psychologic adaptation of children to epilepsy in a parent. *Epilepsia, 25*(1), 40.

Loiseau, P., Strube, E., Broustet, D., et al. (1983). Learning impairment in epileptic patients. *Epilepsia, 24*, 183.

Marston, M.V. (1970). Compliance with medical regimens: A review of the literature. *Nursing Research, 19*(4), 312.

Mungus, D., Ehlers, C., Walton, N., & McCutcheon, C. (1985). Verbal learning differences in epileptic patients with left and right temporal lobe foci. *Epilepsia, 26*(4), 340.

National Spokesman, newsletter of the Epilepsy Foundation of America, Washington DC, 1985, *18* (3–5).

Ozuna, J. (1979). Psychosocial aspects of epilepsy. *Journal of Neurosurgical Nursing, 11*(4), 242.

Ozuna, J., & Cammermeyer, M. (1982). Learning needs of the epilepsy patient. In M.J. VanMeter (Ed.), Neurologic care: A guide for patient education (p. 133). New York: Appleton-Century-Crofts.

Pippenger, C.E. (1979). Therapeutic drug monitoring: An overview. *Therapeutic Drug Monitoring, 1*, 3.

Risch, F., & Rose, A. (1957). Community plan for epileptics. *Public Health Reports, 72*(9), 813.

Rosenstock, I.M. (1966). Why people use health services. *Milbank Memorial Fund Quarterly, 44*(3), 95.

Sackett, D. (1979). A compliance practicum for the busy practiner. In R.B. Haynes, D.W. Taylor, & D.L. Sackett (Eds.), *Compliance in health care* (p. 286). Baltimore: Johns Hopkins University Press.

Sackett, D. (1977). Why don't patients take their medicine? *Canadian Family Physician, 23*, 462.

Shope, J.T. (1982). The patient's perspective. In R.B. Black, B.P. Hermann, & J.T. Shope (Eds.), *Nursing management of epilepsy* (p. 54). Rockville, MD: Aspen.

Snyder, M. (1983). Effect of relaxation on psychosocial functioning in persons with epilepsy. *Journal of Neurosurgical Nursing, 15*(4), 250.

Trimble, M.R., & Reynolds, E.H. (1976). Anticonvulsant drugs and mental symptoms: A review. *Psychological Medicine, 6*, 169.

Voeller, K.K., & Rothenberg, M.B. (1973). Psychosocial aspects of the management of seizures in children. *Pediatrics, 51*(6), 1072.

9

Rhythmic Alterations in Consciousness: Sleep

Mary A. Chuman

The rhythmic nature of sleep and wakefulness has fascinated humans from antiquity to the present. Attempts to uncover the mysteries of sleep have led to the observation and measurement of the sleep-wake cycle under various conditions. Many variables are known to influence the sleep-wake cycle, such as neurochemical, physiologic, psychologic, developmental, and temporal factors. As humans have searched for the mechanisms responsible for sleep, many theories have been proposed to account for the necessity of this time-consuming behavior. These theories describe the purpose of sleep as restorative, energy conserving, protective, instinctive, or ethologically adaptive. The purpose of this chapter is to review the physiologic, psychologic, anatomic, and biochemical correlates of sleep, to describe human responses to disordered sleep, and to describe sleep hygiene interventions appropriate to nursing practice.

PHYSIOLOGIC AND PSYCHOLOGIC CORRELATES OF SLEEP

Throughout the human life span, the body demonstrates a regular alternation between states of wakefulness and states of sleep. Sleep itself has a cyclical organization and can be divided into two main parts: rapid eye movement (REM) sleep and non-REM (NREM) sleep. Thus, the human body alternates among three states: wakefulness, NREM sleep, and REM sleep. Rhythmic alterations in consciousness are associated with each sleep-wake cycle, along with certain biochemical, physiologic, and behavioral changes.

Wakefulness

The frequency of electroencephalogram (EEG) activity is used to classify types of brainwave activity by the number of cycles per second (cps). Four frequency bands are used: delta 1–4 cps, theta 4–8 cps, alpha 8–12 cps, and beta 13–35 cps (Gaillard, 1983). The EEG of an awake person, with eyes open and involved in some activity, is characterized by spontaneous, low-voltage, rapid, beta band electrical activity. In this viligant state, the EEG is random and desynchronized; the desynchrony is associated with the intense cortical activity of the alert or vigilant awakened state.

Electroencephalographic analysis for vigilance assessment indicates that there are rhythmic fluctuations in vigilance during the waking state (Okawa et al., 1984). The vigilance pattern shows large differences from one person to another, with periods of vigilance lasting between 60 and 110 minutes.

Some researchers suggest that there is a circadian rhythm for alertness that is independent of the sleep-wake cycle (Folkard et al., 1985). Evidence from sleep deprivation and shiftwork studies is used to support this suggestion.

Non-Rapid Eye Movement Sleep
Non-REM sleep also is called quiet, slow wave, or S-state sleep. It is subdivided into four stages (stages 1, 2, 3, and 4) based on each stage's characteristic electroencephalogram (EEG), electrooculogram (EOG), and electromyogram (EMG) patterns (Rechtschaffen & Kales, 1968). Frequently, stages 3 and 4 are treated as one stage called slow wave sleep (SWS) or delta sleep. Stage 1 is a transitional phase that is intermediate between full wakefulness and sleep. In normal sleepers, it lasts only a few minutes. Stage 1 is seen as a prelude to sleep onset or after body movements during sleep and is characterized by moderate amplitude theta activity.

Stage 2 is marked by the intermittent appearance of three relatively low amplitude EEG patterns on the background of theta waves: vertex sharp waves that appear at the onset of this stage, sleep spindles, and K-complexes.

Delta sleep (stages 3 and 4) receives its name from the progressively larger and slower delta waves, slow wave sleep (SWS), which must dominate ≥20% of the EEG to characterize this stage. Spindles also may be seen. Somatosensory evoked responses are diminished during SWS; this is compatible with the decreased cerebral responsiveness accompanying the slower, high-voltage, synchronous EEG activity of deep sleep. Eye movements are absent, and EMG activity is low.

Circadian rhythms, behavioral states, and diseases can affect the physiologic changes during sleep states. Under normal conditions, many physiologic parameters decrease during NREM sleep. There is a decrease in blood pressure, cardiac output, core body temperature, gastric acid secretion, heart rate, and heart rate variability (Mancia & Zanchetti, 1980). The lowest heart rate and blood pressure levels are reached during SWS. Periodic variability in minute ventilation is seen in stages 1 and 2. During SWS, there is a small increase in tidal volume and a small decrease in minute ventilation (Sullivan, 1980). Occasional irregular breathing and pauses may be seen. Decreases occur in muscle activity, tone, and oxygen consumption, although people still have enough muscle activity to maintain various sleeping postures. Body position changes are made most frequently during NREM sleep or in transitions from NREM to REM sleep.

Regional cerebral blood flow to the hemispheres decreases during NREM sleep despite a slight elevation in P_{CO_2} (Sakai et al., 1980). Carbon dioxide is a potent vasodilator during normal wakefulness. Cerebral vasomotor responsiveness to carbon dioxide thus appears to be decreased during NREM sleep.

During NREM sleep, growth hormone is secreted in an episodic, pulsatile pattern from the anterior pituitary gland. Although this secretion also occurs during wakefulness (after meals, physical exertion, or psychologic stress), the peak plasma growth hormone concentration occurs during the first SWS stage after the onset of nocturnal sleep (Takahashi, 1979). Growth hormone is known to enhance amino acid transport across cell membranes and to promote protein synthesis. Observations on the sleep-dependent nature of growth hormone secretion have led to speculation that SWS promotes tissue restoration. Luteinizing hormone and follicle-stimulating hormone show a sleep dependency around the age of puberty, but this association does not persist into adulthood. In contrast, testosterone shows a pubertal sleep dependency and continues to show peak plasma levels during sleep into adulthood. This peak accompanies phase shifts in sleep. Possibly, the transition from NREM to REM sleep is associated with testosterone secretion (Roffwarg et al., 1982).

Rapid Eye Movement Sleep

Rapid eye movement (REM) sleep is identified by relatively low voltage, asynchronous, mixed-frequency EEG activity resembling stage 1 sleep, except for the occasional appearance of sawtooth waves. Rapid eye movements and muscle atonia, or a greatly reduced level of EMG activity, are only some of the physiologic characteristics of this sleep state. REM sleep is subdivided into two components: tonic events and phasic events. Whereas SWS is sometimes referred to as orthodox sleep, REM is sometimes called paradoxical sleep. The paradox is that REM sleep is very deep, with higher waking thresholds than in SWS, yet fast asynchronous cortical EEG activity is present (generally a sign of wakefulness) along with diminished muscle tone (an indication of deep sleep). Individuals awakened during paradoxical sleep usually report that they were dreaming.

The tonic or continuous events of REM sleep include desynchronization of the cortical EEG, hippocampal theta waves, diminished or absent deep tendon reflexes, and greatly diminished or absent skeletal muscle tone, especially in the neck and chin (also known as postural atonia). The phasic or intermittent component of REM sleep includes conjugate rapid eye movements, muscle twitches of the limbs and face, penile tumescence, increased brain temperature, and in some experimental animals, high voltage EEG spikes in the pons, lateral geniculate nucleus, and occipital cortex (PGO waves). The pupils can dilate and constrict phasically. Oxygen consumption is elevated, and the vital signs are highly variable. Increased variability in blood pressure and heart rate is seen with transient elevation of up to 40 mm Hg in blood pressure (Mancia & Zanchetti, 1980). Respiration is altered. Minute ventilation, tidal volume, and $PaCO_2$ approach waking levels (Sullivan, 1980). Rapid eye movement bursts and other phasic REM events are associated with irregular breathing episodes (Orem, 1980). In normal children, breathing pauses, oxygen desaturation, and elevated diaphragmatic workload occur especially during REM sleep (Gaultier et al., 1985). It has been speculated that the phasic excitation of body systems during REM sleep may trigger pathophysiologic events in susceptible individuals (e.g., cardiac arrhythmias, sudden infant death syndrome).

During REM sleep, although the cerebral vasomotor responsiveness (vasodilation) to carbon dioxide is decreased, the regional cerebral blood flow increases in both hemispheres of the brain (Ingvar, 1979). These changes do not influence intracranial pressure (ICP) under normal conditions. In people with intracranial pathology, however, REM sleep can precipitate large elevations in ICP (Ross et al., 1975). The association of REM sleep with increased cerebral blood flow, increased brain temperature, and the appearance of a REM rebound phenomenon after sleep deprivation has led to speculation that REM sleep is linked with protein synthesis, memory storage, memory consolidation, and learning (Fishbein & Gutwein, 1981; Squire & Davis, 1981). Further support for this idea comes from animal studies in which protein synthesis inhibitors have been shown to disrupt REM sleep and learning (Drucker-Colin & Espejel, 1980).

SLEEP PATTERNS

For an adult, a typical night of sleep begins with a brief period of stage 1 followed by stage 2 sleep and SWS. NREM sleep continues for approximately 70 to 100 minutes, and then the first period of REM sleep begins. This first REM sleep lasts only about 5 minutes. This sequence of sleep stages (beginning with stages 1–4 NREM and ending with a REM period) is called a sleep cycle. The average sleep cycle is 90 minutes in adults and 60 minutes in infants. An adult's sleep cycle is repeated four to six times each night, depending on the total length of time spent sleeping (total sleep time). In the early part of the night, SWS is most prevalent within the sleep cycle; it is less prevalent toward the end of the total sleep period. REM periods lengthen as the night progresses and the percentage of SWS within a cycle diminishes. The transition from NREM to REM sleep is smoother than the reverse transition at the end of a REM episode (Gaillard, 1983). In fact, dreaming sleep sometimes appears to disrupt sleep continuity; some insomniacs complain of agitated sleep from too much dreaming in the late hours of the night. The adult total sleep period is composed of REM: 20% to 25%, stage 1: 5% to 10%, stage 2: 50% to 60%, and SWS: 10% to 20% (Kales & Kales, 1984).

In infants under 1 year of age, the classification of sleep stages by EEG does not correlate well with other sleep signs (eye movements and muscle tone). Instead, the behavioral state of the sleeping infant can be observed directly. Active and quiet sleeping behaviors, with cycles lasting 40 to 60 minutes, tend to be stable around 36 weeks gestational age. Behavioral states are identified using the infant's muscle tone, motor activity, respirations, eye opening, and eye movement (Thoman, 1975). The criteria of active sleep are irregular (uneven) respirations that are primarily costal in nature, eyes closed, intermittent rapid eye movements, and sporadic motor movements with low muscle tone between movements. The criteria of quiet sleep are eyes closed, respirations relatively slow and abdominal in nature, and tonic level of muscle tone and motor activity limited to occasional startles or sigh sobs. Preterm and small-for-gestational-age infants have greater rates of behavioral state changes than do term infants. This altered rate in sleep behavior cycles persists for 4 weeks postdischarge and can affect maternal perceptions of preterm infants (Watt & Strongman, 1985).

Age affects many sleep patterns: total sleep time, percentage of sleep stages, and sleep disturbances. Individual sleep requirements for the healthy adult can vary widely; sleep needs may be from 3 hours to up to 12 hours per night. In general, total sleep time decreases as people grow older. Newborns and infants sleep approximately 17 to 18 hours in a 24-hour period. This time decreases to 10 to 12 hours around age 4, and to 9 to 10 hours at age 10. Adolescents and adults average 7.5 hours of sleep; older aged adults sleep about 6.5 hours per day (Hauri, 1982b). Older children and adults tend to consolidate sleep time into one sleep period; napping is usually not a regular habit, although napping becomes more common with advanced age. Children spend a larger percentage of sleep time in REM (50%) and SWS (20% to 25%) than do adults. Very little SWS is seen in elderly people, and stages 1 and 2 gradually increase with age.

Circadian Sleep-Wake Cycle
Human beings live in a rhythmic world and are exposed to many external perioidicities. These rhythmic influences range from events occurring on a time scale of years (e.g., sunspot cycles) to annual, monthly, and daily oscillations. The dominant rhythm in humans shows a period of 24 hours in synchrony with the light-dark cycle of the solar day. Rhythms that follow this periodicity of about 24 hours are termed circadian.

A circadian rhythm is seen in human behavioral patterns (e.g., activity, food intake, rest, and sleep) as well as physiologic patterns (e.g., body temperature, endocrine secretions, and metabolism).

In healthy people who conform to a regular sleep-wake and rest-activity cycle, there is a circadian periodicity in plasma cortisol levels and urinary 17-hydroxycorticosteroid (17-OHCS) excretion, as well as in plasma ACTH, thyrotropin, renin, corticotropin and prolactin, urinary potassium, catecholamine, and aldosterone levels (Reinberg & Smolensky, 1983). These rhythmic variations in plasma biochemical levels persist even during sleep deprivation or a shift in the sleep-wake cycle. Currently, researchers are studying circadian rhythms in performance, vigilance, mood, pain threshold, cell proliferation, and responses to drugs and toxins.

Body temperature fluctuates with circadian rhythmicity around a mean of 36.8°C. Normally, temperatures are low during sleep, rise after waking, and peak with an individual's maximum efficiency level. Sleep duration and sleep structure appear to be closely related to circadian rhythms for body temperature. Sleep duration depends more on the circadian phase of body temperature than on the prior amount of wakefulness (Czeisler et al., 1980a). A maximum sleep time is obtained when sleep onset occurs at the maximum core body temperature. The composition of sleep cycles changes with temperature fluctuations; the propensity for REM sleep is increased when sleep onset occurs after the low point of the temperature cycle (Czeisler et al., 1980b). Thus, REM sleep is usually enhanced during a few hours in the morning. Changes in daytime body temperature also can affect sleep cycles. Passive body heating (90 minute waterbath at 41°C) in the late afternoon (2:30 to 5:30 PM) produces an increase in presleep tiredness and SWS (Horne & Reid, 1985). The amount of body heating during exercise, rather than the amount of energy expended, appears to be important in causing increases in total NREM sleep time and SWS (Horne & Moore, 1985). When body cooling accompanies exercise, there is no increase in SWS. Sleep is disturbed by a fever or an elevated ambient temperature; the number and duration of awakenings during sleep are increased. Fever also decreases the amount of REM and SWS (Karacan et al., 1968, 1978).

Sleep Deprivation

Sleep-wake cycle disturbances can result from total or partial sleep deprivation. Researchers have found that, after 48 to 72 hours of total sleep deprivation, it is impossible to prevent sleep completely. Episodes of "minisleeps," which last a few seconds, begin to intrude on wakefulness. Lapses of attention accompany minisleeps. The EEG shows stage 1 or other NREM or REM waves. As the total sleep deprivation time increases, the frequency and duration of minisleeps increase. Sleep-deprived individuals complain of fatigue and sleepiness (which follow a diurnal rhythm). They may appear irritable, serious, or listless. In rare cases, individuals experience visual or tactile hallucinations, personality disorders, or a loss of emotional control. In contrast to the majority of people, patients with endogenous depression often experience an elevation in mood after a night of total sleep deprivation (Van den Burg & Van den Hoofdakker, 1975).

After 24 to 48 hours of deprivation, cognitive task performance, vigilance, mood, and motor skills deteriorate (Haslam, 1984; Opstad et al., 1978), and people report that it takes greater effort to perform tasks requiring speed or perseverance. The behavioral and psychologic effects of sleep deprivation can diminish performance measurably, although recovery to baseline performance levels usually occurs after only 4 hours of sleep. The performance of simple, well-learned physical tasks appears to be unaffected by sleep deprivation (Kolka et al., 1984; Haslam, 1984). In preparation for a period of total sleep deprivation, relatively short periods of sleep (about 4 hours) have been shown to have a beneficial effect on subsequent performance, even in the absence of a prior sleep debt (Nicholson et al., 1985).

Some investigators report that total sleep deprivation disturbs metabolic indices and elevates corticosteroid and catecholamine levels (Kant et al., 1984), whereas others found no significant biologic effects with total sleep deprivation (Ahnve et al., 1981; Horne, 1978). The psychologic state of the individual (e.g., frustration, anxiety, situational or anticipatory uncertainty) may be responsible for many of the changes seen with sleep deprivation (Francesconi et al., 1978).

Partial sleep deprivation may involve a curtailment in the total amount of sleep time or a selective deprivation of sleep stages (REM or NREM). Restricting sleep to fewer than 4 hours of sleep per night results in reduced amounts of stage 2 and REM sleep; the amount of SWS is usually unaltered (Akerstedt & Torsvall, 1985). Vigilance, mood, and the performance of more difficult cognitive tasks decrease rapidly the first 4 days of sleep curtailment (4 hours of total sleep) and then level out (Haslam, 1984). Physical fitness remains adequate. A less severe reduction in sleep time appears to be more easily tolerated. Horne and Wilkinson (1985) report that chronic moderate sleep reduction (reduced from 8 hours per night to 6) can be learned easily and tolerated by young, healthy adults. Overall, subjects accomplished this reduction by strictly adhering to bed and arising times for 6 weeks; daytime mood and performance were unaffected.

The most striking feature of REM sleep deprivation is REM rebound (Dement et al., 1967). When REM-deprived individuals are allowed to sleep, the time to REM sleep is reduced and the intensity of REM phenomena is increased. Large individual differences in the degree of REM rebound are seen (Antonioli et al., 1981), and the selective deprivation of REM sleep appears to affect mood and motivational behavior (Vogel, 1975). Most common are reports of agitation, hyperactivity, emotional lability, and decreased impulse control (Naitoh et al., 1971). In contrast, people with selective NREM sleep deprivation tend to be hyporesponsive, withdrawn, and more physically uncomfortable (Agnew et al., 1967). Delta sleep (SWS) deprivation also produces a delta rebound, which is less intense and intrusive than REM rebound.

Certain agents (e.g., drugs, alcohol, anesthetics), procedures (e.g., surgery), or diseases (e.g., Alzheimer's disease, Morvan's chorea) may produce sleep deprivation through a fundamental disarrangement of the sleep-wake regulating system. For example, surgical intensive care patients continue to experience sleep deprivation despite constant pain relief and minimal environmental disturbances (Aurell & Elmqvist, 1985; Dohno et al., 1979). Under presumed optimal conditions for sleep, the mean cumulative sleep time was less than 2 hours for a minimum of 2 days (Aurell & Elmqvist, 1985). Notably, nurses grossly misjudged and consistently overestimated sleep time as compared with parallel EEG evidence. Stage 3 and 4 and REM sleep were severely or completely suppressed.

ANATOMIC AND BIOCHEMICAL CORRELATES OF SLEEP

The states of sleep and wakefulness have reciprocal interacting, complementary mechanisms; both states are active rather than passive physiologic and biochemical processes. As described in Chapter 5, the state of wakefulness is maintained by intact cerebral hemispheres interacting with the thalamus, hypothalmus, and brainstem. An activated ascending reticular activating system (ARAS), as well as intact neuroanatomic structures, is required for wakefulness. Decreased ARAS activity (low levels of sensory, motor, and mental input), however, does not cause sleep onset automatically. A deactivation of the ARAS is required, along with an active initiation of the sleep process. This hypnogenic or sleep-producing system consists of neuronal areas in the bulbar part of the lower brainstem, the raphe median nuclear complex of the middle brainstem, the ventromedian central thalamus, and the preoptic region of the anteromedian hypothalamus (Monnier, 1983). The neuronal systems that regulate sleep and wakefulness are functionally interacting.

The anatomic neuronal pathways required for sleep and wakefulness are subject also to biochemical regulation. Neurotransmitters alter the excitability of postsynaptic nerve cells (depolarize or hyperpolarize). Other chemical substances have a more general effect on neurons by altering or modulating the baseline metabolic activity or response to other neuronal input. The transmitters and modulators involved in the biochemical regulation of sleep and wakefulness include serotonin, norepinephrine, dopamine, acetylcholine, amino acids (e.g., tryptophan, L-glutamate, glycine, aspartate, taurine, gamma-aminobutyric acid), steroid hormones, neuropeptides and related factors (e.g., beta-endorphin, enkephalin, angiotensin, somatostatin).

There are two major groups of theories that attempt to describe the phenomenon of sleep: the *monoamine theory* of sleep and the *general interaction chemical theory* of sleep. The *monoaminergic theory* of Jouvet (1969) attempts to correlate specific behavioral states, biochemical activity, and neuroanatomic sites of activity. In this theory, the sleep-wake cycle is postulated to be modulated by the balance between serotonergic neuron activity and catecholaminergic neuron activity. The catecholaminergic systems and cholinergic systems are involved in the behavioral and cortical activation of tonic arousal and the execution of REM sleep (Bremer, 1977; Monnier & Gaillard, 1980). The serotonergic median raphe nuclei in the midbrain, pons, and medulla are involved with sleep induction, the maintenance of SWS, and the priming of the brain for transition to REM sleep. REM onset is associated with the secretion of norepinephrine by the locus coeruleus.

In the monoamine theory, specific neurotransmitters and neuroanatomic sites are considered responsible for active mechanisms that initiate and maintain wakefulness (acetylcholine, norepinephrine, dopamine), NREM sleep (serotonin), and REM sleep (norepinephrine). A large number of research findings, however, challenge this mechanistic view and propose a general interaction chemical theory of sleep (Morgane, 1981; Jones, 1979; Ramm, 1980). These researchers describe sleep and wakefulness as the result of multiple independently converging influences involving all areas of the nervous system. The discharge rate, timing, and input–output organization of neurons are studied. Reciprocal interactions between specialized brainstem cells are used to build integrative models of sleep and waking (McCarley & Hobson, 1975; Pompeiano & Valentinuzzi, 1976).

Sleep-inducing or hypnogenic factors, including factor S (Pappenheimer, 1979), delta sleep-inducing peptide (Monnier et al., 1975), and a REM-triggering protein substance R (Drucker-Colin et al., 1980) have been isolated in animals. Peptides and humoral factors are postulated sleep producers in humans, but as yet no endogenous sleep factor has been discovered. The nocturnal administration of L-tryptophan, a precursor of serotonin, is sometimes recommended for use as a soporific. Hartmann and Spinweber (1979) reported that this agent reduces sleep latency and increases the amount of SWS. Other researchers, however, have found that L-tryptophan, in doses up to 1 g, fails to alter sleep latency or sleep stages (Adam & Oswald, 1979; Small et al., 1979).

HUMAN RESPONSES TO ALTERATIONS IN SLEEP-WAKE PATTERNS

Human sleep is influenced by many endogenous and environmental factors. Modern sleep-wake problems are further exacerbated by changing lifestyles, work patterns, noise, pollution, stress, and many other environmental conditions. Sleep disorders are common in the United States and many other industrialized countries. Each year, over 10 million Americans consult a physician about the quality of their sleep, and approximately 50 million adults report sleep difficulties (Institute of Medicine, 1979). Many more people suffer from excessive daytime somnolence and sleep-related problems (e.g., nightmares, nocturnal myoclonus).

Age Factors in Responses

The type and frequency of sleep disturbances vary with age. About 20% to 30% of children in the first 4 years of life have regular sleeping difficulties (e.g., bedtime fears or struggles, night waking, enuresis). Frequently, these difficulties are transient, developmental, or parental management problems. Some sleep problems, however, can be associated with more pervasive disturbances in the child or family. In a study by Lozoff et al. (1985), pediatric sleep problems were defined as night waking involving parents or bedtime struggles occurring 3 or more times per week for at least 1 month, accompanied by conflict or stress. Five experiences distinguished children with persistent sleep problems from those without: family illness or accident, unaccustomed daytime maternal absence, depressed maternal mood(s), sleeping in the parental bed, and ambivalent maternal attitude toward the child. The investigators noted that if pediatric practitioners did not question families routinely about sleep difficulties, the undetected childhood sleep problems could persist for 1 or more years.

After middle adulthood, the quality and temporal organization of sleep appears to be much more easily disrupted. There is an increase in the number of awakenings after sleep onset, as well as greater difficulty in returning to sleep after waking. Complaints of less restful sleep increase. Affectively charged or mood-disturbing events can modify REM sleep characteristics (Cartwright, 1983). The incidence of sleep apneas, nocturnal myoclonus, and other sleep disorders increases markedly with age.

Disorders of Sleep-Wake Pattern
In 1979, the Association of Sleep Disorders Centers (ASDC) published a diagnostic classification of sleep and arousal disorders (Table 9-1). This classification is more precise than the one category regarding sleep problems in North American Nursing Diagnosis Association classification (e.g., sleep pattern disturbance). Further, it separates problems underlying difficulty falling asleep from those associated with lack of feeling rested and excessive sleepiness. The ASDC classification includes disorders that require medical diagnosis and treatment as well as those appropriately managed entirely within the scope of nursing practice.

Four types of disorders are recognized: disorders of initiating and maintaining sleep (DIMS), disorders of excessive somnolence (DOES), disorders of sleep-wake schedule, and dysfunctions associated with sleep, sleep stages, or partial arousals (parasomnias). The patient's chief complaint is used to categorize disorders. This avoids confusion in the use of the term "insomnia," which has been used frequently to refer to any difficulty in sleeping and has encompassed all gradations and types of sleep loss. Thus, a chief complaint of poor sleep places a patient in the DIMS (insomnias) category, whereas a pathologic tendency toward sleep when wakefulness is needed places the person in the DOES category (despite concurrent nocturnal sleep distruption). Disorders of the sleep-wake cycle refer to sleep problems that arise from either disturbances in the individual's endogenous biologic clock (e.g., non-24 hour cycle) or changes in the external environment that do not follow the individual's own biologic rhythm (e.g., jet lag, shiftwork). Disturbances that are coincident with sleep are called parasomnias. The category "not otherwise specified" is included under each classification to allow for both undiagnosed (unknown cause) and additional conditions that may be described in the future.

Only selected disorders are discussed in this chapter. A full description of the structure and guidelines for diagnoses is given by the ASDC and Association of the Psychophysiological Study of Sleep (1979). The collective experience of the ASDC shows that of the patient population treated for sleep disorders, the diagnoses were 51% DOES, 31% DIMS (insomnias), and 15% parasomnias. Of the DOES patients, the subclassifications were 43% sleep apnea, 25% narcolepsy, and 9% idiopathic central nervous system hypersomnolence (Coleman et al., 1982).

☐ **Disorders of Initiating and Maintaining Sleep**

Most transient and situational disorders in initiating and maintaining sleep (DIMS) are triggered by an unfamiliar sleep environment, emotional shock, loss or threat, conflict or acute emotional arousal. The appearance of DIMS correlates with increased life stress measures (Cernovsky, 1984). Usually, a precipitating event is easily identifiable, and the insomnia lasts less than 3 weeks. Sometimes, hypnotics are indicated to allow the patient to rest (decrease sleep onset time and decrease nocturnal or early morning awakenings) and to prevent reinforced learning or conditioned negative associations that can lead to a persistent insomnia. Relaxation exercises and sleep hygiene are helpful. In postoperative patients with mild or moderate pain, a combination of

TABLE 9-1. DIAGNOSTIC CLASSIFICATION OF SLEEP AND AROUSAL DISORDERS.

DIMS: Disorders of initiating and maintaining sleep (insomnias)
- Psychophysiologic
  Transient and situational
  Persistent
- Associated with psychiatric disorders
  Symptoms and personality disorders
  Affective disorders
  Other functional psychoses
- Associated with use of drugs and alcohol
  Tolerance to or withdrawal from CNS depressants
  Sustained use of CNS stimulants
  Sustained use of or withdrawal from other drugs
  Chronic alcoholism
- Associated with sleep-induced respiratory impairment
  Sleep apnea DIMS syndrome
  Alveolar hypoventilation DIMS syndrome
- Associated with sleep-related (nocturnal) myoclonus and restless legs
  Sleep-related (nocturnal) myoclonus DIMS syndrome
  Restless legs DIMS syndrome
- Associated with other medical, toxic, and environmental conditions
- Childhood-onset DIMS
- Associated with other DIMS conditions
  Repeated REM sleep interruptions
  Atypical polysomnographic features
  Not otherwise specified

DOES: Disorders of excessive somnolence
- Psychophysiologic
  Transient and situational
  Persistent
- Associated with psychiatric disorders
  Affective disorders
  Other functional disorders
- Associated with use of drugs and alcohol
  Tolerance to or withdrawal from CNS stimulants
  Sustained use of CNS depressants
- Associated with sleep-induced respiratory impairment
  Sleep apnea DOES syndrome
  Alveolar hypoventilation DOES syndrome
- Associated with sleep-related (nocturnal) myoclonus and restless legs
  Sleep-related (nocturnal) myoclonus DOES syndrome
  Restless legs DOES syndrome
- Narcolepsy
- Idiopathic CNS hypersomnolence

DOES: Disorders of excessive somnolence (continued)
- Associated with other medical, toxic, and environmental conditions
- Associated with other DOES conditions
  Intermittent DOES (periodic) syndromes
    Kleine-Levin syndrome
    Menstrual-associated syndrome
  Insufficient sleep
  Sleep drunkenness
  Not otherwise specified
- No DOES abnormality
  Longer sleeper
  Subjective DOES complaint without objective findings
  Not otherwise specified

Disorders of the sleep-wake schedule
- Transient
  Rapid time zone change (jet lag) syndrome
  Work shift change in conventional sleep-wake schedule
- Persistent
  Frequently changing sleep-wake schedule
  Delayed sleep phase syndrome
  Advanced sleep phase syndrome
  Non-24-hour sleep-wake syndrome
  Irregular sleep-wake pattern
  Not otherwise specified

Dysfunctions associated with sleep, sleep stages, or partial arousals (parasomnias)
- Sleepwalking (somnambulism)
- Sleep terror (pavor nocturnus, incubus)
- Sleep-related enuresis (bedwetting)
- Other dysfunctions
  Dream anxiety attacks (nightmares)
  Sleep-related epileptic seizures
  Sleep-related bruxism
  Sleep-related headbanging (jactatio capitis nocturnus)
  Familial sleep paralysis
  Impaired sleep-related penile tumescence
  Sleep-related painful erections
  Sleep-related cluster headaches and chronic paroxysmal hemicrania
  Sleep-related abnormal swallowing syndrome
  Sleep-related asthma
  Sleep-related cardiovascular symptoms
  Sleep-related gastroesophageal reflux
  Sleep-related hemolysis (paroxysmal nocturnal hemoglobinuria)
  Asymptomatic polysomnographic finding
  Not otherwise specified

From Association of Sleep Disorders Centers, 1979.

an analgesic and a sedative may enhance sleep more than the use of one drug alone (Smith & Smith, 1985).

A more serious and chronic complaint of DIMS requires assessment. This includes problems that last longer than 3 weeks, interfere significantly with daytime performance and mood, remain unchanged by strong attempts at treatment, and are not secondary to ongoing, diagnosed medical or psychiatric problems. A *sleep history* is the first step in understanding the complaint. The following issues are usually explored: (1) chief sleep complaint, including time course, relationship to stress, and initial triggering events, (2) self-treatment measures used for the problem, medication, and nondrug therapies, (3) daytime performance and mood, (4) other complaints associated with sleep, (5) prior sleep history throughout the patient's life cycle, and (6) the patient's view of the problem, its meaning, its possible cause, and its chance of being treated (Hauri, 1982a).

A *sleep log* may supplement the initial history. For 7 to 14 days, the patient records the time of sleep onset, sleep latency, nocturnal awakenings, total sleep time, time of arising, and feelings on awakening. Drug intake, coffee and alcohol intake, and naps are recorded. An interview with the patient's bed partner often provides helpful information. DIMS may stem from medical, psychiatric, or environmental problems, and a complete medical diagnostic work-up is necessary to differentiate medical from environmental problems. Medical causes may include sleep apnea or myoclonus.

Sleep apneic patients who complain of frequent nocturnal awakenings usually show predominantly central apneas. Although DIMS is the predominant subjective report, mixed apneas and excessive daytime somnolence also may be present. Sleep apnea syndromes are discussed in the section "Disorders of Excessive Somnolence" in this chapter.

DIMS associated with sleep-related myoclonus is characterized by muscle contractions in the form of jerks or twitches that repeat every 20 to 40 seconds. Episodes occur primarily in the flexor groups in the lower extremities and last from 5 minutes to 2 hours. In contrast, restless legs syndrome occurs during wakefulness as well as sleep. An unpleasant creeping sensation appears during rest and produces an irresistible urge to move the limbs (primarily dorsiflexion of the feet and flexion of the legs at the hip and knee). This syndrome may arise from motoneuron disease, diseases causing neuropathies, or genetic inheritance (Montplaisir et al., 1985).

In the medical treatment of DIMS complaints, hypnotics initially are effective but lose their efficacy when used chronically. Habituation may be prevented by episodic use (only once or twice weekly) for the more serious, chronic DIMS patients. Nursing judgment in administering hypnotics includes recognition that rebound insomnia can occur on withdrawal, gradual withdrawal (not increased dosage) is required when habituation is present, hypnotics and alcohol interact, and respiratory centers may be depressed (especially in heavy snorers). Sleep hygiene, relaxation and meditation training, and follow-up on psychosocial issues are important. Sleep hygiene needs to be reinforced repeatedly; these measures include regular wake-up time, no daytime naps, no coffee after lunchtime, no evening alcohol, moderate regular exercise, and adequate relaxation time before sleep onset.

☐ Disorders of Excessive Somnolence

Identifying disorders of excessive somnolence (DOES) can be difficult, since complaints of daytime sleepiness are common and present the practitioner with a complex differential diagnosis. Differentiating pathologic sleepiness from normal daily sleepiness (e.g., after meals, warm monotonous setting) depends on: (1) the circumstances and frequency of the sleepiness and (2) ruling out other causes of sleepiness, such as endocrine, metabolic, infectious, and neoplastic diseases. The defining characteristic is repeated instances of inappropriate sleep (e.g., while driving, eating, conversing, engaging in athletic competition). Physical fatigue and diminished mental alertness, without an increase in sleep behavior, should not be categorized as DOES. Patients must actually be sleepy and easily fall asleep whenever left alone; the sleepiness is daily, inappropriate, and unrelenting (Orr et al., 1982). An objective *assessment* of excessive daytime sleepiness (EDS) is possible using the Multiple Sleep Latency Test (MSLT). Using polysomnographic monitoring, a patient is allowed to fall asleep when put to bed for three to five daytime naps (Richardson et al., 1978). In general, patients with EDS fall asleep in 5 minutes or less, whereas normal subjects average a sleep onset latency of 10 minutes. The appearance of several sleep-onset REM periods is usually diagnostic of narcolepsy (see Case Study 1).

The diagnostic classification of DOES includes a varied group of functional and organic conditions in which the chief symptoms may include sleep attacks, excessive sleeping, inappropriate and unavoidable sleepiness and napping, decreased mental and physical performance, increased total sleep time in a 24-hour period, and difficulty in achieving wakefulness or full arousal (e.g., automatic behaviors, subwakefulness, or sleep drunkenness). Psychophysiologic DOES may develop when a person responds to overwhelming stress, conflicts, or losses with sleepiness, napping, and increased total sleep time. This response is rare; certain people may use it as a withdrawal or passive coping measure.

Usually, a precipitating event is linked easily to the onset of EDS. Problems persisting beyond 3 weeks may be, in fact, DOES-associated psychiatric disorders, chronic toxic and allergic reactions, nocturnal myoclonus, or drug abuse. The manifestation of sleepiness in cases of DOES associated with other medical, neurologic, toxic, and environmental conditions can be variable. For example, EDS can be associated with hypothyroidism, liver failure, hypercapnia associated with chronic pulmonary disease, pregnancy, and many central nervous system disorders. This EDS must be differentiated from conditions that are mistakenly labeled sleepiness, for example, fatigue, lethargy, exhaustion, and signs of disordered consciousness (e.g., stupor, coma, intoxication, confusion).

A definitive diagnosis of DOES associated with sleep-induced respiratory impairment is a medical diagnosis and requires a sophisticated sleep, breathing, oxygen saturation, and cardiac status evaluation. Referral to a respiratory specialist, neurologist–sleep researcher, or sleep disorders center is made once the clinical symptomatology has been identified. Apnea is defined as the cessation of airflow at the nose and mouth of greater than 10 seconds duration; shorter respiratory pauses are not counted. Normal adults may have up to four apneas per hour of sleep. Sleep apnea syndrome is diagnosed if at least 30 apneic episodes are observed during both REM and NREM periods (some of which must appear in a repetitive sequence during NREM) over 7 hours of nocturnal sleep (Guilleminault et al., 1976). Single apneas may last from 10 to 120 seconds and end with partial arousal of the individual.

Central apnea is defined as cessation of airflow past buccal and nasal thermistors along with cessation of abdominal and thoracic respiratory movements measured on strain gauges. Airflow ceases due to a lack of diaphragmatic muscle movement. Pure central apneas are uncommon, and usually patients complain of frequent nocturnal awakenings (DIMS). In *obstructive or upper airway apneas*, airflow past thermistors is absent despite measured thoracic breathing movements and exaggerated inspiratory efforts. Sleep is associated with the relaxation of upper airway muscles, and the airway can become smaller (e.g., snoring is due to compromised airflow) or collapse (obstruction). *Mixed apneas* are a combination of the other two types; a central apnea appears and is followed by an obstructive phase. These apneic episodes during sleep lead to decreased arterial oxygen saturation; levels can be as low as 50% to 60% when measured via ear oximeter. Hypoxemia can lead to EDS, cardiac arrhythmias, pulmonary arterial and systemic hypertension, other cardiovascular abnormalities, early morning headache or confusion, automatic behaviors, personality changes, and deterioration in memory and judgment.

Some sleep apnea DOES syndromes have been associated with upper airway abnormalities: obesity, a short thick neck, retrognathia, micrognathia, genetic components, sleeping position, hypothyroidism, and acromegaly. Sleep apnea is seen predominantly among males and postmenopausal women; the male to female ratio for the occurrence of sleep apneas is about 15:1 (Ingbar & Gee, 1985). Although the mechanisms underlying the sleep apnea syndromes are unknown, sleep-induced brainstem abnormalities are implicated. Sleep apneas are longer during REM and NREM sleep in obstructive apnea patients; hypoxemia is greater during REM than NREM sleep in apneic and normal people (Findley et al., 1985). In asymptomatic men, alcohol ingestion increases the frequency of disordered breathing and apneic episodes (Tassan et al., 1981).

Medical therapeutic measures for a sleep apnea syndrome include weight reduction in obese patients, repair of existing oropharyngeal or mandibular abnormalities, discontinuation of all potential sedating drugs (including alcohol), and avoidance of sleep fragmentation or deprivation (Ingbar & Gee, 1985). Other medical measures include drug therapy, continuous positive airway pressure (CPAP), a tongue-retraining device, and tracheostomy.

Nursing *interventions* are educational and supportive. They include advice about safety and the potential for injury if the person should fall asleep while driving, smoking, or working in dangerous job settings and assisting the person to develop a support system to maintain normal social and occupational activity. The interaction of medical and nursing therapy is illustrated in Case Study 1.

Narcolepsy is a syndrome of unknown origin characterized by excessive daytime sleepiness associated with abnormal manifestations of REM sleep. It occurs in approximately 0.06% to 0.1% of the U.S. population (Dement et al., 1973). The main symptoms of narcolepsy are sleep attacks, cataplexy, sleep paralysis, and hypnagogic hallucinations. Any of the four symptoms can occur alone or in combination with the others. In addition to sleep attacks, narcoleptics suffer from a high level of sleepiness throughout the entire day. In some people, episodes of excessive sleepiness are combined with automatic behaviors and amnesia (Van den Hoed et al., 1981). Narcolepsy is differentiated from other disorders of EDS by the appearance, on EEG, of a sleep-onset REM period (SOREMP) within 1 to 15 minutes of sleep onset (Zarcone, 1973). SOREMPs are a rare occurrence in normal people (e.g., after sleep deprivation, REM-suppressant drug withdrawal, endogenous depression). Ambulatory sleep-wake polygraphy may be used to confirm a clinical diagnosis of narcolepsy and exclude nonnarcoleptic disorders of excessive somnolence or disturbances of consciousness (e.g., psychiatric disorders, epilepsy). A long-standing history of EDS (since the teen years or the 20s) and the presence of auxiliary symptoms (e.g., cataplexy, sleep paralysis, and hypnagogic hallucinations) also help establish the diagnosis of narcolepsy. Familial concentrations of the disorder suggest the involvement of a genetic component (Kessler, 1976).

Cataplexy is the brief (seconds or minutes) sudden loss or weakness of skeletal muscle tone without the loss of consciousness. Cataplectic attacks are usually precipitated by a sudden emotional stimulus, such as laughter, joy, or anger. The safety and social problems posed by these attacks may prove more troublesome to narcoleptics than EDS.

Sleep paralysis occurs in some narcoleptics during the transition between sleep and wakefulness. When falling asleep or waking from sleep, the individual experiences a temporary paralysis of all striated muscles. The person is unable to move any muscles other than the muscles of respiration. The episode usually lasts a few minutes and may be accompanied by intense fear or hypnagogic hallucinations. Sleep paralysis ends spontaneously or terminates immediately when the individual is touched or spoken to by another. The frequency of episodes is highly individual; sleep paralysis may occur daily, weekly, or once or twice in a lifetime. Nonnarcoleptics may have occasional episodes of sleep paralysis when awakening. People often are reluctant to report these attacks for fear they will be labeled as having psychiatric problems. Sleep paralysis is attributed to a disturbance in the production and maintenance of wakefulness and the mechanisms producing the muscle atonia of REM sleep.

Hypnagogic hallucinations are vivid, dreamlike sensory experiences that appear as a person is falling asleep but still conscious. The visual, auditory, or tactile hallucinations occur for approximately 1 to 15 minutes. Hypnagogic hallucinations are thought to arise from a SOREMP; the dream component of REM sleep is experienced during a state of wakefulness.

Case Study 1
Ms. C was a 31-year-old sales representative for an industrial supplies company referred to a medical center neurology clinic for evaluation and management of narcolepsy–cataplexy. She recently had moved to the city and experienced difficulty obtaining prescriptions for the stimulants used to treat narcolepsy. She reported the onset of EDS at about age 20. Inappropriate sleep began occurring during driving, college examinations, and sexual activity. The problem had caused her to switch her career choice from accounting to marketing. She felt that misunderstandings over her symptoms were the major cause of a divorce. Her strategies for coping with EDS and sleep attacks included informing her employer about the illness, scheduling two naps each day of about 20 minutes duration, scheduling sales calls after naps, and choosing a nonsedentary, flexible, independent job with productivity measured by output rather than hours spent in the office. She limited driving to short distances, took extra medication beforehand, rolled the car windows down, and drank cold water to fend off any drowsiness. She stopped driving whenever she became sleepy; walking around or a short nap were used to increase alertness.

At about age 28, Ms. C noticed that during laughter or intense emotions, her knees and neck muscles became weak. Her knees would buckle slightly, and her head and jaw dropped downward for 2 to 5 seconds. The examiner observed several of these episodes while taking the history. Ms. C found these cataplectic attacks socially embarrassing and increasingly bothersome at work. She never went to parties ("I can't relax and I absolutely can't drink alcohol") and had a very limited social life. Thinking about a joke or enjoying a beautiful piece of music would trigger attacks. She reported viewing "life in a peculiar distanced way" in order to prevent precipitating attacks. On further questioning, she revealed that driving sometimes was accompanied by automatic behaviors (e.g., driving to an unknown place and not remembering how she got there). Near-accidents had caused her to rely more on public transportation; her new job required less independent travel. Symptoms of sleep paralysis and hypnagogic hallucinations were not reported.

Other than the observed sudden, brief muscle atonia, Ms. C's physical and neurologic examination were essentially negative. Tests performed by her previous physician had revealed a mean sleep-onset latency of 2.5 minutes and SOREMP's during naps. These confirmed the medical diagnosis of narcolepsy. After the evaluation, Ms. C's physician renewed prescriptions of methylphenidate 20 mg twice a day and imipramine 25 mg three times a day. Nursing diagnoses were potential for injury related to daytime sleepiness and cataplexy, and social isolation related to embarrassment about cataplexy. Regular return to clinic appointments was emphasized and scheduled. Nursing *interventions* included discussion of driving, safety, social activities, and emotional support, with continued follow-up planning. The clinician and Ms. C maintained telephone contact between clinic visits; numerous adjustments in prescription dosage were made. Over time, Ms. C continued to show resourcefulness in managing disease-related problems and developing coping strategies. At present, she is an active member of a peer support group.

Narcolepsy is a lifelong disorder that significantly affects an individual's quality of life. Although medical management may provide drug therapy, nursing *intervention* is also needed to provide accurate information and practical coping strategies for adaptation to the illness. Problems and coping strategies identified by narcoleptics cluster around six areas: driving, education, work, family, social life, and medical care (Rogers, 1984). Driving, household, and smoking accidents and near-accidents are significantly higher among narcoleptics (Broughton & Ghanem, 1981). In some, automatic behavior is associated with driving. Sleep attacks and a drowsy appearance often affect occupational, academic, and social performance. Family and friends may show a lack of understanding or negative reactions to EDS, sleep attacks, or cataplexy. Narcoleptics report that their symptoms limit their choice of education major, occupation, leisure time activities, social events, close friends, and scheduling of daily activities. Other problems are fear of addiction, medication compliance, social isolation, scheduling of naps, pregnancy, and denial of the illness. Narcoleptic patients benefit from accurate information about their disease and its treatment, assistance in identifying periods of peak alertness or intense drowsiness, assistance in identifying factors that precipitate or aggravate symptoms, emotional support, and practical strategies for minimizing the effects of the disease on their quality of life (Rogers, 1984). Individuals may wish to contact the American Narcolepsy Association (P.O. Box 5846, Stanford, CA 94305) for additional information and local patient support groups.

☐ Disorders of Sleep-Wake Schedule

A sudden shift in the phase of environmental rhythms occurs when air travellers cross time zones and are suddenly confronted with a new nighttime. The various exogenous and endogenous rhythms of the individual are confronted with the same phase shift, but each rhythm takes a different amount of time to become entrained into the new circadian rhythm. At certain times of the day, a marked feeling of fatigue occurs (late afternoon after westward travel, morning after eastward travel). Furthermore, sleep taken out of phase with the individual's normal circadian rhythm is often disturbed and less refreshing. Researchers are continuing to study the efficacy and residual effects of selected hypnotics in an effort to find palliative therapies. Brief out-of-phase sleeps (about 4 hours) aided by medication that is rapidly eliminated are possible and beneficial in reducing the disruption of waking function associated with circadian rhythm disturbances and insomnia. In one study, short-term use of midazolam significantly increased total sleep time, reduced the number of sleep awakenings, and reduced the amount of time of each awakening (Roth et al., 1985). There were no daytime residual drug effects on performance or daytime sleep latency.

Sleep is disturbed by work schedules that interfere with the normal night sleep hours. The types of schedules encompassed by the term shiftwork are permanent night shift, regular rotation through 8-hour periods of a 24-hour work day, less regular and less strict rotation through a 24-hour work day, and irregular work hours (Akerstedt, 1984). Sleep problems occur mainly in connection with night shift and very early morning work (Foret & Lantin, 1972; Torsvall et al., 1981). Day sleep after night shift work is shortened, averaging only about 4.3 hours, with most of the reduction being in stage 2 and REM sleep time. The amount of SWS is usually adequate. Sleep length after the afternoon shift tends to be longer than postdayshift sleep.

Workers who show good tolerance to shiftwork have a prominent 24-hour circadian time period for body temperature, whereas those with free-running rhythms complain of persistent sleep disturbances, mood changes, fatigue, and digestive troubles (Reinberg et al., 1984). General fatigue is the major disturbance reported by shiftworkers. Fatigue is maximal during the night and may cause people to be overcome by sleep during work (Kogi & Ohta, 1975). This fatigue increases, rather than decreases, with more night shift experience; it diminishes when the night shift is eliminated (Tune, 1969; Akerstedt & Torsvall, 1978). Night shiftworkers often compensate for lost sleep by napping (50% of workers) and extended sleeping time on their days off (Akerstedt & Torsvall, 1985). The majority of night shiftworkers choose to revert to a rest–activity daytime pattern on their days off work. This appears to happen no matter how many years they have been working a regular night shift.

☐ Parasomnias

The parasomnias are dysfunctions associated with sleep, sleep stages, or partial arousals. The processes responsible for the actual sleeping and waking states are not disturbed. The undesirable clinical phenomena may be either exclusively associated with sleep (e.g., sleepwalking) or aggravated by sleep (e.g., asthma).

Sleepwalking, or somnabulism, frequently begins in the first third of the night, during paroxysmal bursts of high amplitude delta waves (SWS). Individuals may sit up in bed, perform perseverative motor acts, walk, and perform automatisms (e.g., open doors, dress, eat). Although objects in the person's path can be avoided, coordination is poor. Speech is avoided or unintelligible. Episodes may last a few minutes to an hour, and the person is amnesic of the event. Occasional sleepwalking is normal in childhood (15% incidence) and early adolescence; often there is a family history of sleepwalking. During periods of major life stress and emotional tension, some adults may sleepwalk. The major concern for the sleepwalker is physical safety (e.g., remove dangerous objects from room, lock windows and doors), since falls and other accidents can occur.

Sleep terrors occur in the first third of the night during delta sleep. Onset is usually a piercing scream, with behavioral manifestations of intense distress (perspiring, rapid breathing and heart rate, frightened expression). Establishing full consciousness may take several minutes even when the individual is physically shaken by another. If the person is fully aroused, a sense of terror or dread is recalled, although vivid dream content is absent. If not aroused, morning amnesia is common. Occasional sleep terrors are considered normal in children ages 4 to 7. Sleep terrors in adults may suggest more serious physical or psychologic problems (Kales et al., 1980). Rarely is medication used for children or adults. Low doses of diazepam are used only when it is absolutely certain that sleep terrors are not triggered by sleep apnea. With sleep apneas, diazepam is contraindicated because of its depression of respiratory functions.

Distinct from night terrors are dream anxiety attacks, although both are called nightmares. Dream anxiety attacks (DAA) generally occur in the late portion of the nocturnal sleep period and arise during REM sleep. They can be experienced also in naps lasting longer than 1 hour. On awakening, recall of the experience is vivid and detailed. Arousal to full consciousness is quick, and behavioral manifestations of anxiety or threat are mild as compared to those with night terrors. The greater the quantity and intensity of REM sleep in a given night, the greater the probability of DAA. Precipitators of DAAs include fever, pharmacologic agents (e.g., reserpine), and abrupt cessation of REM-suppressing drugs (e.g., sleeping pills, alcohol, amphetamines). DAAs tend to be more prevalent at times of stressful life events, emotional turmoil, and after painful, real events.

Nursing Interventions: Sleep Hygiene

Poor sleep is associated with a wide variety of factors that cause and contribute to sleep disturbances: the aging process, drugs, medical conditions, environment, psychologic variables, and life event problems. The differential diagnosis of sleep complaints, such as insomnia or daytime sleepiness, and the treatment of neurologically induced sleep disorders are primarily in the realm of medical diagnosis and management. However, mild or moderate complaints of poor sleep may be appropriate for nursing diagnosis and may be improved with nondrug sleep hygiene (Hauri, 1982b; Maxmen, 1981).

Before discussion of the behavior and guidelines of good sleep hygiene, three general qualifications about sleep are necessary. Sleep and dreaming are usually disturbed the first night a person sleeps in an unfamiliar environment (Browman & Cartwright, 1980), although some insomniacs find it easier to initiate sleep under these first night conditions. Since the first night is atypical, any therapeutic intervention should be used and evaluated after several nights' sleep. Second, individual differences and routines are important. Events surrounding the preparation for sleep can facilitate or inhibit sleep onset. Some people require a steady noise in the background (e.g., television, music); others must have absolute silence. Reading before sleep onset may deepen the sleep of some people, whereas others may find sleep delayed and disrupted by this activity. Third, beliefs about the success or failure of achieving sleep may act as self-fulfilling prophecies. Poor sleep may result from worries, conflict, or anxiety that the person associates with sleep itself.

Environmental Factors Influencing Sleep.
Reducing nighttime *noise* results in an overall improvement in sleep organization, subjective sleep quality, and morning performance. There is no long-term physiologic adaptation to nighttime noise (Vallet & Mouret, 1984). Isolated noise events (e.g., aircraft overflight, trucks) produce a greater arousal from sleep than constant background noise of comparable magnitude (e.g., air conditioner). Intermittent intense noise produces increased nocturnal awakenings and stage 1 sleep. Sleep is disturbed even in people who do not remember the event in the morning. The awakening threshold of a noise varies with the sleep stage and the personal sensitivity of the individual. Women and the elderly tend to be more sensitive to environmental noise. The meaning attached to a specific noise is as important as the noise intensity in inducing arousal reactions. Sleep may be improved in noisy environments by sound attenuation measures, noise screening by providing a constant background noise, and wearing earplugs.

The preferred *ambient sleep temperature* for humans is around 19°C, with a microclimate temperature inside the bed (provided by pajamas, sheets, and blanket) of 28.6°C to 30.9°C (Muzet et al., 1984). Increases or decreases in ambient temperature from this thermal comfort zone result in more frequent and longer awakenings, more body movements, and decreased REM cycle length. Febrile conditions reduce the amount of REM sleep and SWS. Core body temperature influences sleep duration; within the normal temperature range the higher the core body temperature at the time of sleep onset, the greater the length of total sleep time (Czeisler et al., 1980a).

Food intake as a soporific or producer of postprandial sleepiness has variable effects on people (Adam, 1980; Porter & Horne, 1981). A light snack may facilitate sleep for some people, but a change in bedtime food supplements may actually disrupt sleep. Postprandial sleepiness appears to be affected by a multitude of variables, including stomach emptying and digestion time, prior sleep debt, meal volume, time of day, and protein and carbohydrate contents (Stahl et al., 1983). During periods of weight loss, individuals may complain of poor sleep and more frequent nocturnal awakenings.

A single drink of alcohol is sometimes used as self-medication to relieve tension and permit sleep onset. Alcohol, however, does not increase the total sleep time. After alcohol consumption, sleep is fragmented, and the numerous partial awakenings cause a decrease in total sleep time. REM periods are fragmented and reduced, and the person more frequently awakens early and feels unrested. The repeated use of a nightcap may cause rather than alleviate poor sleep. Nicotine, caffeine, and other central nervous system stimulants disturb sleep, and the presence of caffeine is pervasive and often unrecognized (e.g., coffee, tea, colas, chocolate, many over-the-counter and some prescription medications). The long-term use of tobacco and the ingestion of caffeinated beverages after lunchtime disturbs sleep, even in those who believe their sleep is not disturbed (Hauri, 1982b).

Regular heavy *physical exercise*, in an adapted individual, increases total sleep duration and the amount of SWS (Montgomery et al., 1982). The effects of sudden, short-term, intermittent, or heavy exercise, however, are variable and difficult to predict. Moderate exercise, if used consistently, can extend and deepen sleep. Restful sleep is promoted by a reasonable amount of daily exercise at an individual's appropriate capacity and preferred time of day.

Many people follow a routine of nighttime activities that put the mind at rest and prepare them for sleep. These include relaxing in a warm bath, pleasant reading, light activity (e.g., a hobby), meditating, praying, or listening to peaceful music. Sleep onset is aided by relaxing 15 to 60 minutes before retiring.

Behavioral Factors Influencing Sleep. Hauri (1982b) describes four groups of behaviors that may initiate or aggravate sleep problems: trying too hard to sleep, conditioned wakefulness, disruption of the sleep-wake rhythm, and fear of insomnia. Stressful, tense, and ruminative presleep thoughts and behaviors can overstimulate people, thus producing arousal rather than sleepiness at bedtime. Anxiety about the lack of sleep can lead to a preoccupation with "trying hard" to sleep. A vicious cycle can develop; hyperalertness results the more an individual's mind concentrates on the need for sleep and the detrimental consequences attributed to sleep loss (e.g., poor daytime performance, lethargy, irritability). Usually, these people can fall asleep easily under other circumstances (e.g., at a concert or lecture or watching television). Distraction (reading, television, listening to music), relaxation training, or EMG biofeedback therapy may improve sleep (Hauri, 1982b).

Sleeping alone may eliminate sleep disturbances accompanying a bed partner's body movements. When awakened by noise or some other event, the person should allow sleep to return by remaining calm and relaxed in bed. If lying awake in bed produces anger, anxiety, or frustration, the person should change activities (e.g., read, get out of bed, perform some quiet relaxing task). The success of these measures is dependent on strict adherence to a rigid wakeup time. Evening sleep onset should be attempted only when the person feels sleepy.

A maladaptive conditioned wakefulness may arise from frequent stressful episodes of lying awake in bed. Bedtime rituals (e.g., toothbrushing) and the physical bedroom environment (e.g., sight of the bed, feel of the pillow, darkness) may become associated with negative feelings of anxiety, frustration, and anger. Such negative associations may trigger arousal and tension rather than sleepiness. Frequently, the person sleeps better away from the usual bedroom (e.g., on the floor, in another room). Reassociation of sleep with the bedroom setting is required. This is accomplished using the behavior techniques recommended by Bootzin and Nicassio (1978):

1. Go to bed only when you are sleepy.
2. Use the bed only for sexual activity and sleeping; do not do anything else in the bedroom (no reading, listening to music, television watching).
3. If you are unable to fall asleep in about 15 minutes, get up, go to another room, and do something relaxing until you are sleepy. Return to bed only when you are sleepy; if sleep still does not come easily, get up again. Turn the clock toward the wall, since concern for time will only exacerbate the problem. The goal is to associate lying in bed with rapid sleep onset.
4. With nocturnal wakefulness, return to bed only when you feel sleepy.
5. Awake at the same time every day and do not take daytime naps.

In order to maintain this pattern of behavior, most people need support and regular contact with a therapist. A daily sleep log and graph of sleep behavior are helpful to reinforce the behavior pattern and provide tangible evidence of improvement.

Transient stressful life events can lead to changes in an individual's sleep pattern and a disruption of the sleep-wake rhythm. Increased work hours, jet lag, or stress may prevent sleep onset until the early morning hours. People who tend to fall asleep toward the morning frequently oversleep and also compensate by taking naps. A desynchronization of the circadian rhythm can occur. Rigid adherence to a regular wakeup time and avoidance of daytime naps are required.

Transient stressful life events can produce an occasional night of insomnia. If baseline sleep is adequate, the individual usually handles this episode well and may need reassurance that this sleep loss does not cause bodily harm. These basically sound sleepers gradually overcome any maladaptive conditioning and poor sleep habits that accompanied the stressful episode and insomnia. With other people (e.g., chronically poor sleepers), the insomnia accompanying a stressful episode may reinforce maladaptive patterns. A poor night of sleep may trigger fears of insomnia, which become a self-fulfilling prophecy. Without therapeutic intervention, the poor sleep habits and insomnia may persist for years.

REFERENCES

Adam, K. (1980). Dietary habits and sleep after bedtime food and drinks. *Sleep, 3,* 47.

Adam, K., & Oswald, I. (1979). One gram of L-tryptophan fails to alter the time taken to fall asleep. *Neuropharmacology, 18,* 1025.

Agnew, H.W., Webb, W.B., & Williams, R.L. (1967). Comparison of stage 4 and REM sleep deprivation. *Perceptual and Motor Skills, 24,* 851.

Ahnve, S., Theorel, T., Akerstedt, T., Froberg, J., & Halberg, F. (1981). Circadian variations in cardiovascular parameters during sleep deprivation. *European Journal of Applied Physiology and Occupational Physiology, 46,* 9.

Akerstedt, T. (1984). Work schedules and sleep. *Experientia, 40,* 417.

Akerstedt, T., & Torsvall, L. (1978). Experimental changes in shift schedules—Their effects on well-being. *Ergonomics, 21,* 849.

Akerstedt, T., & Torsvall, L. (1985). Napping in shift work. *Sleep, 8,* 105.

Antonioli, M., Solano, L., Torre, A., Violanti, C., Costa, M., & Bertini, M. (1981). Independence of REM density from other REM sleep parameters before and after REM deprivation. *Sleep, 4,* 221.

Association of Sleep Disorders Centers. (1979). Diagnostic classification of sleep and arousal disorders (1st ed.), prepared by the Sleep Disorders Classification Committee, H.P. Roffwarg, Chairman, *Sleep, 2,* 1.

Aurell, J., & Elmqvist, D. (1985). Sleep in the surgical intensive care unit: Continuous polygraphic recording of sleep in nine patients receiving postoperative care. *British Journal of Medicine, 290,* 1029.

Bootzin, R.R., & Nicassio, P.N. (1978). Behavioral treatments for insomnia. In M. Hersen, R. Eisler, & P. Miller (Eds.), *Progress in behavior modification.* New York: Academic Press.

Bremer, F. (1977). Cerebral hypnogenic centers. *Annals of Neurology, 2,* 1.

Broughton, R., Ghanem, Q., Hishikawa, S., et al. (1981). Life effects of narcolepsy in 180 patients from North America, Asia, and Europe compared to matched controls. *Canadian Journal of Neurological Sciences, 8,* 199.

Browman, C.P., & Cartwright, R.D. (1980). The first-night effect on sleep and dreams. *Biological Psychiatry, 15,* 809.

Cartwright, R.D. (1983). Rapid eye movement sleep characteristics during and after mood-disturbing events. *Archives of General Psychiatry, 40,* 197.

Cernovsky, Z.Z. (1984). Life stress measures and reported frequency of sleep disorders. *Perceptual and Motor Skills, 58,* 39.

Coleman, R.M., Roffwarg, H.P., Kennedy, S.J., et al. (1982). Sleep-wake disorders based on a polysomnographic diagnosis. *Journal of the American Medical Association, 27,* 997.

Czeisler, C.A., Weitzman, E.D., Moore-Ede, M.C., Zimmerman, J.C., & Knauer, R.S. (1980a). Human sleep: Its duration and organization depend on its circadian phase. *Science, 210,* 1264.

Czeisler, C.A., Zimmerman, J.C., Ronda, J., Moore-Ede, M.C., & Weitzman, E.D. (1980b). Timing of REM sleep is coupled to the circadian rhythm of body temperature in man. *Sleep, 2,* 329.

Dement, W., Carskadon, M., & Rey, R. (1973). The prevalence of narcolepsy. *Sleep Research, 2,* 147.

Dement, W., Henry, P., Cohen, H., & Ferguson, J. (1967). Studies on the effect of REM deprivation in humans and in animals. *Research Publications—Association for Research in Nervous and Mental Disease, 45,* 319.

Dohno, S., Paskewitz, D.A., Lynch, J.J., Gimbel, K.S., & Thomas. S.A. (1979). Some aspects of sleep disturbance in coronary patients. *Perceptual and Motor Skills, 48,* 199.

Drucker-Colin, R., de Gomez-Puyou, M.T., Gutierrez, M.C., et al. (1980). Immunological approach to the study of neurohumoral sleep factors: Effects on REM sleep of antibodies to brainstem proteins. *Experimental Neurology, 69,* 563.

Drucker-Colin, R., & Espejel, R.M. (1980). Chronic administration of chloramphenicol, a protein synthesis inhibitor, selectively decreases REM sleep. *Behavioral and Neural Biology, 29,* 410.

Findley, L.J., Wilhout, S.C., & Suratt, P.M. (1985). Apnea duration and hypoxemia during REM sleep in patients with obstructive sleep apnea. *Chest, 87,* 432.

Fishbein, W., & Gutwein, B.M. (1981). Paradoxical sleep and a theory of long-term memory. In W. Fishbein (Ed.), *Sleep, dreams and memory* (p. 147). New York: Spectrum Publications.

Folkard, S., Hume, K.I., Minors, D.S., Waterhouse, J.M., & Watson, F.L. (1985). Independence of the circadian rhythm in alertness from the sleep/wake cycle. *Nature, 313,* 678.

Foret, J., & Lantin, G. (1972). The sleep of train drivers: An example of effects of irregular work schedules on sleep. In W.P. Colquhoun (Ed.), *Aspects of human efficiency* (p. 273). London: English Universities Press.

Francesconi, R.P., Stokes, J.W., Banderet, L.E., & Kowal, D.M. (1978). Sustained operations and sleep deprivation: Effects on indices of stress. *Aviation, Space and Environmental Medicine, 49,* 1271.

Gaillard, J.-M. (1983). Mental activity during sleep. In M. Monnier & M. Meulders (Eds.), *Functions of the nervous system* (p. 275). New York: Elsevier.

Gaultier, C., Praud, J.P., Clement, A., D'Allest, A.M., Khiati, M., Tournier, G., & Girard, F. (1985). Respiration during sleep in children with COPD. *Chest, 87,* 168.

Guilleminault, C., Tilkian, A., & Dement, W. (1976). The sleep apnea syndrome. *Annual Review of Medicine, 27,* 465.

Hartmann, E., & Spinweber, C. (1979). Sleep induced by L-tryptophan. *Journal of Nervous and Mental Disease, 167,* 497.

Haslam, D.R. (1984). Military performance of soldiers in sustained operations. *Aviation, Space and Environmental Medicine, 55,* 216.

Hauri, P.J. (1982a). Evaluating disorders of initiating and maintaining sleep (DIMS). In C. Guilleminault (Ed.), *Sleeping and waking disorders: Indications and techniques* (p. 225). Menlo Park, NJ: Addison-Wesley.

Hauri, P.J. (1982b). *The sleep disorders.* Kalamazoo, MI: Upjohn.

Horne, J. (1978). A review of the biological effects of total sleep deprivation in man. *Biological Psychology, 7,* 55.

Horne, J.A., & Moore, V.J. (1985). Sleep EEG effects of exercise with and without additional body cooling. *Electroencephalography and Clinical Neurophysiology, 60,* 33.

Horne, J.A., & Reid, A.J. (1985). Night-time sleep EEG changes following body heating in a warm bath. *Electroencephalography and Clinical Neurophysiology, 60,* 154.

Horne, J.A., & Wilkinson, S. (1985). Chronic sleep reduction: Daytime vigilance performance and EEG measures of sleepiness, with particular reference to "practice" effects. *Psychophysiology, 22,* 69.

Ingbar, D.H., & Gee, J.B.L. (1985). Pathophysiology and treatment of sleep apnea. *Annual Review of Medicine, 36,* 369.

Ingvar, D.H. (1979). Cerebral circulation and metabolism in sleep. In R. Priest, A. Pletscher, & J. Ward (Eds.), *Sleep research* (p. 13). Baltimore: University Park Press.

Institute of Medicine. (1979). *Report of a study: Sleeping pills, insomnia and medical practice.* Washington, DC: U.S. National Academy of Sciences.

Jones, B. (1979). Elimination of paradoxical sleep by lesions of the pontine gigantocellular tegmental field in the cat. *Neuroscience Letters, 13,* 285.

Jouvet, M. (1969). Biogenic amines and the state of sleep. *Science, 163,* 39.

Kales, A., & Kales, J.D. (1984). *Evaluation and treatment of insomnia.* New York: Oxford University Press.

Kales, J.D., Kales, A., Soldatos, C.R., et al. (1980). Night terrors: Clinical characteristics and personality patterns. *Archives of General Psychiatry, 37,* 1413.

Kant, G.J., Genser, S.G., Thorne, D.R., Pfalser, J., & Mougey, E.H. (1984). Effects of 72 hour sleep deprivation on urinary cortisol and indices of metabolism. *Sleep, 7,* 142.

Karacan, I., Thornby, J.I., Anch, A.M., Williams, R.L., & Perkins, H.M. (1978). Effects of high ambient temperature on sleep in young men. *Aviation, Space and Environmental Medicine, 49,* 855.

Karacan, I., Wolff, S.M., Williams, R.L., Hursch, C.J., & Webb, W.B. (1968). The effect of fever on sleep and dream patterns. *Psychosomatics, 9,* 331.

Kessler, S. (1976). Genetic factors in narcolepsy. In C. Guilleminault, W.C. Dement, & P. Passouant (Eds.), *Narcolepsy* (p. 285). New York: Spectrum.

Kogi, K., & Ohta, T. (1975). Incidence of near accidental drowsing in locomotive driving during a period of rotation. *Journal of Human Ergology, 4,* 65.

Kolka, M.A., Martin, B.J., & Elizondo, R.S. (1984). Exercise in a cold environment after sleep deprivation. *European Journal of Applied Physiology and Occupational Physiology, 53,* 282.

Lozoff, B., Wolf, A., & Davis, N.S. (1985). Sleep problems seen in pediatric practice. *Pediatrics, 75,* 477.

Mancia, G., & Zanchetti, A. (1980). Cardiovascular regulation during sleep. In J. Orem & C.D. Barnes (Eds.), *Physiology in sleep* (p. 43). New York: Academic Press.

Maxmen, J.S. (1981). *A good night's sleep.* New York: Norton.

McCarley, R.W., & Hobson, J.A. (1975). Neuronal excitability modulation over the sleep cycle: A structural and mathematical model. *Science, 189,* 58.

Monnier, M. (1983). Sleep, dream and waking as an integral function. In M. Monnier & M. Meulders (Eds.), *Functions of the nervous system* (p. 7). New York: Elsevier.

Monnier, M., & Gaillard, J. (1980). Biochemical regulation of sleep. *Experientia, 36,* 22.

Monnier, M., Schoenenberger, G., Dudler, L., & Herkert, B. (1975). Production, isolation and further characteristics of the sleep peptide delta. In P. Levin & W. Koella (Eds.), *Sleep 1974* (p. 41). New York: Karger.

Montgomery, I., Trinder, J., & Paxton, S.J. (1982). Energy expenditure and total sleep time: effect of physical exercise. *Sleep, 5,* 159.

Montplaisir, J., Godbout, M.A., Boghen, D., DeChamplain, J., Young, S.N., Lapierre, G., & Ing, M. (1985). Familial restless legs with periodic movements in sleep: Electrophysiologic, biochemical, and pharmacologic study. *Neurology, 35,* 130.

Morgane, P.J. (1981). Monoamine theories of sleep: The role of serotonin—A review. *Psychopharmacology Bulletin, 17,* 13.

Muzet, A., Libert, J.-P., & Candas, V. (1984). Ambient temperature and human sleep. *Experientia, 40,* 425.

Naitoh, P., Pasnau, R., & Kollar, E. (1971). Psychophysiological changes after prolonged deprivation of sleep. *Biological Psychiatry, 3.* 309.

Nicholson, A.N., Pascoe, P.A., Roehrs, T., Roth, T., Spencer, M.B., Stone, B.M., & Zorick, F. (1985). *Aviation, Space and Environmental Medicine 56,* 105.

Okawa, M., Matousek, M., & Petersen, I. (1984). Spontaneous vigilance fluctuations in the daytime. *Psychophysiology, 21,* 207.

Opstad, P.K., Ekanger, R., Nummestad, M., & Raabe, N. (1978). Performance, mood and clinical symptoms in men exposed to prolonged, severe physical work and sleep deprivation. *Aviation, Space and Environmental Medicine, 49,* 1065.

Orem, J. (1980). Neuronal mechanisms of respiration in REM sleep. *Sleep, 3,* 251.

Orr, W.C., Altshuler, K.Z., & Stahl, M.L. (1982). *Managing sleep complaints.* Chicago: Year Book.

Pappenheimer, J.R. (1979). "Nature's soft nurse": A sleep-promoting factor isolated from brain. *Johns Hopkins Medical Journal 145,* 49.

Pompeiano, O., & Valentinuzzi, M. (1976). A mathematical model for the mechanism of rapid eye movements induced by an anticholinesterase in the decerebrate cat. *Archives Italiennes de Biologie, 114,* 103.

Porter, J.M., & Horne, J.A. (1981). Bed-time food supplements and sleep: Effects of different carbohydrate levels. *Electroencephlography and Clinical Neurophysiology, 51,* 426.

Ramm, P. (1980). The locus coeruleus, catecholamines, and REM sleep: A critical review. *Behavioral and Neural Biology, 29,* 410.

Rechtschaffen, A., & Kales, A. (Eds.). (1968). *A manual of standardized terminology, techniques and scoring system for sleep stages of human subjects.* Los Angeles: Brain Information Service/Brain Research Institute, UCLA.

Reinberg, A., Andlauer, P., De Prins, J., Malberg, W., et al. (1984). Desynchronization of the oral temperature circadian rhythm and intolerance to shift work. *Nature, 308,* 272.

Reinberg, A., & Smolensky, M.H. (Eds.). (1983). *Biological rhythms and medicine.* New York: Springer-Verlag.

Richardson, G.S., Carskadon, M.A., Flagg, W., et al. (1978). Excessive daytime sleepiness in man: Multiple sleep latency measurement in narcoleptic and control subjects. *Clinical Neurophysiology, 45,* 621.

Roffwarg, H.P., Sachar, E.J., Halpern, F., & Hellman, L. (1982). Plasma testosterone and sleep: Relationship to sleep stage variables. *Psychosomatic Medicine, 44,* 73.

Rogers, A.E. (1984). Problems and coping strategies identified by narcoleptic patients. *Journal of Neurosurgical Nursing, 16,* 326.

Ross, G., Maira, G., & Vignati, A. (1975). Intracranial pressure during sleep in man. In P. Levin & W. Koella (Eds.), *Sleep 1974* (p. 169). New York: Karger.

Roth, T., Hauri, P., Zorick, F., Sateia, M., Roehrs, T., & Kipp, J. (1985). The effects of midazolam and temazepam on sleep and performance when administered in the middle of the night. *Journal of Clinical Psychopharmacology, 5,* 66.

Sakai, F., Meyer, J., Karacan, I., Derman, S., & Yamamoto, M. (1980). Normal human sleep: Regional cerebral hemo dynamics. *Annals of Neurology, 7,* 471.

Small, J.G., Milstein, V., & Golay, S. (1979). L-Tryptophan and other agents for sleep EEG. *Clinical Electroencephalography and Neurophysiology, 10,* 426.

Smith, G.M., & Smith, P.H. (1985). Effects of doxylamine and acetaminophen on postoperative sleep. *Clinical Pharmacology and Therapeutics, 37,* 549.

Squire, L.R., & Davis, H.P. (1981). The pharmacology of memory: A neurobiological perspective. *Annual Review of Pharmacology and Toxicology, 21,* 331.

Stahl, M.L., Orr, W.C., & Bollinger, C. (1983). Postprandial sleepiness. *Sleep, 6,* 29.

Sullivan, C.E. (1980). Breathing in sleep. In J. Orem & C.D. Barnes (Eds.), *Physiology in sleep* (p. 214). New York: Academic Press.

Takahashi, Y. (1979). Growth hormone secretion related to the sleep and waking rhythm. In R. Drucker-Colin, M. Shkurovich, & M. Sterman (Eds.), *The function of sleep* (p. 113). New York: Academic Press.

Tassan, V.C., Block, A.J., Boysen, P.G., et al. (1981). Alcohol increases sleep apnea and oxygen desaturation in asymptomatic men. *American Journal of Medicine, 71,* 240.

Thoman, E.B. (1975). Early development of sleeping behaviors in infants. In N.R. Ellis (Ed.), *Aberrant development in infancy: Human and animal studies* (p. 122). New York, Wiley.

Torsvall, L., Akerstedt, T., & Gilberg, M. (1981). Age, sleep, and irregular work hours: A field study with EEG recording, catecholamine excretion, and self-ratings. *Scandinavian Journal of Work, Environment and Health, 7,* 196.

Tune, G.S. (1969). Sleep and wakefulness in a group of shift workers. *British Journal of Industrial Medicine, 26,* 54.

Vallet, M., & Mouret, J. (1984). Sleep disturbance due to transportation noise: Ear plugs vs oral drugs. *Experientia, 40,* 429.

Van den Burg, W., & Van den Hoofdakker, R.H. (1975). Total sleep deprivation in endogenous depression. *Archives of General Psychiatry, 32,* 1121.

Van den Hoed, J., Kraemer, H., Guilleminault, C., Zarcone, V.P., Miles, L.E., Dement, W., & Mitler, M.M. (1981). Disorders of excessive daytime somnolence: Polygraphic and clinical data for 100 patients. *Sleep, 4,* 23.

Vogel, G.W. (1975). A review of REM sleep deprivation. *Archives of General Psychiatry, 32,* 749.

Watt, J.E., & Strongman, K.T. (1985). The organization and stability of sleep states in fullterm, preterm, and small-for-gestational-age infants: A comparative study. *Developmental Psychobiology, 18,* 151.

Zarcone, V. (1973). Narcolepsy. *New England Journal of Medicine, 288,* 1156.

SECTION 2. COGNITION PHENOMENA

10

Cognition: An Overview

Barbara Boss

DEFINITIONS, CONCEPTS, AND THEORIES

Cognition is a complex concept, comprised of a number of relevent phenomena, including memory, learning, thinking or thoughts, judgment, reasoning, and insight.

Memory is the process in which learned information is stored and retrieved, whereas *learning* is the process whereby behavior is modified as a result of experience. Kupfermann argues that the neural basis of learning and memory can be summarized in four principles that relate to the anatomic and physiologic correlates of memory: (1) memory develops in stages, and change in memory is continual, (2) physical changes occur in the brain to produce long-term memory, (3) memory traces are stored widely throughout the nervous system, and (4) the hippocampus and temporal lobes have special functions related to memory storage and retrieval (Kupfermann, 1985).

Thinking may be defined as "the process of logic and reasoning assumed to exist inside the individual and accessible through a study of verbalized associations and actions," and a *thought* may be defined as "the act or power of thinking, cogitation or meditation" (English Language Institute of America, 1967). The neurophysiologic substrate of thought is proposed to involve simultaneous activation (nerve impulse transmissions) in the cerebral cortex, thalamus, limbic system, and reticular formation of the brainstem. The activated limbic system, thalamus, and reticular formation areas are believed to determine the general nature of the thought—including its qualities, such as pleasant or unpleasant and painful or comfortable—the crude modalities of sensation, the gross localization to a body area, and other such characteristics. The activated cortical areas are believed to discriminate specific features of the thought, such as specific body part location of sensations or exact location of objects in the visual field, distinct sensory patterns, and specific characteristics, all of which are reaching awareness at any one time (Guyton, 1987). It is recognized that some primitive thoughts may be mediated entirely by lower brain centers. A person with destruction of large areas of the cerebral cortex is still able to have thoughts.

The degree of awareness of surroundings is reduced after such an injury.

Reasoning is defined as "the process of drawing conclusions or inferences from facts or premises," and *judgment* is defined as "the act of deciding or passing decision on something." *Insight* has been defined as the understanding of oneself, self-understanding (English Language Institute of America, 1967; Armstrong et al., 1979).

Complex cognitive (intellectual) operations, that is, operations of the brain requiring analysis and interpretation, are yet to be explained neurophysiologically. The mechanisms have not been determined, but a few facts are known. The brain focuses attention on specific types of information. The different qualities of each set of information signals, that is, each sensory experience, are dissected away from the central signal and transmitted to the various areas of the brain that are designed specifically for analyzing the quality or qualities of the sensory experiences. New information is compared to old information in the memory stores by the brain through determining patterns of stimulation. Previous experiences of the same or similar types are thus recognized and associated. How the comparisons are made is not known (Guyton, 1987).

Relationships Between Brain Anatomy and Cognition

There are two major theoretical views of cognition: the aggregate field view and the localization view. The *aggregate field view* argues that all brain areas have equal potential in function and that for many cognitive functions, as well as other functions, any part of the brain could substitute for any other part. This viewpoint was dominant throughout the late nineteenth and first part of the twentieth century, and its proponents included British neurologist Henry Head, German neuropsychologist Karl Goldstein, and American psychologist Karl Lashley from Harvard. Lashley (1929) formulated the "mass action" theory of brain function, which proposed that brain mass is the relevant feature for cognitive function, rather than individual neurons and specific neuronal connections. The aggregate field view is closely related to the theory of intelligence first proposed by Spearman that suggests that there is a general factor of intelligence that contributes to all human performance. Proponents point to the positive correlation among all tests of cognitive ability as evidence to support this view (Kandel, 1985a).

The *localization view* proposes that the neuronal architecture, with its individual neurons and specific neuronal connections, is of primary importance to brain function, including cognition. The areas are not equipotential as to function. The great neuroscientists Broca, Wernicke, and Penfield have been proponents of this view. Again, this view is closely aligned with the psychologic theory of intelligence that holds intelligence to be the sum total of a number of primary cognitive abilities, such as memory, verbal skill, numerical ability, and visual–spatial perception first proposed by Thurstone. Proponents do not accept the existence of a general cognitive factor.

Neuropathologic studies have offered no support to the aggregate field theory nor to the existence of a general factor of intelligence. These viewpoints, if true, would lead to the assumption that diffuse cortical brain injury would impair cognition (or g factor) proportionally to the brain mass involved. Pathologic studies of damaged brains across all age groups never have demonstrated a universal cognitive deficit associated with degree of brain injury, nor has this general cognitive ability been demonstrated to decrease consistently with age (Kandel, 1985a).

Neuropathologic studies do support the relationship between specific cognitive deficits and injury and dysfunction in particular parts of the cerebral hemispheres. However, neuropathologists have never been able to localize general reasoning and thinking. In addition, the findings from clinical and laboratory studies are more consistent with the localization theory. The evidence weighs in favor of localization and even in favor of asymmetrical representation of function in the human cerebral cortex (Ferris et al., 1981).

Left and Right Brain Distinction. Dramatic evidence for the support of asymmetry of hemispheric localization of function to one hemisphere has arisen since the early 1960s from the split-brain research initiated by Sperry and his associates. It has been demonstrated clearly that both hemispheres perform sensory analysis, have memory, are able to learn, form thoughts, and make judgments (Kandel, 1985a). Much of the analysis, memory, learning, and thoughts, however, appear to be different. The two hemispheres have different interpretative capacities.

The *left hemisphere* demonstrates a superior ability for tasks requiring an orderly, logical, systematic assessment of components, such as language, mathematical calculations, complex abstraction, and reasoning. The left hemisphere functions in an analytic mode using sequential analysis. Memories are thought to be stored as component parts and in language format (Blakesless, 1980; Finn, 1983; Kandel, 1985a).

The *right hemisphere* is superior at spatial–visual tasks. It is vital for the analysis and interpretation of nonlanguage sounds, such as music, of visual experiences, and of spatial relationships. The right hemisphere functions to process whole sensory experiences simultaneously (input). This hemisphere functions on a holistic level. Memories apparently are stored in a holistic fashion as the auditory, visual, and spatial stimuli are experienced. In addition, the right hemisphere orchestrates holistic performance, such as athletic or ballet performance (Finn, 1983; Kandel, 1985a).

Clearly, the right and left hemispheres mediate different types of cognition (intelligence). Thus, overall research findings support the concept that cognition is a gestalt of multiple primary abilities, which have some degree of anatomic localization. Certain regions are more concerned with one cognitive ability than others, although these cognitive abilities are not mediated exclusively by only one area. Cognition, then, is the result of integrated action of neurons located in different regions (Adams & Victor, 1985; Kandel, 1985a).

COGNITION: NORMAL DEVELOPMENT

Nervous system development is characterized by differentiation and cell multiplication during early prenatal life. Differentiation involves three phrases: proliferation and generation of specific classes of neurons, migration of cells to characteristic positions, and maturation of cells with specific connections (Table 10–1).

During development, especially at times of rapid biochemical differentiation, the nervous system is sensitive to environmental influences that play a significant role in advancing or hampering normal development. Nutrition, hormones, oxygen levels, and external stimulation have been identified as factors that affect normal development. Protein is necessary to maintain the rates of proliferation of developing neurons and glial cells from the second trimester through the first year of life. Undernourishment during fetal life and early postnatal life results in a decreased number of neurons and glial cells (Schacher, 1985). The normal nervous system maturation sequence requires availability of vitamins, minerals, and calories during fetal development and in the first postnatal year. Exposure to androgens at a critical period appears to be necessary to activate the neural components that mediate male sexual orientation and behavior. Androgens at this critical period effect a permanent change in certain brain tissues that probably sensitizes these tissues to future androgen stimulation. Thyroid hormone is essential during the late stages of fetal life for (1) development of normal neuronal cell size, normal axon and dendrite size and number, and axodendritic synapses, (2) normal neuronal protein and nucleic acid metabolism, and (3) normal electrical activity (Noback & Demarst, 1975). Continuous oxy-

TABLE 10–1. MACROSCOPIC AND MICROSCOPIC DEVELOPMENTAL CHANGES.

Time Period	Developmental Changes
Approximately 18 days postconception	*Macroscopic:* None. *Microscopic:* Ectoderm along that which becomes the back differentiates and thickens to form neural plate. Ectoderm in head region differentiates and thickens to form placodes (origin of special senses).
Approximately 25 days postconception	*Macroscopic:* None. *Microscopic:* Lateral edges of neural plate rise and grow medially until they unite to form the neural tube (the primordial structure that gives rise to the CNS, including all neurons and glial cells). Tube detaches from skin and slips beneath surface.
Before 1 month postconception	*Macroscopic:* Cephalic end of neural tube differentiates and enlarges into three dilations (primary brain vesicles): rhombencephalon (hindbrain), mesencephalon (midbrain), and prosencephalon (forebrain). *Microscopic:* Upper portion of the neural tube proliferates into four concentric zones: 1. Ventricular zone, composed of ventricular cells (pseudostratified columnar epithelium), is the germinal zone where cell proliferation generally occurs; 2. Subventricular zone, next to the ventricular zone, derives certain classes of neurons and all the macroglia of the CNS; 3. Intermediate (mantle) zone, formed from migrating cells of the ventricular and subventricular zones, appears to evolve into gray matter of the CNS; 4. Marginal zone, the outermost zone, has no primary cells of its own, is cell sparse, and eventually forms much of the white matter of the CNS.
Second fetal month	*Macroscopic:* Differentiation into a five-vesicle brain: prosencephalon divides into a telencephalon and diencephalon; Telencephalon surrounds diencephalon. *Microscopic:* Neurons of neocortex originate from ventricular zone as postmitotic cells with an exception. Some cortical cells migrate to subventricular zone and proliferate again. Cortical cells from the ventricular and subventricular zones migrate through the intermediate zone to the cortical plate in an inside-out migration. Deeper layers of cortex are formed before more superficial layers. The initial wave of cells migrates as far as possible between the marginal layer and the white matter. Succeeding waves migrate past these cells and come to lie in the middle third of the mature cortex. Later cells migrate to the superficial layers of the cortex. Differentiation of cortical neurons progresses in the following sequence: 1. Efferent cells (pyramidal cells), 2. Primary afferent neurons (thalamic afferent fibers), 3. Instrinsic interneurons of the major neuronal pathways (stellate cells),

TABLE 10–1. MACROSCOPIC AND MICROSCOPIC DEVELOPMENTAL CHANGES *(Cont.)*

Time Period	Developmental Changes
	4. Lateral interactions by intrinsic interneurons (horizontal cells and pyramidal axon collaterals). 5. Secondary extrinsic afferent neurons (callosal and associational neurons). Glial cells develop after neurons. Neuronal maturation, which takes place in four stages, begins with stage 1: growth and elongation of axons.
Third fetal month	*Macroscopic:* Lateral sulci appear. *Microscopic:* Neuronal maturation continues to stage 2: elaboration of dendritic processes.
Fifth fetal month	*Macroscopic:* Central sulci, calcarine sulci, and parieto-occipital sulci appear. *Microscopic:* Neuronal maturation continues to stage 3: expression of appropriate biochemical properties.
Seventh fetal month	*Macroscopic:* All gyri and major sulci are present. *Microscopic:* Neuronal maturation continues to stage 4: formation of synaptic connections.
Eighth fetal month	*Macroscopic:* Precentral and postcentral gyri are prominent. Lateral sulci are wide, and the insula is visible. Secondary sulci develop. Occipital lobes override the cerebellum. *Microscopic:* Apical dendritic system of cortical pyramidal cells develops in the following progression: apical dendrites, basilar dendrites, axodendritic synapses, axosomatic synapses, and axodendritic synapses on spines. Initial formation and orientation of dendrites appear to be determined by instrinsic factors (called developmental programmed maturation). Final shape and morphologic specialization appear to be dependent on local interactions with afferent synaptic input (called environmentally arranged learning).
Term	*Macroscopic:* Brain weight is 350 g. Frontal and temporal lobes are short. Insula covered by overlying structures. Few tertiary sulci exist. Subcortical white matter tracts are unmyelinated except for a few somatic afferent tracts (general somatic, auditory, and visual systems). *Microscopic:* None.
First postnatal year	*Macroscopic:* None. *Microscopic:* Basilar dendritic system of the pyramidal cells develops

TABLE 10–1. MACROSCOPIC AND MICROSCOPIC DEVELOPMENTAL CHANGES *(Cont.)*

Time Period	Developmental Changes
1 year of age	*Macroscopic:* Brain weights 1,000 g (extremely rapid growth rate). *Microscopic:* None.
Second postnatal year	*Macroscopic:* Slightly slower growth rate. *Microscopic:* None.
2 years of age	*Macroscopic:* Relative size and proportions to adult. Gray matter is demarcated from myelinated subcortical white matter. Tertiary sulci are predominant. *Microscopic:* None.
Up to third year of life	*Macroscopic:* Female brain grows more rapidly, and myelination takes place at a faster rate. *Microscopic:* None.
After third year of life	*Macroscopic:* Male brain grows more rapidly. *Microscopic:* None.
At puberty	*Macroscopic:* Female brain weighs approximately 1,250 g. Male brain weighs approximately 1,375 g. *Microscopic:* None.

gen availability is essential for nervous system development.

Synaptic connections are stabilized by the appropriate environmental conditions in prenatal life. Reinforcement by environmental stimuli is required for complete development of each pathway (Boss, in press; Schacher, 1985). Environmental agents may impair or prevent normal nervous system development. Such environmental factors include infectious agents (such as rubella and syphilis), excessive radiation, various chemical toxins, and trauma.

Reinforcement by environmental stimuli postnatally is required for normal nervous system development, but current evidence supports a relatively strict constructionist view related to this requirement. The major connections within the nervous system are established primarily under genetic and developmental control. The initial establishment of connections occurs in the absence of learning. Learning is important for subsequent fine tuning and maintenance and for regulating the strength of the connections, as in the case of memory.

NEUROANATOMY AND NEUROPHYSIOLOGY OF PRIMARY COGNITIVE ABILITIES

The study of neural correlates of cognition is begun by examining the specific facts and current theories related to the primary abilities involved in cognition. These primary abilities include the memory systems, goal-oriented behavior, analysis and interpretation of sensory data, and elaboration of thought.

The Memory Systems

Memory is fundamental to the cognitive process. Two memory systems have been demonstrated on the basis of the mechanism of memory storage: short-term memory and long-term memory (Guyton, 1987; Kupfermann, 1985). Three memory systems have been used for evaluation on a clinical basis: immediate memory, recent memory, and remote memory. The short-term memory system and the immediate memory system are essentially the same neuroanatomically and neurophysiologically. The long-term memory system is subdivided into long-term secondary memory, which is somewhat equivalent to the recent memory system, and long-term tertiary memory, which includes most of the remote memory system.

Short-Term Memory System. Short-term memory (immediate memory) is "the memory of a few facts, words, numbers, letters, or other bits of information for a few seconds to a minute or more at a time" (Boss, 1982; Guyton, 1987). Neuroanatomically, the immediate memory system is thought to require the activity of the reticular formation of the high brainstem, which is defined as being medial to the cranial nerve nuclei and extending from the thalamus to the entry point of the fifth cranial nerve (Fig. 10–1), because neurophysiologically the immediate memory system is activated when a person recognizes and attends to a stimulus. The stored information is referred to as "immediate recall." This memory system has a very limited storage capacity. For example, the average person cannot maintain more than five to nine digits in the immediate memory system. Immediate recall seems to be dependent partly on rehearsal of the information and is, therefore, very distraction labile. If another stimulus interrupts the rehearsal, the information is not held in the immediate memory system.

Several neural mechanisms have been proposed to mediate immediate memory. All these mechanisms have the potential to hold specific information for several seconds to a minute or more: reverberating circuits, posttetanic potentiation, and direct current (DC) potential. The *reverberating circuit theory* holds that sensory signals set up reverberating oscillations, the signals passing through a multistage circuit of neurons in the local area of the cortex itself or between the cortex and thalamus. The *posttetanic potential theory* proposes that the change in the excitability of the synapse is the basis of immediate memory. The *DC potential theory* states that the basis for immediate memory is a prolonged decrease in the membrane potential of the neuron that lasts for seconds to minutes after a period of excitation (Guyton, 1987). Visual afterimages have been demonstrated to be a mechanism of immediate memory in the visual system. The development of such visual images is thought to occur because of photochemical processes in the retina (Kandel, 1985b). Thus, one very simple form of immediate memory appears to be encoded by a transient physical change in the peripheral receptors.

A reduction in or loss of immediate recall appears to be the result of dysfunction in the reticular formation itself or in the tracts that arise from this area and synapse with cortical neurons in the parietal, temporal, and occipital association areas (Boss, 1982; Guyton, 1987).

Long-Term Memory System. For a memory to be retained, it must be transferred from short-term to long-term memory. Long-term memory (fixed memory, permanent memory) is the storage of information which may be recalled at a later time—minutes, hours, or days later, for example (Guyton, 1987). Long-term

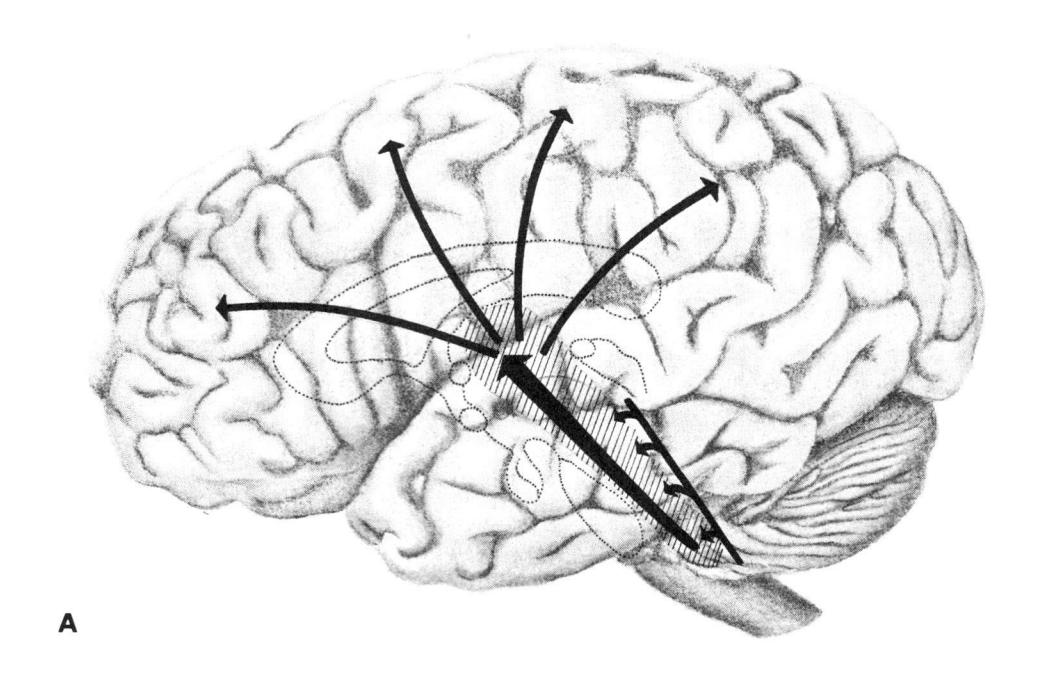

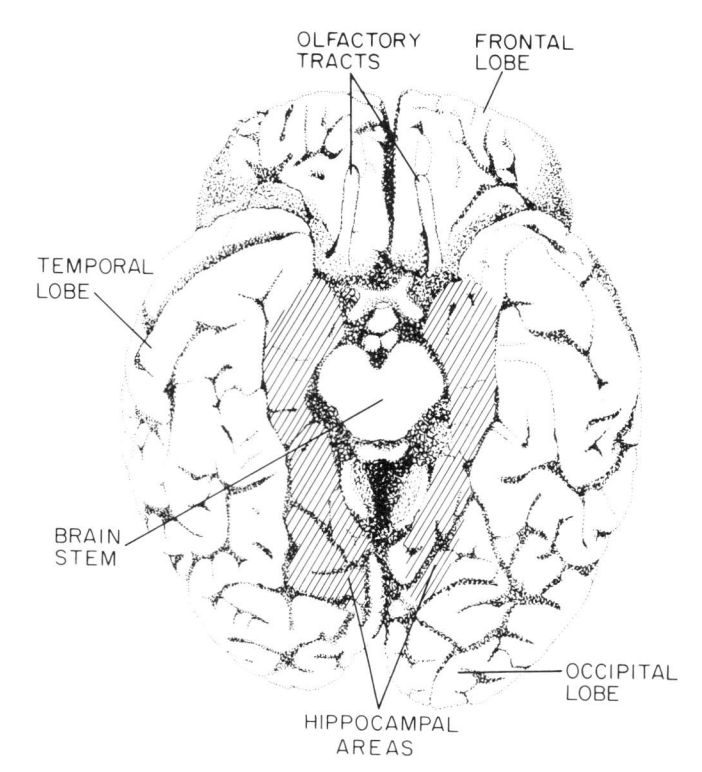

Figure 10–1. (A) The location of the reticular formation is indicated by the widest arrow in the figure. The branching, small arrows are the sensory input for the reticular formation, whereas the narrow, longer arrows represent diffuse projections from the core of the reticular formation to the cortex. The reticular formation in the brainstem is believed to participate in short-term memory. (B) The hippocampal formation. This structure is believed to play an important role in retrieval of long-term memory. *(From P.H. Mitchell et al. [1984]. Neurological assessment for nursing practice. New York: Appleton-Century-Crofts.)*

secondary memory is a long-term memory that may be easily forgotten and very difficult to recall (Guyton, 1987). A long-term tertiary memory has a very strong memory trace and usually persists throughout life (Guyton, 1987).

All parts of the nervous system appear to have the type of plastic neuronal properties required for memory storage. Long-term memory is not mediated in a localized area, but memories are stored throughout the association areas (Fig. 10–2). Although the hippocampus and adjacent temporal lobe areas do not store memories, they are involved in the process by which memories are stored and retrieved from storage. The hippocampus and its adjacent areas are now thought to play a role in sorting important information from nonessential information, coding this information, and rehearsing the memory store to consolidate it into a long-term memory store (Fig. 10–1b) (Guyton, 1987; Kupfermann, 1985).

Long-term memory is not dependent on continued activity of the brain, as is the case in short-term memory. Long-term memory has been demonstrated via electron microscopy to be associated with an anatomic change in the synapse (Guyton, 1987; Kupfermann, 1985). The synaptic changes probably enhance (facilitate) specific neuronal circuits. Nerve impulses thus pass through the neuronal circuits with increasing ease. The terms memory engram and memory trace refer to a facilitated circuit.

Because long-term secondary memory is not dependent on rehearsal, a person may attend to other stimuli without loss of the previous memory store. Long-term secondary memory is stable to distraction, but recent memory stores may be disrupted by extreme stimuli, such as head trauma, electroconvulsive shock therapy, and extreme psychologic stress, causing *retrograde amnesia*.

If the memory is to last so that it may be retrieved and recalled days later, the synapse must become permanently facilitated, a process referred to as consolidation. The process of consolidation and the time required for a memory trace to undergo consolidation are probably due to rehearsal of the short-term memory (Guyton, 1987). The brain is thought to rehearse new information so that the important aspects of the sensory experiences become more and more fixed in long-term memory stores. An essential feature of consolidation is codifying of the sensory experiences into different classes of information. Similar patterns are retrieved and recalled from the memory stores to help codify the new information. Information about similarities and differences of the old and new information is stored, not the unprocessed information in the original sensory experience. Thus, memory stores are dynamic and changing over time. The thalamus is thought to play a role in directing the person's attention to relevant information in different association areas. Change from a secondary memory (a weak trace type) into a tertiary memory (a strong trace type) is thought to be accomplished by rehearsal. Each time a memory is retrieved or the sensory experience is repeated, a more permanently facilitated synapse develops. The degree of facilitation may become so high that the information is recalled within a fraction of a second and will last for a lifetime (Guyton, 1987).

Long-term memory may be affected by a failure in (1) transferring information from short-term to long-term memory, (2) consolidating the long-term memory store, or (3) retrieving and recalling the memory or by a physical loss of the memory stores (Fig. 10–3). Bilateral failure (destruction) of the hippocampus and associated temporal lobe structures results in a profound recent memory deficit that is irreversible (Engel & Romano, 1959; Wells, 1977). There is a loss of ability to form new long-term memories, called *anterograde amnesia*, although previously acquired long-term memories remain intact and short-term memory is unaffected. The transition from short-term to long-term memory appears to be affected in many types of learning. In Korsakoff's psychosis, the severe recent memory deficit appears to be an inability to suppress interfering memories from previously learned material. Thus, the

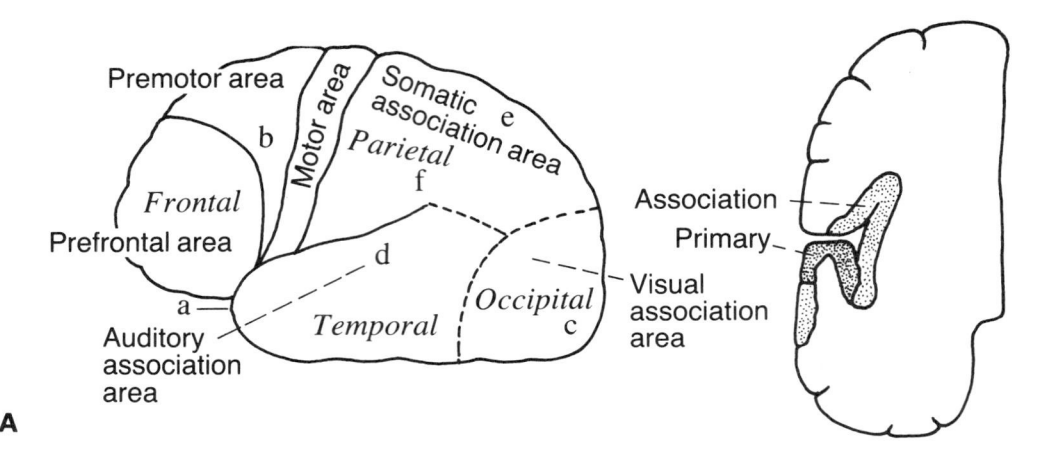

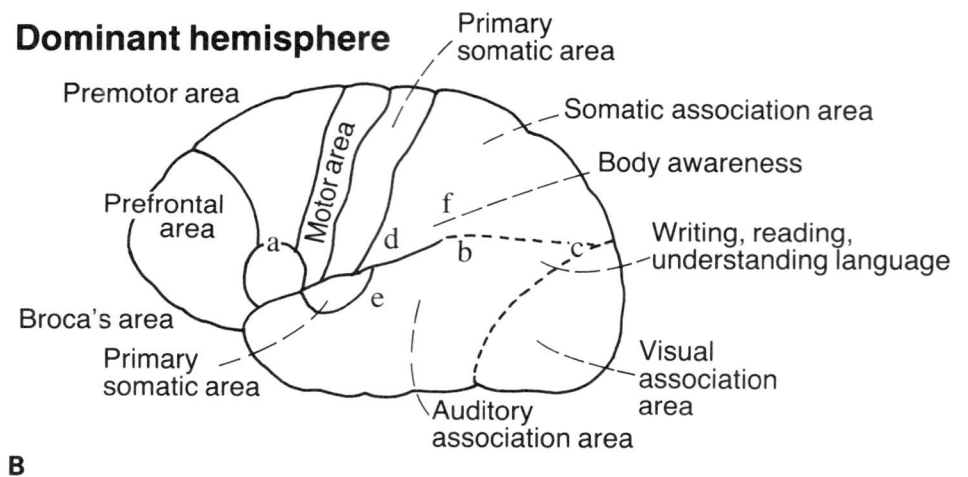

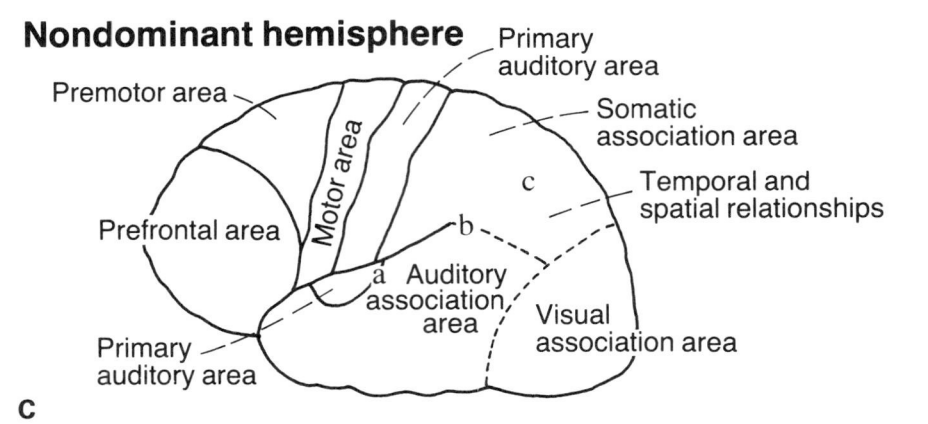

Figure 10–2. Organization of the cerebral cortex and anatomic correlates for cortical deficits (see Table 10–2). *(Adapted from Boss, B. J. [1983]. The dementias.* Journal of Neurosurgical Nursing, 15*(2), 73.)*

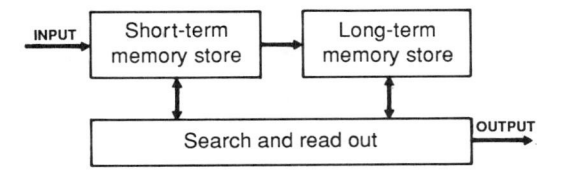

```
INPUT → [Short-term      ] → [Long-term       ]
         [memory store   ]    [memory store    ]
              ↕                     ↕
         [    Search and read out        ] → OUTPUT
```

Figure 10–3. Input into the brain is processed in short-term memory, forming a short-term memory store. At a slightly later point in time, information is transferred into a more permanent long-term store. In this model, there is also a system that functions to search the memory store and to read out the information as demanded by specific tasks. *(From Kandel & Schwartz. Principles of Neural Science, 1985. Courtesy of Elsevier/North Holland.)*

defect in at least some of the anterograde amnesias may be in memory retrieval rather than memory storage (Kupfermann, 1985). Consolidation may be impaired by trauma or other stressors. Physical loss of the memory stores may result from compression, injury, ischemic injury, surgical resection, or many of the dementing illnesses. Failure to retrieve and recall memories accounts for the retrograde amnesia.

Goal-Oriented Behavior

Equally as important as the memory systems for cognitive function is the individual's ability to maintain focus of attention so that long-term memories may be consolidated. The prefrontal areas of the cerebral cortex appear to enable an individual to concentrate on a sequence of memories or thoughts (Guyton, 1987). Being able to maintain one's focus of attention on a thought sequence is essential. Otherwise, the person is distracted and loses the train of thought and consolidation is not able to occur. This ability is referred to as maintaining goal-oriented behavior. Cognitive functioning is directed toward a goal, for example, learning some new material, solving a particular problem, or determining what response is called for.

Clinically, the inability to maintain concentration is manifested as easy distractibility from a thought sequence. The person can perform simple cognitive tasks, such as solving basic mathematical calculations or answering short uncomplicated questions, but cannot maintain concentration to carry out a more complex cognitive task, such as answering a complex question or a series of questions.

Analysis of Sensory Information

The primary and secondary receptive areas of the cortex identify, localize, and begin to analyze sensory stimuli. The association areas (interpretative areas) of the cerebral cortex perform more in-depth analysis and interpretation of sensory stimuli (Fig. 10–2). By comparing the new sensory information with stored memories that are of a similar nature, new sensory experiences are analyzed (Guyton, 1987).

In the analysis process, the individual aspects of the sensory experience are separated, then each aspect is analyzed by comparing it to past sensory experiences. The exact mechanisms by which this is done are not well understood, but in analyzing sensory information, patterns of stimulation seem to be of primary importance. One of the predominant methods of analysis appears to be dissecting information into its component patterns. Sensory information is apparently processed to determine patterns, yet how such patterns of sensations are detected is not known.

The different areas of the cortex reacting to specific types of sensory information include the somesthetic cortical areas, the visual cortical areas, and the auditory cortical areas (Fig. 10–2, Table 10–2).

Somesthetic Cortex. The parietal cortex plays a principal role in the higher level processing of somatic sensory information. The primary somesthetic areas, located in the postcentral gyri, receive somatic sensory input from the ventroposterior thalamus areas. These primary somesthetic areas are believed to analyze only the simple aspects of sensations. They mediate the analysis of localization of sensations, appreciation of movement and position sense, and identification of cutaneous stimuli. This gives the individual the

TABLE 10-2. ANATOMIC CORRELATES FOR CORTICAL DEFICITS.[a]

Area of the Hemisphere	Cortical Deficits
A. Cortical Areas of the Hemispheres	
a. Medial temporal lobes	Impaired recent memory
b. Frontal lobes	Paratonia
	Flexion posturing
	Bladder dysfunction
Motor areas	Pathologic reflexes
Premotor areas	Gait dyspraxias
	Facial dyspraxia
Prefrontal areas	Distractibility
	Loss of social graces
	Impulsiveness
	Mood shifts
c. Visual association areas	Impaired remote visual memories
	Visual agnosia
	Visual neglect syndrome
d. Auditory association areas	Impaired remote auditory memories
	Auditory agnosias
	Auditory neglect syndrome
e. Somatic association areas	Impaired remote somatic memories
	Somatic agnosias (astereognosia)
	Somatic neglect syndrome
f. Inferior posterior parietal lobe	Ideational dyspraxia
B. Cortical Areas of the Dominant Hemisphere	
a. Broca's area	Motor (anterior, expressive) dysphasias
	Speech dyspraxia
b. Superior temporal–inferior parietal area	Sensory (posterior, Wernicke's) dysphasia
	Anomia
c. Posterior hemisphere	Impaired reading
	Acalculia
d. Inferior parietal area	Conductive dysphasia
e. Auditory association area	Word deafness
f. Inferior parietal–temporal area	Perseveration
C. Cortical Areas of the Nondominant Hemisphere	
a. Superior posterior temporal area	Agnosia for nonlanguage sounds
b. Posterior temporal-inferior parietal area	Constructional dyspraxia
	Dressing dyspraxia
c. Parietal lobe	Impaired nonverbal ideation (ideational dyspraxia)
	Impaired drawing or construction of simple and complex figures (spatial construction impairment)
	Impersistence

From Boss, B. J. (1983). The dementias. *Journal of Neurosurgical Nursing, 15*(2), 93.
[a] See corresponding visual representation in Fig. 10-2.

ability to appreciate weight, texture, or temperature. The contribution of the secondary somesthetic areas, located at the base of the postcentral gyri, have not been demonstrated in man (Guyton, 1987; Noback & Demarst, 1975).

The somesthetic association areas of the parietal cortex, occupying the superior parietal lobes posterior to the postcentral gyri, receive input from the primary and secondary somesthetic areas and the lateral thalami. These areas function to interpret somesthetic sensations and store memories of sensory experiences. The discriminative aspects of the primary somesthetic senses are integrated in the somesthetic association cortex. The somesthetic areas provide an individual with the ability to conceptualize qualities of objects, such as shape, form, texture, size, and smoothness. Quantity estimates, such as weight, degree of pressure applied, and temperature change also may be made. Not only may this information be drawn from manual manipulation of an object, but such qualitative and quantitative information may be given by the person even in the absence of the direct sensory stimulus. For example, if an individual is asked to give sensory component information about a pen, a coin, or a leather armchair, that person is able to draw up the sensory images from the association area long-term memory stores. Dysfunction of the somesthetic association areas reduces the person's ability to analyze and interpret different characteristics of somatic sensory experiences. The ability to recognize complex objects and forms by touch is impaired, and the person loses the sense of body form.

Visual Cortex. The primary visual areas, located on the medial portion of each occipital lobe, the striate area, are the primary receptive areas for visual stimuli (Figs. 10–1, 10–2). Here initial perception of the visual stimulus, such as form, brightness, and shading, takes place. Color is thought to be partially analyzed by the primary visual cortices, although initial recognition of color is at the subcortical level. Unlike somesthetic sensation, there is no conscious perception of visual stimuli at a subcortical level. An individual is functionally blind without an intact primary visual cortex (Guyton, 1987).

The visual association areas, that is, the secondary visual areas, receive input from the striate area and mediate further processing of visual information, responding to more complex patterns than do the primary visual areas, and thus are involved in analysis of complicated visual patterns of stimuli. Dysfunction of the visual association areas (visual interpretative areas) does not result in blindness but does diminish the person's ability to recognize and interpret what is seen, that is, to perceive forms, size, and meaning of objects. Loss or impaired function of the visual association area in the left (dominant) hemisphere produces an inability to comprehend written language, referred to as "dyslexia" or "word blindness." Loss of written language comprehension does not occur with dysfunction of the right (nondominant) hemisphere, but performance of tasks requiring visual–spatial perception, such as drawing, is impaired markedly.

From the secondary visual cortices, the processed visual information is projected to the posterior portions of the temporal lobes, where the highest level of visual image integration is thought to take place. Here, tasks that require visual perception are learned, such as using vision to cue eating, to drive, or to read this chapter. Impaired function in this area of the left (dominant) hemisphere begins to impair language comprehension and all cognitive functions that rely heavily on language comprehension. Impairment of this area within the right (nondominant) hemisphere impairs all visual–perceptual comprehension and all cognitive functions that rely on accurate visual–spatial appreciation.

Auditory Cortex. The auditory cortices, that is, primary auditory areas and secondary auditory areas (the auditory association areas), are located in the posterior superior temporal gyri and extend over the lateral border onto the insular cortex and onto the most lateral portion of the parietal lobe (Fig. 10–2). The primary and secondary auditory areas of the left (dominant) hemisphere mediate language comprehension. The primary and secondary auditory areas of the right (nondominant) hemisphere mediate nonlanguage sound analysis and interpretation.

The primary auditory areas, which receive input directly from the medial geniculate body, detect individual elements, that is, pitches and patterns of the auditory stimuli. For example, a simple sound may be identified as being weak or loud (low or high intensity) or of low or high frequency. Simple patterns can be interpreted. However, the primary auditory cortex alone cannot provide normal auditory experiences. The meaning of the sound cannot be interpreted, and there is no perception of words or intelligible sounds. Dysfunction in the auditory cortex results in hearing loss (Guyton, 1987).

The primary auditory areas working in conjunction with their respective secondary auditory areas provide for the analysis of complicated sounds. The primary auditory cortex and the thalamic association areas adjacent to the medial geniculate body provide input to the auditory association areas. Dysfunction in the secondary auditory areas does not result in the loss of hearing but produces difficulty in interpreting sounds, that is, a reduced ability to understand the meaning of the auditory stimuli. If there is dysfunction in the left (dominant) hemisphere's auditory association area, language comprehension is seriously impaired. The individual has a reduced ability to understand spoken language. If the dysfunction is in the right auditory association area, the individual has a reduced ability to appreciate and interpret nonlanguage sounds, such as music.

General Interpretive Area. The somesthetic, visual, and auditory association areas merge in the inferior portion of the parietal lobe, the angular gyrus, and the supramarginal gyrus. The supramarginal gyrus and the posterior temporal lobe are often labeled the general interpretive area (or general association area). This area integrates processed sensory information and correlates input associated with the somesthetic modalities and those associated with auditory and visual senses. Complex memory patterns involving more than one sensory modality are believed to be stored at least partially in this area. This integration of input from all sensory association areas allows synthesis of a common thought.

A person with dysfunction in the general interpretive area is able to hear without difficulty, read printed words, and has no loss of sensation but is unable to recognize the thought conveyed or the meaning of the sensory experiences. Such dysfunction in terms of interpretation leaves a person with a tremendous cognitive deficit.

The general interpretive area of the left hemisphere is usually very highly developed and, because it mediates complex language, plays the largest single role of any area of the cerebral cortex in the higher levels of brain function that are referred to as cognition. A majority of our sensory experiences are converted into language equivalents, then analyzed, interpreted, and stored in the left general interpretive area.

Dysfunction in the left general interpretive area leaves the person not only with a Wernicke's (sensory, receptive, posterior) dysphasia but also with a loss of cognitive functions associated with language or symbolism, such as the ability to perform mathematical calculations and to think through logical problems.

The general interpretative area of the right (nondominant) hemisphere mediates understanding and interpretation of music, nonverbal visual experiences, spatial relationships between the person and the surroundings, and probably somatic experiences related to hand and extremity use. People with dysfunction in the right general interpretive area lose cognitive functions associated with nonlanguage sounds, such as appreciation of tone and delivery of speech, as well as those functions associated with visual–spatial dimensions, such as drawing, art appreciation, and athletic performance. They may exhibit a neglect syndrome, varying in severity to the point of denial of illness, and a constructional dyspraxia.

Dysfunction in the supramarginal gyrus results in astereognosis, the inability to recognize common objects on the basis of somatic sensory information. The person is unable to appreciate the meaning of the sensory stimuli. For example, when a person with a supramarginal area dysfunction on the right side has a comb placed in the contralateral hand, he or she is not able to recognize the object as a comb or visualize it in imagination through manual examination of the object. The person is able to state isolated qualities about the object but is unable to integrate the bits of information into the concept of a comb.

Elaboration of Thought

As has been discussed previously, cognitive function is not simply the maintenance of attention and placing the information in a long-term memory store. Cognitive function involves consolidating the long-term memory store that requires retrieving and recalling pieces of the sensory information for reprocessing on the basis of later sensory data entered into the memory system. The prefrontal areas appear to enable this type of storage of many bits of sequential information in various cortical association areas. Thus, the information is retrieved and recalled again and again as the thought sequence is carried on, permitting what is called elaboration of thought. Elaboration of thought is defined as an "increase in depth and abstractness of the different thoughts" (Guyton, 1987). Guyton suggests that abilities associated with human intelligence, such as the ability to plan or solve complicated mathematical problems, may be possible because of the prefrontal ability to bring about the simultaneous storage of many types of information (Guyton, 1987).

A person with dysfunction in elaboration of thought acts impulsively without apparent consideration to the consequences of the behavior or the appropriate degree of responses that is called for. This impulsiveness contributes to the emergence of socially unacceptable behavior (Boss, 1982).

COGNITION: NORMAL AGE-RELATED CHANGES

Neurons begin to age at 30 years. Aging is manifested by a decrease in the number of neurons and an increase in size and number of neuroglial cells. Dendrites and dendritic spines decrease in number (Boss, in press). Striking changes in the somatodendritic apparatus lead to this loss of dendrites with age. Initially, these changes appear to begin as swelling and distortion of the somatodendrite, followed by dendritic loss. Axon diameter thins, as does the myelin sheath. In addition, special and general receptors decrease in number.

Lipofuscin, granulovacuolar organelles, and neurofibrillary tangles may be found in some cells (Cote, 1985). Lipofuscin is thought to be composed of large end-stage lysosomes that have accumulated, recycled membranes, and other cellular debris that cannot be catabolized further by the neuron. Lipofuscin granules have not been demonstrated to impair neuronal function. Different types of neurons appear to accumulate lipofuscin at different rates. Degenerating neurons of the hippocampus and adjacent cortex accumulate granulovacuolar organelles in their cytoplasm and dendrites. These vacuoles are encapsulated by membrane and possess a dense small granule in the center. Neurofibrillary tangles (Alzheimer's bodies) are large bundles of twisted tubules composed of a pair of filaments.

Neuritic (senile) plaques may be seen extracellularly. The plaque is composed of a central amyloid core that is surrounded by degenerating neuronal processes and an outer covering of glial cells. Plaques are anywhere from 5 to 100 µm in diameter and are most densely found in the hippocampus but are common in the neocortex as well (Cote, 1985).

Macroscopic changes include a decrease in brain weight and a volume of less than 15% by age 80. Atrophy of portions of the cerebral cortex, especially in the limbic lobe, insula, and orbital gyri of the frontal lobe, is present. Thus, the gyri narrow in width and the sulci widen. There is an increase in ventricular size and an increased volume of cerebrospinal fluid to fill the space vacated by cortical neurons. The white matter tracts become thinner, and the meninges thicken (Boss, in press).

Biochemically, total brain protein is reduced by 30%, but total brain DNA is increased, presumably because of glial cell proliferation. Lipid content of the brain is only minimally changed. The amount of available neurotransmitters is decreased probably as a result of changes in enzymes. The enzymes required for dopamine and norepinephrine synthesis are drastically reduced. A less severe reduction occurs in the enzymes that catalyze acetylcholine and glutamic acid production. Neuronal activity is decreased, evidenced by a decreased frequency and amplitude of brain waves on an electroencephalogram. There is about a 20% reduction in cerebral blood flow and a decreased oxygen consumption. There is about a 10% decrease in conduction velocity (speed of transmission), thus increasing response time (Cote, 1985; Guyton, 1987).

Functionally, recent memory decreases with normal aging to some small degree. Learning time is increased, and reaction time and response time increase.

SUMMARY

What is the neurophysiologic basis of thinking, reasoning, forming judgments, or gaining insight? The neurophysiology of cognition (e.g., mentation, intellectual activity), even the neuroanatomic structures involved in cognition, have not been definitely established. It has been demonstrated that different parts of the brain, predominantly in the cerebral cortices, focus on specific aspects of sensory experiences. Patterns of sensory stimulation are compared to patterns already stored in memory. Data support the localization view proposing that cognition is the result of primary cortical processes carried out by the specific neurons and their specifically developed interneuronal connections. Cognition is the integration of primary cortical abilities that have some degree of anatomic localization.

Development of the neuroanatomic structures necessary for cognition starts early in the prenatal period with the proliferation and generation of classes of neurons and other cells that shortly thereafter migrate to their appropriate location and begin the process of cell maturation with the establishment of specific interneuronal connections. These processes are probably genetically and developmentally determined. The presence of internal environmental influences, such as specific nutrients, oxygen and hormones, and external environmental influences, such as external stimulation, exert a definite influence on the developing cortical areas and their primary abilities prenatally and postnatally. Final cortical development appears to result from environmentally induced learning, which enables the strengthening and fine tuning of certain primary abilities.

The specific primary abilities of certain cortical structures have been established through laboratory and clinical studies. The primary abilities relevant to cognition are the memory systems permitting analysis and interpretation of sensory data, goal-oriented behavior, and elaboration of thought. The neuroanatomy and neurophysiology of memory and its relationship to learning are more clearly understood than the neuroanatomy and neurophysiology of cognition.

Memory is fundamental to learning and cognition. The ability to establish, retain (consolidate), retrieve, and recall long-term memory stores is the basis of all learning. A memory trace is actually a facilitated neuronal circuit that, if it becomes permanently facilitated (consolidated), permits retrieval and recall of long-term memory stores. Through retrieval and recall, all components of the new information are examined in the various cortical areas for patterns of similarity and dissimilarity to previously stored long-term memories. The hippocampus and its adjacent areas play a major role in the establishment, retaining, and retrieval of memories. The cortical association areas are the predominant storage areas for long-term memories. Memory is impaired if there is a failure or impairment in the ability to establish, consolidate, or retrieve and recall long-term memory stores.

The prefrontal areas contribute to memory and cognition by mediating goal-oriented behavior and elaboration of thought. Through the primary ability of goal-oriented behavior, a person is able to concentrate on a sequence of memories or thoughts that enhances the consolidation process. Elaboration of thought is believed to enabie the retrieval and recall of individual components of sequential sensory experiences in the various cortical association areas again and again as a thought sequence progresses, permitting an increase in the depth and abstractness of the thoughts. Failure of or impairment in goal-oriented behavior and elaboration of thought results in distractibility, lack of concentration, impulsiveness, concreteness, and poor decision making.

Neuroanatomically, neurons age by decreasing the number and size of the neuronal cell bodies and neuronal processes and the thickness of their myelin sheaths. Neuronal metabolic processes decrease, and therefore neuronal functions slow. Neurophysiologically, recent memory is slightly decreased, learning time is somewhat increased, and reaction and response time are increased. Exaggerated neuronal aging may be manifest as dementia.

REFERENCES

Adams, R.A., & Victor, M. (1977). *Principles of neurology*. New York: McGraw-Hill.

Armstrong, M.E., Howe, J., Smith, A.P., Smith, M.M., & Snider, M.J. (1979). *McGraw-Hill nursing dictionary*. New York: McGraw-Hill.

Blakesless, T.R. (1980). *The right brain*. Garden City, NY: Doubleday.

Boss, B.J. (1982). Acute mood and behavior disturbances of neurological origin: Acute confusional states. *Journal of Neurosurgical Nursing, 14*, 61.

Boss, B.J. (in press). Neuroanatomy and neurophysiology. In K. McCance & S. Huether (Eds.), *Pathophysiology*. Menlo Park, CA: Addison-Wesley.

Cote, L. (1985). Aging of the brain and dementia. In E.R. Kandel & J.H. Schwartz (Eds.), *Principles of neural science* (2nd ed., p. 784). New York: Elsevier/North Holland.

Engel, G.L., & Romano, J. (1959). Delirium: a syndrome of cerebral insufficiency. *Journal of Chronic Disease, 9*, 260.

English Language Institute of America. (1967). *The living Webster encyclopedia dictionary of the English language*. Chicago: Author.

Ferris, S.H., deLeon, M.J., Wolf, A.P., George, A.E., Reisberg, B., Christman, D.R., Yonekura, Y., & Fowler, J.S. (1981). Positron emission tomography in dementia. In R. Mayeux & W.B. Rosen (Eds.), *The dementias (p. 123)*. New York: Raven Press.

Finn, R. (1983). New split-brain research divides scientists. *Science Digest, 19*(12), 54, 103.

Guyton, A.C. (1987). *Basic human neurophysiology* (3rd ed.). Philadelphia: W.B. Saunders Company.

Kandel, E.R. (1985a). Brain and behavior. In E.R. Kandel & J.H. Schwartz (Eds.), *Principles of neural science* (2d ed., p. 3). New York: Elsevier/North Holland.

Kandel, E.R. (1985b). Synapse formation, trophic interactions between neurons, and the development of behavior. In E.R. Kandel & J.H. Schwartz (Eds.), *Principles of neural science* (2nd ed., p. 743). New York: Elsevier/North Holland.

Kupfermann, I. (1985). Learning. In E.R. Kandel & J.H. Schwartz Eds.), *Principles of neural science* (2nd ed., p. 805). New York: Elsevier/North Holland.

Lashley, K.S. (1929). *Brain mechanisms and intelligence: a quantitative study of injuries to the brain*. Chicago: University of Chicago.

Noback, C.R., & Demarst, R.J. (1975). *The human nervous system: Basic principles of neurobiology* (2nd ed.). New York: McGraw-Hill.

Schacher, S. (1985). Determination and differentiation in the development of the nervous system. In E.R. Kandel & J.H. Schwartz (Eds.), *Principles of neural science* (2nd ed., p. 729). New York: Elsevier/North Holland.

Wells, C.E. (1977). *Dementia*. Philadelphia: Davis.

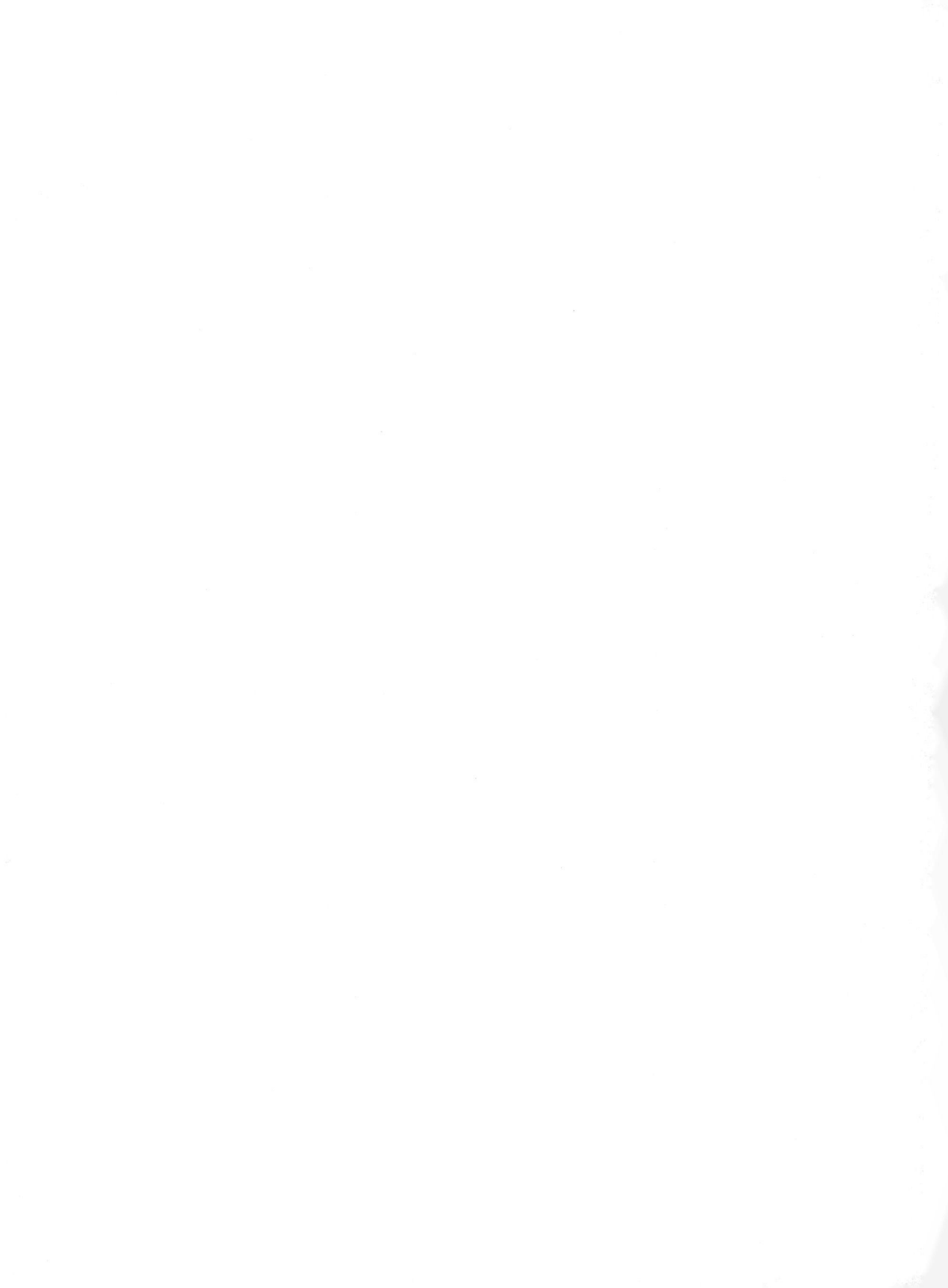

11

Assessment of Cognition

Margarethe Cammermeyer

ASSESSMENT OF COGNITIVE FUNCTION IN THE CLINICAL SETTING

Assessment of cognitive function is an assessment of integrated brain function and occurs with each verbal and nonverbal interaction. It may be formal or informal, conscious or unconscious, or part of a social or professional interaction. For example, a family determines, from daily contact, that a member is no longer capable of performing activities of daily living. In contrast, a neuropsychologist uses formal tests to identify impaired cognitive functioning. Both family and professional identify impaired cognition, but the methods of assessment differ.

This chapter focuses on methods of assessing cognitive processes, such as memory, information processing, and goal-oriented behaviors. It does not assess primary sensory functions, such as hearing (not to be confused with understanding), vision (not to be confused with spatial–perceptual ability), or primary motor functioning (not to be confused with apraxia). Such assessment is described in Chapter 23. The presumption in this chapter is that the peripheral organs, such as the eyes and ears, are working properly.

Nursing assessment of cognition is directed toward discovering dysfunctions that have an impact on daily living. It is, therefore, useful to consider an organizational framework that emphasizes brain functioning.

FUNCTIONAL ORGANIZATION OF THE BRAIN

Luria (1973) organizes the brain into three primary functional units. The first functional unit includes the brainstem, mesial cortex, and diencephalon and is the seat of *arousal* (*alertness*), *memory*, and *emotion*. This first unit is, therefore, the center for "regulating and modifying the body's tone and control over inclinations and emotions of the person . . . they are the center for memory and consciousness" (pp. 60, 67). Anatomically, this area comprises the reticular activating system of the brainstem.

The second functional unit is the seat for *reception, analysis,* and *storage of sensory information.* Peripheral sensory organs of hearing, vision, smell, and touch enable information from the environment to be transmitted through the sensory system into the second functional unit. The sensory information is processed by integration with information received from the first functional unit. The diencephalon must be intact, and the person must be aroused or alert to receive and process the incoming information. Some input from the third functional unit also enters into this information processing. For example, memory and emotional processing of the information occur in response to the sensory stimulus. Anatomically, the second functional unit comprises the posterior cerebral hemispheres and the temporal, parietal, and occipital areas (Luria, 1973).

The third functional unit described by Luria (1973) *programs, regulates,* and *verifies input.* The anterior portions of the brain from the premotor cortex receive information from the first and second functional units and respond to the information, culminating in some motor output or autonomic response. The output may take the form of movement or speech or may be limited to cortical integration of information considered "thought" or "emotion." The limbic system and deeper cortical structures are presumed to encompass the third functional unit.

In contrast to Luria (1973), Plum and Posner (1980) consider cognition to be a part of consciousness. They ascribe cognitive functions to the content of consciousness, as contrasted with the arousal functions of consciousness. As described in Chapter 5, arousal is measured by the observable responsiveness of a person to a variety of stimuli. Cognitive functioning, or the content of consciousness, cannot be tested adequately in people with altered arousal.

Functionally, the content of consciousness, as defined by Plum and Posner (1980), includes higher cortical activities, such as receiving, processing, organizing, and storing information. The content of consciousness can also be measured, in part, through determination of a person's orientation in time and space, reasoning, abstract thinking, and goal-oriented behaviors. These are behaviors comparable to those that are mediated by Luria's third functional unit: information about what a person can do and how much a person knows. In addition, Lezak (1983, p. 38) describes cognitive "executive functions" that determine whether and how a person cares for oneself, is employable, or maintains normal social relationships.

Both structural and metabolic processes may alter cognition or information processing. For example, a mass in the left parietal region results in communication difficulties. Metabolic imbalance alters the chemical substrate of brain metabolism and produces changes in cognitive functioning; for example, low blood glucose, severe hypoxemia, and sudden hyponatremia can all produce confusion and loss of consciousness.

TYPES OF COGNITIVE ASSESSMENT

Cognitive functions are presumed to be measurable. The kinds of higher level executive functions that have an impact on people's lives include communication, perception, visual and manual praxis, memory, orientation, attention, self-regulation, and personality (Lezak, 1983). These functions are determined by evaluating individual ability to perform specific actions or responses purported to reflect specific cognitive processes. These areas and useful assessments are shown in Table 11-1.

Both the kinds of questions or tasks assessed in Table 11-1 and the ongoing observations of patients or clients in clinical settings provide some indication of cognitive functioning as it influences everyday life. The methods and tools used to assess cortical functioning, however, cannot capture the full dimensions of cognitive processes or how those processes interact to create the "humanity" of an individual. The methods used to evaluate cognitive function are derived from neuropsychology and tend to measure cortical functioning in isolation, that is, not in the context of the activities of daily living. Nursing can make a useful contribution to the evaluation

TABLE 11–1. COGNITIVE FUNCTIONS AND THEIR GENERAL EVALUATION.

Function	Evaluation
Orientation	To time, place, person, situation, ability to self-regulate, impulse control, and grasp of gestalt of situation
Verbal function	Verbal fluency, repetition of words, fluency of making and understanding spoken and written language
Perceptual function	Visual: Recognize object from visual cues; picture recognition Auditory: Evaluated by asking to repeat a sentence Tactile: Construction with tiles or identifying objects; following sequence of commands using objects
Visuospatial functions and dexterity	Entails creating designs from two dimensional pictures
Memory function	Broad area requiring evaluation of visual, auditory, immediate, short-term and long-term memory; evaluated through historical interview, repetition of words, numbers, and nonsense words, sentences, or stories at various time intervals after first presentation; pictures may be drawn from visual memory or stories repeated from auditory recall
General fund of knowledge and gestalt for situations	Assimilation in general areas of evaluation
Construct formation and reasoning ability	Using judgment and using previous life experiences; become encompassed in backdrop of memory functioning

of cognitive functioning by integrating understanding of the neuropsychologic assessment with evaluation of the impact of cognitive dysfunction on everyday living.

Cognitive functioning can be evaluated by using formal neurobehavioral batteries, screening neuropsychologic tests, or tests that evaluate specific cognitive functions.

Formal Neurobehavioral Batteries

Formal neurobehavioral batteries are useful in that they

1. Systematically evaluate numerous areas of cognitive function
2. Provide a complete evaluation
3. Have established interrater reliability among administrators
4. Have been used repeatedly and show stability
5. Have been validated against other measures of brain function.

The major disadvantages of such batteries are that they are time consuming and costly; they require that patients be highly attentive and cooperative; and they have a high level of specificity in dealing with both normal and abnormal areas of cognitive function. Further, they require specialty training to administer and evaluate results and are difficult to administer in acute care settings (Lezak, 1983). Examples of such batteries include personality inventories, intelligence tests, and neuropsychologic tests.

There are no adequate or specific measures of personality, only measures of behavioral traits. Traits commonly described as components of personality include somatization, obsessive–compulsive behavior, interpersonal sensitivity, depression, anxiety, hostility, phobic anxiety, paranoid ideation, and psychoticism. Tests such as the Minnesota Multiphasic Personality Inventory (MMPI) and the Symptom Checklist-90, Revised (SCL-90 R) are used as measures of these behavioral traits (Derogatis, 1977) and have been used to describe *personality traits*. The MMPI takes several hours to complete and may be offensive to people who feel it is a test to see if they are "crazy." The MMPI does not assist in localizing diseases per se, but it provides a pattern of responses noted in subjects with psychiatric or neurologic disorders. There are 566 questions in the MMPI, with no time limit to complete. It is scored by computer, which may delay receipt of results. It is, therefore, of limited value in the acute care setting.

The SCL-90 R is a brief, 90-item self-report symptom inventory designed to reflect *psychologic symptom patterns*. Each item is rated on 5-point scale from "not at all" to "extremely" distressed response. The test takes from 15 to 20 minutes to complete and is not offensive, yet provides useful information that assists in identifying personality patterns of behavior. Personality, emotions, social stresses, and hospitalization affect the results of neuropsychologic testing.

The most commonly used test of general *intellectual ability* is the Wechsler Adult Intelligence Scale (WAIS). An adjusted version has been developed for children of preschool and primary school age that is similar to the adult version but downgraded and revised as appropriate to developmental age. The three versions of the Wechsler Intelligence Scale evaluate verbal and performance ability. The verbal scale includes general information, comprehension, arithmetic, similarities, digit span, and vocabulary. The performance scale includes digit symbols, picture completion, block design, picture arrangement, and object assembly. The results provide information about verbal comprehension, perceptual organization, and memory. Numerous studies have been performed to standardize the tests and establish reliability and validity (Buron, 1978). The major limitation of the WAIS is that it takes from 6 to 8 hours to administer. The written report accompanying the WAIS score provides specific information of how the person performed on each subtest, but the final result is expressed in a single number.

Another commonly used formal neuropsychologic test is the Halstead-Reitan Battery. The Halstead Battery is comprised of six tests including a category test, tactual performance test, rhythm test, speech sounds, perception test, and fingertapping test. To the battery Reitan added the Trail Making Test, an aphasia screening test, sensory examination, and motor strength evaluation. The entire test takes from 6 to 8 hours to administer.

Although the Halstead-Reitan Battery has limited value in patients with a dense motor or sensory deficit, it is useful as a neuropsychologic test of cognitive deficits (Reitan, 1955; Reitan & Tarshes, 1959).

Neuropsychologic Screening Tests

Administration of formal test batteries often is not practical for acutely ill patients because of their physical disabilities and limited attention span. Under such conditions, an abbreviated screening assessment tool is more useful. Such tools assess several areas of functioning in a brief time and can be performed by people without formal neuropsychologic training. Nurses, speech therapists, rehabilitation specialists, and others are developing screening instruments for use in the acute care setting. The objectives of such an instrument are that it must be able to assess multiple areas of cognitive function, be able to identify cognitive dysfunction, be reliable, reproducible, and valid, be clinically relevant for patient care, safety, autonomy, and self-esteem, and be administered practically.

Screening assessment is begun during the admission interview to a medical facility. The assessment includes evaluating the patient's ability to hear, and to communicate, and to maintain visual contact and affective interaction. The content of responses allows for additional evaluation of communication skills, coping, orientation, judgment, and emotional and social interaction. The screening neuropsychologic assessment instrument is used to corroborate initial clinical impressions. One such screening tool, adapted from the Reitan-Indiana Aphasia Screen, can be adapted for bedside administration. It is comprised of six components:

1. Copy these figures:

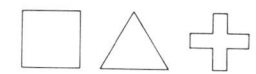

   □ △ ✛

2. Name these figures.
3. Spell the names of the figures.
4. Repeat the sentence: "He shouted the warning."

5. Explain the meaning of the sentence.
6. Write the sentence.

These questions explore the patient's visual–spatial ability, the ability to communicate, repeat words, understand, use abstract reasoning, and write. Other screening neuropsychologic tools can be used that corroborate the identification of cognitive dysfunction detected in the initial interview.

The Mini-Mental State (MMS) (Folstein et al., 1975; Anthony et al., 1982) is a general neuropsychologic screening tool used in such clinical areas as medicine, psychiatry, and geriatrics. The MMS tests orientation, registration, attention, calculations, recall, and language. Subtest scores are summed for one final score. A total scores of less than 23 is noted in patients with dementia and psychiatric disorders with 80% to 90% reliability. The test focuses on communication ability and does not deal with spatial–perceptual skills or other right brain functions. When using the MMS, the quality of the answers may have more pragmatic value than the single number score. Difficulty with orientation, attention, recall, and language will interfere with ability for self-care. The MMS takes 5 minutes to administer. The WAIS IQ and MMS show general agreement when compared in psychiatric and neurologically impaired populations. A 39% false-positive result was noted by Dick et al. (1984) in people with less formal education and in older patients.

Another brief neuropsychologic screening instrument is the Portable Short Mental Status Questionnaire (PSMSQ) (Pfeiffer, 1975). This is a 10-item test of orientation, recent and long-term memory, and serial calculations. The total score is a single number that purports to measure intelligence or mild, moderate, or severe impairment. The test employs commonly used questions and quantifies the patient's answers. The test has a normative score for the geriatric population, and results are affected by the educational preparation of the subject.

A widely used neuropsychologic tool is the Trail Making Test (Reitan, 1955). Originally, this was called the Taylor Number Series and was used by the Army in 1945 to test general ability, since it requires attention to detail and ability to alternate sequencing of events. The Trail Making Test has two sections, A and B. Trail Making A consists of 25 consecutively numbered circles spread out over an 11 by 8½ inch paper. The purpose of this test is to draw a line as rapidly as possible from circle to circle in consecutive sequence. Trail Making B consists of alternating number and letter sequences. The Trail Making Test has been used to evaluate organic brain damage. A patient with a metabolic disorder may be able to complete both Trail Making A and B but do so very slowly. With structural changes in the brain, the patient may be totally unable to organize thoughts sufficiently to follow through on the sequencing of the numbers or be unable to alternate between numbers and letters. Translated into real world situations, this means that the patient may have difficulty with self-care activities that require organizing sequential activities. The Trail Making Test has normative data and is age normed (Brown et al., 1958; Conn, 1977; Reitan, 1955).

The Reitan-Indiana Aphasia Screen is a test in which the subject is shown a series of pictures, words, and numbers on a small, handheld flip chart. Each question purports to evaluate a specific cognitive skill. The person is asked to draw a square and if unable to do so is considered to have constructional apraxia. If unable to name a pictured object, the person is considered to have an anomia. As the person is unable to respond appropriately to a command, the cognitive deficit is defined on the flip chart. The second half of the Reitan-Indiana Aphasia Screen evaluates sensory– and spatial–perceptual function. The subject is asked to identify objects by touch and to identify where they are touched when their eyes are closed. The test also evaluates the patient's visual field perception. The Reitan-Indiana Aphasia Screen is used as a screening tool to evaluate cognitive abilities, such as communication skills, spatial–perceptual intactness, gestalt of a situation, judgment, and abstract thinking. There are no scores when the screen is completed. The major drawback of the test is the inability to quantify results or document decrements of change, which makes serial evaluations difficult. The test is useful, however, because it can identify specific cognitive deficits and can be administered with minimal training.

Another brief neuropsychologic instrument is the Neurobehavioral Cognitive Status Examination (NCSE) (Kiernan et al., 1987; Mueller, 1984). The NCSE provides information in 10 areas: level of consciousness, orientation, attention, communication, memory, constructional ability, calculations, reasoning, abstraction, and similarities. Specific questions are asked as screening questions. If the screening questions are answered accurately, the next area of cognitive functioning is evaluated. If the person does not pass the screen, a metric portion of the subset of questions is asked. The questions are progressively more difficult until the person is no longer able to answer the metric questions or until the question reaches the same level of complexity as the screening question. The scores are tabulated and recorded on a visual graph. Normative ranges are noted in the shaded portion of the graph (Appendix 11–1).

The NCSE takes 20 minutes to administer, requires several props (tiles, pencil, stopwatch, key, coin, flash cards), and a manual. Tabulating the scores in each category is simple. The rating of mild, moderate, or severe impairnent does not necessarily reflect a patient's ability to function in the real world. Information obtained from this and other neuropsychologic instruments cannot be generalized to all people, although the information obtained is useful to determine areas of cognitive impairment. Interviewing the patient and family will provide the additional information required to incorporate the results on the NCSE into real world situations to develop strategies for intervention.

A major advantage of the NCSE is that it evaluates a full range of cognitive abilities, is inexpensive, and can be repeated readily on serial assessment. Little test–retest effect has been noted in patients with neurologic dysfunction. The test can be administered by people with minimal previous training. The major drawbacks include the inability of the test to evaluate impulsive responses and reliance on verbal ability to respond to questions. Patients with dysphasia will do poorly on this test, as is the case with other screening neuropsychologic tests.

Specific Tests of Cognitive Function

A third method of neuropsychologic evaluation involves administering specific tests addressing only selected areas of cognitive functioning. For example, the patient with Alzheimer's disease may be given only memory tests. Serial administration of these tests can then document changes in memory over time. These specific tests are efficient and less demanding of the patient's and examiner's time and concentration. The integration, however, of the specific cognitive function into the total social functioning of the person may be missed with selected function testing.

The Galveston Orientation and Amnesia Test (GOAT) (Levin et al., 1979) is a brief quantitative scale that measures orientation and memory. It is used specifically for evaluation of posttraumatic and retrograde amnesia. Questions address orientation to time, place, person, and present and past events. It is a 10-item scale, with one total sum as the score obtained. Deficits in memory and orientation exist if the score is less than 66. A negative total score of −100 is possible.

A comparison of functions evaluated in a variety of neuropsychologic tests is shown in Table 11–2.

INTEGRATION OF NURSING AND NEUROPSYCHOLOGIC ASSESSMENT

The most basic, yet essential, aspect of assessing cognitive processing is in the nursing interview and through observations made during that interview with the patient. The interview includes determining the patient's fund of knowledge based on expectation by

TABLE 11-2. COMPARISON OF MENTAL STATUS EXAMINATIONS WITH FUNCTIONS TESTED.

	Ori[a]	Att	Calc	Lang	Const	Mem	Reas
Mental Status Questionnaire	+						
Portable Short Mental Status Questionnaire	+		+				
Mini-Mental State	+	+	+	+	+	+	
Galveston Orientation and Amnesia Test	+					+	
Cognitive Capacity Screening Examination	+	+	+	+		+	+
Neurobehavioral Cognitive Status Examination	+	+	+	+	+	+	+

[a]Ori, orientation; Att, attention; Calc, calculation; Lang, Language; Const, construction; Mem, memory; Reas, reasoning.

age, culture, and educational background. The history the person and family describe and observations of the patient's interactions provide extensive information for further evaluations. Subsequent evaluations can be viewed in the following context from the interview:

- Communication: Ability to speak, understand, and respond appropriately
- Orientation: Alert and aware of time, place, and person at all times
- Judgment: Decision making governed by insight into self and situation
- Emoting: Able to express full range of emotions
- Coping: Presence of major stressors resulting in anxiety, tension headache, irritability
- Social interaction: Has family and support; able to form relationships

If the interview suggests cognitive deficits (Table 11-3), further evaluation often is useful. The briefer neurobehavioral screening tests have pragmatic value in such clinical settings. Some tests are more specific than others; for example, the GOAT is useful when evaluating memory function. If orientation and dementia are the areas of interest, the PSMSQ or MMS may be more useful. The NCSE is useful as a broader tool for assessing cognitive functioning in the acute care setting. These tests are easy to administer, inexpensive to score, take little time to administer, and can be used in test–retest situations with the patient as his or her own control. The information obtained from these tests is communicated easily to other health care providers and is useful for patient care and planning.

If the screening evaluation is considered incomplete to derive an effective evaluative plan, specialized evaluation is warranted. Formal neuropsychologic tests are administered by neuropsychologists to obtain extensive information about the cognitive process of the brain. Such testing is time consuming and costly and has limited clinical value in acute care settings. The tests are useful, however, to obtain specific information on all aspects of cognition not available by cursory evaluation using less sophisticated measures.

The value of effective, accurate assessment cannot be overemphasized to ensure appropriate patient assessment and to develop effective patient diagnosis and appropriate interventions. The nurse is in the unique posi-

TABLE 11-3. GUIDELINES OF INDICATIONS TO FORMALIZE NEUROPSYCHOLOGIC ASSESSMENTS.

- Patient or family describes changes in mental status or cognition.
- Behavior and responses aberrant to situation in view of age, education, culture.
- There is evidence or concern about learning disabilities.
- There are difficulties with behavioral or psychologic problems or developmental psychosocial difficulties.
- There is evidence of difficulty adapting to change.

162 II. 2. COGNITION PHENOMENA

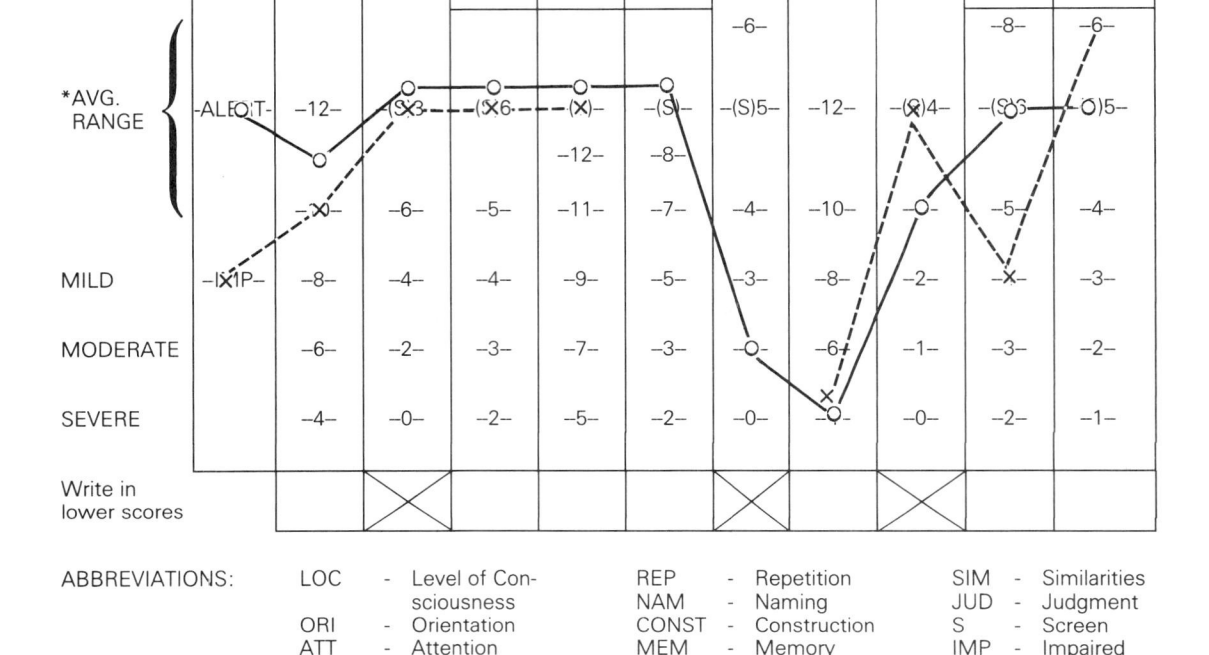

| | LOC | ORI | ATT | LANGUAGE ||| CONST | MEM | CALC | REASONING ||
				COMP	REP	NAM				SIM	JUD
							–6–			–8–	–6–
*AVG. RANGE	-ALE⊗T-	–12–	–(S)3–	–(X)6–	–(X)–	–(S)–	–(S)5–	–12–	–(X)4–	–(S)○3–	○5–
					–12–	–8–					
		–X–	–6–	–5–	–11–	–7–	–4–	–10–	–○–	–5–	–4–
MILD	–IX1P–	–8–	–4–	–4–	–9–	–5–	–3–	–8–	–2–	–X–	–3–
MODERATE	–6–	–2–	–3–	–7–	–3–	–○–	–6–	–1–	–3–	–2–	
SEVERE	–4–	–0–	–2–	–5–	–2–	–0–	–○–	–0–	–2–	–1–	
Write in lower scores											

ABBREVIATIONS:
- LOC - Level of Consciousness
- ORI - Orientation
- ATT - Attention
- COMP - Comprehension
- REP - Repetition
- NAM - Naming
- CONST - Construction
- MEM - Memory
- CALC - Calculations
- SIM - Similarities
- JUD - Judgment
- S - Screen
- IMP - Impaired

Figure 11–1. The cognitive status profile of a patient diagnosed with an aneurysm. The x—x path indicates the preoperative aneurysm clipping profile; the o—o path indicates the profile 2 weeks after the aneurysm clipping.

tion of spending more time than any other health professional with the patient and family. The nurse makes the initial interview assessment, may perform brief specific or screening neuropsychologic tests, and observes the moment by moment behavior of the patient. After further evaluation, the nurse can integrate the findings of the neuropsychologic assessment into real life interventions to improve the quality of patient care, self-esteem, and realistic long-term planning for and with the patient and family. The utility of integrating formal testing and everyday observation can best be demonstrated through a case study.

Case Study 1
Mr. G is a 53-year-old self-employed furniture upholsterer in good health except for a history of alcohol abuse. Two days before admission, he had complained of a severe headache and confusion. Later that day he was found obtunded by his wife. A computerized tomography (CT) scan and angiogram confirmed a subarachnoid hemorrhage, with an aneurysm located at the most caudal portion of the basilar artery.

On admission, Mr. G was drowsy but would open his eyes, respond appropriately to commands, and move all extremities. He was oriented to time, place, and person. He was aware that he had had an abnormal bleeding around his brain and that his condition was serious. His reduced attention span necessitated reiteration of his treatment and restrictions each time he was awakened. Although he smiled and was superficially socially appropriate, he did not appear unduly concerned about his life-threatening situation and slept most of the time. When questioned, he was able to describe the events leading up to his hospitalization as he drifted in and out of sleep. When awake, he recognized his family and would talk with them briefly. Attempts were made to administer the NCSE on three occasions, but he was so drowsy that the test could never be completed.

A week after his subarachnoid hemorrhage, Mr. G had a craniotomy with clipping of a basilar artery aneurysm. Postoperatively, his only noticeable neurologic deficit was a third cranial nerve palsy (eyelid ptosis, dilated pupil, loss of adduction of right eye). Subsequent CT scans and arteriogram confirmed that the aneurysm had been clipped adequately.

The implications of any behavioral changes that the family may have noted in his behavior were masked by their relief in his having survived surgery. They verbalized that he was a little slower in his thinking and did not talk as spontaneously as before surgery, but they thought that these changes would improve after he went home and recovered. The nursing staff had noticed changes in Mr. G's behavior after surgery; the preoperative gleam in his eyes had dulled, and his face was not as expressive. He was less spontaneous and did not initiate conversations as he had done before surgery. He required instructions to complete self-care activities, was passive in planning his care, and was more dependent than preoperatively.

The postoperative NCSE evaluation identified cognitive dysfunction in the areas of construction, memory calculations and sequencing, and set changes (Fig. 11-1). Discharge planning and family teaching centered on incorporating information from the NCSE and the Trail Making Test with potential problems at home. He was discharged from the hospital neurologically stable and expected to improve in cognitive functioning.

One month after surgery, Mr. G was evaluated by a physician who concluded that the patient's mental status had returned to normal limits. Yet his family discussed his persistent difficulty in dressing himself, particularly tying his shoes. On many days he would not even get out of bed. Mr. G did not acknowledge these as problems but attributed his difficulties to poor vision. His wife and mother-in-law had to attend to his upholstery business because he was unable to resume work.

In view of the family history and lack of expected recovery of cognitive functioning, a repeat NCSE was performed. Mr. G's verbal communication and verbal judgment were within normal limits, but construction and ability to follow through to complete tasks were markedly impaired. Since the NCSE results had not improved, a repeat CT scan was performed that demonstrated enlarged ventricles and communicating hydrocephalus. He was admitted to the hospital, and a lumboperitoneal shunt was placed surgically.

Six weeks after shunting, Mr. G returned to the clinic with a gleam in his eye and an engaging smile. He was back at work full time, did not require assistance, and was taking care of himself. The follow-up CT scan confirmed resolution of the hydrocephalus, and the follow-up NCSE had returned to the normal range (Fig. 11-2).

For Mr. G, the neuropsychologic tests guided family discharge planning initially. When he continued not to improve as expected, the NCSE confirmed the persistence of cognitive impairment beyond what had been expected. The resulting medical evaluation and surgical intervention corrected the underlying medical problem. Subsequently, the NCSE, on repeated testing, confirmed the return of cognitive functioning, which was substantiated by Mr. G's return to work and ability to function independently.

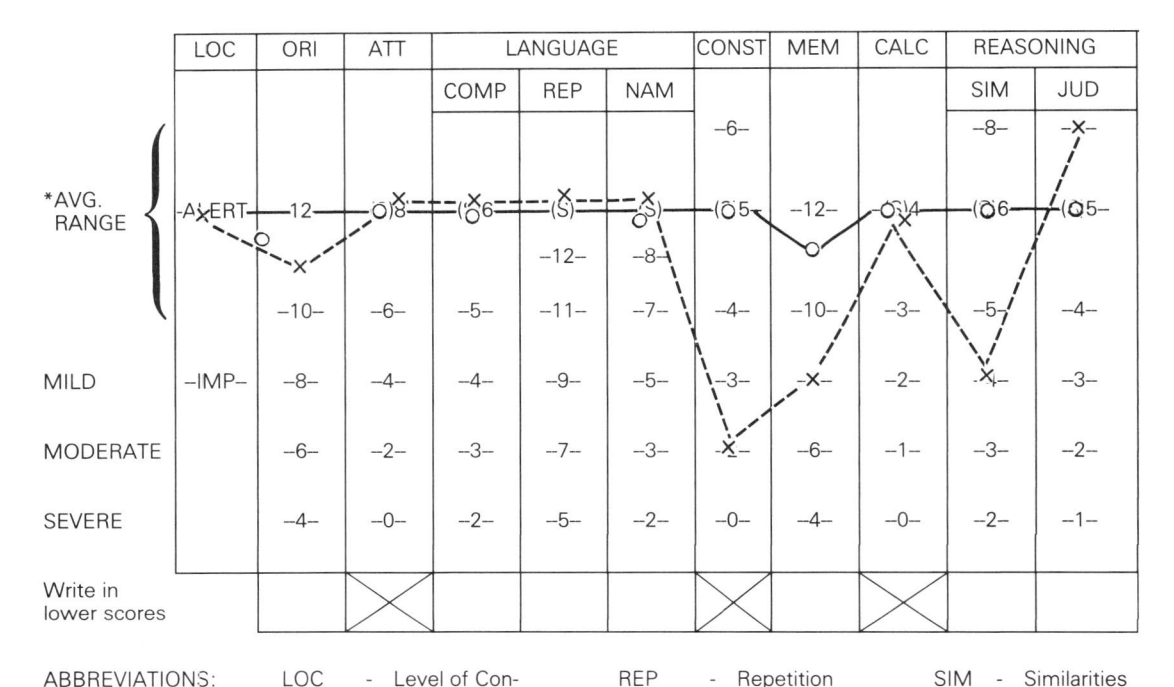

	LOC	ORI	ATT	LANGUAGE			CONST	MEM	CALC	REASONING	
				COMP	REP	NAM				SIM	JUD
							–6–			–8–	–X–
*AVG. RANGE	-A⤬ERT-	–12–	Ⓞ8	(Ⓞ6	(S)	(S)	(Ⓞ5	–12–	Ⓞ4	(Ⓞ6	(Ⓞ5
					–12–	–8–					
		–10–	–6–	–5–	–11–	–7–	–4–	–10–	–3–	–5–	–4–
MILD	–IMP–	–8–	–4–	–4–	–9–	–5–	–3–	–X–	–2–	–X–	–3–
MODERATE		–6–	–2–	–3–	–7–	–3–	–X–	–6–	–1–	–3–	–2–
SEVERE		–4–	–0–	–2–	–5–	–2–	–0–	–4–	–0–	–2–	–1–
Write in lower scores											

ABBREVIATIONS:
LOC - Level of Consciousness
ORI - Orientation
ATT - Attention
COMP - Comprehension
REP - Repetition
NAM - Naming
CONST - Construction
MEM - Memory
CALC - Calculations
SIM - Similarities
JUD - Judgment
S - Screen
IMP - Impaired

Figure 11–2. The cognitive status profile of a patient diagnosed with hydrocephalus. The ×—× path indicates the preoperative shunting profile; the o—o path indicates the profile 10 weeks after shunting.

REFERENCES

Anthony, J. C., LeResche, L., Niaz, U., Von Korff, M. R., & Folstein, M. F. (1982). Limits of the Mini-Mental State, a screening test for dementia and delirium among hospital patients. *Psychological Medicine, 12* 397.

Brown, E. C., Casey, A., Fisch, R.I., & Neuringer, C. (1958). Trailmaking test as a screening device for the detection of brain damage. *Journal of Consulting Psychology, 22*(6), 469.

Buron, O. K. (Ed.). (1978). *The eighth mental measurement yearbook.* Birmingham, AL: Gryphon Press.

Conn, H.O. (1977). Trailmaking and number-connection tests in the assessment of mental state in portal systemic encephalopathy. *Digestive Diseases, 22*(6), 541.

Derogatis, L.R. (1977). *SCL-90 manual for the revised version.* Baltimore: Johns Hopkins University Press.

Dick, J.P.R., Gjuiloff, R.J.H., Steward, A., Blackstock, J., Bielawska, C., Paul, E.A., & Marsden, C.D. (1984). Mini-Mental State examination in neurological patients. *Journal of Neurology, Neurosurgery, and Psychiatry, 47,* 496.

Folstein, M. F., Folstein, S. E., & McHugh, P.R. (1975). "Mini-Mental State," a practical method for grading the cognitive state of patients for the clinician. *Journal of Psychiatric Research, 12,* 189.

Kiernan, R.J., Mueller, J., Langston, J.W., & VanDyke, C. (1987). The Neurobehavioral Cognitive Status Examination: A brief but differentiated approach to cognitive assessment. *Annals of Internal Medicine, 107,* 481.

Levin, H. S., O'Donnell, V. M., & Grossman, R. G. (1979). The Galveston Orientation and Amnesia Test. *Journal of Nervous and Mental Disease, 167*(11), 675.

Lezak, M. (1983). *Neuropsychological assessment* (2nd ed.) New York: Oxford University Press.

Luria, A.R. (1973). *The working brain.* New York: Basic Books.

Mueller, J. (1984). The Mental Status Examination. In H. H. Goldman (Ed.), *A review of general psychiatry,* (Chap. 18, p. 206). Los Altos, CA: Lange.

Pfeiffer, R. (1975). A short portable mental status questionnaire for the assessment of organic brain deficit in elderly patients. *Jornal of American Geriatrics Society, 23,*(10), 433.

Plum, F., & Posner, J.B. (1980). *Diagnosis of stupor and coma* (2nd ed.), Contemporary Neurology Series. Philadelphia: Davis.

Reitan, R. M. (1955). The relation of the Trail Making Test to organic brain damage. *Journal of Consulting Psychology, 19*(5), 393.

Reitan, R. M. & Tarshes, E. L. (1959). Differential effects of lateralized brain lesions on the Trail Making Test. *Journal of Nervous and Mental Disease, 129,* 257.

BIBLIOGRAPHY

Jacobs, J. W., Bernhard, M.R., Delgado, A., & Strain, J. J. (1977). Screening for organic mental syndromes in the medically ill. *Annals of Internal Medicine, 86*(1), 42.

Kahn, R. L., Goldfarb, A. I., Pollack, M., & Peck, A. (1960). Brief objective measures for the determination of mental status in the aged. *American Journal of Psychiatry, 117,* 326.

Mitchell, P., Cammermeyer, M., Ozuna, J., & Woods, N. F. (1984). Neurological assessment. Reston, VA: Reston.

Strub, R. L., & Black, F. W. (1977). *The mental status examination in neurology.* Philadelphia: Davis.

APPENDIX 11-1.

NEUROBEHAVIORAL COGNITIVE STATUS EXAMINATION TEXT BOOKLET[a]

	Addressograph

NAME: _____ OCCUPATIONAL STATUS: _____
AGE AND DATE OF BIRTH: _____ DATE: _____
NATIVE LANGUAGE: _____ TIME: _____
HANDEDNESS (circle):   L   R EXAMINER: _____
LEVEL OF EDUCATION: _____ EXAMINATION LOCATION: _____

COGNITIVE STATUS PROFILE[b]

	LOC	ORI	ATT	LANGUAGE			CONST	MEM	CALC	REASONING	
				COMP	REP	NAM				SIM	JUD
*AVG. RANGE	-ALERT-	-12-	-(S)8-	-(S)6-	-(S)- -12-	-(S)- -8-	-6- -(S)5-	-12-	-(S)4-	-8- -(S)6-	-6- -(S)5-
		-10-	-6-	-5-	-11-	-7-	-4-	-10-	-3-	-5-	-4-
MILD	-IMP-	-8-	-4-	-4-	-9-	-5-	-3-	-8-	-2-	-4-	-3-
MODERATE		-6-	-2-	-3-	-7-	-3-	-2-	-6-	-1-	-3-	-2-
SEVERE		-4-	-0-	-2-	-5-	-2-	-0-	-4-	-0-	-2-	-1-
Write in lower scores											

ABBREVIATIONS:
- S - Screen
- LOC - Level of Consciousness
- IMP - Impaired
- ORI - Orientation
- ATT - Attention
- COMP - Comprehension
- MEM - Memory
- REP - Repetition
- NAM - Naming
- CALC - Calculations
- CONST - Construction
- SIM - Similarities
- JUD - Judgment

Note: The validity of this examination depends on administration in strict accordance with the Neurobehavioral Cognitive Status Examination Manual.

* For patients over age 65 the average range extends to the "mild impairment level" for Constructions, Memory and Similarities.

[a] From the Northern California Neurobehavioral Group, Inc. 1983.
[b] See Figures 11-1 and 11-2 for examples of specific cognitive status profiles.

NEUROBEHAVIORAL COGNITIVE STATUS EXAMINATION (NCSE) Record patient's responses verbatim.

I. LEVEL OF CONSCIOUSNESS: Alert _____ Lethargic _____ Fluctuating _____
   Describe patient's condition: _____
   _____

II. ORIENTATION (Score 2, 1, or 0.)
                                            Response   Score
   A. Person   1. Name (0 pts.)   _____   _____
               2. Age (2 pts.)   _____   _____
   B. Place   1. Current location (2 pts.) _____   _____
               2. City (2 pts.)   _____   _____
   C. Time   1. Date: mo. (1 pt.)_____ day (1 pt.)_____ yr. (2 pts.)_____ _____
               2. Day of week (1 pt.)   _____   _____
               3. Time of day within one hour (1 pt.) _____   _____
                                                            Total Score   _____

III. ATTENTION
   A. Digit Repetition
      1. Screen: 8-3-5-2-9-1   Pass _____   Fail _____
      2. Metric: Graded digit repetition (Score 1 or 0; discontinue after 2 misses at one level.)
             Score   Score   Score   Score
         3-7-2 _____   5-1-4-9 _____   8-3-5-2-9 _____   2-8-5-1-6-4 _____
         4-9-5 _____   9-2-7-4 _____   6-1-7-3-8 _____   9-1-7-5-8-2 _____
                                                            Total Score   _____

   B. Four Word Memory Task
      Give the four unrelated words from Section VI: robin, carrot, piano, green. (Alternate
      list: table, lion, orange, glove.) Have patient repeat the four words twice correctly
      (see manual) and record the number of trials required to do this: _____.

IV. LANGUAGE
   A. Speech Sample
      1. Fishing Picture (Record patient's response verbatim.)
      _____
      _____
      _____
      _____

   B. Comprehension (Be sure to have at least 3 other objects in front of the patient for this
      test.) If a, b, and c are successfully completed, praxis for these tasks is assumed
      normal.
      1. Screen: 3-step command: "Turn over the paper, hand me the pen, and point to your
                  nose."   Pass _____   Fail _____
      2. Metric: (Score 1 or 0.) If incorrect, describe behavior.
                                            Response   Score
         a. Pick up the pen.   _____   _____
         b. Point to the floor.   _____   _____
         c. Hand me the keys.   _____   _____
         d. Point to the pen and pick up
            the keys.   _____   _____
         e. Hand me the paper and point
            to the coin.   _____   _____
         f. Point to the keys, hand me
            the pen, and pick up the coin. _____   _____
                                                            Total Score   _____

   C. Repetition
      1. Screen: The beginning movement revealed the composer's intention.
                                                    Pass _____   Fail _____
      2. Metric: (Score 2 if first try correct; 1 if second try correct; 0 if incorrect.)
                                            Response   Score
         a. Out the window.   _____   _____
         b. He swam across the lake.   _____   _____
         c. The winding road led to the
            village.   _____   _____
         d. He left the latch open.   _____   _____
         e. The honeycomb drew a swarm
            of bees.   _____   _____
         f. No ifs, ands, or buts.   _____   _____
                                                            Total Score   _____

NEUROBEHAVIOR COGNITIVE STATUS EXAMINATION TEXT BOOKLET *(cont.)*

IV. Language *(cont.)*

D. Naming
  1. Screen: a) Pen_____ b) Cap or Top_____ c) Clip_____ d) Point, Tip, or Nib_____
     Pass _____ Fail _____
  2. Metric: (Score 1 or 0.)

	Response	Score		Response	Score
a. Shoe	_____	_____	e. Horseshoe	_____	_____
b. Bus	_____	_____	f. Anchor	_____	_____
c. Ladder	_____	_____	g. Octopus	_____	_____
d. Kite	_____	_____	h. Xylophone	_____	_____

Total Score _____

V. CONSTRUCTIONAL ABILITY

A. Screen: Visual Memory Task (Present stimulus sheet for 10 seconds, then have patient draw from memory. Must be perfect to pass. The examiner may wish to have patients who fail the screen copy the two figures).
  Pass _____ Fail _____

B. Metric: Design Constructions (Score 2 if correct in 0-30 seconds; 1 if correct in 31-60 seconds; 0 if correct in greater than 60 seconds or incorrect.)

Record incorrect attempts below _____ Time _____ Score _____

Place squares in front of patient as shown here:

1. Design 1:
2. Design 2:
3. Design 3:

Total Score _____

VI. MEMORY
(Score 3 if recalled without prompting; 2 if recalled with category prompt; 1 if recognized from list; 0 if not recognized.) Check if correct.

Words	Check	Category Prompt	Check or Response	List (circle)	Score
Robin	_____	Bird	_____	Sparrow, robin, bluejay	_____
Carrot	_____	Vegetable	_____	Carrot, potato, onion	_____
Piano	_____	Musical instrument	_____	Violin, guitar, piano	_____
Green	_____	Color	_____	Red, green, yellow	_____

Incorrect initial responses:_____ Total Score _____

VII. CALCULATIONS

A. Screen: 5 x 13   Response:_____   Time:_____   (Must be correct within 20 seconds.)
  Pass _____ Fail _____

B. Metric: (Score 1 point if correct within 20 seconds.) Problems may be repeated, but time runs continuously from first presentation.

	Response	Time	Score
1. How much is 5 + 3?	_____	_____	_____
2. How much is 15 + 7?	_____	_____	_____
3. How much is 39 ÷ 3?	_____	_____	_____
4. How much is 31 - 8?	_____	_____	_____

Total Score _____

VIII. REASONING

A. Similarities (Explain: "A hat and a coat are alike because they are both articles of clothing." If patient does not respond, encourage; if patient gives differences, score 0.)
  1. Screen: Painting-Music (Must be abstract - only art, artistic, or forms of art are acceptable.)
     _____   Pass _____ Fail _____
  2. Metric: (Score 2 if abstract; 1 if imprecisely abstract or concrete; 0 if incorrect.) See manual for examples. Check if abstract.

	Check	Abstract Concept	Other Responses	Score
a. Rose-Tulip	_____	Flowers	_____	_____
b. Bicycle-Train	_____	Transportation	_____	_____
c. Watch-Ruler	_____	Measurement	_____	_____
d. Corkscrew-Hammer	_____	Tools	_____	_____

Total Score _____

B. Judgment
   1. Screen: What would you do if you were stranded in the Denver Airport with only $1.00 in your pocket?
   _____
   _____
                                      Pass _____   Fail _____
   2. Metric: (Score 2 if correct; 1 if partially correct; 0 if incorrect.)
      a. What would you do if you woke up 1 minute before 8 o'clock and remembered an important appointment downtown at 8?
      _____
      _____
                                                    Score_____
      b. What would you do if while walking beside a lake you saw a 2 year old child playing alone at the end of a pier?
      _____
      _____
                                                    Score_____
      c. What would you do if you came home and found that a broken pipe was flooding the kitchen?
      _____
      _____
                                                    Score_____
                                               Total Score_____

List all current medications and dosages:
1._____ 2._____ 3._____ 4._____
5._____ 6._____ 7._____ 8._____

Note any known or observed motor, sensory or perceptual deficits that may affect test performance (e.g., impaired visual or auditory acuity, tremor, apraxia, dysarthria):
_____
_____
_____

General Comments (e.g., distractability, frustration, exhaustion, cooperation, patient's impression of performance):
_____
_____
_____
_____

Space for Visual Memory Task

12

Alterations in Memory

Rebecca Sisson

A frequent sequela of brain disturbances is a change in the ability to remember. Loss of memory for events concurrent with a traumatic injury or disease onset is a consistent clinical feature. Alteration in memory is categorized as a cognitive deficit and is a complex phenomenon that encompasses a variety of higher cortical functions. Intact memory is evidence of higher cortical functioning. Loss of memory, or *amnesia*, is a symptom of either a physiologic or a psychologic disturbance.

In physiologic disturbances, the symptom indicates a change in the usual function and rarely occurs in isolation. The person with amnesia probably also has other symptoms, such as weakness, sensory loss, or mood swings. The nature of these associated problems will vary according to the location of the lesion. Physiologically based memory problems can originate at the storage or retrieval stage of memory development, with different pathologies producing one or both disturbances in memory processing.

Memory traces are not localized to any one brain structure. All parts of the nervous system appear to have the types of plastic properties needed for memory storage (Kupfermann, 1985). The hippocampus and temporal lobes, however, seem to be the most important in human memory processing.

In disorders of psychologic function, the symptom of memory loss is a clue to the organization of the patient's world (Brown, 1977). Memory loss is very disorganizing whether the cause is physiologic or psychologic.

THEORIES OF MEMORY

According to Brown (1977), memory is a type of reproductive thinking, and thought is a kind of productive memory. Both memory and thinking are components of cognition. Retention and recall are associated with learning, and memory loss can affect either or both of these functions. Learning can thus be a problem for patients with alterations in memory.

An important principle to remember is that memory has stages and is constantly changing (Kupfermann, 1985). Once something has been learned, the ability to remember varies depending on the task, the retrieval effectiveness, and the individual's current physiologic state. For learning to occur, the experience must be imprinted. If this does not happen, the memory is not stored.

Memory storage is thought to be short-term and long-term. Research indicates that information is initially processed in the short-term memory store and then, by some process yet unknown, is stored in long-term memory. A third component of memory is the "search and readout," or retrieval. This is the system that is most frequently affected by a physiologic disturbance.

Short-Term Memory
Also known as *primary memory* to some researchers, short-term memory is said to be immediate—the information is reproduced rapidly, having never left consciousness. Recall is easy for a limited amount of information, and there is a tendency for rapid decay, for example, looking up a telephone number and remembering it just long enough to dial the number. For short-term memory store, attention is necessary.

The coding method for short-term memory is thought to be neuronal activity and a physical change in peripheral receptors. This physiologic change is not believed to result in imprinting unless the information or experience has meaning to the individual.

Working Memory
Baddeley and Hitch (1974) have proposed the idea of a working memory that is more complex than short-term memory, being an alliance between several temporary storage systems and an attentional component. They suggest that working memory involves this attentional component or central processor and an articulatory loop that permits transient storage of a limited amount of information. Baddeley (1984) states that working memory uses a range of parallel subsidiary systems. He describes two of these systems as involving sensory components: one subvocal speech and the other a visual–spatial sketch pad. These are used by the individual to "hear" or "visualize" information and, therefore, better process the data for storage.

Working memory is not an accepted concept to many researchers. It is new and not applied widely in clinical practice or research. Further study is needed to provide convincing evidence to support this theory.

Long-Term Memory
Frequently called secondary or remote memory, this memory store has been shown to effect actual structural change in the brain, probably by means of protein synthesis. Research postulates that this physical change is what allows memories from 10 years or longer to be retained. Meaning seems to influence whether something is retained in long-term memory. This is a complex system and, according to Baddeley (1984), has two major divisions: *visual and verbal memory* and *semantic and episodic memory*.

Visual appearance and the name of an object, both given at the same time, tend to make remembering easier. Visual alone is better than verbal alone—"A picture is worth a thousand words." This has obvious implications for memory therapy and indicates the importance of testing both visual and verbal capabilities.

Semantic memory is used to refer to memory of knowledge, and *episodic memory* is more situational or autobiographic in nature. Patients with amnesia seem to have a breakdown in episodic memory but retain semantic memory. This is probably because information learned years before the memory problem is easily retained, whereas trying to remember what you had for breakfast may be more difficult.

Sensory Memory
This type of memory is of interest to some researchers who study memory systems. Baddeley (1984) describes this as the sensory system's ability to store sensory information for brief periods of time. The system most frequently studied is visual. The fact that visual images are briefly retained is what makes cinematography possible. A series of still pic-

tures received rapidly is perceived as a moving object because of this brief storage of images. Many researchers do not agree that this is a memory system but instead label this phenomenon *perception*.

Many theories of memory have been proposed. Since the research is recent, no consensus has been reached. The only two accepted theories are those for short-term and long-term memory. Future research may provide evidence of other memory systems.

PATHOPHYSIOLOGY OF MEMORY LOSS

An alteration in memory can result from a variety of central nervous system pathologies, including infection, tumors, seizure disorders, cerebrovascular accidents, toxicity, metabolic response, or trauma. The mechanisms producing change in the structure of nervous tissue that result in memory loss are usually compression, hemorrhage, herniation, ischemia, or actual removal of tissue. The temporal lobes and hippocampi are the major regions of the brain involved. Damage to the right hemisphere temporal lobe frequently impairs visual–spatial memory. Damage to the left hemisphere results in verbal long-term memory impairment. Diffuse brain injury after blunt trauma also will produce loss of memory to varying degrees.

Types of Memory Loss
There are three basic causes of memory loss: *trauma*, which disrupts blood flow and alters neurotransmission, *degeneration of brain tissue*, and *tissue loss* from surgical removal.

Trauma
The most common cause of memory loss is trauma. Included as trauma are closed head injuries, skull fractures, strokes, and missile injuries. *Posttraumatic amnesia (PTA)*, as defined by Russell and Nathan (1946), is the interval from the time of injury to the time the person is sufficiently aware of his or her surroundings to commit them to memory. During PTA, the person may be confused and disoriented and lack the capacity to store and retrieve new information. The criteria for determining PTA and its extent have not been consistent in research reports. Many researchers, however, use Russell's definition and criteria. Anterograde and retrograde amnesia are considered components of PTA.

Anterograde amnesia is the loss of memory for events after the onset of trauma or disease. During this period, the person may be aware of his or her surroundings but be unable to store the events. Disorientation has been shown in some studies to coincide with anterograde amnesia (Levin et al., 1982). Retrograde amnesia refers to the period of time before the injury of which the person has no recollection (Russell, 1971). Usually, retrograde amnesia is of a few minutes to 30 minutes duration. This memory rarely returns, and it is believed that the events are not stored as a result of the physiologic disruption associated with trauma. Although retrograde amnesia tends to be relatively short, there are cases in which the amnesia extends back several months. As PTA resolves, the retrograde amnesia shrinks. There is generally believed to be a correlation between resolution of PTA and the return of memory before the injury. There may be brief periods of amnesia within periods of recall, often referred to as "islands" of memory loss. Resolution of the amnesia generally occurs to the point that the moment of injury is the only missing piece.

Degeneration of Brain Tissue
Korsakoff's syndrome frequently is used as the term to categorize all amnesias caused by degenerative brain pathology. This syndrome includes impaired recent memory, impaired learning, and confabulation. It can be seen in patients with brain tumors involving the thalamus and the mamillary bodies, in alcoholic patients and those with other drug-related pathologies, and in other degenerative confusional states.

Surgical Loss of Brain Tissue

In the literature, this type of memory loss is related to the surgical removal of the temporal lobes. Surgical amnesia also occurs from the use of anesthetic drugs. These are very different types, since the lobectomy affects all future memory storage and learning, whereas the drugs produce an amnesia only for the period of time just before the surgery.

Diagnoses of Specific Pathophysiology

When local brain lesions can be identified, it appears that memory disturbances are specific to regions of the brain. According to Luria (1976), certain memory functions are located in specific regions (Table 12–1). General diffuse brain damage resulting in an oculovestibular deficit seems to be associated with poor memory function (Levin et al., 1979). It is difficult to localize the region of injury in many cases of brain trauma, however, especially in the severely injured with coma lasting longer than a week. Frequently, it is not possible to assess memory function accurately after brain injury because of associated depression, distractibility, and poor concentration. It is best to assess each patient individually, since no true pattern of memory disturbance can be identified according to location of lesion.

Three categories of neuropathology are used in this chapter to organize and illustrate the nursing management when there is an alteration in memory. These are cerebrovascular accident, head injury, and brain tumor. Although there are other pathologies producing memory loss, these are the most common. The principles used to intervene when these conditions exist can be applied to other neuropathologic disturbances.

☐ Impaired Remote Memory and Recall Ability

Case Study 1: Stroke

Mrs. L, a 78-year-old woman was admitted with the diagnosis of cerebrovascular accident (CVA), right hemiparesis. She was stuporous and appeared dehydrated. She responded to pain, moved her left side spontaneously, and opened her eyes when she heard her name. The pupils were equal and reactive, and cranial nerves were normal. Mrs. L became aware, in several days, that she was in the hospital. She was confused by her surroundings and did not remember coming to the hospital. She did not know what day it was or how much time had passed. When the nurse came into her room, Mrs. L tried to ask what had happened. The words would not come, and the sounds that she heard herself making were strange. The nurse, in a loud voice, told Mrs. L that she had had a stroke and was going to be all right. Mrs. L was very upset—she could not remember anything.

Gradually, in the course of a week, Mrs. L began to make herself understood, and some words were becoming easy to remember. She was still confused about many things.

A general physical *assessment* and neurologic examination revealed a well-nourished but slightly dehydrated female. All findings were essentially normal except for right upper

TABLE 12–1. REGIONS OF SPECIFIC MEMORY ALTERATION.[a]

Area of Lesion	Memory Disturbance
Medial zone of frontal lobe	Loss of orientation to time, place, and state of self
Left temporal lobe	Audioverbal memory impaired; lack of word retention
Left parieto-occipital	Spatial agnosia and speech structure difficulty; problems learning written material
Right hemisphere	Disturbance in imprinting and recalling visual material (e.g., recognizing faces)
Thalamus/hippocampus	Severe memory problems with Korsakoff's syndrome-like symptoms

[a]Localization based on Luria (1976).

extremity weakness and decreased sensation to light touch. The right lower extremity could perform gross motor movement; sensation was intact.

To assess memory, orientation, and other cognitive abilities, the Galveston Orientation and Amnesia Test (GOAT) and Neurobehavioral Rating Scale (NRS) were used. The GOAT score was 54, indicating an impairment (a score of 65 or less indicates impairment). The NRS score showed a moderately severe rating on conceptional disorganization, memory deficit, and decreased initiative; a moderate rating on expressive deficit and poor planning; and a mild rating on anxiety, agitation, depressed mood, and inaccurate insight and self-appraisal.

Observations and direct questions revealed that Mrs. L could not remember her address and did not know where she was, except that she was at a hospital (no name). She stated that she remembered nothing before awakening in the hospital room. She was able to name three articles correctly after 5 minutes and describe her sister's visit the previous evening. She could not describe the exercise taught her by the physical therapist. Appropriate nursing *diagnoses* were impaired remote memory and impaired recall ability.

At this stage of recovery the most important nursing *intervention* is to provide reality orientation and memory cues. The sister, who is the only relative, should be included in the planning, teaching, and reorienting. A calendar and clock can be used to reinforce time and date orientation. The large printed name of the hospital and room number near the bedside would orient her to place. Personal belongings and reminders of home would provide the stimuli to remind her of where she lives. A daily schedule should be posted to remind Mrs. L of mealtimes, physical therapy, speech therapy, and occupational therapy.

Most important is a consistent approach. All staff and the patient's sister should use the same cues. Short, simple phrases are best for giving instructions, and positive reinforcement will provide encouragement. The *outcome criteria* for this patient are that she will remember the day, time, and place, recall her home and address, and relate her daily routine schedule.

☐ **Impaired Remote Memory and Retention Ability**

Case Study 2: Closed Head Injury

Mike is recovering from a head injury. He also had abdominal injuries, requiring a splenectomy, and a lumbar fracture that was fused. The critical period is past, and he is now in a rehabilitation program. The physical weakness in his right arm and leg has greatly improved, and he is able to walk without a cane. There is still a slight problem with fine motor movement and coordination in his right hand.

It has been 3 months since the automobile accident that resulted in Mike's head injury, and he had been in a coma for 6 days. Since regaining consciousness, he has made remarkable recovery, and his prognosis is favorable. In talking with Mike, it becomes evident that there are areas of memory difficulty. He has no memory of the events just before the accident; his last memory is of a friend's wedding 1 month before the accident.

The physical and neurologic examination *assessments* are essentially normal except for right side weakness of the face, arm, and leg. The computerized tomography (CT) scan done after the injury revealed a left cerebral contusion with temporal lobe hemorrhage. A mental status evaluation revealed good short-term memory but retrograde amnesia for 1 month before the injury and posttraumatic amnesia of approximately 1 month. The GOAT score was 75, which is in the borderline range.

Mike describes his memory as "not good" and says he has trouble concentrating, especially when reading. He denies headaches or dizziness. He states that his right arm and leg are weak, and he has decreased vision in his right eye. The rating on the NRS indicates a moderate expressive deficit, memory deficit, and inaccurate insight and self-appraisal. Mike is a dentist and says he plans to go back to work soon after returning home. The nursing *diagnoses* made were impaired remote memory and impaired memory retention ability.

Family involvement is critical in the planning and use of selected techniques in *intervention*. Mike will require many memory cues from his family and friends. Reminders of home, such as pictures, letters, and personal items, will help resolve the posttraumatic amnesia. Practicing activities of daily living in a realistic setting will be beneficial in reminding Mike of his previous routines. Gaining skill in reading and following instructions will mean practice in short sessions to decrease tiring and loss of concentration. A notebook may be helpful for note taking.

The lack of insight into his deficiency is a difficult problem. Reviewing books of dental procedures and practice may help Mike; however, his alteration in memory may not become evident to him until he actually tries to go back to work. The family should be prepared to cope with this situation.

The *outcome criteria* for this client are that he will recall home and describe the setting, describe the acute care hospital before the rehabilitation unit, demonstrate the ability to recall events and retain information, and discuss decisions related to his future plans.

☐ Impaired Short-Term Memory and Retention Ability

Case Study 3: Brain Lesion
Mr. S is a 71-year-old man admitted with a diagnosis of left frontoparietotemporal mass, possibly a cyst. Over the past several months he had progressively developed temporal area headaches, personality change, loss of short-term memory, and dementia. The CT scan localized a large, fluid-filled cyst, and surgery was performed to remove it.

In the postoperative *assessment*, Mr. S had essentially normal physical and neurologic findings. Some right homonymous hemianopia persisted, and he remained disoriented and confused.

Mental status examination revealed a GOAT score of 50, which is in the impaired range. He was not oriented to time and place and could not remember events before surgery. When questioned about his memory he stated that it "wasn't too good." He could not remember what he had for breakfast or if the doctor had visited.

When the family was interviewed, they were very concerned about Mr. S's memory. He constantly repeated himself and did not seem able to retain anything he was told. He would get lost just as soon as he left his room. The family expressed apprehension about Mr. S's return home. The nursing *diagnosis* was impaired short-term memory with impaired retention.

Initially, Mr. S needs constant reality orientation. Nursing *intervention* includes reminding him of the time, date, and place whenever possible. A large calendar near the bed and a clock can be used as aids.

Mr. S will need aids to remind him of personal hygiene routines and daily schedules. It often is helpful to label drawers, cabinets, and closets with the contents; for example, the bathroom cabinet could have a label (e.g., *Razor*). Another helpful aid is a list of activities or instructions in the appropriate room at home. The family could be instructed to post lists in the bathroom—wash face and hands, brush teeth, shave—and in the kitchen—instructions for making coffee.

Mr. S can be helped to learn to write everything in a notebook, especially messages, appointments, and names. Important telephone numbers should be posted by the phone along with the names.

Involve the family from the beginning in suggesting interventions and in learning about techniques to aid memory. The family must understand the importance of allowing Mr. S to be as independent as possible; he should be encouraged to do as much as he is able and gradually to increase the complexity of his activities.

The *outcome criteria* are that Mr. S will be able to state day and time, relate information about activities of the day, and carry out personal hygiene.

HUMAN RESPONSES TO BRAIN DAMAGE: MEMORY ALTERATIONS

The three Case Studies illustrate that similar problems can arise from brain damage that occurs in a variety of ways and that there can be dissimilarities in behavioral responses of individuals. These dissimilarities occur because of differences in brain function affected by the basic pathology, differences in stage of recovery, differences in age, and differences in the preinjury cognitive function of people. The following discussion provides information to help nurses to determine accurately the nature and extent of alterations in memory associated with brain disorders and to intervene appropriately, based on the nursing diagnosis.

Manifestations of Memory Deficit

In the past, there has not been an emphasis on assessment of mental status, including memory, by nurses. One reason has been the lack of instruments or assessment guides. Because little has been studied or reported in the nursing literature, the area of mental assessment has been left to the psychologists. With increased knowledge and advanced training, the neuroscience nurse has begun to develop tools for assessing cognitive function, communication skills, and memory.

There are several reports in the literature of tools developed and used by nurses to assess cognitive function after head trauma (Cammermeyer, 1983; Dowling, 1985; Parsons & Crosby, 1985; Turner et al., 1984; Warren et al., 1984). Such general assessment of cognitive function is described in Chapter 11. Specific memory assessment aids are discussed in this chapter.

The generalist in neuroscience nursing has the knowledge and skill to assess patients' neurologic function accurately. Physical and mental assessment are required to plan appropriate nursing care. Baseline and ongoing physiologic assessment is accepted practice in neuroscience nursing. Psychologic and mental assessment has become part of many nurses' practice, but no guidelines for this assessment are available for general use.

The specialist in neuroscience nursing can fill this gap by developing guidelines and specific tools to measure emotional and behavioral changes in patients. The experienced nurse has the knowledge and competence gained from practice to design assessment protocols that can be used by the generalist. Several neuroscience nurse specialists currently are developing and testing tools for mental and behavioral assessment. Such tools can greatly enhance the data-gathering phase of the nursing process.

Behavioral Observations

In the day-to-day interaction with a patient, the neuroscience nurse can make many observations that provide evidence of a memory problem. The most obvious manifestation is forgetting—names, dates, events, activities, current news, appointments, or visitors. Casual conversation with some specific questions interjected can disclose gaps in memory. It is important to determine whether new (recent) or old (remote) memory is affected. Such questions as When were your born? What time did you wake up today? Where did you go on vacation last year? Who were the visitors here yesterday? When is your physical therapy appointment? What year did you graduate from school? are helpful in determining which type of memory loss is present. Another manifestation of memory alteration is losing items or getting lost. Not remembering where items were placed or where personal articles are stored or which door is to the bathroom or what direction to take to physical therapy or how to find one's room are all common occurrences for persons who suffer from memory deficits.

Determining whether a patient can follow through on a series of activities of self-care identifies areas of memory loss. Does the person remember when to get up, bathe, dress appropriately, and eat breakfast, or does he or she forget some items in the sequence? It is particularly important when discharge is anticipated to determine if the deficit affects activities of daily living. An ongoing assessment and observations of memory function will provide the nurse with valuable data for making a nursing diagnosis and planning interventions.

Formal Assessment Tools

Another method for assessing memory is the use of tools developed by nurses and other health professionals for this purpose. Objective data can be obtained that may help pinpoint specific problem areas of memory function. Several such tools are listed in Table 12–2.

The author, in collaboration with Levin et al. (1982), developed a Neurobehavioral Rating Scale (NRS) designed to assess 27 areas of cognitive and behavioral sequelae of head trauma. It was first tested on 108 head-injured patients and is being tested currently on stroke victims. Memory loss is one item for which the NRS is very sensitive. A brief structured interview is used by the clinician to obtain data, followed by the rating, which is done without the patient's presence. The interview and rating take less than 30 minutes. This rating scale soon will be available for use by the trained clinician. A nurse specialist can easily use this tool to assess outcomes after various types of head trauma.

Another tool, the Galveston Orientation and Amnesia Test (GOAT) (Levin et al., 1979), is useful during the early stages after head trauma to document the resolution of PTA (Fig. 12–1). The author has used it to assess recovering stroke victims.

Mental Status examinations are another source of data for the nurse in making a comprehensive assessment. These tests identify which aspects of memory are affected and which are intact. Usually such testing is done by a neuropsychologist, but others, including nurses, can be trained to administer these tests. One such test that has been used by nurses is the Neurobehavioral Mental Status Examination (NMSE) (Kiernan et al., 1984). This test, which has been revised and is now called the Neurobehavioral Cognitive Status Examination (NCSE) (Kiernan et al., 1987), is discussed in detail in Chapter 11.

TABLE 12–2. TOOLS TO ASSESS MEMORY AND COGNITIVE DEFICITS.

Tool	Author
Wechsler Memory Scale	Wechsler (1945)
Galveston Orientation and Amnesia Test (GOAT)	Levin et al. (1979)
Disability Rating Scale	Rappaport et al. (1982)
Neurobehavioral Rating Scale (NRS)	Levin et al. (1982)
Brief Neuropsychological Mental Status Examination	Turner et al. (1984)
Neurobehavioral Cognitive Status Examination (NCSE)	Kiernan et al. (1987)

The widely used Wechsler Memory Scale has seven subtests used to provide a summary score (memory quotient). This scale is not particularly sensitive to impairment of memory for visual material; thus, another test should be used to assess this component. The test batteries chosen for use should contain verbal and visual memory assessment (Brooks & Lincoln, 1984).

Some neuropsychologists prefer to use a collection of specific tests rather than one battery. This allows the clinician to assess particular aspects of memory. Such a collection should include:

1. Logical recall: A story is read to the patient, who is asked to explain it.
2. Word pairs association learning: A word pair is read, then one word is given to the patient and he or she is asked to name the other.
3. Visual memory tests: The patient is shown geometric shapes and then asked to reproduce them from memory.
4. Delayed recall (verbal or visual): The patient is told a story or shown pictures, and

Name _____	Date of Test └──┴──┘
Age _____ Sex M F	mo day yr
Date of Birth └──┴──┘	Day of the week s m t w th f s
mo day yr	Time AM PM
Diagnosis _____	Date of injury └──┴──┘
	mo day yr

GALVESTON ORIENTATION & AMNESIA TEST (GOAT)

Error Points

1. What is your name? (2) _____ When were you born? (4) _____   └──┴──┘
   Where do you live? (4) _____
2. Where are you now? (5) city _____ (5) hospital _____   └──┴──┘
   (unnecessary to state name of hospital)
3. On what date were you admitted to this hospital? (5) _____   └──┴──┘
   How did you get here? (5) _____   └──┴──┘
4. What is the first event you can remember *after* the injury? (5) _____   └──┴──┘
   Can you describe in detail (e.g., date, time, companions) the first event you can recall after injury? (5) _____
5. Can you describe the last event you recall *before* the accident? (5) _____   └──┴──┘
   _____ Can you describe in detail (e.g., date, time, companions) the first event you can recall *before* the injury? (5) _____
6. What time is it now? _____ (1 for each ½ hour removed from correct time to maximum of 5)   └──┴──┘
7. What day of the week is it? _____ (1 for each day removed from correct one)   └──┴──┘
8. What day of the month is it? _____ (1 for each day removed from correct date to maximum of 5)   └──┴──┘
9. What is the month? _____ (5 for each month removed from correct one to maximum of 15)   └──┴──┘
10. What is the year? _____ (10 for each year removed from correct one to maximum of 30)   └──┴──┘

Total Error Points   └──┴──┘
Total Goat Score (100-total error points)   └──┴──┘

Figure 12–1. The Galveston Orientation and Amnesia Test (GOAT) form. *From: Levin, H.S., O'Donnell, V.M., & Grossman, R.G. The Galveston Orientation and Amnesia Test.* Journal of Nervous and Mental Disease, *167(11), 675–684,* © *by Williams & Wilkins, 1979.*

after a time lapse, usually 30 minutes, is asked to tell the story or draw the picture.

There are many other tests, and each psychologist will have a preference. The major disadvantage to most tests of mental status is that they are not related very closely to difficulties encountered in daily life.

The initial assessment also involves obtaining a detailed history, including baseline data and input from family members. The nursing history should obtain information in the following areas: (1) individual's description of present problem, (2) past illnesses and injuries, (3) coping mechanisms, (4) education level, (5) occupation, (6) family, interpersonal, and social information, and (7) usual daily activities—sleeping, waking, eating, and activity patterns. The baseline data are gathered by a thorough neurologic examination. Any information gaps or additional data should be obtained from family members. It is especially important to have the family's perspective on the patient's personality and previous coping mechanisms. Alteration in memory is very frustrating, and it is helpful to have family input and involvement from the beginning.

The more comprehensive the assessment, the more likely it is that the neuroscience nurse will arrive at an accurate diagnosis and treatment plan. Many creative and individualized aids could be developed by the nurse to identify problems in remembering daily routines.

Nursing Diagnoses for the Individual

After the in-depth assessment, the neuroscience nurse will be able to arrive at the specific problem or nursing diagnosis. These identified deficits are functional in nature and reflect an inability of the patient to cope with aspects of daily living activities. The following are possible nursing diagnoses when an alteration in memory is present:

- Impaired short-term memory: Evidenced by problems with recalling or recognizing events that occurred in the immediate past (0 to 5 minutes) and can be either auditory or visual
- Impaired remote memory: Evidenced by inability to recall or recognize events of remote past (months to years)
- Impaired recall ability: Evidenced by problems with recalling material or procedures learned in practice sessions, such as an exercise procedure, making coffee, or how to use public transportation
- Impaired retention: Evidenced by problems with remembering short instructions, basic routines of daily life, assignments or appointments, and personal decisions

There are many concurrent and related problems that the brain-injured person might experience. These frequently influence and compound the diagnoses. Problems with attention, concentration, language, and judgment affect the person's ability to cope with memory deficits. It is unusual for any one of these deficits to appear alone. The memory deficits and related problems may serve as etiologies for three general nursing diagnoses: potential for injury related to impaired recall, self-care deficit, and alterations in family processes.

Nursing Intervention

The neuroscience nurse generalist has the knowledge and skill to adapt intervention techniques to meet the needs of a patient population. Specific methods could be tested with the diagnostic categories using variations of the techniques tested in the laboratory setting. The nurse is in the perfect situation to design strategies for improving memory function in the real life setting. Having the most frequent contact with patients and their families, the nurse can develop more meaningful and individualized intervention techniques and strategies.

The neuroscience nurse specialist can develop new specific intervention techniques to assist patients who have memory loss and other cognitive dysfunctions. Modification of current clinical laboratory techniques for memory retraining could be useful in the intervention plans by nurses. The continued testing of various nursing strategies by the nurse specialist will provide neuroscience nursing with a much needed knowledge base for practice.

When there is a memory deficit, the goals of nursing may be to improve the specific memory deficit but are more likely to reflect the more general problems that are caused by memory deficits: potential for injury, self-care deficits and disruptions in family relationships. Thus nursing care *goals* are likely to be in the following areas: promotion of safety, provision of memory aids and self-help devices, inclusion of the family in problem identification and in teaching.

Initially, the focus is on in-hospital activities. The neuroscience nurse can design activities and provide memory aids that promote memory retraining. Of course, this is not done in isolation. The nurse should incorporate in her interventions the goals and activities of the other health team members, for example, encouraging the patient to practice exercises learned in physical therapy or skills learned in occupational therapy.

There are three principles to be remembered when planning activities to improve memory function (Moffat, 1984):

1. Make tasks simple and measurable so that progress is evaluated easily.
2. Space out the learning sessions and make them brief.
3. Provide positive reinforcement of appropriate behaviors.

The literature on memory retraining is very recent, and the methods often are useful in the clinical setting but not appropriate for preparing the patient for the real world. The nurse has a great challenge in trying to design memory aids that will help the patient deal with everyday activities. When there is permanent brain damage, the return of function is slow and often minimal. The latest research indicates that there may be some recovery of function or transfer of function to other areas of the brain. For the present, the nurse must use creativity to work with the patient with a memory deficit.

Several researchers (Harris, 1984; Moffat, 1984) have described external memory aids as the most useful. These include notebooks, calendars, charts, lists, alarms, timers, and prompt cards. These aids can be used by the patient and the family to remind them of schedules, appointments, and activities.

Internal memory aids described in the literature include visual imagery and verbal strategies (Lewinsohn et al., 1977; Glasgow et al., 1977; Moffat, 1984; Zarit et al., 1982). Most of these have been tested only in laboratory settings and offer little for rehabilitation of the patient with memory loss due to brain injury.

A therapy that was developed for use with psychiatric and geriatric patients has been found to be useful with the head-injured patient. Reality orientation aims to retrain a person's awareness of time, place, and current events. It is a process of continuous stimulation and repetition of basic orientation information (Cerny & McNeny, 1983). To be effective, reality orientation must be used on a 24-hour basis by all members of the staff. The program should begin as soon as the patient arouses from coma. The two basic components of the therapy are consistency and repetition. Whenever any staff member interacts with the patient, he or she should provide some orientation information. The family must be involved and can provide valuable information as well as bringing personal and familiar objects from home. Photographs, posters, clothing, clocks, calendars, radios, and other favorite personal possessions can be used in reality orientation. A daily schedule board should be posted in full view to remind the patient of activities and therapies. It also helps the family and staff to reinforce the schedule and encourage the patient to follow it.

In keeping with the goals of nursing intervention, the outcomes should reflect behaviors by the patient that indicate that the goals have been met. The areas to be evaluated are:

1. Safety: The patient will not injure himself.
2. Use of memory aids: The patient will use the self-help techniques.
3. Family involvement: The family will encourage the use of self-help techniques.
4. Independence: The family will allow the patient to be as independent as possible.

SUMMARY

The challenge to neuroscience nurses is to assess the patient accurately and plan interventions that assist in adjustment to the disabilities that accompany neurologic disorders. Mental alterations present a particularly difficult task. Memory loss is distressful to the patient and the family and is the problem dealt with least by nurses. Often the inability to remember is viewed as the result of hospitalization and, therefore, expected to improve when the person returns to familiar surroundings. Unfortunately, this is usually not the case when there has been an intracranial insult.

With the development and use of specific assessment tools, the neuroscience nurse can better determine the extent of neurologic deficit. Once a memory loss has been determined, the nurse can begin a realistic plan to help the patient and family adjust.

REFERENCES

Baddeley, A.D. (1984). Memory theory and memory therapy. In B. Wilson & N. Moffat (Eds.), *Clinical management of memory problems*. Rockville, MD: Aspen.

Baddeley, A.D., & Hitch, G. (1974). Working memory. In G.H. Bower, (Ed.), *The psychology of learning and motivation* (Vol. 8). New York: Academic Press.

Brooks, D.N. (1983). *Outcome of severe head injury*. Oxford: Oxford University Press.

Brooks, N., & Lincoln, N.B. (1984). Assessment for rehabilitation. In B. Wilson & N. Moffat (Eds.), *Clinical management of memory problems*. Rockville, MD: Aspen.

Brown, J. (1977). *Mind, brain and consciousness*. New York: Academic Press.

Cammermeyer, M. (1983). A growth model of self-care for neurologically impaired people. *Journal of Neurosurgical Nursing, 15*(5); 299.

Cerny, J. & McNeny, R. (1983). Reality orientation therapy. In M. Rosenthal, E.R. Griffith, M. Bond, & J.D. Miller (Eds.), *Rehabilitation of the head-injured adult*. Philadelphia: Davis.

Dowling, G.A. (1985). Levels of cognitive functioning: Evaluation of interrater reliability. *Journal of Neurosurgical Nursing, 17*(2), 129.

Glasgow, R.E., Zeiss, R.A., Barrera, M., & Lewinsohn, P.M. (1977). Case studies on remediating memory deficits in brain-damaged individuals. *Journal of Clinical Psychology, 33*(4), 1049.

Harris, J. (1984). Methods of improving memory. In B. Wilson & N. Moffat (Eds.), *Clinical management of memory problems*. Rockville, MD: Aspen.

Kiernan, R., Mueller, J., & Langston, J.W. (1984). Mental status examination. In H. Goldman (Ed.), *Review of general psychology*. Los Altos, CA: Lange.

Kiernan, R.J., Mueller, J., Langston, J.W., & Van Dyke, C. (1987). The Neurobehavioral Cognitive Status Examination: A brief but differentiated approach to cognitive assessment. *Annals of Internal Medicine, 107*, 481.

Kupfermann, I. (1985). Learning. In E. Kandel & J. Schwartz (Eds.), *Principles of neural science* (2nd ed.). New York: Elsevier/North-Holland.

Levin, H.S., Benton, A.L., & Grossman, R.G. (1982). *Neurobehavioral consequences of closed head injury*. New York: Oxford University Press.

Levin, H.S., O'Donnell, V.M., & Grossman, R.G. (1979). The Galveston Orientation and Amnesia Test: A practical scale to assess cognition after head injury. *Journal of Nervous and Mental Disease, 167*(11), 675.

Lewinsohn, P.M., Danaher, B.G., & Kikel, S. (1977). Visual imagery as a mnemonic aid for brain-injured persons. *Journal of Consulting and Clinical Psychology, 45*(5), 717.

Luria, A.R. (1976). *The neuropsychology of memory*. Washington, DC: V.H. Winston & Sons.

Moffat, N. (1984). Strategies of memory therapy. In B. Wilson, & N. Moffat (Eds.), *Clinical management of memory problems*. Rockville, MD: Aspen.

Parsons, L.C., & Crosby, L.J. (1985). Development of a nurse neurologic assessment tool. Presented at University of Maryland Tool Development Conference, New Orleans, 1985.

Rappaport, M., Hall, K.M., Hopkins, K., Belleza, T., & Cope, D.N. (1982). Disability rating scale for severe head trauma: Coma to community. *Archives of Physical Medicine and Rehabilitation, 63*, 118.

Russell, W.R. (1971). *The traumatic amnesias*. London: Oxford University Press.

Russell, W.R., & Nathan, P.W. (1946). Traumatic amnesia. *Brain, 69*, 183.

Turner, H.B., Kreutzer, J.S., Lent, B., & Brockett, C.A. (1984). Developing a brief neuropsychological mental status exam: A pilot study. *Journal of Neurosurgical Nursing, 16*(5), 257.

Warren, J.B., Goethe, K.E., & Peck, E.A. (1984). Neuropsychological abnormalities associated with severe head injury. *Journal of Neurosurgical Nursing, 16*(1), 30.

Wechsler, D. (1945). A standard memory scale for clinical use. *Journal of Psychology 19*, 87.

Zarit, S.H., Zarit, J.M., & Reever, K.E. (1982). Memory training for severe memory loss: Effects on senile dementia patients and their families. *The Gerontologist, 22*(4), 373.

BIBLIOGRAPHY

Cermak, L.S. (Ed.). (1982). *Human memory and amnesia*. Hillsdale, NJ: Lawrence Erlbaum.

Clites, J. (1984). Maximizing memory retention in the aged. *Journal of Gerontological Nursing, 10*(8), 34.

Eysenck, M.W. (1982). *Attention and arousal: Cognition and performance.* London: Springer-Verlag.

Jennett, B., & Teasdale, G. (1981). *Management of head injuries* (Chap. 12). Philadelphia: Davis.

Kintsch, W. (1977). *Memory and cognition.* New York: Wiley.

Roberts, A.M. (1979). *Severe accidental head injury* (Chap. 6). London: Macmillan.

Rosenthal, M., Griffith, E.R., Bond, M., & Miller, J.D. (Eds.). (1983). *Rehabilitation of the head-injured adult.* Philadelphia: Davis.

Rusk, H.A., Block, J.M., & Lowman, E.W. (1969). Rehabilitation of the brain-injured patient. In E. Walker, W. Caveness, & M. Critchley (Eds.), *The late effects of head injury.* Springfield, IL: Thomas.

Schacter, D.L., & Crovitz, H.F. (1977). Memory function after closed head injury: A review of quantitative research. *Cortex, 13,* 150.

Wilson, B.A., & Moffat, N. (Eds.). (1984). *Clinical management of memory problems.* Rockville, MD: Aspen.

13

Alterations in Cognitive Processing

Sister Callista Roy

Cognitive processing is a significant and distinctive human life process. Cognitive deficits are crucial for all patients, particularly the patients encountered in neuroscience nursing practice. How people think and act has been a subject for philosophic and scientific study through the ages. Aristotle divided mental functions into the cognitive, or thought, processes and the emotional and moral aspects. Today neurobiologists, neuropsychologists, and others chart the relationship between brain organization and mental activities. The postindustrial society is marked by major structural changes. A pivotal change is that information is rapidly replacing energy as society's main resource. Martel (1986) notes that information, unlike energy, is infinite and does not disappear. One can thus postulate that how people process information is the key to the future. Moving into the next century, we are an information processing society. As a major profession within the society, nursing focuses on understanding all human life processes and will accept the challenge of the future to understand and enhance how people process their environment. Clinical practice in neuroscience nursing both provides and calls for developing this specific knowledge.

MODELS OF COGNITIVE PROCESSING

The literature on intelligence and communication theory provides models for understanding cognitive processes. Guilford (1956) described the structure of the intellect as involving memory and thinking. Thinking, in turn, involved cognition, production, and evaluation and could use both convergent and divergent operations. According to this view, intelligence tests measured basic abilities. Gradually, the study of intelligence changed to consider processes underlying behavior. Hunt (1980) integrated the earlier literature and looked at intelligence as an information processing concept with three components: structure, process, and knowledge base. Models of intelligence either attempted to explain mental processes in terms of perception and short-term memory or concerned themselves with the manner in which problems are solved. To explain memory search and reaction time response, Sternberg (1966) proposed a sequential model in a linear chain of boxes. The processing sequence starts with a presentation of the stimulus, which leads to stimulus encoding, which then leads to serial comparison, binary decision, translation, and response organization, and finally to the activation of response.

Haber (1974) describes the origins and types of another approach to information-processing models. A general model of communication was developed in the 1940s to apply to telephone switchboard systems. It described a system with statistical concepts of information source, transmitter, signal, noise source, receiver, message, destination, and received signal. Information content could be specified in terms of uncertainty reduction or a change in the number of alternative possibilities that the events being communicated could represent. This made it possible to measure information processing without depending on the events themselves. Information from different sources, arriving through different sense modalities, could then be compared to make more general statements about perceptual processes. The arrival of digital computers as a computational and analogic device greatly facilitated description and experimentation (particularly in laboratory psychology) of the mechanisms, stages, processes, and models of information processing.

The types of information processing models are distinguished on the basis of attention to a given aspect of the information processing continuum. At the input side of the continuum, there are models that deal with perception, such as visual or auditory stimulation held in memory then recoded. Another group of theorists has focused on memory-related information processing models and their empirical consequences. They denote such stages as rehearsal, recognition, acoustic representation for linguistic material, the processes that underlie forgetting or memory loss, and responding as distinct from storage. These models pay little attention to input variables, recognizing only that stimulation precedes storage. The third type of model focuses on problem-solving behavior and verbal associative learning and does not pay much attention to perceptual or memory processes as such. These models have given rise to the whole field of computer applications called artificial intelligence.

Das (1984) noted that if we want to understand how information is processed by human beings, we must comprehend how processing occurs in the brain rather than in the computer. Following Hunt's three components of intelligence, he proposed an information integration model in which the structure is the brain, the processes are neuropsychologic, and the knowledge base is provided by the experience and education of the person. Das' work is based on the clinical studies of Luria (1973, 1980), who worked for more than 40 years with Soviet neurologists and psychologists to describe disturbances of the higher cortical functions in the presence of local brain lesions. Detailed and insightful observations of victims of World War II resulted in systematic treatment to restore brain functions deranged by head injuries.

Luria conceptualized three main functional divisions of the brain: one to control arousal, one for coding, and one for planning and decision making. The theory was distinct in that it emphasized functional units of the brain. The functional units, according to Luria, have both depth, cortically and subcortically, and spread, that is, across hemispheres. Processing of information in simultaneous quasispatial arrays, for example, is spread over a large area comprising the occipital and parietal lobes. Successive information processing, that is, ordering information temporally, also is located widely, mainly in the temporal and frontotemporal areas of the brain. Planning and decision making seem to involve the whole of the frontal lobes. At the same time, depth is involved, in that coding, such as coding of visual information, passes through hierarchical levels of the brain consistent with its topography.

Luria's theory of the holistic function of the cerebral hemispheres rejected traditional views of localization. If there were not discrete centers for aspects of language, of calculation, or of writing, there must be a reanalysis of such conditions as agnosia and apraxia. Today, Luria's more holistic view is supported in both the scientific and popular literature. For example, Buffington (1986) notes that the pop psychology myth of the left side of the brain controlling only logic and language and the right side solely creativity and intuition has been reduced from fact to fiction. With recent work stemming from technologic advances in research, scientists are back to considering that the whole brain theory may be correct.

A combination of approaches has been used to obtain functional maps of the brain. These involved topographic studies of the effects of brain damage, stimulation of the exposed cortex during surgery, microelectrode recordings of cortical activity evoked by behavior or sensory stimuli, and radioactive isotope techniques to measure the enhanced blood supply to cortical areas that are activated by the performance of specific sensory, motor, and mental tasks. In reviewing a century of this work, Mountcastle (1979) concludes that each neocortical area has a distinctive cytoarchitecture and a distinctive function; however, it also possesses its own unique set of extrinsic connections. He supports Luria's earlier insights and emphasizes that "the brain is a complex of widely and reciprocally interconnected systems and that the dynamic interplay of neural activity within and between these systems is the very essence of brain function" (p. 21).

Although the past decade has seen great advances in neuroanatomy and neurophysiology, still it must be recognized that the neural substrates related to cognition are poorly known. Willis and Grossman (1981) summarize current knowledge by saying that participation and interaction of many brain areas appear to be involved in most of these processes, that cortical and subcortical areas are involved, and that the processes of consciousness, attention, and perception are intimately interrelated.

Nursing assessments and interventions related to patient cognitive processes are influenced greatly by these holistic formulations of cerebral function. Figure 13–1 proposes a model for nursing's view of cognition processing. The inner circle lists basic internal processes of arousal–attention, sensation–perception, coding–concept formation, memory, language, planning, and motor response. These functions are dependent on the brain structure, neurologically and neurochemically, and they occur within the field of consciousness (Willis & Grossman, 1981, p. 447). The next circle represents the situation that the person is immediately confronting and processing. Roy (1984; Andrews & Roy, 1986) refers to this as the focal stimulus. The outer circle represents the education and experience of the person within which the current processing situation is embedded. In terms taken from the Roy Adaptation Model of Nursing, these are considered contextual and residual stimuli. The broken lines in the figure indicate the permeability between the stimulus fields. The clinical discussion that follows is based on the developing knowledge of integrated brain function presented here and the nursing model derived from it.

DOMAINS OF COGNITIVE PROCESSING

Lezak (1983) notes that as more is learned about how the brain processes information, it becomes more difficult to make theoretically acceptable distinctions between the different functions involved in human information processing.

INPUT ⟶	CENTRAL PROCESSING ⟶	OUTPUT
Arousal–Attention	Coding–Concept Formation	Planning
Sensation–Perception	Memory Language	Motor Response

Information processing system.

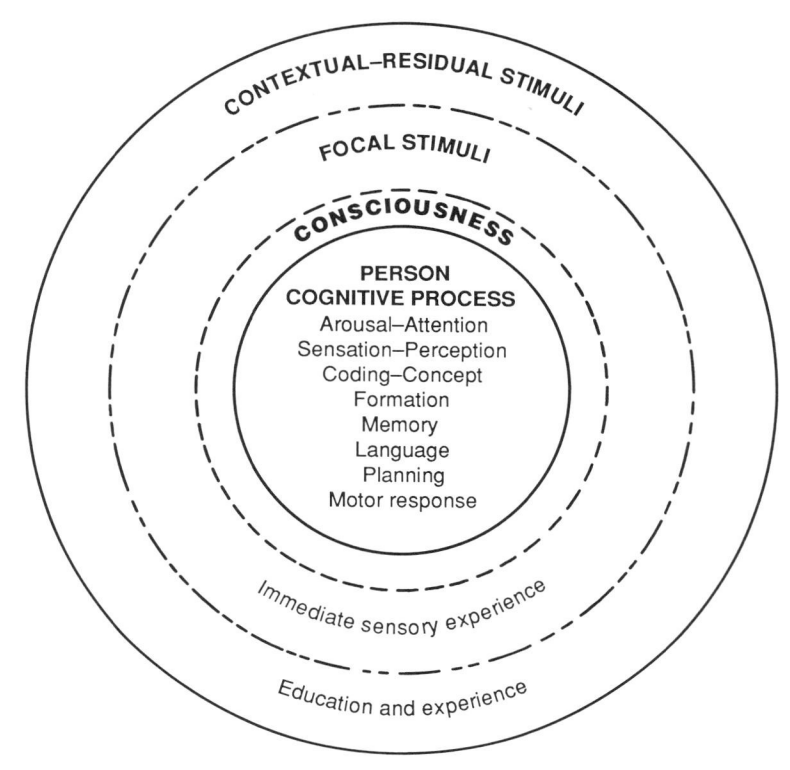

Figure 13-1. Nursing model for cognitive processing.

It is useful for the purposes of this chapter, however, to organize a person's cognitive processing according to functions within each stage of the information processing system (see p. 187). The *input stage* of processing involves the functions of arousal and attention as well as sensation and perception. *Central processing* includes the functions of coding and concept formation, memory, and language. Functions that can be examined at the *output stage* are planning and motor response.

HUMAN RESPONSES TO ALTERED COGNITIVE PROCESSING

In various conditions affecting the central nervous system, there are changes in all or some of these domains of cognitive processing. The section that follows discusses these deficits, which may be considered nursing diagnoses, their clinical manifestations, and the nursing interventions that are based on an understanding of the specific deficit (Table 13-1).

Diagnoses for the Individual

☐ Impaired Cognitive Input Function

Deficits related to the person's ability to take in information occur within the domains of arousal–attention and sensation–perception.

Arousal and Attention. In the domain of arousal and attention, deficits occur in relation to selective attention, speed of process-

TABLE 13-1. DEFICITS OF COGNITIVE INPUT PROCESSES.

Deficits by Function	Behavioral Manifestations	Interventions
A. Arousal–Attention		
1. Selective attention		
a. Focused attention deficit (FAD)	Automatic response to stimulus and inability to modify response	• Remove the stimulus that is eliciting the automatic response
	Perseveration	• Change the stimulus–response bond through behavioral modification
	Inability to establish a new focus of attention	• Include the automatic response in a desired behavior pattern
b. Divided attention deficit (DAD)	Inability to maintain a focus of attention to the immediate situation in context of ordinary background stimuli	• Use verbal cues to maintain focus
	Decrease in number of pieces of information consciously held in mind	• Minimize distractions • Give information in small amounts and complexity
	Slowness in following instructions or learning new tasks	• Patiently wait for series of cognitive operations to be made
	Frustration with environment	• Encourage efforts in spite of frustration
c. Unilateral neglect	Impaired ability to attend to both left and right hemispaces, shown by hemiinattention, hemiinintention, and hemineglect	• Teach safety awareness • Teach compensation techniques to the individual, family, significant others, and health care providers
2. Speed of processing	As in DAD	• As in DAD
3. Alertness		
a. Receptivity deficit	Decreased general receptivity to stimulation shown by somnolence, drowsiness, passivity	• Use verbal, tactile, pain stimulation to rouse to desired level of response
b. Phasic alertness deficit	Decreased expectancy response shown in facial expression, posture, or EEG	• Provide verbal cues to increase readiness to respond
c. Tonic alertness deficit	Impaired ability to sustain a specific focus of attention over an extended period of time	• Recognize limits of extended alertness and divide learning or performance tasks to fit within limits
B. Sensation–Perception		
1. Primary sense processing		
a. Partial or complete blindness	Inability to detect things in the visual environment	• Maintain safety and integrity of body parts without sensation
b. Hearing disorders	Impaired reception of sound	• Preserve optimal sensory function
c. Olfactory or gustatory disorder	Impaired sense of smell or taste	• Develop and use a systematic method to compensate for lost sensation

TABLE 13-1. DEFICITS OF COGNITIVE INPUT PROCESSES. *(Cont.)*

Deficits by Function	Behavioral Manifestations	Interventions
d. Disorders related to touch, temperature, position and discriminating sense, vibration, and pain	Impaired somatic sensation	• Develop and use a systematic method to compensate for lost sensation

2. Pattern recognition
   a. Visual, tactile, acoustic agnosia
   b. Alexia
   c. Topographic disorientation
	Loss of ability for identification, recognition, discrimination, or classification of stimuli that is out of proportion to the loss of perception of the existence of the stimuli	• Simplify the environment
		• Encourage patient to use alternate senses and cues for identifying objects
		• Use exercises to reactivate patient's comprehension of words
		• Provide aids for reading, e.g., ruler, large print
		• Accompany patient to any new location and provide written instruction even in familiar places

3. Naming and association a. Naming and association deficits	Inability to name and associate correctly	• Teach to recognize deficits and to compensate for them • Simplify the environment
b. Disorders of color naming c. Disorders of color association	Loss of color vision	• Use exercises that construct visual images and practice charades
d. Spatial analysis deficits	Inability to grasp the whole visual field Unstable useful visual field Difficulty perceiving moving objects Misjudgments of depth	• Simplify the environment • Maintain safety • Develop and use a systematic method to compensate for deficits

ing, and alertness. Arousal and attention direct perceptual mechanisms to stimuli in the field of consciousness. Behaviorally, arousal is defined by the orienting of sensory receptors to a stimulus. This orienting may be produced by (1) a change in stimulus level, for example, in attempting to arouse a patient the nurse raises her voice above the level of the background noise in the intensive care unit, (2) presentation of a novel stimulus, for example, a speaker may use cartoons to illustrate highly theoretical material, and (3) presentation of a stimulus that has been learned as a signal for reward or punishment, for example, the announcement of a fire drill orients all hospital personnel to that stimulus. For research purposes, electrophysiologic signs of the process of paying attention can be observed by recording sensory evoked potentials from the cerebral cortex.

A continuous stream of stimulation reaches the senses and a vast amount of information is present in the memory system. Yet actual behavior, of the patient or nurse, is determined by only a fraction of this information. A number of theories of selective attention have been developed to explain the process of attending to one stimulus and stopping all others below the level of awareness. Early theories assumed that information could be filtered by the person according to how meaningful or pertinent it was. A later theory (Schneider & Shiffrin, 1977) proposed that selectivity was not structually connected to any fixed level of abstraction, that is, not to the process of giving meaning to the stimulus. If one views processing as both automatic and controlled by the individual, there are different kinds of attention deficits. This theory is particularly useful in describing problems of neuroscience patients.

Shiffrin and Schneider (1977) describe two forms of processing. *Automatic processing* does not demand conscious effort, but rather is the result of learning and practice, for example, the skill of driving a car regularly. *Controlled processing*, on the other hand, is the temporary activation of a sequence of elements that can be set up quickly and easily but requires attention, like driving an unfamiliar car. The capacity for controlled processing is limited; it usually occurs in serial steps and typically in new situations. All information entering the system is processed automatically up to the highest level possible without conscious control. Processing is initiated by the appropriate input, is based on activation of a learned sequence of long-term memory elements, then proceeds automatically to the response. This framework specifies two kinds of limitations of selective attention, that is, focused attention deficits and divided attention deficits.

Focused attention deficits (FADs) result from automatic response tendencies conflicting with responses required by the task at hand. There is a conflicting stimulus–response bond. The nurse who has always used emergency equipment from a certain cupboard will, therefore, reach in that direction when an emergency occurs, even though she has been transferred to another unit where emergency equipment is stored in a different place. If the person cannot interrupt a learned automatic process, FAD occurs.

Divided attention deficits (DADs), however, result from speed limitations of consciously controlled processing. Controlled processing makes use of results of automatic processing and operates on this information by means of a strategy formed on the basis of instruction, prior learning, and context. Transformations of the input information are carried out, and responses have to be selected from the behavioral repertoire. Since this processing is speed limited, the available processing capacity must be divided over several cognitive operations required for the task. For example, if a nurse being oriented to a new job gets a detailed list of instructions when asking for directions to the cafeteria, she is likely to answer politely, "Thank you," and go on to ask another person who may have a shorter list of instructions. Limitations of rate of processing are discussed subsequently.

Unilateral neglect has been described as a specific type of selective attention deficit (Mesulam, 1985). This composite phenomenon can be analyzed from the perspective of complex perceptual, motor, and motivational aspects. Yet it appears that this phenomenon represents a fundamental disturbance in a vector aspect of attention—namely the spatial distribution of directed sensory attention. Mesulam notes that the possibility of unilateral neglect merely reflecting a combination of elementary sensory motor deficits can be dismissed. Repeated studies have shown that the extent of sensory loss does not correlate with the severity of neglect. Some patients with intact visual fields may still show neglect, whereas patients with hemianopia do not necessarily neglect the blind field but rather move their head and eyes to take in the field on the visually impaired side.

Mesulam (1985, p. 156) developed a hypothetical model of a neural network for the distribution of attention based on observations of the three regions of the entire cortex that consistently lead to unilateral neglect when damaged (Fig. 13–2). In this model, the distribution of directed attention is coordinated by a neural network that contains three independent but interacting representations of the extrapersonal world. The posterior parietal cortex may contain a sensory template of the extrapersonal world. The frontal eye fields and related cortex may contain a motor map for the distribution of orienting and exploratory movements with the extrapersonal space.

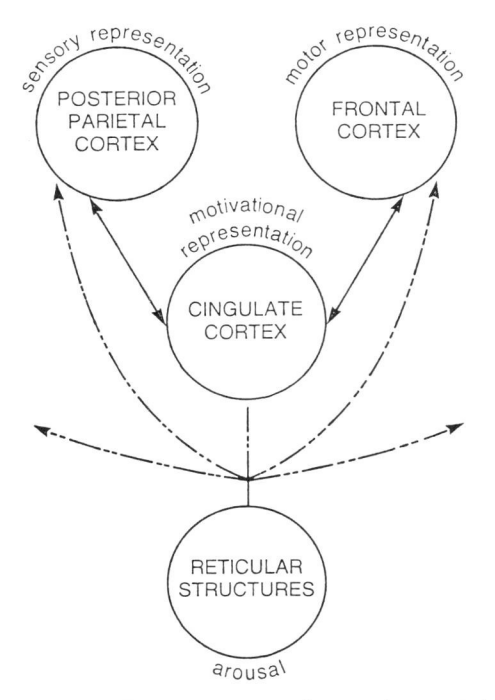

Figure 13–2. The components of a neural network involved in modulating directed attention. *(From Mesulam, 1981.)*

Mesulam's model shows a third representation to contain a map for the distribution of expectancy and relevance, perhaps centered on cingulate cortex. Arousal tone may be given by reticular structures that provide input for each of the three representations. Finally, each representation has specific connections with the striatum and thalamus. Assuming this mechanism, the effective distribution of attention within the extrapersonal space requires a flexible interaction among the three representations. This model, based on empiric and clinical data, is consistent with Luria's notion of functional systems of the brain that have both depth and spread. In discussing unilateral neglect, the integrity of the entire network or, as Mountcastle called it, the complex of reciprocally interconnected systems is more relevant than theories of cortical localization.

A second major category of deficits in the cognitive functions of arousal and attention relates to *speed of processing*. The speed with which the person can process information will determine partly what will be noticed and how much will go unnoticed. As described earlier in Schneider and Shiffrin's notion of controlled processing, the number of operations possible in a certain time unit is finite. Whenever controlled processing fails to deal with all information that should be processed for optimal task performance, a DAD occurs. A dramatic example of this type of deficit seemed apparent in the decision to launch the space shuttle Challenger in January 1986. In the months of investigation that followed the fatal explosion of the spacecraft, details of information were laid out that were not processed adequately during the much shorter timespan of the launch decision.

In head injury patients, several studies provide convincing evidence that there is a slowing down of controlled processing of information. The person must expend even greater energy paying attention because he or she has less attention to pay. Because of this speed of processing deficit, these patients are influenced greatly by the number of stimulus alternatives. With more things to pay attention to and less attention to pay, they are easily distracted and then feel frustrated when their efforts to take in their environment prove unsuccessful. Using the Paced Auditory Serial Addition Task, or PASAT, Gronwall and Sampson (1974) compared hospital controls and head injury patients classified in two degrees of severity. The nature of errors did not discriminate patients from control subjects, and without time pressure, both patients and controls could do the task almost perfectly. They concluded that the poor performance of head injury patients in the usual testing condition is probably the result of a slow, but qualitatively normal processing strategy.

The third type of arousal–attention deficit is related to alertness. Posner (1975) uses the term alertness to refer to a hypothetical state of the central nervous system that affects general receptivity to stimulation, for example, variations in sleep and wakefulness. The half-asleep patient may not readily take in and process a list of instructions in the same way that he or she would when fully awake. Human performance is not constant over time, and researchers describe fluctuations in efficiency that have both phasic and tonic shifts. Phasic changes occur rapidly and depend on the person's interests and intentions. Such changes have been described by the expectancy wave (EW) on the electroencephalogram (EEG). It is as if the brain of a person driving a car and waiting for a traffic light to change is idling like the car engine. When cues are noted that the light is about to change, such as the cross traffic stopping, the EW wave occurs. Tonic changes of alertness, on the other hand, occur slowly and involuntarily. Since tonic changes cover minutes or hours, they are studied by viligance tasks that measure the person's efficiency at detecting a signal. These lapses of attention also are measured by changes in the EEG. Such research on alertness is used to guide decisions related to safety standards in certain occupations, for example, the number of consecutive hours an airline pilot may fly.

It often is assumed that patients with various neurologic or neurosurgical conditions have deficits of sustained attention. Decreased EWs were found in some early studies of alertness in head injury patients, suggesting that the basic deficit after head injury is the inability to sustain attention of a level required for normal performance on some tests. In recent studies using more precise measures, however, this hypothesis was not supported. A research group in Holland (Brooks, 1984) reported studies of control subjects and head injury patients on auditory vigilance tasks lasting 30 minutes. Every 4 seconds, a click is presented by means of headphones, with one of five clicks being 4 decibels weaker that the standard clicks. Normal subjects show clear performance decrements during the second half of the session. Their EEGs indicated signs of drowsiness. In the severe head injury patients tested, a relationship between EEG and performance was not found.

In fact, these patients showed persistently alert EEGs during the task, whereas their heart rates were higher. Their signal detection performance was decidedly poorer but was steady over time. These investigators find some evidence that phasic alertness may be nonoptimal after head injury, but they note that these patients may have higher tonic levels of alertness.

Patients may show clinical signs of attention and arousal deficits (Table 13–1, A). As noted earlier, FADs involve automatic response tendencies based on already established stimulus–response bonds, a behavior recognized in the patient who makes automatic responses to stimuli and is unable to modify that response. Behaviorally, perseverations may occur, such as always repeating the name of a certain person regardless of the specific question asked about people the patient has known. The persistence of overlearned behaviors inhibits the person's ability to establish a new focus of attention. Thus, the stroke patient whose bathroom at home was to the left of the bed may continue to go in that direction seeking the bathroom in spite of efforts to teach him or her to go in the other direction.

In general, the nurse's *interventions* with this type of attention deficit include (1) removing the stimulus that is eliciting the automatic responses, (2) changing the stimulus–response bond through behavioral modification techniques, or (3) including the automatic response in a desired behavioral pattern. In the example of the stroke patient, the first approach is not appropriate, and modifying the behavior might take a great deal of time and effort for both the patient and the nurse. The third approach might be most useful; for example the patient's bed may be turned to face the other direction so that turning left becomes the desired response, that is, the correct direction to the bathroom.

Assessment of DADs indicates an inability to maintain a focus of attention to the immediate situation in the context of ordinary background stimuli. The patient shows a decrease in the number of pieces of information that can be held consciously in mind and a slowness in following instructions or learning new tasks. The patient's awareness of this deficit or the reactions of others often result in feelings of frustration for the patient.

Nursing *interventions* for patients with this attention deficit include managing the environment and their own input to the patient. When the patient must attend to a given task, the nurse uses verbal cues to maintain focus, for example, "It's lunchtime now, and you are to keep eating." At the same time, background distractions can be minimized by, for example, turning the television off and limiting interaction with other patients in the room during mealtime. Any information given to the patient should be provided in simple terms and in small amounts at a time. Recognizing that the patient is going through a series of cognitive operations to complete processing of the information, the nurse will wait patiently for the process to be completed. She will watch for cues that the patient has successfully processed the input or has not done so. Her response will be to encourage the patient's efforts in either case. She continues to modify the amount of information to match the patient's speed of processing ability.

We noted Mesulam's description of *unilateral neglect* as a disturbance in the spatial distribution of directed attention. Given that the patient does not have the necessary intact neural network, he or she will show an impaired ability to attend to both left and right hemispaces, as shown by hemiinattention, or hemineglect. *Interventions* for this condition involve teaching safety awareness and teaching compensation techniques. The patient, the family and significant others, and the health care staff will learn these techniques.

Speed of processing was discussed as a dimension of attention and arousal separate from selective attention. Deficits in this area are reflected in divided attention deficits, since a limitation in the speed of processing results in attention having to be divided over the total amount of input. The *assessment* and the appropriate *interventions* are, therefore, the same as those for divided attention deficits. Again, the nurse is aware of the great amount of energy the patient must expend to accomplish a series of cognitive operations slowly. In a busy neurounit, it is not always easy to wait for the patient response, but the nurse's use of this knowledge can provide the patient with the opportunity to be a thinking person.

The category of deficits listed in Table 13–1 (A, 3) relates to alertness. This deficit may be manifested by a *decreased general receptivity* to stimulation. When a patient seems not to be responding to stimulation, the nurse uses verbal, tactile, and, if necessary, pain stimulation as *interventions* to arouse the person. This category of deficit overlaps somewhat with consciousness, yet refers to the person who is conscious but has a decreased level of alertness.

In *assessing phasic alertness deficits*, one notes a decreased expectancy response, as shown in a nonalert or vacant facial expression. Posture may be slumped and appear unready for a response, and it may be possible to identify an alertness deficit on an EEG by use of average evoked potentials. If there is a *tonic alertness deficit*, the patient will show also an impaired ability to sustain a specific focus of attention over an extended period of time. In providing care, the nurse uses verbal cues to increase readiness to respond; for example, the nurse may address the patient by name and tell the patient that she or he is there to help the patient get ready for the family's visit. The patient may still look bewildered, but with the patient aroused, the nurse may proceed with the task. In doing this, the nurse uses another basic *intervention* for alertness deficits. The nurse recognizes limitations and divides the task into timeframes that match the patient's tonic alertness; for example, helping the patient dress may take 10 minutes. Since this is the limit of the patient's alertness ability, the nurse will return later to help the patient ambulate to the sunroom during another short period of alertness.

Sensation and Perception

The second domain of cognitive functions related to the person's ability to take in information is that of sensation and perception. The model of integrated brain function implies that all cognitive processes are interrelated. The process of sensation and perception presuppose arousal and attention, and they provide the initial step for central processing by coding, memory, and language. For purposes of describing cognitive deficits and their clinical implications, however, these functions can be considered separately.

Kolb and Whishaw (1980) make the simple distinction that sensation is the result of activity of receptors and their associated afferent pathways to the corresponding neocortical sensory areas, whereas perception is the result of activity of cells in the cortex beyond the first synapse in the sensory cortex. From the nursing model of information processing proposed in this chapter (Fig. 13–1), we might consider that immediate sensory experience is transformed into a percept in the neocortex by such factors as education and experience; that is, the focal stimulus is processed in the light of contextual and residual stimuli. For example, if during a fire, smoke covers the last two letters of the exit sign, it will still be preceived as **EXIT** even though the sense perception was only **EX**. Sensation is a more passive process; for example, light on the retina creates the visual *sensation* of the outline of two letters, but *perception* is the active process of encoding the impulses transmitted by the aroused retina into a pattern of letters that make a word that has meaning in the current situation. That is, the person perceives the exit as a way to leave the burning building.

Researchers have described the relationship between sensory experience during development and the forming of perceptual mechanisms. Deprivation of visual experience has been shown to result in malformation of a proportion of the dendritic spines of mouse visual cortex neurons, although some spines develop normally in the absence of vision. Visual deprivation also produces changes in the shapes of the receptive fields of cat visual cortex neurons (Willis & Grossman, 1981). Studies of perception examine the way in which the physical characteristics of stimuli, such as intensity, quality, and position in space, are encoded by neural activity. Transformations in the neural activity at each relay station in the sensory pathway are studied throughout the somatosensory system. Laws are described that relate the physical property of the intensity of the stimulus to the psychologic property of the intensity of the percept. For example, a power function best describes the transformation of stimulus energy to the intensity of the percept. The intensity of a series of stimuli, then, must increase exponentially to produce equally spaced increments of sensation and thus the person's report of the perception of the sensation.

There are several important properties of normal sensation and perception that help in understanding deficits of these cognitive functions. Intact visual perception is characterized by the constancy of the percepts. An example of this phenomenon is size constancy: A bed observed from a distance of 5 feet does not look twice as large as a bed observed from a distance of 10 feet, even though its retinal image is twice as large as the one seen from 5 feet. Learning plays a role in developing such constancies. There is a sensation of stability of the external world that is important in being able to manipulate the environment. Another significant aspect of perception is the recognition of objects. This aspect of perception is related to the philosophic notion of the knowledge of universals. We can recognize (classify) a particular object, such as a bed, that we have never seen before as an example of a class of objects (beds) even when the object is presented to us in a different spatial orientation, such as upside down. By perceptual mechanisms, we tend to group objects into patterns. It is not known, however, to what extent organizational tendencies in perception are innate and to what extent they are learned.

Willis and Grossman (1981) indicate that there may be a considerable degree of inherent, or "prewired," organization of responses to particular types of stimuli built into the nervous system. They cite work of recordings from single neurons at various levels of the visual system in amphibia and in mammals that reveal the presence of neurons that act as detectors for certain properties of the stimulus, such as motion detectors, edge detectors, or contour detectors. Mesulam (1985) likewise draws heavily on relevant evidence in nonhuman primates to describe neural connectivity in the cortex that includes primary sensory and motor areas, modality-specific (unimodal) association areas, and high-order (heteromodal) association areas. This description of cortical zones of the human brain is consistent with Luria's concept of functional divisions described earlier in this chapter. Within and across these zones and their depth projections into the paralimbic and limbic areas, sensory signals are transformed into complex percepts. For example, facial recognition is a complex nonverbal perceptual task performed by the whole right hemisphere. It is the extensive cortical distribution and complexity of perceptual activities that make them highly vulnerable to brain injury, yet also perhaps more available for recovery processes.

The distinction between sensation and perception and the descriptions of peripheral and central neural networks are useful because they allow understanding of the effects of lesions to lower (sensory) and upper (perceptual) components of the somatosensory system. Clinically, nurses in neuroscience practice will encounter patients with deficits in at least four categories: primary sensory deficits, such as blindness and deafness, disorders of pattern recognition, acquired disorders of naming and association, and disorders of spatial analysis. Primary sensory deficits and their nursing interventions are discussed in Chapters 23 and 24.

☐ **Disorders of Pattern Recognition**

The presence of normal primary sensation in itself does not mean that the person can use the information obtained by the senses. The discriminative functions involve pattern recognition and study the ability of the sensory cortex to correlate, analyze, and interpret sensations. The term *agnosia* is used to describe, in Teuber's words, "a normal percept stripped of its meanings" (Teuber, 1968). Damasio (1985) provides an operational definition of visual agnosia that further clarifies the distinction between primary sensory deficits and pattern recognition deficits:

> a disorder of higher behavior confined to the visual realm, in which an alert, attentive, intelligent, and nonaphasic patient with normal visual perception gives evidence of not knowing the meaning of those stimuli—that is of not recognizing them. (Damasio, 1985, p. 259)

Damasio maintains that although perception and recognition are part of a continuum, it is possible to identify both behaviorally and neurophysiologically some components of the process that are related mainly to perception and some that are related mainly to recognition. The painstaking search for supporting evidence of effective perception precedes the identification of an agnosia. Furthermore, the correct identification of a deficit as one of sense processing or of pattern recognition affects the design of appropriate nursing interventions.

Agnosias occur in the visual, auditory, and somatosensory realms. It is difficult to isolate a disturbance to a given realm, just as it is difficult to distinguish agnosias from sensory deficits. Still, the types of major agnosias and the deficits involved may be summarized (based on classification and discussion by Kolb & Whishaw, 1985, p. 205) as follows:

Type	Deficit
Visual agnosias	
Object agnosia	Naming, using, or recognizing objects
Agnosia for drawings	Recognition of drawn stimuli
Prosopagnosia	Recognition of faces
Color agnosia	Association of colors with objects
Color anomia	Naming colors
Achromatopsia	Distinguishing hues
Visual–spatial agnosia	Stereoscopic vision, topographic concepts

Type *(cont.)*	Deficit *(cont.)*
Auditory agnosias	
Amusia	Tone deafness; melody deafness; disorders of rhythm, measure, or tempo
Agnosia for sounds	Identifying meaning of nonverbal sounds
Somatosensory agnosias	
Asterognosia	Recognition of objects by touch
Anosognosia	Awareness of illness
Anosodiaphoria	Response to illness
Autotopagnosia	Localization and naming of body parts
Asymbolia for pain	Reaction to pain

Alexia is a particular disorder of visual pattern recognition, and in the pure form is called alexia-without-agraphia or word blindness. This deficit is manifested by severe impairment of the ability to read most words and sentences, and in many patients, even the reading of single letters is defective. The patient can see sentences, words, and letters and can copy them but cannot read them. Research on the mechanisms of this deficit and how it relates to agnosia and to aphasia is ongoing. Much progress in the understanding of the visual function has taken place in the past two decades (Mountcastle et al., 1975; Hubel, 1982). Formulations that have been hinted in neuropsychologic investigations are supported by current experimental work in animals. Refinements of neuroimaging techniques—computerized tomography (CT), positron emission tomography (PET), single photon emission tomography (SPET), nuclear magnetic resonance imaging (MRI)—will permit more elaborate clinical and experimental work related to the processing of complex visual information in the human brain. This work provides significant implications for interventions with visual deficits of perception, as well as helping to understand better ways of studying other deficits of pattern recognition.

A variety of disorders involving spatial orientation are included in the designation *topographic disorientation*. The acquired inability to locate a public building in a city, to find one's room at home, or to describe either verbally or by means of a map how to get to a specific room or place are all behavioral manifestations of this deficit. The cause of this deficit is based on unilateral hemispatial neglect or on a global amnestic syndrome.

In *assessment* of the three types of pattern recognition deficits discussed—agnosia, alexia, and topographic disorientation—the behavioral manifestations in general involve the loss of or impaired ability to identify, recognize, discriminate, or classify stimuli that is out of proportion to the loss of perception of the stimuli. *Interventions* related to these deficits focus first on simplifying the environment. Since the person has difficulty making sense of the perceptual world, the task of taking it in is simplified by having fewer stimuli and ensuring that the stimuli present are meaningful. For example, only one dish at a time is placed in front of the person, and another is added only when the first is empty. Taylor and Ballenger (1980) recommend a structured environment with the key elements of simplicy, order, and routine for brain-damaged patients, and these suggestions are relevant particularly for people with pattern recognition deficits.

Second, the patient can be encouraged to establish awareness of the deficit and then to use alternate senses or cues for identifying and recognizing a stimulus. For example, the patient with prosopagnosia may be taught to touch his or her eye and face saying, "I don't see faces." Then he or she practices relying on voices, mannerisms, uniforms, and so forth to identify health care personnel. Specific learning exercises may help reactivate a person's comprehension of words. These exercises often are included in handbooks for families of stroke or head injury patients. One example (from a handbook published by Pi Lambda Theta, 1983) is to use fairly large, colorful pictures and a list of words related to the pictures, as well as words unrelated to the pictures. The person is shown a group of words and a picture and asked to point to the word or words that go with the picture. The task may be reversed, and the person is shown a group of pictures and a word, then asked to point to the pictures that go with the word. Another variation is to show the person a group of words, all but one of which belong in the same category, for example, animals, and then ask the person to pick out the one that does not belong.

Aids for reading, such as a ruler to follow the line and large print, may help some patients improve pattern recognition. The person with topographic disorientation should be accompanied to any new location and will need written instructions even in familiar places. It is clear that an infinite amount of patience is required of the person with a pattern recognition deficit, as well as of the family and of all health care providers, in adapting lifestyle and the need for independence within the context of the remaining abilities.

Luria (1973) discusses the fact that perceptual ability is not confined to the processes of perception. Rather, for example, visual perceptual activity necessarily includes the active formation of visual images corresponding to a single word meaning. In this active perceptual process, there is a search for the most important elements of information, their comparison with each other, the creation of a hypothesis concerning the meaning for the information as a whole, and the verification of this hypothesis by comparing it with the original features of the object perceived. A person may have an intact ability to create a visual synthesis of an object or a picture, yet be unable to relate it to past experience—in other words, not be able to associate it in memory. The mechanisms underlying *naming and association deficits* is not entirely clear. Geschwind (1965; Benson & Geschwind 1985) suggests a disturbance that effectively separates a primary sensory or sensory association area from the dominant hemisphere language area.

Luria (1973, p. 239) provides clinical observations showing the behavioral characteristics of such deficits. These patients still can see clearly an object or a picture of it. However, either the patients cannot relate the object to their personal experience (e.g., when looking at a picture of a group of soldiers on a tank, one patient said, "This is my family, my father, sisters and children") or will assess the meaning of a picture on the basis of irrelevant associations (e.g., a patient interpreted the picture of a boy who had broken a window and had been caught by the owner of the house as, "Someone from Buryat Republic has won a competition (!), and they are presenting him with a cup").

Disorders of color naming and color association are particular types of this perceptual deficit. Damasio (1985) differentiates *disorders of color naming* from achromatopsia, or loss of color vision. This deficit occurs when otherwise nonaphasic patients can experience the sensation of color and can match colors according to hue but are unable to name those colors that they perceive apparently without difficulty. The author's discussion of efforts to analyze the lesion that leads to this deficit provides further insight into the complexities of the neurophysiology of human sensual–perceptual processing.

Studying an extensive series of patients, Damasio concluded that the lesion necessary for color-naming defects is located in the left hemisphere, mesially, in the transition between the occipital and temporal lobes, in a subsplenial position. The right homonymous hemianopia that also is present in these patients is caused by an additional lesion either in the geniculate body, visual cortex, or optic radiations. Damasio notes that, regardless of the lesion that causes it, the net effect of a right field cut is to circumscribe visual information to the right visual cortex. The effect of the occipitotemporal lesion is to interfere with the ability of language areas in the left hemisphere to receive visual information related to color. This lesion may simply disconnect color information conveyed by the corpus callosum. Another possibility is that some crucial step in the processing of that information takes place in the occipitotemporal transition cortex. Other types of visual information still reach the remainder of the left visual association cortices, thus explaining the preservation of other aspects of visual naming.

In his discussion of *disorders of color association*, Damasio further notes that the cognitive basis of the concept of color is fragile, being principally dependent on (1) the association of a verbal tag with a given color and (2) the association of a given color with the objects that commonly carry it (an association that must be, at least in part, verbally mediated). The author suggests that a functional dissociation between visual and verbal processes is likely to prevent the concomitant arousal of verbal and visual memory traces on which the attribution of meaning to a normal color perception must depend.

Deficits of naming and association as described here and all the variations reported in the literature have the common behavioral manifestation of inability to name and associate correctly. *Interventions* for such deficits are similar to those given for the primary sensory and pattern recognition deficits. Simplification of the environment is key, as is developing an awareness of the deficit and assisting the person to use his or her remaining abilities. Exercises that have the person construct visual images may be useful; for example, ask the patient to describe a house he has been in, then a house he has never been in; a familiar bird, then a strange bird; a person he knows well, then someone he has never met. The nurse or family member can use magazine pictures, naming words for various things seen. The patient repeats each word to help build association of words and pictures. Charades may be used to recall and name words.

The fourth type of deficit of sensation and perception is that of *spatial analysis*. Damasio (1985) describes one of the most striking of these disorders called *Balint's syndrome*, an acquired disturbance of the ability to perceive the visual field as a whole, resulting in the unpredictable perception and recognition of only parts of it (simultanagnosia), which is accompanied by an impairment of target pointing under visual guidance (optic ataxia) and an inability to shift gaze at will toward new visual stimuli (ocular apraxia).

Essentially, these patients become unable to grasp the field of vision in its entirety and will report seeing clearly in only a small fraction of the panorama, with vision outside that spot described as hazy. The subjective problem becomes more difficult because this fragment of useful field is not stable and moves erratically from quadrant to quadrant. Such patients commonly fail to detect and orient to new stimuli that may appear in the periphery of the visual field. An object that is seen clearly at a given moment may disappear suddenly from view as the center of vision shifts. Patients will complain about objects vanishing from the scene they are inspecting and an inability to report more than one or two components of the visual field at any one time. They may find that moving objects are especially difficult to perceive. With the optic ataxia, these patients can point with accuracy to targets in their own body or clothing, using somatosensory information, and also to a source of sound. Depending on vision, however, there is marked difficulty reaching toward small targets and in finger pointing. These patients are unable to direct gaze voluntarily toward a new stimulus appearing in the periphery of the visual field. Even if told that the stimulus has entered the field, they will not orient to it, or if they do, the gaze is inaccurate.

Related visual disturbances are the inability to discriminate depth on the basis of binocular visual information and the inability to judge directional orientation of lines. Disorders of auditory–spatial analysis are considered inconsequential in relation to the visual ones, although these also can be distressing to a person and can present threats to safety. For example, a woman suffering recent one-sided hearing loss after acoustic neuroma surgery reported spending an inordinate amount of time trying to locate visually the source of an annoying tinny sound in her office. In desperation, she called a colleague in the office next door to ask if the noise was outside the window. This person responded that there was not an unusual noise coming from outside the window, but she would come and investigate the sound. Entering the office, the colleague pointed directly to an electric typewriter in the corner and said, "That machine is on."

The main behavioral feature of these deficits is inaccurate and distorted perception. Clinically, *interventions* are designed as they are for people with primary sensory losses, particularly partial or complete blindness. The nurse focuses on maintaining safety and developing a systematic method to compensate for the deficit. In addition, the patient and family must learn to adapt their lifestyles and the patient's need for independence within the constraints of the deficit.

The person's ability to use arousal, attention, sensation, and perception to take in the environment is a preparation for central processing. This aspect of cognitive processing and the deficits of central processing are described in the next section.

☐ Impaired Function of Central Cognitive Processing

The person's relationship to the environment has been described in terms of arousal and attention directing perceptual mechanisms to take in immediate sensory experience. At this point in human information processing, the central processes become primary. Input stimuli are processed further by way of coding and concept formation, memory, and language. Since memory and language are such significant areas of deficit for neuroscience patients, they have been discussed more extensively in Chapters 12 and 14.

Coding

The brain's unique power is due mainly to its ability to store information, that is, to code a representation of experience for future use. In Luria's description of functional units of the brain, the second of these complex working systems is for the reception, coding, and storage of information (1973, p. 67). Some years ago Lashley (in Pribram, 1969b) reviewed the experimental evidence related to how the brain performs storage and retrieval. He then stated that, on the basis of the available evidence, learning and remembering obviously were impossible. Scientists continue to pursue the intractable question of how information is stored. Pribram (1969a) noted that what appears to happen is that the nervous system is so constructed that it analyzes from the complexities of the receptive mechanisms some sort of alphabet that can be used as a code to represent the input. He used the notion of the neural hologram analogously to photographic holograms. In this photographic process, a record of wave patterns emitted or reflected from an object is frozen until it is read out by a process called wavefront reconstruction. Work on understanding central cognitive processing focuses on how the brain functions to code, store, and use information.

Willis and Grossman (1981) summarize the work in the field. They note that central functions are thought of as producing a structural or electrophysiologic change in the brain. This change has been called the memory trace even though no particular type of localization or mechanisms of storage are identified. Various models are used to study the processes that produce the memory trace, for gaining access to the trace, for recalling it to consciousness, and for producing motor activity. The general principles that these authors provide for the clinical neurosciences include:

1. Storage of information is a function of the brain as a whole.
2. The hippocampus may be involved in processes of sorting, assembling, and supplying information, for example, with sensory information that is emotionally significant.
3. Such processes in the broadest sense can be thought of as plasticity, or modifiability of synaptic function.
4. Short-term changes in synaptic function have been identified in work on habituation and conditioning, but how such short-

term changes might be converted into long-term learning or memory lasting for years is not known.
5. Such changes in synaptic function imply either growth of new synaptic connections or a change in the functional effectiveness of synapses.
6. Metabolic activity or protein synthesis might be important in the processes under consideration.

Woody (1982) discusses the chemical forms that theoretically are available for controlling engram or code formation, that is, subionic particles, ions and molecules, macromolecules, and complex molecular aggregates.

Since cognitive central processing is a function of the brain as a whole, it is most sensitive to the effects of changes in the brain regardless of site. For example, significant changes in memory storage following anesthesia have been noted (White & Wolf-Wilets, 1977), as have persistent disorders of learning and memory as long as 10 to 20 years after head injury (Brooks, 1984). Clinicians use various ways to classify deficits of processing so that they may plan care for patients with these deficits. The extensive disorders specifically noted in the central processing functions of memory and language are discussed in Chapters 12 and 14. Coding and concept formation, however, are viewed as additional functions of central processing that are requisite for memory and language functions. The deficits observed in these domains along with their behavioral manifestations and relevant nursing interventions are listed in Table 13–2.

Based on the theoretical and empirical view of brain function being presented, we might describe coding as involving the registration of incoming stimuli, the consolidation of it into a form for storage, and the synthesis of consolidated elements with previous brain codings or engrams. Lezak (1983) describes registration as the holding of large amounts of incoming information briefly (1 or 2 seconds at most) in sensory store. It is neither strictly a memory function nor a perceptual function but rather a selecting and recording process by which perceptions enter the memory system. It has been called the valve to determine which memories are stored. Acquired sensory response patterns, perceptual and response predispositions, and attention-focusing components of perception play an integral role in the registration process. As indicated in the nursing model for cognitive processing (Fig. 13–1), immediate sensory experience takes place within a field of consciousness, with the permeable boundaries of the contextual and residual stimuli, that is, education and experience, also available to the processing person. A key deficit in the domain of coding might be called *altered level of consciousness* (Table 13–2, A). Consciousness has been defined as an awareness of the internal and external environment. Crigger and Strickland (1985) provide the distinction that, theoretically, consciousness includes two components: arousal, the awakeness of the person, and content, the interpretation of the internal and external environment. If a person is having difficulty registering immediate sensory experience, the difficulty may be in either the arousal or the content component; that is, the person may not be alert enough to register or the person's content storage may be disrupted in such a way that new information cannot enter. Behaviorally, the deficit is manifested by minimal, no, or nonproportionate responses to stimuli. Confusion, delirium, and agitation are further manifestations of changes in levels of consciousness. *Assessment* and nursing *interventions* of decreased and increased behavior at arousal are discussed in Chapters 6 and 7.

Concept Formation

The process of concept formation is essential to the person's ability to process and cope effectively with the world. Concept formation adds qualitatively different functions to the coding process. Specifically, these functions include integrated recognition, abstraction and flexibility, and calculation (Table 13–3).

Pattern recognition is the ability of the sensory cortex to correlate, analyze, and interpret sensations. Just as Damasio (1985) be-

TABLE 13–2. DEFICITS OF COGNITIVE CENTRAL PROCESSES.

Deficits by Function	Behavioral Manifestations	Interventions

A. Coding
  1. Registration
      Altered level of consciousness
	Minimal, no, or nonproportionate response to stimuli	• Use verbal, tactile, pain stimulation to rouse to desired level of response
		• Provide for safety and meeting basic needs
		• Simplify the environment
		• Converse as if patient can register information

	Confusion, delirium, agitation	• Develop a sense of trust and confidence • Help family to understand patient's behavior • Use calm, matter-of-fact, nonpunitive approach to reassure patient of protection • Firm, consistent, personal restraint temporarily with reassurance
2. Consolidation Defective information storage	Impaired ability to use prior experience to benefit future actions Defective spontaneous recall	• Help patient and family recognize the deficit • Provide continuous flow of useful, orienting information • Develop and use routine for daily living care • Structure the environment for simplicity and safety • Encourage and support patient and family • Be patient with problems inherent in limitations
3. Synthesis Lack of perspective	Impaired ability to differentiate and identify common elements in past, present, and future sets of information; to identify differences and relationships among these elements; and to integrate such information into a whole as a basis for a modulated response	• Provide protection and supportive supervision • Structure the environment for safety and psychologic comfort • Provide for relief of caregivers • Assist family with issues related to long-term institutional care

B. Concept formation
  1. Integrated recognition
      Fractionated recognition
	Lack of subjective familiarity with stimulus
	Absence of responses adequate to the stimulus
	Loss of the ability to identify stimuli
		• Provide structured, controlled environment
		• Help deal with feelings of perplexity and fear of unfamiliar

2. Abstraction and flexibility a. Conceptual concreteness	Inability to form concepts and use categories	• Limit the need to abstract or symbolize

TABLE 13–2. DEFICITS OF COGNITIVE CENTRAL PROCESSES. *(Cont.)*

Deficits by Function	Behavioral Manifestations	Interventions
	Inability to generalize from a single instance	• Maintain same environment
	Inability to apply procedural rules and general principles	• Show rather than explain
	Preference for obvious, superficial solutions	• Avoid confusing the patient with details beyond the immediate
	Inability to make distinctions related to relevancy, essences, appropriateness	• Avoid joking and teasing
b. Conceptual inflexibility	Inability to shift a course of thought or action according to the demands of the situation	
3. Calculation		
Acquired disorders of calculation	Impaired ability to identify values of digits in a counting system	• Teach to recognize the deficit and make plans for meeting needs that require calculation
	Impaired ability to identify or use symbols or elements of mathematical operations	• Reassure patient that this is an understood phenomenon, but is still being studied further
		• Encourage patient about likelihood of recovery
C. Memory	Amnesias (see Chap. 12)	
D. Language	Aphasias (see Chaps. 14, 15)	

lieves that perception and recognition are part of a continuum, so here it is maintained that integrated recognition is a further point along that continuum. It is, then, within the domain of concept formation.

Some critics claim that agnosic failures, or pattern recognition deficits, can be understood as the combined result of a primary sensory processing disturbance and generalized mental deterioration or as a complex mixture of disturbed perception and faulty sensorimotor exploration. Geschwind (1965) has stated that recognition is not a unitary process and has suggested that agnosic errors result from disconnection of intact cortical sensory regions from an intact speech area. The term, according to Geschwind, covers the totality of all the associations aroused by any object. Recognition at the central process end of the contiuum encompasses a broad range of behaviors, including attention, feature extraction, exploratory behavior, pattern and form perception, temporal resolution, and memory. Damasio et al. (1982) expand this thesis by adding that recognition is a combined evocation of pertinent multimodal memories that permit the experience of familiarity. With advances in studying sensory systems, recognition of sensorially presented stimuli is now understood as a complex outcome of parallel processing occurring simultaneously at the cortical and subcortical levels. Bauer and Rubens (1985) review these advances and note that much of the problem of agnosia can be reduced to the problem of fractionated recognition abilities. In dealing with the central cognitive processes, we refer to one deficit of concept formation as *fractionated recognition*. Behaviorally, this deficit is manifested by a lack of subjective familiarity with the stimulus

TABLE 13-3. DEFICITS OF COGNITIVE OUTPUT PROCESSING.

Deficits by Function	Behavioral Manifestations	Interventions
A. Planning		
1. Impaired problem solving	Inability to order systematically an internally generated, temporally distributed sequence of activity	• Identify nature and extent of deficit and provide for safety
2. Impaired means–end analysis	Failure to identify a group of subgoals and organization of those goals into a set of acts leading to attainment of larger goal Patient report of poor functioning because of problems with "concentration and following instructions"	• Provide supervision and support for routine activities • Guide toward productive and satisfying activity after routines completed
3. Impaired judgment	Inability to act appropriately in an ambiguous situation	
B. Motor response		
1. Motor planning		
a. Sequencing disorder	Impaired ability to put together coherent sets of movements and progress from one component to the next	• Plan to meet needs of activities of daily living • Maintain sensitivity to thinking and feeling person
b. Dyspraxia	Impaired ability to generate individual, goal-oriented skilled movements	
2. Initiating Action Deficit of intentional movement	Impaired ability to initiate planned action	
3. Regulating action Deficit of monitoring, modulating, and regulating responses or actions	Evidence that errors of action are not perceived or that, if perceived, do not lead to correction, e.g., missed lines in account book	

and an absence of responses adequate to the stimulus, as well as by a simple loss of ability to identify stimuli. In nursing *interventions*, a structured and controlled environment is important for these patients, as it is for patients with other cognitive processing deficits. Since familiarity with the environment is lacking, the nurse will help the person cope with the resulting feelings of perplexity and fear.

Another stage of concept formation involves abstraction and flexibility. Woody (1982) notes that perception involves primary image construction and arises from uncomplicated processing of sensory-coded information. Conceptualization and language, on the other hand, appear to involve extended secondary image construction. An extended image implies some inference drawn from perception. It is an image of an image and may not correspond to physical reality. Such abstracted conceptualizations seem to depend on similarities being detected between primary images.

Woody (1982) defines a primary image as an aggregate of sensory-coded information distributed among a commonly line labeled set of neurons. Extended imagery is the process whereby the central nervous system, with all its stored information, orders the matter of primary images in space and time and supplies the concepts whereby we understand experience. For example, a fish would go through the following sequence: (1) sensation—"I see something," (2) primary image–"worm shaped," (3) extended image—"Is it food or bait?" Although the use of language is closely related to abstract conceptualization, this does not mean that words are necessary for abstract thinking. The example is often given of Helen Keller, who was blind and deaf but after learning language could explain: "Ideas derived from material objects appear to me first in ideas similar to those of touch. Instantly, they pass into intellectual meanings. Afterwards, the meaning finds expression in what is called inner speech" (1954).

A deficit of the functions of abstraction and flexibility is called *conceptual concreteness* and mental inflexibility. Behaviorally, the person who is having difficulty thinking abstractly shows an inability to form concepts, use categories, generalize from a single instance, or apply procedural rules and general principles, such as grammar or conduct. There is a preference for obvious, superficial solutions. The person cannot comprehend subtle underlying or intrinsic aspects of a situation and, therefore, is unable to distinguish what is relevant from what is irrelevant, essential from unessential, and appropriate from inappropriate. With this deficit, since the person cannot generalize, he or she deals with each event as if it were novel, an isolated experience with its own set of rules.

Conceptual inflexibility often occurs with concrete thinking, and the effects of each are mutually reinforcing. In some people, however, particularly when there is frontal lobe involvement, conceptual inflexibility can be present to a significant degree without much impairment of the ability to form and apply abstract concepts. The key feature of this deficit is the inability to shift a course of thought or action according to the demands of the situation.

Interventions for people showing concrete thinking or conceptual inflexibility focus on limiting the need to abstract or symbolize and maintaining sameness in the environment. It is better to show these patients than to try to explain; for example, "This is a picture of the rehabilitation hospital." Procedures are described as they are occurring rather than in advance, using simple and concrete language; for example, "You are going to have a spinal tap. I'll help you. First turn on your side like this. Now the doctor will clean your back. It will feel cold." Conversations generally focus on the patient and present concerns. Trying to broaden the focus of attention may confuse the patient. Family members can limit their talk to simple, familiar things happening at home or in the person's neighborhood. In particular, Taylor and Ballenger (1980) note that the patient who cannot deal with abstractions takes everything literally, including teasing or joking statements. Humor and sarcasm are readily misunderstood and must be avoided until the patient can handle them. Showing appreciation for a humorous remark may be an early sign of recovering central processing functions.

Calculation is a specialized function of abstraction. It involves operations of ordering and compounding using numbers. As with other central processes, observations of people with deficits of calculation show that this is not a unitary function that can be lateralized and localized specifically. The process of calculation is understood as similar to language. There is no unitary aphasia or lesion localization that produces a generalized language disturbance. Rather language is differentially disrupted by compromise of its various neural substrates. These different lesions produce different patterns of language errors. Recent contributions to the classification of acalculia (disturbances in calculation) show a trend toward more detailed analysis of errors, just as in the analysis of aphasia.

Levin and Spiers (1985) note that this type of analysis can be combined with improved methods of lesion localization by CT scans and new techniques to measure regional cerebral blood flow and metabolism to understand better the cerebral organization of calculation. They point to Warrington's study of a physician whose language fully recovered within 1 month of a left posterior parieto-occipital intracerebral hematoma. Even though the patient's acute aphasia subsided, he exhibited a residual decline in efficiency and accuracy of calculation for all oral and written arithmetical operations, whereas his capacity to follow procedural rules (e.g., borrowing) in solutions to mathematical problems, provide numerical cognitive estimates (e.g., how tall is the average Englishwoman?), and select the larger of two numbers was relatively well preserved. The case analysis demonstrates several points about calculation as a central process. First, it is possible to identify a dissociation between arithmetic processing in general and accurate retrieval of specific computational values. Second, calculation represents a major category of semantic knowledge within which it is possible to identify various subcategories that may become disrupted. Third, there is further evidence that the left hemisphere is preferentially involved in mediating the fundamental calculation process.

Based on current understanding of this central function, acquired *disorders of calculation* are divided into three categories: acalculia secondary to alexia and agraphia for numbers, acalculia resulting from spatial disorganization of numbers, and anarithmetria, or impaired calculation in the strict sense. The major behavioral manifestations of these deficits that the nurse will assess are (1) the impaired ability to identify values of digits in a counting system and (2) impaired ability to identify or use symbols or elements of mathematical operations. *Interventions* are aimed at having the person recognize the deficit so that alternate plans can be made for meeting needs that require calculation. The management of a checkbook is a common example. An understanding of the problem can be comforting to the patient. He or she may be told the nature of the disturbance and reassured that it is a phenomenon that is understood but still being studied. The person can be encouraged by being told that abilities in this area are likely to improve as the disease condition improves.

The reception, coding, and storage of conceptual information constitute only a phase of human cognitive processes. This central processing acts in preparation for the phase in which conscious activity is organized and carried out.

□ **Impaired Cognitive Functions of Output Processing**

Luria (1973, p. 79) describes the third functional system of the brain as the one responsible for programming, regulating, and verifying activity. Lezak (1983) discusses such processes in terms of the executive functions and motor performance. The executive functions include four components: goal formulation, planning, carrying out goal-directed plans, and effective performance. Each of these components is necessary for appropriate social responsibility and for effective self-serving adult conduct.

Insight into the significance of human output is provided by Sacks' descriptions (1983) of postencephalitic patients emerging from parkinsonian inactivity when treated with the drug L-Dopa. Observing patients who were suddenly mobile after years of virtually total immobility led the neurologist to reflect on the truth of Leibniz's dictum "Quod non agit non existit"—What does not act does not exist. He comments, "We are critically dependent on a continual flow of impulses and information to and from all the sensory and motor organs of the body. We must be active or we cease to exist: activity and actuality are one and the same" (p. 302). Sacks called the experiences he was witnessing in his patients "awakenings."

Executive functioning is effected by intactness of the frontal lobes and subcortical areas, particularly the limbic structures, including the thalamic nuclei. The system of executive functions can break down at any stage in the behavioral sequence that makes up planned or intentional activity. Furthermore, when a person's capacity for these functions is defective, it involves typically a cluster of deficiencies, with one or two components especially prominent. The outlet channel for executive functions is the motor cortex, but, as Luria notes, the motor projection cortex cannot work in isolation; all a person's movements require, to some extent, a tonic background. This background is provided by the basal motor ganglia and the fibers of the extrapyramidal system. The prefrontal cortex plays an essential role in regulating the state of activity. Activity changes in accordance with the person's complex intentions and plans formulated with the aid of language. This sequence is key to the organization of human behavior. Luria cites investigations that identify a feedback mechanism as an essential component of any organized action. He concludes that the frontal lobes perform not only the function of synthesis of external stimuli, preparation for action, and formation of programs, but also the function of allowing for the effect of the action carried out and verification that it has taken the proper course. The deficits involved in the output functions of cognitive processing are described in relation to the two major functions of planning and motor response (Table 13–3).

Planning

Planning involves formulating a goal and determining the steps needed to achieve that goal. Goal formulation is a complex process of determining what one needs or wants and conceptualizing some kind of future realization of that need or want. Lezak (1983) points out that the capacity to formulate a goal relates to one's motivations and psychologic awareness of self. This is true even at the less well-conceptualized level of forming an intention.

People who lack the capacity to formulate goals simply do not think of things to do. They may be capable of performing complex activities, such as swatting away an annoying fly, or responding to internal stimuli, such as a full bladder. They cannot, however, initiate such activity unless instructed to do so. Even simple activities, such as eating, can be done only with continuing explicit instructions. If deficits are less severe, people may be able to eat what is set before them without the verbal direction to eat but will not seek out food spontaneously, even when they are hungry. With mild impairment of planning functions, patients can do their usual chores and engage in familiar activities and hobbies without prompting. These people however, typically are unable to assume responsibilities that require long-term or abstract goals, and they do not enter new activities independently.

Lezak (1983) notes that in order to plan, a person must be able to conceptualize change from present circumstances, deal objectively with self in relation to the environment, and view the environment objectively. This ability relates to the functions of abstraction and flexibility discussed as part of central cognitive processing. The person must be able to conceive of alternatives, weigh and make choices, and evolve a conceptual framework or structure that will give direction to carrying out the plan conceptualized. Judgment is the particular weighing of one type of behavior against another. It involves the use of foresight and anticipating the outcome of one's actions.

Specific deficits of the planning function include impairments of problem solving, means–end analysis, and judgment (Table 13–3, A). *Impaired problem solving* is manifested behaviorally by the person's inability to order systematically an internally generated, temporally distributed sequence of activity. *Impaired means–end* analysis refers to failures in identification of a group of subgoals and organization of those goals into a set of acts leading to the attainment of the larger goal. For verbally related means–end analysis, the critical point is the temporal ordering of the subgoals—what the person does first, second, and so forth. Nonverbally, deficits in this processing may appear as difficulty solving a visually presented maze. *Impaired judgment* is seen behaviorally as inability to act appropriately in an ambiquous situation. A commonly used assessment of judgment is to ask patients what they would do if they found a sealed stamped addressed envelope on the street. Weintraub and Mesulam (1981), however, caution that taking into account studies of moral development, there are distinctions among knowing what to do, knowing why you are doing it, and actually acting in a real situation. A person may be able to respond appropriately to the examiner but might act in an entirely different way that is clearly inappropriate. They suggest that a more reliable way to assess judgment is by direct observation of behavior or by interviewing family members carefully about the patient's behavior in situations requiring judgment.

These authors note that much knowledge about frontal lobe functions remains elusive; patients with selective frontal lobe damage usually exhibit two features. First, functions attributed to the other three lobes of the brain, such as motor dexterity, perceptual abilities, memory, and language, are relatively preserved, and second, there are deficits in judgment, insight, mental flexibility, reasoning, abstraction, planning, sequencing, and in testing of attentional tone—especially those tests that depend on response inhibition and on the ability to sustain behavioral output.

Patients with more subtle deficits of planning can be *assessed* in the workplace and in the home. They will report that they can no longer function well because they cannot concentrate or cannot follow complex instructions. Penfield (in Mesulam, 1985) reported that at the end of the acute postoperative period, his sister, on whom he had had to perform a right-sided prefrontal lobectomy, had preserved abilities of judgment, insight, social graces, and cognitive abilities. When he visited her home as a dinner guest, however, he noticed a diminished capacity for planned preparation and administration of the meal and a slowing of thinking. Mesulam (1985) notes that such subtle changes are characteristic of unilateral prefrontal lesions and that bilateral involvement leads to the more dramatic disturbances of motivation, insight, judgment, and comportment seen as highly inappropriate behavior.

Since people with planning deficits cannot generate and carry out a plan for their own daily activities, they need guidance to avoid aimless wandering once they have finished their routine activities. Again, as with other cognitive deficits, *interventions* are directed toward identifying the nature and extent of the deficit and providing the supervision and supportive care needed for safety and for leading as productive and satisfying a life as possible.

Motor Response

The final stage of human information processing is the translation of cognitive activity into overt behavior. Lezak (1983) notes that this stage requires a response modality sufficiently integrated with central cortical activity to transform conceptual experience into manifest behavior. In addition, following Luria's emphasis on self-regulation, the person needs a well-functioning response feedback system for continuous monitoring and modulation of output. Since the distinguishing features of complex movement have not been described adequately, it is more difficult to discuss this as a basic process and to outline the deficits of functioning.

Willis and Grossman (1981) discuss willed movement and note that it appears to be characterized by the act of initiating the movement. Once the movement is started, it is possible that it may be carried on by centrally programmed or reflex mechanisms. Willed movements have the second characteristic that their purpose is to reach some goal. This may be a goal in the person's sensory field or one that is represented in the person's memory store of information. The motivational aspect of voluntary movement suggests that the descending motor systems are being driven from a core of the person that is related to consciousness, emotion, and memory. Structures with projections to large portions of context are important in the initiation of movement, and, therefore, Willis and Grossman (1981) suggest that the nonspecific thalamic system might function in voluntary movement. Limbic structures and their thalamic and frontal lobe projections that apparently are involved in emotion, motivation, and memory may also be important.

As listed in Table 13–3 (B), the major functions of motor response include motor planning, initiating action, and regulating action. Considering motor planning first, major deficits are sequencing disorders and dyspraxia. *Sequencing disorder* is recognized behaviorally as an impaired ability to put together coherent sets of movements and progress from one component to the next. *Dyspraxia* refers to an impairment of the ability to generate individual, goal-oriented skilled movements. Apraxia can be defined as the inability to carry out a motor act despite intact motor and sensory systems, good comprehension, and full cooperation. Deficits of motor planning are not a result of impaired comprehension, motivation, or other such factors. Posture and movement are normal, but skill is lost. Rather than a disorder of movement per se, it is a disorder of the systems that command movement or, in other words, a failure in output transmission. With such disorders, automatic or habitual movements frequently are preserved. Initiating action is a specific function of motor response. Difficulties with this function can be termed *deficits of intentional movement*. Brooks (1986) discusses models of intended movement and provides details of the neural basis of motor control. He describes learned tasks, such as hitting a golf ball, as an action sequence produced by overall plans that create smooth, fast, skillful action. Such motor programs are a set of muscle commands that are structured before the motor action begins, and in the neurologically intact person they can be sent to the muscles with the correct timing so that the entire sequence can be performed. Behaviorally, deficits in this function are seen as impaired initiation of planned action.

In discussing the function of regulating action, Lezak (1983) notes that an activity is as effective as the performer's ability to monitor, self-correct, and regulate the intensity, tempo, and other qualitative aspects of performance. Abilities for self-correction and self-monitoring are vulnerable to many different kinds of brain damage. Some patients cannot correct their mistakes because they do not perceive them. Other patients may perceive their errors, even identify them yet, because of other output deficits, not be able to initiate action to correct them. Behaviorally, this deficit shows up in many ways, for example, in a missed line in an account book or shoelaces that break because of too much pressure. Cramped writing may leave little or no space between words; responses on paper and pencil tests or questionnaires may be skipped.

Impairments related to motor response greatly disrupt the integrated functioning needed for carrying out activities of daily living. *Interventions* will be aimed specifically at meeting these needs. At the same time, the nurse will be aware that it may be only the output of cognitive functioning that is a difficulty for the patient. Except that these people cannot execute what they intend, they are normally thinking and feeling people.

SUMMARY

This chapter has highlighted cognitive function from an information processing approach. Based on works in the neural and behavioral sciences, a nursing model of information processing was offered. Clinical applications of the model outlined the cognitive functions of each stage of the model. Deficits of these functions were described, and interventions useful in working with people with the deficits were identified. The whole area of cognitive processing and its neural basis is rapidly developing. Brooks (1986) offers the analogy that we need a simple map to board a fast-moving train so that we may recognize the landscape as it flits by the windows. This chapter is an attempt to provide this simple map, with the understanding that the detailed charting of the rich landscape is a challenge that still lies before us.

REFERENCE

Andrews, H.A., & Roy C. (1986). *Essentials of the Roy adaptation model*. E. Norwalk, CT: Appleton-Century-Crofts.

Bauer, R.M., & Rubens, A.B. (1985). Agnosia. In K.M. Heilman & E. Valenstein (Eds.), *Clinical neuropsychology* (2nd ed., p. 187). New York: Oxford University Press.

Benson, D.F., & Geschwind, N. (1985). Aphasia and related disorders: A clinical approach. In Mesulam, M. (Ed.), *Principles of behavioral Neurology* (p. 193). Philadelphia: Davis.

Brooks, N. (1984). Cognitive deficits after head injury. In Brooks, N. (Ed.) *Closed head injury: Psychological, social, and family consequences* (p. 44). Oxford: Oxford University Press.

Brooks, V. (1986). *The neural basis of motor control*. New York: Oxford University Press.

Buffington, P. W. (1986). In our right (and left) minds. *SKY* (March), 33.

Crigger, N.J., & Strickland, C.C. (1985). Selecting a nursing diagnosis for changes in consciousness. *Dimensions of Critical Care Nursing, 4*(3), 156.

Damasio, A.R. (1985). Disorders of complex visual processing: Agnosias, achromatopsia, Balint's syndrome, and related difficulties of orientation and construction. In Mesulam, M. (Ed.) *Principles of behavioral neurology* (p. 259). Philadelphia: Davis.

Damasio, A.R., Damasio, H., & Van Hoesen, G.W. (1982). Prosopagnosia: Anatomic basis and behavioral mechanisms. *Neurology, 32,* 331.

Das, J.P. (1984). Intelligence and information integration. In J. Kirby (Ed.), *Cognitive strategies and educational performance* (p. 13). New York: Academic Press.

Geschwind, N. (1965). Disconnection syndromes in animals and man. *Brain, 88,* 237, 585.

Gronwall, D.M.A., & Sampson, H. (1974). *The psychological effects of concussion*. Auckland: Auckland University Press.

Guilford, J.P. (1956). The structure of the intellect. *Psychological Bulletin, 53,* 267.

Haber, R.N. (1974). Information processing. In E.C. Carterette & M.P. Friedman (Eds.), *Handbook of perception* (Vol. 1, p. 313). New York: Academic Press.

Hubel, D. (1982). Exploration of the primary visual cortex, 1955–78. *Nature, 299,* 515.

Hunt, E. (1980). Intelligence as an information-processing concept. *British Journal of Psychology, 71,* 449.

Keller, H. (1954) *Story of my life*. NY: Doubleday.

Kolb, B., & Whishaw, I.Q. (1985). *Fundamentals of human neuropsychology* (2nd ed.). New York: W.H. Freeman.

Levin, H.S., & Spiers, P.A. (1985). Acalculia. In K.M. Heilman & E. Valenstein (Eds.), *Clinical neuropsychology* (2nd ed., p. 97. New York: Oxford University Press.

Lezak, M.D. (1983). *Neuropsychological assessment* (2nd ed.). New York: Oxford University Press.

Luria, A.R. (1973). *The working brain: An introduction to neuropsychology*. New York: Basic Books.

Luria, A.R. (1980). *Higher cortical functions in man*. New York: Basic Books.

Martel, L. (1986). *Mastering change: The key to business success*. New York: Simon & Schuster.

Mesulam, M. (1981). A cortical network for directed attention and unilateral neglect. *Annals of Neurology, 10*(4), 309.

Mesulam, M. (1985). Attention, confusional states, and neglect. In M. Mesulam (Ed.), *Principles of Behavioral Neurology* (p. 125). Philadelphia: Davis

Mountcastle, V.B. (1979). An organizing principle for cerebral function: The unit module and the distributed system. In F.O. Schmitt & F.G. Worden (Eds.), *The neurosciences* (p. 21). Cambridge: MIT Press.

Mountcastle, V.B., Lynch, J.C., & Georgopoulos, A. (1975). Posterior parietal association cortex of the monkey: Command functions for operations within extrapersonal space. *Journal of Neurophysiology, 38,* 871.

Pi Lambda Theta, San Jose Area Chapter. (1983). *Helping head injury and stroke patients at home: A handbook for families*. San Jose, CA: Author.

Posner, M. I. (1975). The psychobiology of attention. In M. S. Gazzaniga & C. Blakemore (Eds.), *Handbook of psychobiology* (p. 441). New York: Academic Press.

Pribram, K.H. (1969a). *Brain and behavior 2: Perception and action*. Middlesex, England: Penguin Books.

Pribram, K. H. (1969b). *Brain and behavior 3: Memory mechanisms*. Middlesex, England: Penguin Books.

Roy, C. (1984). *Introduction to nursing: An adaptation model*. (2nd ed.). Englewood Cliffs, NJ: Prentice-Hall.

Sacks, O. (1983). *Awakenings*. New York: Dutton.

Schneider, W., & Shiffrin, R. M. (1977). Controlled and automatic human information processing: I. Detection, search and attention. *Psychology Review, 84,* 1.

Shiffrin, R. M., & Schneider, W. (1977). Controlled and automatic human information processing: II. Perceptual learning, automatic attending and a general theory. *Psychology Review, 84,* 127.

Sternberg, S. (1966). High-speed scanning in human memory. *Science, 153,* 652.

Taylor, J. W., & Ballenger, S. (1980). *Neurological dysfunctions and nursing intervention.* New York: McGraw-Hill.

Teuber, H. L. (1968). Alteration of perception and memory in man. In L. Weiskrantz (Ed.), *Analysis of behavioral change.* New York: Harper & Row.

Weintraub, S., Mesulam, M.-M., & Kramer, L. (1981). Disturbances in prosody. A right-hemisphere contribution to language. *Archives of Neurology, 38,* 742.

White, M.J., & Wolf-Wilets, V. (1977). Memory loss following halothane anesthesia. *AORN, 26,* 1053.

Willis, W.D., & Grossman, R.G. (1981). *Medical neurobiology* (3rd ed.). St. Louis: Mosby.

Woody, C. D. (1982). *Memory, learning, and higher function.* New York: Springer-Verlag.

SECTION 3: COMMUNICATION PHENOMENA

14

Communication Disorders: An Overview

Roberta Schwartz-Cowley and William R. Roth

Human communication is often taken for granted despite the fact that it is a tremendously complex process. It represents a sophisticated interplay of language, memory, and reasoning that permits the exchange of ideas, emotions, and desires within one person or among many people. The very foundations of present society, the means of maintaining information from the past, and the projection of plans and aspirations for the future are direct results of this ability to communicate interpersonally and intrapersonally. Impairment or loss of this ability can be catastrophic for an individual and also has implications for the impaired person's family and community.

Communication is a learned system of symbols and codes used to represent thoughts and ideas. When the same group of symbols and codes is learned by more than one individual (shared system), each can understand what the other expresses. This system is most often called *language*.

LANGUAGE: DEFINITION AND ACQUISITION

According to Bloom and Leahy (1978), "a language is a code whereby ideas about the world are represented through a conventional system of arbitrary signals for communication" (p. 10).

Definition

Language is a code in the sense that strict rules govern how its signals are formed and used. These signals (symbols) are arbitrary rather than innate. Symbols, such as speech sounds, spoken and written words, and gestures, were originally invented, maintained, or changed over time by choice. Language is also arbitrary by nature of the cultural variations around the world. For example, the English language varies significantly from the Chinese language, but the English language also varies within itself (Bollinger, 1975).

Language is informative, directive, and expressive: it allows for the exchange of information intrapersonally and interpersonally and over time (informative), it can be used to cause a person to perform or not perform a specific action (directive), and it conveys feelings and emotions and serves to provide reinforcement and encouragement or the opposite (expressive) (Liles, 1975).

Linguist Noam Chomsky (1968) referred to the fact that, despite a relatively small number of sounds, letters, and gestures, humans have an infinite number of ways to express themselves. This is because the rules for language that govern the content, form, and use of the expressions also allow for creativity and innovation (Perkins, 1971).

Acquisition

Language and its rules are acquired through exposure. A child will learn his or her native language given sufficient exposure to it unless the child is restricted by sensory impairment or learning disabilities (Devilliers & Devilliers, 1978).

Initially, a child learns how to put sounds together to form words. By 1 to 1½ years, a child will normally have absorbed and begun to use a vocabulary of as many as 50 to 100 words and will have begun to understand sentences spoken by others. Learning and using sounds for verbal expression generally continues until age 7 or 8 years. During that time, the child will learn to combine words to convey more meaning than would be possible with simple word utterances. The child will learn rules that control how these words are used and sentences for appropriate and efficient communication. This overall learning occurs as a gradual acquisition, overgeneralization, and refinement of the symbols of language (Devilliers & Devilliers, 1978; Leonard, 1982; Moskowitz, 1981). Language acquisition at this time is largely passive, reflecting assimilation, modification, or trial and error.

Learning a written language is an active process of associating printed symbols with meaning and verbal correspondents. This learning is achieved through active assistance from others. Gestural communication tends to be learned both passively and actively through recognition, association, assimilation, and inquiry (Hughes, 1962; Knapp, 1981).

Language acquisition, however, is not merely a matter of learning symbols. According to Devilliers and Devilliers (1978), "some changes in child's speech and understanding reflect the growth of linguistic knowledge; others reflect the development of memory capacity, attention span, or reasoning ability" (p. 5).

This fact is important to consider because a person learns the basic rules of word formation and grammar in childhood, but language learning continues throughout life. This continued learning is a result of the growth of concept development, better understanding of context, setting, and interpersonal relationships, and increased use of abstraction and problem-solving abilities. This learning is expected to continue passively but may be accelerated or expanded when an individual actively attempts to develop and refine personal language skills as certain needs are encountered.

As people age and mature, they display a high degree of variability in their development of both intrapersonal and interpersonal communication skills. When these people grow older, their acquisition and improved use of language seems to slow down; this decline can be related to a concomitant decline in older people's physiology and auditory capability. Obler and Albert (1981), for example, believe that deterioration of language comprehension and expression with age is likely a manifestation of reduced hearing acuity, attenuation of attending and memory skills, and changes in neuroanatomy and neurophysiology. Expressive language may be further compromised by anatomic and physiologic changes associated with speech, writing, and gestural mechanisms (Kahane, 1981).

Reductions in communication ability during the normal aging process are not predestined, however, and when they do occur, they tend to be individual, like the learning process itself. Obler and Albert (1981) also note that, for many older people, communication skills (and, thus, language) do not deteriorate. Language efficiency and growth may continue because of improved narrative skills, increased ability to encode thought into language and communicate effectively, and a better understanding of what others intend. Furthermore, perceived changes in cognitive skills and memory may not reflect neurophysiologic decline but, rather, adaptation to the different circumstances and requirements encountered by the geriatric population (Denny, 1981; Smith & Fullerton, 1981).

The likelihood of disrupted language acquisition, therefore, appears to occur on a highly individualized basis and not be related directly to age considerations. Disorders in language acquisition and use are more readily related to abnormalities that disrupt a person's ability to express and understand. These abnormalities involve anatomic or physiologic changes secondary to vascular, degenerative, and metabolic disorders or to trauma, tumors, infections, or other disorders.

ANATOMY: SPEECH, HEARING, AND LANGUAGE MECHANISMS

A brief review of the structure and physiology of the speech, language, and hearing mechanisms will enhance the discussion of specific communication disorders.

Speech Mechanism

The speech act is a highly complex process involving the coordination of respiratory, laryngeal, palatopharyngeal, lingual, labial, and mandibular musculature. The channel through or adjacent to these structures is the vocal tract, essentially a tube with valves and filters to modify the outgoing airstream (Zemlin, 1968). Principal valving or constriction of the tract occurs at the level of the vocal folds, at the palatopharyngeal sphincter, at various positions of the tongue as it approximates areas within the oral cavity, and at the lips. The quality of sound is related to the sound frequencies generated by the airstream. These frequencies are filtered or modified within the vocal tract by resonance, the characteristic of sound in which existing sound frequencies are magnified or diminished as they pass through the vocal tract (Fry, 1980) (Fig. 14-1).

Respiration is the force for speech production. Cooperative interaction of the thoracic and abdominal musculature produces inhalation and exhalation. The exhaled airstream is directed through the bronchial tree and trachea to the larynx. The airstream has no purposeful sound quality until it reaches the larynx. Speech breathing involves quick inhalation and prolonged or extended exhalation; thus, respiration for speech is anticipatory and linquistically conditioned (Perkins, 1971; Zemlin, 1968).

The larynx, a collection of muscles and cartilaginous structures that serves as the first valve in the vocal tract, is suspended between the hyoid bone and the trachea by the exterior or extrinsic laryngeal muscles. The principal cartilages of the larynx for speech purposes are the thyroid, the cricoid, and the paired arytenoids. The interior or intrinsic laryngeal muscles are innervated by cranial nerve X (vagus) and are responsible for phonation or the voicing of speech sounds.

Phonation, an aerodynamic process, occurs through vibration of the vocal folds as air passes through the opening between the vocal folds (the glottis). The vocal folds are adducted or approximated by contractions of the lateral cricoarytenoid muscles, resulting in increased subglottic pressure as the exhaled airstream gathers below the closed folds. The pressure overcomes the resistance of the elastic vocal folds and forces the folds apart, releasing the airstream and vibrating the vocal folds, which produces phonation or voicing. (The airstream will ascend without voicing if the exhaled air passes through the glottis when the vocal folds are abducted or opened away from each other. Both voiced and unvoiced air is directed upward to the oropharynx for further modification.) The pitch or frequency of the vibrations is relative to the length, mass, and tension of the individual's vocal folds and how these are varied (Fry, 1980; Zemlin, 1968). Finally, air pressure changes and elastic recoil draw the folds back together again.

The second vocal tract valve is the palatopharyngeal sphincter. Most speech

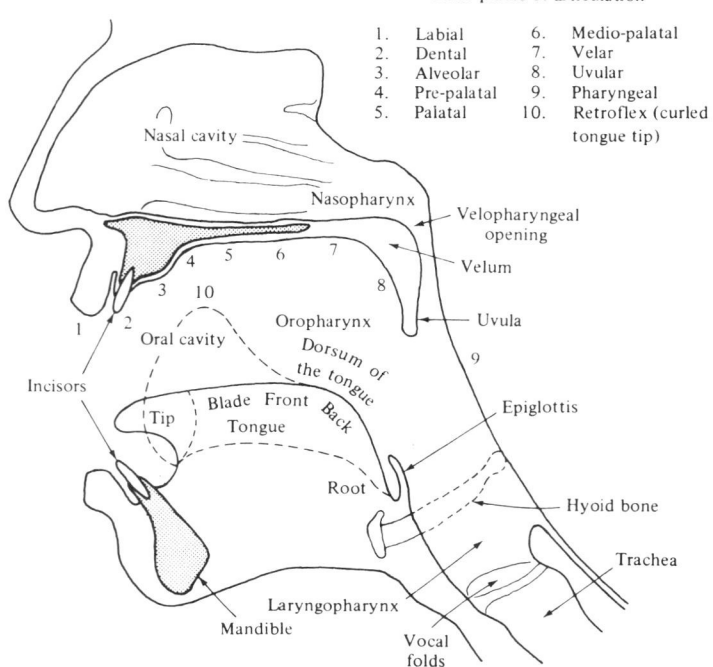

Figure 14–1. The vocal tract and points of articulation: (1) labial, (2) dental, (3) alveolar, (4) prepalatal, (5) palatal, (6) mediopalatal, (7) velar, (8) uvular, (9) pharyngeal, and (10) retroflex (curled tongue tip).

sounds are produced in or are directed through the oral cavity because the nasopharynx has been sealed off, directing the exhaled airstream through the oropharynx to the oral cavity. The nasopharyngeal port is sealed off by sphincteric closing of the palatopharyngeal isthmus by elevation and tension of the soft palate and approximation of the soft palate by the posterior and lateral pharyngeal walls of the superior constrictor muscles. (The nasopharyngeal port is open for only three speech sounds, the nasal sounds of "M," "N," and "NG.") This palatopharyngeal action is due to innervation by cranial nerve X (vagus), with the contribution of motor fibers from cranial nerve V (trigeminal) (Bateman, 1977; Perkins, 1971; Zemlin, 1968).

The airstream receives most of its modification within and as it leaves the oral cavity. The shape of the oral cavity, due to the size of the mouth and the amount of space the tongue takes up as it is positioned in different ways, will cause some frequencies to be amplified, some frequencies to diminish, and some new frequencies to be created secondary to resonance. In addition, specific vowel sounds and consonants will be formed by (1) positioning the tongue, (2) positioning the lips, and (3) moving the lips and jaw. These oral modifications constitute the final valves of the vocal tract.

The complex movements of the tongue are based on interplay of both extrinsic and intrinsic musculature. These movements are principally caused by innervation from cranial nerve XII (hypoglossal). Labial or lip movements are variations on sphincteric action due to cranial nerve VII (facial) innervation. Mouth opening adjustments are related to mandibular or jaw movements secondary to innervation from the motor branch of cranial nerve V (trigeminal). Damage to these structures or disruption of cranial nerve innervation could be catastrophic to speech production.

Hearing Mechanism

Speech and other sounds are *heard* by way of acoustic, mechanical, and electrical energy that is transmitted through the outer, middle, and inner portions of the ear and through the ascending neural pathways to the cortical association areas (Newby, 1979). The anatomy of hearing is reviewed in Chapter 23.

Language Mechanism

Reception and comprehension of linguistic symbols, association and integration of these symbols, and the formulation and programming of expression are associated with activity in the cerebral cortex. Typically, these functions are attributed to the left hemisphere of the cerebrum, although exceptions have been reported. For purposes of this discussion, the left hemisphere is considered the dominant hemisphere for language. Language is a cooperative process that involves many areas of the dominant hemisphere. It also relies on intact assistance from the nondominant (right) hemisphere and subcortical areas for maximal function and efficiency (Bayles, 1979).

The areas of the brain most often associated with language are located in the temporal and frontal lobes (see Fig. 10–2). The primary auditory cortex (Heschl's gyrus) and Wernicke's area, located in the superior temporal gyrus, are of primary importance for the reception and comprehension of spoken language. The primary speech cortex (Broca's area) is responsible for motor programming of the intended speech message and also is associated with adherence to rules for word and sentence construction. Located in the inferior portion of the third frontal gyrus, Broca's area is adjacent to the precentral gyrus of the frontal lobe, often called the "motor strip" or "motor cortex." The lower portion of the motor cortex, which is responsible for actions of the larynx, tongue, jaw, lips, and face, is situated closest to Broca's area. Transmission between Wernicke's area and Broca's area is accomplished by a tract of nerve fibers called the arcuate fasciculus. Transmission of information from the primary visual cortex to Wernicke's area is accomplished by the angular gyrus of the parietal lobe. This fact is particularly relevant because comprehension of the written word depends on auditory association; that is, auditory symbols are associated with written symbols to allow accurate interpretation and comprehension through reading (Benson, 1979; Benson & Geshwind, 1983).

From a neuroanatomic and neurophysiologic viewpoint, a language model involves a highly complex, cooperative process. It is important to consider the brain's language activities as a diffuse, integrative process involving not isolated, specialized areas but interrelated areas that complement each other for maximal communication adequacy and efficiency.

Motor–Speech Mechanism

Once programmed, the motor–speech act must be transmitted to the appropriate speech musculature to achieve the intended speech production. The speech program is delivered to the motor cortex. The direct pathway of motor activity involves upper motor neurons and is referred to as the pyramidal system. Messages are transmitted to the final common motor pathway (lower motor neurons) comprised of the motor nuclei of the cranial nerves, the myoneural junctions, and the muscles themselves. These direct or voluntary processes are regulated by three other more indirect processes: (1) the extrapyramidal system, which is comprised of neural pathways descending from the basal ganglia and other subcortical bodies to effect involuntary subconscious and automatic monitoring and regulation of the direct processes, (2) the cerebellum, which also influences the coordination and accuracy of control functions; and (3) vestibular–reticular centers in the brainstem, which give rise to pathways projecting to the lower motor neurons for the purpose of regulating reflex activity at the level of the lower motor neurons (Darley et al., 1975).

COMMUNICATION DISORDERS

A detailed discussion of communication disorders is best begun with a framework or categorization for accurate description and differentiation. Communication can be over-simplified, but presented correctly, as the transmission and integration of language. *Transmission* entails both expressive characteristics of language and the means by which the linguistic symbols are received. *Integration* includes the process of association, interpretation, and formulation for the purpose of decoding and encoding language.

Disorders may occur at the periphery of receptive or expressive transmission, or they may affect specific structures that reduce transmission. For example, trauma or a disease process could impair hearing at the level of the outer or middle ear, yet sensory and neural components of hearing would remain intact. Likewise, dysarthria secondary to cerebral vascular accident could impair verbal expression markedly, yet the language centers of the brain would remain unimpaired.

Disorders of Transmission

Disorders of transmission should be viewed with regard to (1) structure (e.g., muscle, bone, cartilage), (2) the means of innervating these structures (e.g., motor–speech mechanism), and (3) the central system required for adequate recognition before comprehension and adequate programming of the motor acts after linguistic formulation for expressive purposes.

The patient with communication impairment due to a neurogenic disorder may have one or more of the following expressive or receptive transmission disorders: the dysarthrias, dyspraxia, dysgraphia, dyslexia, agnosia, or hearing impairment secondary to conduction, sensorineural, or retrocochlear disorders (Tables 14–1 and 14–2).

☐ **Expressive Disorders of Transmission**

Expressive disorders of transmission include the dysarthrias, dyspraxis of speech, and dysgraphia.

Dysarthrias
Dysarthria comprises a group of speech disorders resulting from disturbances in muscular control. Because there has been damage to the central or peripheral nervous system, some degree of weakness, slowness, incoordination, or altered muscle tone characterizes the activity of the speech mechanism. The term encompasses coexisting motor disorders of respiration, phonation, articulation, resonance, and prosody (Darley et al., 1975).

In the past, dysarthrias have been classified with regard to neuroanatomy or neurophysiology (Froeschels, 1943; Grewel, 1957). A more recent classification relates a described muscular dysfunction to a specific form of dysarthria (Darley et al., 1969; 1975). The dysarthrias are differentiated as flaccid, spastic, ataxic, hypokinetic, hyperkinetic, and mixed.

Flaccid dysarthria results from damage to any portion of a lower motor unit. This unit is comprised of the lower motor neuron's body and axon, the myoneural junction, and the muscle itself. Damage may be a result of widespread injury, specific nerve impairment, impairment of the myoneural junction, or damage to the muscle fibers themselves. The speech quality of the person with flaccid dysarthria varies, depending on the specific area of disruption, but is typically characterized by breathy voice, audible inspiration, and hypernasality (Darley et al., 1975; Wertz, 1978).

Spastic dysarthria results from suprasegmental (upper motor neuron) damage. These pathways are closely approximated through their courses, and lesions to the pyramidal tracts are more often than not accompanied by lesions to the extrapyramidal tracts (Darley et al., 1975). Unilateral lesions to upper motor neurons will produce remarkable, but typically mild, impairment of speech. Spastic dysarthria involving bilateral upper motor neuron damage is usually associated with widespread damage to the central nervous system. Spastic dysarthria due to bilateral involvement causes marked speech deficits, chiefly characterized by markedly imprecise articulation of speech and a harsh voice quality (Darley et al., 1975; Rosenbeck & LaPointe, 1978).

TABLE 14-1. DISORDERS OF TRANSMISSION.

Disorder	Anatomic Area Affected	Etiology
Receptive		
Hearing impairment	Outer, middle, or inner ear, auditory nerve, and subcortical tracts to cortex	Trauma, disease, CVA,[a] tumors, presbycusis
Auditory verbal agnosia	Auditory association area of cortex in superior temporal gyrus	CVA, trauma, disease, tumors, diffuse encephalopathy, degenerative disorder
Dyslexia	Angular gyrus, left occipital lobe with concomitant lesion to splenium of corpus collosum	CVA, trauma, disease, diffuse degenerative disorders
Expressive		
Dysarthrias:		
• Flaccid	Lower motor neuron and motor unit	CVA, trauma, bulbar palsy, myasthenia gravis, trauma
• Spastic	Upper motor neurons (pyramidal tracts)	CVA, trauma, pseudobulbar palsy
• Ataxic	Cerebellum	CVA, trauma, tumors, intoxication, degeneration or demyelinating processes
• Hypokinetic	Basal ganglia, substantia nigra, subthalamic nuclei (extrapyramidal tracts)	Reductions in dopamine production secondary to Parkinson's disease
• Hyperkinetic	Basal ganglia, substantia nigra, subthalamic nuclei (extrapyramidal tracts)	Reductions in acetylcholine production secondary to CVA, tumors, trauma, dystonia, chorea, torticollis, tardive dyskinesia, infection
• Mixed	Combinations of above lesion sites	Variable (e.g., amyotrophic lateral sclerosis, multiple sclerosis, Wilson's disease)
Dyspraxia of speech	Area of third frontal gyrus of left hemisphere adjacent to motor cortex	CVA, trauma, tumors
Dysgraphia	Frontal lobe, parietal–temporal lobes of left hemisphere, posterior areas of right hemisphere	CVA, trauma, tumors, diffuse cortical lesions

[a]CVA, cardiovascular accident.

A familiar manifestation of bilateral upper motor neuron impairment is pseudobulbar palsy, which results in spastic dysarthria with characteristic symptomatology similar to that of bulbar palsy. Differentiating between the two involves identifying the areas affected and remembering that spastic dysarthria affects overall movement patterns, whereas flaccid dysarthria secondary to bulbar palsy affects individual motor units (Darley et al., 1969). Increased incidence of emotional lability is also associated with pseudobulbar palsy (Darley et al., 1975).

Ataxic dysarthria is associated with bilateral or widespread damage to the cerebellum (Darley et al., 1975). The predominant role of the cerebellum appears to involve regulating and attenuating the descending cortical speech program (Brown et al., 1970). Ataxic dysarthria is related, like other central nervous system disorders, to a variety of injuries. Friedreich's ataxia is a disease process commonly associated with ataxic dysarthria. Speech characteristics include marked speech misarticulations, stress changes, and prolongations. These manifestations are thought to be symptoms of overall reduced coordination and inhibition of the motor–speech program (Darley et al., 1975). The characteristics of ataxic dysarthria are commonly associated with, and at times mistakenly attributed to, alcohol intoxication ("drunk speech").

TABLE 14-2. DISORDERS OF TRANSMISSION–CHARACTERISTICS.

Disorder	Characteristics
Hearing disorder	Reduced ability to receive sounds resulting in impaired reception of speech Reduced ability to recognize speech despite intact transmission from ear to cortex
Reading disorder	Reduced ability to recognize letters and words in written or printed form
Speech disorders	Breathy voice and audible inspiration, hypernasality, imprecise consonants, relatively flat pitch and loudness Markedly imprecise speech articulation, slow rate of speech, voice reductions due to strained phonation, low pitch and harsh quality Markedly reduced speech articulation of consonants and vowels, stress changes, prolongations and inappropriate pauses, irregular rhythms and coordination Imprecise consonants, reductions and equalizations of pitch, stress, and loudness, short rushes of speech, inappropriate pauses, rate of speech inappropriately varied: • Slow hyperkinesias result in speech disorder characterized by distorted speech movements, inappropriate prolongations, reduced articulation, strained voice, irregular breakdowns • Quick hyperkinesias result in speech disorder characterized by imprecise speech articulation, prolonged pauses in speech, variable rate and loudness, flat pitch, and harsh voice • Combinations of the above characteristics relative to site of lesion and types of dysarthria presented Impairment in programming speech movements for intended speech act; highly consistent errors of production at any level of the vocal tract; disorder also characterized by faulty compensation attempts
Writing disorder	Mechanical difficulties secondary to reduced motor control; such symbol errors as reversals, omissions, distortions, and misspellings, or visual–spatial difficulties.

Hypokinetic dysarthria is considered to be a manifestation of damage to portions of the extrapyramidal level of the motor–speech program. Disorders of inhibition with regard to the extrapyramidal system, usually associated with reduced production of dopamine, result in hypokinesis and hypokinetic dysarthria (Bateman, 1977; Darley et al., 1975). The most common form of hypokinesia is parkinsonism (Darley et al., 1975; Rosenbeck & LaPointe, 1978; Wertz, 1978). It is important for the neuroscience nursing clinician to remember that parkinsonism-like symptoms have been known to develop in patients using drugs containing reserpine or one of the phenothiazines (Darley et al., 1975).

Marked limitation of range of movement is the characteristic most often associated with speech impairment secondary to hypokinesia (Darley et al., 1975). Speech characteristics tend to encompass flat or reduced aspects, and occasionally short rushes of words are noted (Darley et al., 1975; Wertz, 1978).

Hyperkinesia (and *hyperkinetic dysarthria*) is related to extrapyramidal dysfunction specific to reduced facilitory function and often is attributed to reductions in the production of acetylcholine. The symptomatology involves quick and slow abnormal involuntary movements. These movement disorders should be thought of on a continuum of quickest to slowest, with occasional overlapping (Fig. 14–2).

The quick hyperkinesias are characterized by random, nonpurposeful movements typically accompanying purposeful movement, causing disruption in the normal sequence of motor–speech activity at all levels (respiration, phonation, resonance, articulation, prosody) (Darley et al., 1975).

Characteristics of slow hyperkinesias include twisting and prolonged movement patterns, and gradual increases and subsequent

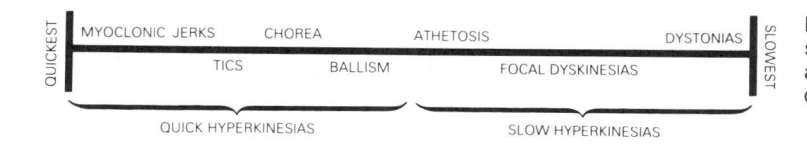

Figure 14–2. Diagrammatic representation of movement disorders associated with hyperkinetic dysarthria.

decreases in muscle tone (Darley et al, 1975; Rosenbeck & LaPointe, 1978; Wertz, 1978). Slow hyperkinesias are associated with extrapyramidal lesions, but more cortical involvement may be present than that noted in other extrapyramidal disorders (Darley et al., 1975).

The dysartharias discussed have been viewed as pure and mutually exclusive disorders. The widespread neuropathology associated with cerebrovasular accident (CVA), head trauma, disease, toxins, and other causes suggests, however, that combinations of disorders, or *mixed dysarthrias*, exist. In fact, they do. Although the potential variety of combinations is limitless, three outstanding disorders traditionally have illustrated the symptomatology of mixed dysarthria.

Amyotrophic lateral sclerosis is a disease characterized by progressive degeneration of both upper and lower motor neurons. Speech gradually deteriorates secondary to increasing combinations of spastic and flaccid dysarthrias. In addition, compromise of the bulbar musculature can lead to difficulties with respiration and swallowing.

Multiple sclerosis, although not completely understood, is a demyelinating condition of the central nervous system. Speech is not always affected, but when it is, variable involvement of spastic, ataxic, and flaccid dysarthrias is noted. The severity of dysarthria is directly related to the severity of the overall neurologic involvement.

Wilson's disease, a genetic and metabolic disorder, affects the body's ability to process mineral intake, specifically copper, in the diet, which eventually leads to neuromotor degeneration. A marked symptom of Wilson's disease is dysarthria, with variable combinations of spastic, ataxic, and hypokinetic involvement. Concomitant disorders involve ataxia, dysphagia, intention tremor, rigidity, and drooling.

Other mixed dysarthrias might result secondary to diffuse head injury, multiple CVA or disseminated tumors, Jacob-Creutzfeldt disease, Shy-Drager disease, hydrocephalus, and other diffuse encephalopathies.

Dyspraxia of Speech

Motor-speech programming is an almost incomprehensibly complex process that is beyond conscious, voluntary control. Critical to this process is the frontal lobe of the brain's left hemisphere; it provides accurate and efficient programming of the motor–speech process after formulation of linguistic content and grammatical form.

Dyspraxia (sometimes called apraxia) of speech, an articulatory disorder differentiated from dysarthria and aphasia, occurs when this motor–speech programmer is impaired by brain damage. It is seen largely as a disorder of motor–speech manifested by errors in articulation and the patient's attempts to compensate for these errors (Darley, 1982; Darley et al., 1975; Rosenbeck, 1978; Wertz, 1978).

The speaker presents a reduced ability to position the different parts of the speech mechanism for speech sound production and a reduced ability to sequence the sounds to produce spoken words. Speech is highly variable, and errors are inconsistent, characterized by groping and frustration of the speaker who knows what he or she wants to say but cannot produce the words as planned. Substitutions are more common than other types of errors (e.g., "dake a take" for "bake a cake") (Rosenbeck, 1978).

Dyspraxic speech is believed to occur secondary to a lesion in the third frontal convolution of the left hemisphere. The lesion is usually secondary to CVA or head trauma (Wertz, 1978). The lesion thus occurs within (or close to) Broca's area, which is considered the principal center for verbal expression of language. Not surprisingly, dyspraxia of speech more often than not occurs along with aphasic involvement.

It is important to remember that dyspraxia of speech is clearly distinguished from dysarthria, aphasia, and oral apraxia. Apraxia of speech is a *speech disorder secondary to programming impairment*; errors are highly inconsistent. Dysarthrias, on the other hand, are *speech disorders related to impaired muscle movement*; errors are consistent. Aphasia deficits involve word choice and linguistic rules, not the actual motor–speech performance. Oral apraxia involves reduced programming of all volitional acts of the oral musculature, whereas dyspraxia of speech is noticed only during speech production (Benson & Geshwind, 1983; Darley, 1982; Darley et al., 1975; Wertz, 1978).

Dysgraphia

Dysgraphia, a transmission disorder that also impairs expression, is defined as loss or impairment of the ability to produce written language secondary to brain damage (Benson, 1979). It is an expressive disorder that occurs after language formulation.

Abnormalities of writing are complex and are difficult to attribute to specific areas of the brain. The most frequently mentioned areas with regard to dysgraphia are (1) the frontal lobe of the dominant hemisphere (impaired motor control), (2) the parietal–temporal area of the dominant hemisphere (symbol errors), and (3) the posterior areas of the right hemisphere (visual–spatial difficulties) (Benson, 1979; Benson & Geshwind, 1983; Darley, 1982).

☐ Receptive Disorders of Transmission

Receptive disorders of transmission include hearing impairment, auditory verbal agnosia, and dyslexia.

Hearing Impairment

The diversity of hearing impairments is enormous. Briefly, impairments typically are associated with middle ear dysfunction (conductive hearing loss), inner ear dysfunction (sensorineural hearing loss), and dysfunction of the neural pathways beyond the cochlea (retrocochlear hearing loss). There impairments can occur in combination and are discussed in Chapters 23 and 24. Also see Newby (1979) and Zemlin (1968).

Auditory Verbal Agnosia

Auditory verbal agnosia is a disorder in which the sensations of speech reach the cortex and are experienced but without recognition or meaning (Darley, 1982; Perkins, 1971; Sies, 1974). It often is associated with reductions in auditory comprehension secondary to aphasia (Sies, 1974) but is considered a sensory deficit rather than an impairment in symbolic language (Darley, 1982).

Dyslexia

Dyslexia is a reading disorder. Dyslexia has both acquired and congenital origins. Simply, it is the loss or impairment of the ability to read (Benson, 1979). Rather than a language disorder of one modality, it is a reduced ability to recognize and interpret written symbols.

Dyslexia is often accompanied by dysgraphia, when the lesion is in the parietal–temporal juncture and, more specifically, the angular gyrus.

Disorders of Language Integration

The language integration disorders include aphasia, cognitive–linguistic impairment, and generalized intellectual impairment (Table 14-3).

☐ Aphasia

Aphasia is an integrative language disorder that affects *all* language modalities. It is secondary to brain damage. It is not attributable to dementia or confusion, sensory or motor dysfunction. It is characterized chiefly by reductions in available vocabulary, reduced verbal retention span, and reductions in the

TABLE 14–3. DISORDERS OF LANGUAGE INTEGRATION.

Disorder	Anatomic Area Affected	Etiology	Characteristics
Aphasia			
• Broca's	Third gyrus of left frontal lobe (Broca's area)	CVA,[a] trauma, tumors	Halting nonfluent speech, restrictions in vocabulary and grammar, reductions in language modalities of comprehension and expression, reduced verbal retention
• Wernicke's	Posterior portion of superior temporal gyrus of left hemisphere (Wernicke's area)	CVA, trauma, tumors	Fluent speech, reduced meaningful content, paraphasia, reduced auditory comprehension, poor error awareness, circumlocutions, word-finding difficulty, reduced reading and writing
• Anomic	Parietal–temporal juncture of left hemisphere, angular gyrus	CVA, trauma, tumors	Fluent speech relatively devoid of substantive words, word-finding difficulty, and circumlocutions, less auditory comprehension impairment and less paraphasia
• Conduction	Arcuate fasciculus	CVA, trauma, tumors	Word-finding difficulty, marked paraphasic errors, fluent speech occasionally disrupted for word retrieval, relatively intact error awareness, grammatically intact
• Transcortical sensory	Periphery of Wernicke's and Broca's areas, isolating intact language areas	CVA, trauma, tumors, anoxia	Adequate speech articulation, marked paraphasia and neologisms, often irrelevant and echolalic, intact repetition, severely reduced reading and writing
• Transcortical motor	Anterior and superior to Broca's area, deep to Broca's area	CVA, trauma, tumors	Reduced initiation of speech, variably nonfluent then fluent, word-finding difficulty, relatively intact articulation, repetition and comprehension, rare paraphasias
Cognitive–Linguistic Impairment	Diffuse cortical and subcortical lesions	Trauma, multiple CVAs, diffuse cerebral metastases or infection	Reduced cognitive functioning, including reductions in arousal and alertness, selective attention and concentration, discrimination and categorization, memory, abstraction and associational abilities, and analysis and reasoning; these reductions subsequently impair language usage
Generalized Intellectual Impairment	Diffuse cortical and subcortical lesions	Dementia secondary to disease, other diffuse degenerative processes	Language impairment relative to severity of intellectual impairment (dementia), characterized by reductions in concentration, memory, generalization and abstraction

[a]CVA, cerebrovascular accident.

ability to use learned linguistic rules (Benson, 1979; Brookshire, 1978; Darley, 1982; Perkins, 1971; Schuell et al., 1964).

Aphasia typically is associated with lesions to the primary linguistic centers (Wernicke's area, Broca's area), but aphasia is noted also in areas adjacent to these in the cortex (Benson & Geshwind, 1983; Wertz, 1978). New information suggests possible subcortical correlations for aphasia (Benson, 1979; Goodglass & Kaplan, 1983).

Aphasia has been described and categorized based on lesion location and linguistic deficit (Darley, 1982; Goodglass & Kaplan, 1972; Schuell et al., 1964). Because the variety of existing adjectives and labels can be confusing, one framework based on lesion location and derived from the research at the Boston Veterans Administration Hospital (Goodglass & Kaplan, 1972) is used here.

Broca's Aphasia

Broca's aphasia has been called verbal, motor, or expressive aphasia. It occurs as a result of a lesion in the third frontal convolution of the left hemisphere. Its characteristics include restricted vocabulary, sparse, poorly articulated words, and restrictions of grammar to the simplest, most automatically used forms (Goodglass & Kaplan, 1983). Written language follows the pattern of speech impairment and often is found to be more impaired than speech. Numerous efforts at self-correction of expression are attempted but are often unsuccessful (Darley, 1982). Productions are essentially halting or nonfluent, and considerable frustration is shown by the speaker, who typically is aware of the difficulties. The individual with Broca's aphasia comprehends spoken and written language better than he or she can speak or write, but comprehension is still impaired. Productions of more than one or two words tend to be telegraphic (e.g., "want . . . water . . . drink").

Wernicke's Aphasia

Wernicke's aphasia has been called sensory, acoustic, or receptive aphasia. This language disorder typically is associated with lesions in the posterior portion of the first temporal gyrus of the left hemisphere. Essential characteristics of Wernicke's aphasia include impaired auditory comprehension and speech that is fluently produced but relatively bereft of content. Productions are often circumlocutious or tangential and frequently are interspersed with paraphasic errors or jargon. For example, in reference to the word "fire," a Wernicke's aphasic might refer to it as "the thing that burns" (circumlocution), "fear" (paraphasia), or "grop" (jargon). The person will make these types of errors because of difficulty comprehending and monitoring his or her own productions as well as comprehending and monitoring the speech of others (Schuell et al., 1964). Such a person has little frustration with his or her own productions, however, since the person has a markedly reduced error awareness (Benson & Geshwind, 1983).

Word-finding difficulty or naming impairment, an important consideration, usually is associated with this type of aphasia. A Wernicke's aphasic may have such severe word-finding difficulty that the person may appear to have an expressive deficit and may be misdiagnosed as an expressive aphasic.

Reading skills are reduced at least as much as listening skills, primarily because Wernicke's area is believed to be within the area where visual and auditory linguistic symbols are associated and integrated for language use (Goodglass & Kaplan, 1983). Writing, as a reflection of speech, also is reduced in meaningful content and exhibits circumlocutious and tangential characteristics, although the mechanics and legibility should be relatively intact. Paraphasic errors are known to intrude into written expression as well (Benson, 1979; Darley, 1982; Goodglass & Kaplan, 1983).

Anomic Aphasia

Anomic aphasia has been called amnesic aphasia. Like Wernicke's aphasia, anomic aphasia is fluent, with intact grammatical structure. The major difference is that the anomic aphasic has more severe word-finding difficulty, but without paraphasic errors and with relatively little auditory comprehension difficulty. The listener begins to notice that the content of the aphasic's speech is relatively devoid of substantive words: Instead of "I went to the store to buy some bread," one might hear "I went over there (points) to get those things, you know what I mean" (Darley, 1982; Goodglass & Kaplan, 1983).

This aphasia is usually associated with parietal–temporal lesions, and the lesion's proximity to the angular gyrus is noteworthy (Goodglass & Kaplan, 1983).

Conduction Aphasia

Conduction aphasia, sometimes referred to as central aphasia, is an aphasic syndrome most notably associated with increased paraphasic errors and the reduced ability to repeat words (Benson & Geshwind, 1983; Goodglass & Kaplan, 1983). It often is attributed to a lesion in the arcuate fasciculus, the fiber pathway that is believed to be the means of linguistic transfer from Wernicke's area to Broca's area, and vice versa (Benson, 1979; Geshwind, 1979; Goodglass & Kaplan, 1983). The fluent conduction aphasic has an anomic component but will usually retrieve paraphasic words in a struggle to recall the correct word. Relatively unimpaired error awareness is manifested by struggle behavior and can be attributed erroneously to the nonfluency of Broca's aphasia. The most language difficulty and the highest incidence of paraphasic intrusion occur primarily in repetition.

Transcortical Sensory Aphasia

Transcortical sensory aphasia is a rare aphasic syndrome that is believed to occur under exceptional circumstances. "Watershed lesions" secondary to CVA or anoxia cause damage about the periphery of the intact Wernicke–Broca language complex (Benson & Geshwind, 1983; Goodglass & Kaplan, 1983). The result is that the language areas function unimpaired, but they are isolated from the higher-level ideation areas of the rest of the brain and from the motor–speech mechanism.

Characteristics include adequate speech articulation but with marked paraphasia and neologisms (new words). Responses are often irrelevant and, occasionally echolalic. Confrontation naming of objects is reduced, but repetition is intact. Reading and writing are severely impaired.

Transcortical Motor Aphasia

Transcortical motor aphasia is another uncommon aphasia syndrome that is associated with lesions located either on the anterior–superior periphery of Broca's area or deep within that area (Goodglass & Kaplan, 1983). The person with this type of aphasia has difficulty initiating communication, and his or her responses are typically disorganized and display word-finding difficulty. Such a person tends to be considered more nonfluent than fluent, but is capable of sporadic fluent speech with intact grammar (Benson & Geshwind, 1983; Goodglass & Kaplan, 1983).

Aphasia is a language disorder that manifests varying degrees of impairment in all language modalities (auditory comprehension, verbal expression, reading, and writing). The classifications given cannot be considered mutually exclusive, but they tend to highlight the language functions that are most impaired or preserved when lesions to the brain affect certain areas. The etiology of the lesion may involve different destructive or degenerative processes, but aphasia typically results from CVA or traumatic head injury. Aphasia is a disorder of the brain's ability to integrate and associate language and linguistic symbols, not a disorder of transmission.

☐ Cognitive–Linguistic Disorders

Cognitive–linguistic disorders are impaired language skills due not to disruption of the previously mentioned language areas but to diffuse cortical or subcortical injuries that affect the person's ability to be alert, to concentrate, to remember, and to reason, which, in turn, reduces the efficiency of the person's language. This debility traditionally has been referred to as the language of confusion (Halpern et al., 1973), but this label refers to only one feature of a vast continuum of cognitive impairment. Lesions may result from space-occupying lesions (e.g., subdural hematoma), contusions, shearing of axon tracts, or open head wounds (such as gunshot wounds). A preliminary study at the Shock Trauma Center of the Maryland Institute for Emergency Medical Services Systems (MIEMSS) has suggested that cognitive–linguistic deficits, ranging from mild to severe, occur secondarily to closed head injury despite negative CT scan results.

In recent years, the area of cognitive–linguistic disorders has received increasing attention as efforts to rehabilitate head injury patients have grown nationally (Levin et al., 1982; Rosenthal et al., 1983). Work during the 1970s at Rancho Los Amigos Hospital (Downey, CA) has given rise to classification systems of cognitive functioning that are beneficial for better understanding of the cognitive–linguistic impairment and for the prediction of recovery (Hagen et al., 1977).

According to Hagen (1983), "the majority of language impairment characteristics, while similar to aphasia disorders, are symptoms of an underlying impairment, release, suppression, and/or disorganization of the cognitive processes which support language processing" (p. 4).

Specifically, it is believed that a hierarchy of cognitive processes are affected relative to (1) the areas of the brain that are injured and (2) the severity of the injuries. The hierarchy begins with the most severe impairment associated with reduced or absent ability to be aroused and alert, followed by deficits in selective attention and concentration. The hierarchy proceeds to consider disruptions of discrimination, separation, and categorization skills. At this point, disorders of memory and association are observed more commonly. Analysis, synthesis, and reasoning are the highest level of cognitive functioning to be impaired. At any level, these deficits would impair the person's ability to use his or her language mechanism maximally, accurately, or efficiently.

Typical language disturbances include varying degrees of impairment for comprehension and expression, the likelihood of confabulation, jargon, or circumlocution, and irrelevant, disinhibited, and tangential expressions. Word-finding difficulty and grammatical disruptions have been reported (Hagen, 1983).

It should be noted that the diffuse nature of the injuries associated with cognitive–linguistic impairment will likely give rise to other speech and language disorders, such as dysarthria, dyspraxia, aphasia, and so forth. Considerable effort is needed to diagnose these overlapping disorders correctly and differentially.

Head injury patients at the MIEMSS Shock Trauma Center typically have cognitive–linguistic deficits secondary to their traumatic brain damage (Speech pathology, 1984). The presence of aphasia, however, is noted frequently as well.

One means of differentiation that is helpful involves observing the appropriateness and relevance of the patient's behavior (Halpern et al., 1973). For example, if the patient displays marked auditory comprehension difficulty after head injury and has difficulties with concentrating, acting appropriately, or reasoning and orientation, it is likely that the comprehension difficulty is part of a diffuse cognitive–linguistic disorder, not aphasia.

This distinction is important because assistance and therapy for the patient with cognitive–linguistic impairment differs from that for the aphasic patient (Chapter 2).

Generalized Intellectual Impairment

The language of generalized intellectual impairment represents a complex of disorders that comprise dementia (Wertz, 1978). Like the cognitive–linguistic disorders described previously, the language deficits secondary to generalized intellectual impairment represent impairment of diffuse areas of the brain. Darley (1982) notes that problems cross all language modalities and that the severity of language impairment reflects the severity of intellectual impairment. Differential diagnosis must include an exacting and detailed premorbid history with a variety of formal and informal evaluations of intellect and language facility.

The location of the lesions responsible for dementia is not as relevant as that for other communication disorders. Typically, large portions of the cortex or the entire brain are involved (Wertz, 1978).

Dementia is associated primarily with disease processes, such as Alzheimer's disease, Pick's disease, Jakob-Creutzfeldt disease, and Huntington's chorea. The severity of the language disorders and the prognosis for recovery are as variable as the wide variety of possible etiologies.

ACUTE AND LONG-TERM IMPLICATIONS

Acquired communication disorders often accompany a variety of debilitating vascular disorders, traumatic injuries, and diseases. These disorders create an enormous potential for crisis and catastrophe in the lives of everyone they affect, be it directly (the patient) or indirectly (the family, the caregiver, the community).

Effects of Communication Disorders

In the *individual*, communication disorders can cause speech, language, and hearing deficits, which can lead to high frustration and anxiety levels as well as to diminished self-image, lack of personal fulfillment, and feelings of pessimism and isolation. In addition, a patient with such a disorder will project his or her deficits and fears beyond the immediate situation: "How will these deficits affect me and my family? My friends? My job?" These reactions may increase the effects of the deficits, laying the groundwork for a strong downward spiral in terms of adjustment and rehabilitation.

In a similar manner, the patient's *family members* also experience these feelings. The family and significant others need to adjust to a change in their lives. The family can be expected to go through a period of denial, anger, and depression. It is not unusual for other marked sequelae of brain injury (e.g., hemiplegia, visual–spatial disturbances, incapacitation) to demoralize and affect the family further. Periods of overreaction and underreaction with unrealistic hopes and doubts are often manifested. The family will need considerable counseling and education to assist in their adjustment. The neuroscience nurse specialist can be of direct assistance in this regard and may serve as the coordinator for other assistance from specialists in the areas of medicine and rehabilitation.

In the *community*, the patient with an acquired communication disorder may have considerable difficulty returning to his or her place of employment, school work, or home responsibilities. Job efficiency in fields that require regular verbal interaction (e.g., sales, management) may be drastically altered. Communication deficits in concentration, memory, or reasoning accurately could be catastrophic for employees or students who must work complex and sophisticated tasks with pressures to succeed and meet deadlines. In addition, such disorders can adversely affect personal interests with friends and social or religious organizations and can exert an adverse impact on the management of home duties and economic responsibilities.

Role of the Neuroscience Nurse

Coordination

Into this potentially disastrous situation steps the neuroscience nurse. In the role of both acute–chronic medical specialist and rehabilitation specialist, the nurse has the responsibility of understanding and modifying the communication disorder's effects not only on the patient but also on the patient's family and community. The patient and family will turn to the nurse specialist for information, assistance, and counseling. The neuroscience nurse must draw on personal expertise and training and on information from the patient, family members, and friends and coordinate input from physicians and rehabilitation specialists to meet this need.

Consultation

It is particularly important for the neuroscience nurse to consult with a communication disorders specialist to obtain maximal diagnostic information and assistance with planning and implementation of treatment. The speech–language pathologist is a trained and accredited specialist in the field of communication disorders with at least a master's education and at least 9 months of supervised clinical practice before being nationally accredited by the American Speech–Language–Hearing Association. The accredited speech–language pathologist holds the certificate of clinical competence that reflects completion of academic and practical experiences and denotes expertise in the field of communication disorders.

Cooperative interaction between the neuroscience nurse and the speech–language pathologist allows two specialists to combine their skills for the benefit of patient, family, and community.

Influence of the Neuroscience Nurse

The neuroscience nurse who understands the process of communication disorders will be able to assist the *patient* in adapting efficiently to the environment to alleviate the effect of the disorder. The nurse must know which language modalities yield the highest results in terms of each patient's comprehension or self-expression.

Family members will need extensive counseling to help them adjust to the changes in their relationship with the patient. They will need to learn those things that will benefit the patient and assist his or her ability to communicate; they must be made aware of those things that should be avoided as potentially harmful to the patient. Because most family members will have little, if any, knowledge of these communication disorders, misinterpretations may occur. The neuroscience nurse can act to prevent such misunderstanding or to correct it early in the patient's care process by providing the family with practical and useful advice and information. The nurse can thus spare both patient and family unnecessary anxiety and fears.

Some communication disorders may necessitate extensive planning before the patient's discharge to ensure the patient's return to maximal function, for example, arrangements with the patient's employer, appropriate education of children and concerned friends, and arrangement for outpatient therapies if necessary.

Plans begun in the acute or chronic phase of care that precede a return home must have long-term goals directed at the *community*. The neuroscience nurse can coordinate family, community, and social service endeavors to help the patient make a maximally functional return to the community.

SUMMARY

Language and communication are highly sophisticated processes in human relationships. Communication has become more critical in daily life as present society places more and more emphasis on the informative, directive, and expressive elements of language and communication. Disorders in communication can markedly disrupt the quality of life for the individual affected as well as that of his or her family and community.

Communication disorders are described in this chapter with regard to transmission and integration impairments. Transmission refers to the sensorimotor activities that permit reception and expression of linguistic symbols, such as speech, written symbols, or gesture. Receptive transmission disorders discussed are (1) acquired hearing impairment, which affects transmission and transmutation of sound through the ear to the auditory nerve portion of cranial nerve VIII, (2) auditory verbal agnosia, which refers to impaired ability to recognize speech, and (3) acquired dyslexia, which refers to impaired ability to recognize written or printed letters or words. Expressive transmission disorders discussed were (1) the dysarthrias, which relate to speech disturbances due to paresis or incoordination of speech movements, (2) dyspraxia of speech, which refers to impairment of the cortical programmer for the complex organization of the motor–speech act, and (3) dysgraphia, which refers to various disorders of the ability to write.

Integration disorders are those language impairments that cause disruption of the brain's ability to associate and process the symbols of language. It is not a disorder of transmission to or from people but a reduction in comprehension, assimilation, and formulation of symbolic language. The disorders discussed are (1) aphasia, which refers to sudden disruption of language secondary to disorders of specific areas of the brain thought to be primarily responsible for language processes, (2) cognitive–linguistic impairment, which refers to diffuse cortical and subcortical lesions (usually secondary to head injury) that reduce cognitive functioning and, consequently, interfere with language adequacy and efficiency, and (3) generalized intellectual impairment, which is also a diffuse impairment of cognitive and language function but which is usually presented as a gradual onset secondary to disease and age-related considerations.

This chapter and Chapter 15 are directed toward a better understanding of communication and communication disorders and the management of these disorders. The neuroscience nurse specialist is highly involved in direct care of the communicatively impaired patient and serves as coordinator of medical and rehabilitation specialists for the family. The understanding the neuroscience nurse carries into this role will assist in improving interdisciplinary cooperation and will help provide maximum benefit for the patient, family, and the community to which the patient returns.

REFERENCES

Bateman, H. (1977). *A clinical approach to speech anatomy and physiology*. Springfield, IL: Thomas.

Bayles, K. (1979). Language and the brain. In A. Akajian et al. (Eds.), *Linguistics: An introduction to language and communication*. Cambridge, MA: MIT Press.

Benson, D. F. (1979). *Aphasia, alexia, and agraphia*. New York: Churchill-Livingstone.

Benson, D. F., & Geshwind, N. (rev. 1983). The aphasias and related disturbances. In A. B. Baker & L. H. Baker (Eds.), *Clinical neurology* (Vol. 1, Chap. 10). Philadelphia: Lippincott (Harper & Row).

Bloom, L., & Leahy, M. (1978). *Language development and language disorders*. New York: Wiley.

Bollinger, D. (1975). The origin of language. In D. Bollinger (Ed.), *The origin of language* (2d ed.). New York: Harcourt, Brace, Jovanovich.

Brookshire, R. H. (1978). Auditory comprehension and the aphasias. In D. F. Johns (Ed.), *Clinical management of neurogenic communicative disorders*. Boston: Little, Brown.

Brown, H. R., Darley, F. L., & Aronson, A. E. (1970). Ataxic dysarthria. *Journal of Neurology, 7*, 302.

Chomsky, N. (1968). *Language and mind*. New York: Harcourt, Brace, Jovanovich.

Darley, F. (1982). *Aphasia*. Philadelphia: Saunders.

Darley, F., Aronson, A., & Brown, J. (1969). Differential diagnostic patterns of dysarthria. *Journal of Speech and Hearing Research, 12*(2), 246.

Darley, F., Aronson, A., & Brown, J. (1975). *Motor speech disorders*. Philadelphia: Saunders.

Denny, N. W. (1981). Adult cognitive development. In D. Beasley & G. A. Davis (Eds.), *Aging: Communication processes and disorders*. New York: Grune & Stratton.

Devilliers, J. G., & Devilliers, P. A. (1978). *Language acquisition*. Cambridge, MA: Harvard University Press.

Froeschels, E. (1943). A contribution to the pathology and therapy of dysarthria due to certain cerebral lesions. *Journal of Speech and Hearing Disorders, 8*, 301.

Fry, D. B. (1980). *The physics of speech*. Cambridge, MA: Cambridge University Press.

Geshwind, N. (1979). Specializations of the human brain. *Scientific American, 241*(3), 180.

Goodglass, H., & Kaplan, E. (1972). *The assessment of aphasia and related disorders*. Philadelphia: Lea & Febiger.

Goodglass, H. & Kaplan, E. (1983). *The assessment of aphasia and related disorders* (2nd ed.). Philadelphia: Lea & Febiger.

Grewel, F. (1957). Classification of dysarthrias. *ACTA Psychiatric Scandinavica (Copenhagen), 32,* 325.

Hagen, C. (1983). *Diagnosis and treatment of language disorders secondary to closed head injury.* Paper presented at the Rehabilitation of the Brain-Injured Young Adult Conference, Leesburg, VA. Unpublished.

Hagen, C., Malkmus, D., & Durham, P. (1977). *Levels of cognitive functioning.* Downey, CA: Professional Staff Association of the Rancho Los Amigos Hospital.

Halpern, H., Darley, F., & Brown, J. (1973). Differential language and neurological characteristics in cerebral involvement. *Journal of Speech and Hearing Disorders, 38*(2), 162.

Hughes, J. P. (1962). *The science of language: An introduction to linguistics.* New York: Random House.

Kahane, J. C. (1981). Anatomic and physiologic changes in the aging peripheral speech mechanism. In D. Beasley & G. A. Davis (Eds.), *Aging: Communication processes and disorders.* New York: Grune & Stratton.

Knapp, M. (1981). A structure for the analysis of nonverbal communication. In V. P. Ciark, P. Escholz, & A. Rosa (Eds.), *Language: Introductory readings* (3rd ed.). New York: St. Martin's Press.

Leonard, L. B. (1982). Early language development and language diseases. In G. H. Shames, & E. H. Luiig (Eds.), *Human communication disorders: An introduction.* Columbus: Merrill.

Levin, H. S., Benton, A. L., & Grossman, R. G. (1982). *Neurobehavioral consequences of closed head injury.* New York: Oxford University Press.

Liles, B. L. (1975). *An introduction to linguistics.* Englewood Cliffs, NJ: Prentice-Hall.

Moskowitz, B. A. (1981). The acquisition of language. In V. P. Ciark, P. Escholz, & A. Rosa (Eds.), *Language: Introductory readings* (3rd ed.). New York: St. Martin's Press.

Newby, H. (1979). *Audiology* (4th ed.). Englewood Cliffs, NJ: Prentice-Hall.

Northern, J., & Lemme, M. (1982). Hearing in auditory disorders. In G. H. Shames & E. H. Luiig (Eds.), *Human communication disorders: An introduction.* Columbus: Merrill.

Obler, L. K., & Albert, M. L. (1981). Language and aging: A neurobehavioral analysis. In D. Beasley & G. A. Davis (Eds.), *Aging: Communication processes and disorders.* New York: Grune & Stratton.

Perkins, W. H. (1971). *Speech pathology: An applied behavioral science.* St. Louis: Mosby.

Rosenbeck, J. C. (1978). Treating apraxia of speech. In D. F. Johns (Ed.), *Clinical management of neurogenic communicative disorders.* Boston: Little, Brown.

Rosenbeck, J. C., & LaPoine, L. L. (1978). The dysarthrias: Description, diagnosis, and treatment. In D. F. Johns (Ed.), *Clinical management of neurogenic communicative disorders.* Boston: Little, Brown.

Rosenthal, M., Griffith, E., Bond, M., & Miller, J. D. (Eds.). (1983). *Rehabilitation of the head-injured adult.* Philadelphia: Davis.

Schuell, H., Jenkins, J., & Jimenez-Pabon, E. (1964). *Aphasia in adults.* New York: Harper & Row.

Sies, L. F. (Ed.). (1974). *Aphasia theory and therapy: Selected lectures and papers of Hildred Schuell.* Baltimore: University Park Press.

Smith, A. D., & Fullerton, A. M. (1981). Age differences in episodic and semantic memory: Implications for language and cognition. In D. Beasley, & G. A. Davis (Eds.), *Aging: Communication processes and disorders.* New York: Grune & Stratton.

Speech pathology: New approach to head injury. (July 1984). *Maryland EMS News, 11*(1).

Wertz, R. (1978). Neuropathologies of speech and language: An introduction to patient management. In D. F. Johns (Ed.), *Clinical management of neurogenic communicative disorders.* Boston: Little, Brown.

Zemlin, W. R. (1968). *Speech and hearing science: Anatomy and physiology.* Englewood Cliffs, NJ: Prentice-Hall.

15

Management of Neurogenic Communication Disorders

Roberta Schwartz-Cowley and Andrew K. Gruen*

Diagnosis and management of patient problems created by communication disorders require an interdisciplinary team effort. Patients admitted to the neuroscience unit of a medical facility often have significant communicative and cognitive–linguistic disorders. High levels of frustration mount on the part of the patient, neuroscience nurse, other members of the medical staff, family members, and significant others when the patient cannot engage adequately in meaningful discourse. The neuroscience nurse becomes a key member of the interdisciplinary team responsible for helping the patient communicate basic personal needs, educating the patient and family about health care concerns, and being a liaison between the patient and other medical personnel.

The importance of clear differentiation between communicative and cognitive–linguistic disorders and the resultant appropriate treatment goals and procedures cannot be overstated. Achievement of such goals often depends on the neuroscience nurse's early intervention. An increase in patient performance and concomitant decrease in overall frustration and maladaptive behaviors that would become increasingly difficult to remedy over time results. In effect, the neuroscience nurse becomes actively involved in the rehabilitation process.

Rehabilitation's goal is to enable the patient to achieve the highest degree of independence through guidance and instruction by trained specialists via an interdisciplinary team approach to patient care. The team seeks to maximize the recovery process and to channel reemerging behavior into purposeful activity through progressive stimulation and modification of observed patient behavior. Specific discipline or specialty boundaries become less apparent and threatening in this type of team interaction, increasing not only the smooth functioning of the team but also the level of care given.

In this collective team approach, a patient's general abilities and problem areas are classified and discussed in terms of how they interface with all professional fields involved

---

*The authors wish to acknowledge Connie P. Walleck, M.S., R.N., CNRN, for her contributions concerning nursing diagnoses of neurogenic communication disorders.

in that patient's care. The neuroscience nurse, physician, speech–language pathologist, occupational therapist, physical therapist, dietician, and family service social worker outline basic capabilities and deficits and collectively determine common consistent environmental, behavioral, and medical modifications needed to maximize the patient's overall recovery process. It is in this same framework, with input from the respective specialized professionals and patient care providers, that the team approaches the patient's communicative and cognitive–linguistic evaluation and treatment implementation.

To maximize nursing interventions for the patient who has such disorders, the neuroscience nurse must develop physical and mental assessment skills, determine realistic goals, and delineate proper, effective therapeutic procedures. Doing so establishes and maintains patient self-esteem, the overall effectiveness of the health care organization, and patient and family satisfaction.

It is imperative, therefore, for the neuroscience nurse to become adept at (1) observing and documenting communicative and cognitive–linguistic disturbances, (2) assessing various physical and mental indices through informal means, and (3) using functional treatment strategies to help the patient overcome the frustrations and disabilities evidenced in the neuroscience unit. The strategies so employed require only minor modification for maximal patient benefit regardless of whether the behavior occurs in the acute, rehabilitative, or chronic care facility.

HUMAN RESPONSES TO ALTERED COMMUNICATION

Receptive Communicative and Cognitive–Linguistic Deficits

Communicative endeavors comprise an intimate relationship among organizing cognitive–linguistic information skills, understanding spoken or written language, and producing verbal or written language. This all-encompassing process can be shattered at any point when a patient suffers acquired neurologic change. Careful observation of *understanding* difficulties becomes a paramount, but often overlooked, aspect of analyzing the communication process. Because comprehension cannot be assessed accurately without *judging* the patient's response to expression, it is difficult to determine objectively whether and how much of an understanding deficit exists.

Assessment for possible receptive communicative or cognitive–linguistic disorders includes both behavioral observation and informal screening. For example, at times, the patient may appear not to hear what is said and may ask for frequent repetition of directions, such as transferring procedures or menu choices. The patient may appear unable to follow commands consistently, especially commands that entail complex, lengthy, or abstract directions. This may be noted in activities, such as dressing change procedures. The patient may appear capable of following certain instructions during various periods of the day or for certain people but not for others or at a different time of day, such as when fatigued. He or she may appear to forget commands or instructions and require repetition of even simple, routine activities. Attention skills may be poor, with little eye contact or personal concentration. The patient may not indicate true understanding of written material, such as the menu, even after reading the words aloud. The patient may seem to contradict himself or herself by responding in an inappropriate manner to questions requiring a yes or no response; for example, "Are you cold?" "No." "Do you want a blanket?" "Yes." The patient may appear to understand commands of varying lengths for short periods of time, followed by intermittent periods of confusion.

This seemingly inconsistent response pattern or unreliability in following commands often distresses those involved with the patient, including nursing personnel and family members. When the confusion continues, they begin to question the patient's motivation and desire for recovery and to wonder whether or not the patient is playing games. Frustration on the part of all parties concerned builds, and a detrimental cycle occurs that leads to and increases additional miscommunication.

Informal assessment of the patient's receptive skills can help identify many of the problem etiologies. Systematic evaluation, careful decision making, and proper referral procedures can expedite effective treatment. The goal of assessment is to provide objective documentation of the strengths and weaknesses of the patient's ability to deal with incoming messages.

The screening tools used by nursing staff should include the following categories. First, the nurse should verbally give the patient *simple, concrete commands*. Care should be taken to minimize accompanying gestures, since they tend to invalidate the assessment. Commands start with simple, one-step instructions: "Make a fist" or "Point to the floor." Identification by pointing—whether body parts, room objects, or specific people in the room—is appropriate. Next, *two-step commands* comprised of combinations of previous commands are given. The nurse must take into account the effects of motor weakness and poor motor initiation or control when providing commands to patients with muscle or nerve deficits. Of particular note is the patient who demonstrates difficulties in following sequential commands in an organized manner or problems in dealing with complex thoughts. These behaviors are indicators of cognitive–linguistic disorganization (Hagen, 1984).

As the third step, *yes–no questions* are asked of the patient. Clinical research suggests that a patient whose comprehension is not consistently intact will respond more often in the affirmative (Gruen, 1982). Ascertainment of a reliable "yes" or "no" response is imperative. (The nurse should have available the correct answers for comparison.) Questions can incorporate information from the patient's care plan or medical record, such as biographical information, family names, and previous medical findings. The patient's response can be verbal, written, or gestural, depending on expressive capabilities. If the accuracy of the patient's yes–no response is questionable, the nurse can provide similar content questions that require both a positive and a negative response; for example, one might ask the patient if he or she is in the hospital (yes) and then ask if he or she is at home (no). Conflicting information so obtained can help to establish that the patient's comprehension of verbal messages is not adequate. Should the patient demonstrate difficulty in understanding verbal input, the nurse can present similar information, either in writing or by gestures, but must be certain to document the modification employed.

Next on the assessment continuum for understanding is *determining the patient's comprehension of the written word*. The nurse may supply short paragraph information, such as newspaper articles or a home instruction packet, for the patient to read and then may question the patient's understanding of what he or she read. Simpler forms of reading assessment would include matching written words to objects in the room.

Other informal assessment considerations include observing the duration of selective attention, determining the possibility of hearing loss (noted especially in geriatric and traumatized populations), and recognizing the presence of a foreign language as determined by observation of the interaction between the patient and family or significant others.

Although it is important for the neuroscience nurse to provide an informal assessment of the patient's receptive abilities, a certified speech-language pathologist should provide careful and complete *formalized assessment* of communicative or cognitive–linguistic behaviors. Objective, standardized evaluative tools, such as the Boston Diagnostic Aphasia Examination, the Western Aphasia Battery, and the Minnesota Test for the Differential Diagnosis of Aphasia, are particularly useful in quantifying and qualifying patient behaviors. Routine readministration of such tools assures documentation of progress over time.

An otolaryngologist and certified audiologist should provide the documentation and formalized evaluation of the patient's hearing status. The otolaryngologist will physically examine the hearing mechanism, including the outer, middle, and inner ear regions, and will recommend medical or surgical interventions. Based on the interpretation of an audiologic evaluation (which might include air conduction, bone conduction, and impedance testing), the certified audiologist may recommend environmental or behavioral modifications, such as hearing aids or sign language instruction, that would serve to maximize the patient's ability to hear and understand verbal communication.

A referral to a neuropsychologist is appropriate for patients who demonstrate cognitive–linguistic disorders. Comprehensive standardized evaluations, such as the Halstead-Reitan Neuropsychological Test Battery and Luria-Nebraska Neuropsychological Battery, commonly are used to help delineate specific deficit areas arising from a cognitive, perceptual, and motor interaction system. Consolidation of the cognitive–linguistic evaluation provided by the certified speech–language pathologist and cognitive–motor perceptual examination provided by the neuropsychologist results in an overall comprehensive interpretation from which functional therapeutic guidelines can be established.

Once a diagnosis of a receptive–communicative or cognitive–linguistic disorder has been established and documented by the specialist, an appropriate *intervention* plan is needed. It is important for the neuroscience nurse to realize that many aspects of daily patient care can be transformed into meaningful, functional, rehabilitative procedures. Modifying the communicative environment, the speaker's utterances, or the patient's behaviors will have a positive effect on comprehension. In addition, the informed family should be encouraged to engage the patient in social discourse (Christo, 1978).

The communicative environment should be as quiet as possible (Boss, 1984) to achieve a conducive, calm setting. Distractions, such as extraneous noises, people, and activity, should be kept to a minimum so that the patient's selective attention skills will be maximized (Broida, 1979). The nurse should remove unnecessary items that could be a source of distraction for the patient.

The patient needs an atmosphere of caring and encouragement; the communicatively impaired patient can easily perceive a threatening atmosphere via the speaker's tone of voice or gestures or through his or her own partial understanding of verbal messages. A one-on-one communication situation uses effective environmental control with only one person speaking at a time (Norman & Baratz, 1979). Above all, the patient should be exposed to controlled, calm discourse from others providing ample opportunities to hear speech, since this may aid increased comprehension (Boss, 1984).

When a speaker addresses a listener who has considerable difficulty in understanding verbal messages, it is imperative that characteristics of the message be carefully monitored and modified. This goal can be accomplished in several ways. Gesturing that a conversation will soon begin helps prepare the patient for communication (Lubinski, 1981), as does initiating statements with the patient's name and establishing direct eye contact (Enderby, 1980; Hagen, 1984). Unless a hearing loss has been identified, using a significantly louder voice or exaggerated mouth movement *does not* enhance comprehension of verbal messages (Norman & Baratz, 1979). Serbin and Sommers (1984) found, on the contrary, that normal voice loudness and intonation patterns present the patient with familiarity and help facilitate comprehension.

Several sources indicate that the addition of gestures, pantomime, and facial expression supplement auditory comprehension (Boss, 1984; Enderby, 1980; Norman & Baratz, 1979; Weinhouse, 1981). Multimodal presentation, that is, the use of various input modalities, such as written cues, pictures, and drawings, is helpful (Ryan, 1982). Consistently maintaining topics of conversation, speaking in short precise statements, and using familiar terminology also have beneficial effects for the patient (Christo, 1978; Enderby, 1980). Excessive slowing of the speech signal may hinder comprehension because of the loss of natural intonation patterns and the effect of short-term recall difficulties (Hooper & Dunkle, 1984). Inserting pauses between phrases has been found to enhance overall comprehension of verbal messages (Christo, 1978; Lasky et al., 1976; Louis & Povse, 1980). Maintaining adult level topics of conversation and frequent repetition of daily nursing procedures while having the patient perform or cooperate with medical treatments also have beneficial results (Ozuna, 1984).

The common inclination is to believe that if the patient has a verbal communication deficit, he or she also has a comprehension deficit. In reality, however, patients can often understand much more than they can communicate expressively. For this reason, the nurse should monitor all bedside conversations. *Nothing* should be said within a patient's hearing range that the patient should not hear even if it appears that he or she does not understand. Many depressing and often embarrassing situations can thus be avoided.

According to Arnst and Purvis (1977), receptive difficulty attributed to hearing loss necessitates several considerations. The nurse should face the patient directly and maintain eye contact. The nurse should not shout or exaggerate facial movements, actions that tend to distort the message and result in confusion. The nurse should also reduce the level of, or remove, if possible, competing stimulation sources, such as television, radio, and visitors. If the patient becomes confused during conversation, the content can be repeated in a slightly different manner. Often the patient can tell the nurse clearly and concisely what he or she can or cannot hear and can provide suggestions for increasing communicative efficiency. The speaker should avoid signs of impatience, since impatience tends to discourage active continued performance (see section "Augmentative Communicative Systems" in this chapter).

Generally, the understanding of a patient with a symbolic language or cognitive–linguistic disorder (and, to a lesser degree, a hearing impairment) can be increased by decreasing the length of utterance, limiting distractions in the environment, decreasing the complexity and abstraction quality of the conversation, increasing the specificity of commands presented, increasing multimodal cues (gestures, pictures, words) and decreasing the number of possible alternatives available to the patient. Although speed of presentation rate has been suggested as a significant variable in auditory comprehension, clinical research data support insertion of pauses rather than lengthening the actual time presentation rate of the stimulus.

Of paramount importance is the need for the speaker to maintain a positive communicative atmosphere with the patient, routinely checking for comprehension in nonthreatening ways. To achieve this goal, the neuroscience nurse may have to modify his or her own speech in terms of length, complexity, and extraneous information. Consider the following command given to a patient who demonstrates decreased understanding abilities: "Turn over part way on your left side so that I can change the 4 by 4 dressing pad that is soaked with blood and could result in an infection if not changed promptly and carefully." If the patient appears confused or indicates that he does not understand, the following modifications are encouraged. "Mr. Smith (tap patient on his shoulder to get his attention). I need to change (pause) your dressing (point to dressing site). Roll this way (gesture to the left and help the patient initiate movement). Thank you."

Case Study 1

Kay, a 62-year-old female, arrived at the emergency room with slurred speech and decreased comprehension, as reported by her husband, Richard. Richard reported that he had found Kay lying on the bathroom floor approximately 2 hours before arrival at the Shock Trauma Center.

Results from a preliminary computerized tomography (CT) scan indicated intracranial hemorrhage encompassing the left temporal, parietal, and occipital areas. Considerable swelling was noted. A cerebral arteriogram later confirmed an aneurysm, which was repaired surgically.

Initial nursing assessment revealed a slightly obese woman who was incontinent and unable to feed herself and who demonstrated right hemiparesis. Kay was unable to follow simple verbal commands such as "Make a fist." She was, however, able to complete simple activities when presented with demonstration by gestures. Kay was initially nonverbal but could indicate basic needs by gesture.

When Richard visited his wife each morning, her responsiveness level tended to increase for short periods of time. The speech-language pathologist was consulted and diagnosed Kay's communicative problems as moderate to severe receptive aphasia accompanied by an expressive aphasic component. Her primary difficulties included sensory overload, perseverative responses, and difficulties in following verbal commands without accompanying gestures. Therapy goals included progression of simple commands from gesture and verbal stimulus to gradual fade of gestural cues. Activities of daily living were reviewed with Kay in a combined speech–language pathology, occupational therapy, and nursing therapy program.

☐ Impaired Verbal Communication Related to Receptive Aphasia with Expressive Component

Accurate identification of the type of communication impairment (Carpenito, 1983) is important in designing an appropriate plan for communicating with the client. Key indicators of the nature of Kay's communication deficit were inability to follow verbal commands, inability to verbalize, and ability to communicate with gestures.

Specific interventions included the following:

- *Alternate methods of communication.* Until the exact problem with communication can be identified, an alternate communication system will allow some interaction with the patient. Pad and pencil, an alphabet board, hand signals, eye blinks, and flash cards with words or pictures can all provide the patient with a communication mechanism.
- *Use simple commands with gestures.* A patient can show a great deal of frustration when comprehension is impaired. Techniques to increase comprehension should be used by the caregivers. Facing the patient and establishing eye contact can help the patient to focus attention on the caregiver and the communication. The use of uncomplicated commands with accompanying gestures will help to increase understanding. Reducing external distractions with only one person speaking at a time can assist the patient in maximizing comprehension.
- *Teach family and significant others means of communicating with the client.* Increasing the understanding of all who communicate with the patient is critical in providing continuity for the patient and decreasing the frustrations of all concerned. Sharing the plan for communication is imperative so that the family can participate in adequate care and can share through the communication plan established.

The outcome criteria are that the patient will (1) demonstrate increased ability to understand, (2) participate in a defined plan for communication, (3) demonstrate improved ability to express needs, and (4) relate decreased frustration with communicating to others.

☐ Sensory–Perceptual Alterations Related to Sensory Overload

The environment plays an important role in increasing barriers to communication. For the patient having difficulty interpreting and understanding the environment, sensory overload can occur quickly. This overload can increase disorientation, agitation, fear, anxiety and an altered ability to problem solve. The overall effect for the patient with a speech deficit is a delay in ability to successfully communicate.

Specific interventions include the following:

- *Reduce or eliminate contributory factors.* The caregivers should create an atmosphere of acceptance and privacy. Providing a nonrushed environment and reducing environmental noise will permit the patient to feel that time will be given for communication to occur. Distractions need to be kept to a minimum when communication is occurring between the patient and caregiver. Encourage the patient to take his or her time when talking.
- *Use techniques to increase understanding.* Decreasing the sensory overload that can increase the client's confusion and delay the establishment of a communication system is necessary. Explanations about the environment can reduce anxiety. Reassurance of the patient's well-being can allow for reduced fear, which will help to decrease sensory overload and frustration.

The *outcome criteria* expected are that the patient will (1) maintain an orientation to reality, (2) experience decreased symptoms of sensory overload, and (3) demonstrate decreased anxiety related to increased understanding of the environment.

Kay initially responded inconsistently to yes–no questions (she answered "yes" by head nod response regardless of truth value). By the end if the second week postonset, Kay was able to respond verbally to yes–no questions with 80% accuracy. When an error was made, Kay responded most often that an erroneous fact was true.

At the time of discharge to a rehabilitation care facility 20 days postonset, Kay was able to follow simple commands with minimal visual–gestural cueing, answer yes–no questions with 85% to 90% accuracy, and indicate basic personal needs via pointing and verbal responses.

Expressive Communicative and Cognitive–Linguistic Deficits

Expressive abilities involve an individual's ability to communicate through speech, writing, or gesture. In the medical field, concern is raised when the patient is unable to communicate basic needs effectively and fluently to the nursing staff. Although Schuell (1953) suggests that all people who have acquired neurologic language deficits demonstrate some degree of comprehension or understanding difficulty, expressive disorders frequently are easier to observe, thus providing a more obvious framework for documentation and assessment. Treatment of expressive disorders relies heavily on the processes involved and general characteristics displayed by the patient.

Expressive communicative or cognitive–linguistic disorders occur in many variations and may reflect significant differences in functional communication difficulties. For some patients, verbal expression is impossible because of tracheostomy or laryngectomy. Some patients appear able to speak but are difficult to understand because of slurring, laborious attempts at speech, reduced volume, lack of vocalization, or groping behavior. Other patients might have significant word–sound substitutions or distortions. Some patients appear able to repeat words but cannot communicate personal needs verbally. At times, the neuroscience nurse may note that the patient sings in his room but is unable to respond verbally to orientation questions and must resort to writing answers or gesturing. The propensity for profanity heard from certain patients tends to concern family members and nursing staff even though the family denies that the patient previously used such language publicly. Often neologisms (inappropriate sound groupings) or jargon (inappropriate word groups) are heard that do not appear to have any purposeful meaning to the specific situation. A patient might demonstrate tip-of-the-tongue syndrome, finding it difficult to retrieve words easily, or might appear to be stuttering, demonstrating significant bouts of dysfluent speech even though no significant dysfluent past history is documented. Perseveration of words or thoughts confuses both the speaker and listener; the listener may note the patient's difficulty in changing topics of discussion without a seemingly mandatory return to previous topic areas.

Such disorders result in frustration for the patient because he or she is unable to communicate basic needs adequately to the nursing staff. Frustration is found in the listener also, who wants to aid the speaker but does not have the necessary strategies or techniques to ensure successful communication attempts with such patients.

Careful, sequential *assessment* of a patient's expressive capabilities will provide valuable information for treatment guidelines. Although the nurse can provide very detailed screening results, referrals to the speech–language pathologist and other professionals are still essential. The following assessment considerations are designed to require verbal responses; however, they can be modified to accommodate written and gestural responses as well.

A short oral peripheral examination, evaluating the structure and function of the lips, tongue, cheeks, and palate, is an essential component in assessing expressive capabilities. Particular note is made of any weakness or asymmetry. Dentition, in terms of intact teeth, presence or absence of dentures or plates, and alignment, is quickly assessed, and the presence of excessive drooling or insufficient saliva in the oral cavity is documented. Rapid repetition of sound sequences (diadochokinesis) is used to determine the integrity of quick tongue movements in anterior, middle, and posterior aspects of the oral cavity.

Once the oral peripheral examination is completed, the sequence of verbal expression is initiated. Assessment requires the repetition of single sounds, words, and phrases and the production of automatic speech acts (verbal sequences that are overlearned, such as counting from 1 to 10 or naming the days of the week). Close-ended phrases, which include antonyms and synonyms, are generated to assess if the patient can determine closure concepts. Visual confrontation naming tasks are completed, including naming objects, body parts, pictures, and words. Open-ended conversation is elicited by having the patient describe pictures, tell a story, or explain the sequence of a particular activity of daily living, such as brushing teeth. Characteristics of perseveration, echolalia and palalia, circumlocution, tangentiality, fluency, fluidity of thought, attention, prosody, confabulation, slurring, voice disturbances, and so on are noted in terms of context of occurrence, frequency of occurrence, and overall effects in functional communication.

A referral to the certified speech–language pathologist is necessary so that all areas of speech–language and cognitive–linguistic performance can be evaluated and so that appropriate, detailed therapy programs can be implemented. The speech–language pathologist will also recommend various referrals to be completed, depending on characteristics observed. A referral to an otolaryngologist is made if the patient's voice is hoarse, breathy, excessively soft, or harsh. A clear diagnosis of vocal cord pathology can be obtained by the physician and needs to be completed before voice therapy initiation because of various ramifications of physiologic and structural components that could predispose to modification of voice therapy procedures (Boone, 1977; Parks & Shanks, 1983). The otolaryngologist can examine the hearing mechanism also to determine if the patient who speaks softly has a hearing loss that interferes with adequate auditory feedback of verbal messages. The otolaryngologist may then refer the patient to a certified audiologist, who will complete the audiometric evaluations.

A referral is made to the neuropsychologist when the patient's expressive content is disorganized and shows signs of significant confusion.

Brookshire (1978) lists eight principles of therapeutic *intervention* for patients with acquired neurologic damage affecting speech and language processes:

1. Structure treatment programs so that most of the patient's experiences are with tasks at levels of difficulty such that performance is slightly deficient but not completely erroneous.
2. Keep stimulus materials used in treatment simple and relevant to the patient's areas of deficit.
3. Elicit large numbers of responses from the patient.
4. Begin each treatment session with familiar tasks in which the patient is generally successful.
5. Introduce new materials and procedures as extensions of familiar materials and procedures.
6. Provide feedback regarding accuracy and appropriateness of the patient's responses where such feedback appears to be beneficial.
7. Show the patient his progress.
8. Direct treatment toward general abilities rather than specific responses whenever possible.

Although these suggestions are designed with the speech–language pathologist in mind, generalizations for routine nursing intervention can be made.

In collaboration with Brookshire's suggestions, many other researchers and clinicians point to various modifications and concepts that serve to enhance the patient's ability to communicate basic needs efficiently and effectively. Manipulation of the communicative environment can benefit many people (Broida, 1979). This can be accomplished by providing opportunities for the patient to speak, such as in group gatherings, in a multibed ward, or in conversational settings with the neuroscience nurse, and can maximize motivation and success in speaking (Norman & Baratz, 1979). Routine nursing procedures can be discussed with the patient, providing another opportunity for the patient to participate in his or her care (Lasky et al., 1976). The nurse should exercise care in helping the patient maintain proper and consistent oral hygiene (Christo, 1978).

The patient's speaking behaviors should be modified and directed toward positive speaking situations. Keeping the conversation focused on topics familiar to the patient will tend to produce word usage more intact than will conversations about unfamiliar subjects. A patient interested in gardening, for example, will achieve more efficient and effective communication if discussion includes topics such as fertilizers or types of vegetable plants, as opposed to discussions about new fashion styles in clothing. The nurse should also stress the "can do" approach to rehabilitative intervention by focusing conversation around the speech and language abilities that remain rather than on the patient's deficits. Such focusing will augment the patient's self-esteem and maintain a positive attitude toward communication. As a listener, the nurse should maintain a positive accepting attitude toward the patient and praise successful attempts at communication. Such patients often exhibit emotional lability, which needs to be accommodated by switching topics of conversation (Lasky et al., 1976). If not dealt with quickly and purposefully, emotional lability tends to be perseverated and, thus, more difficult to modify effectively.

The nurse should allow the patient ample time to produce speech. As discussed previously, human discourse is a cooperative event between two or more people that involves complex sequencing and patterning of thoughts and words. Many patients can participate effectively if they have enough time to process incoming messages and produce outgoing communication. The commonly held principle of quickly aiding the communicatively handicapped person can have deleterious effects (Broida, 1979; Enderby, 1980). Encouraging the patient to express his or her thoughts as independently as possible is essential. The nurse–speaker must exercise care to support, rather than criticize, the patient's attempts at communication (Broida, 1979; Linebaugh, 1984). The nurse can encourage the patient to use spontaneous, overlearned speech, such as "Hi." and "I don't know," so that the patient can become part of the communicative and social setting as much and as soon as possible (Linebaugh, 1984). The patient should be encouraged to use gestures and printed words to augment verbal communicative performance as necessary.

Broida (1979) suggests the concept that it is acceptable to help the patient produce a word or phrase after sufficient time for self-expression has elapsed. Several cueing strategies, including associative, descriptive, phonologic, gestural, and graphic cues, can benefit the patient who demonstrates word-finding problems. Associated cues include providing antonyms, synonyms, category members, and overlearned expressions, such as "A cold hand, a warm _____ (heart)." Descriptive cues may focus on physical attributes, such as "It is tall, green, and has leaves. It is a _____ (tree)." Functions of objects can be provided to aid in word retrieval, such as "You sleep in a _____ (bed)." Phonologic cues provide the patient with part or all of the word, such as "b" or "bed" is given as a cue to "bedpan." Pantomiming actions, directions, descriptions, and qualifiers of words or ideas provide gestural cueing. The neuroscience nurse may ask the patient to demonstrate the use of an object he or she desires. Cues, such as writing the first letter and leaving spaces for subsequent letters of a word or writing the entire word, can often elicit the patient's verbal response through the multimodal presentation conceptual framework.

The neuroscience nurse can maximize the patient's expressive capabilities in other ways, including anticipating the patient's needs, expanding the patient's responses, avoiding continual direct confrontation of the patient's speech errors, and determining what is most important for the patient to communicate with expectation and preparation for responses.

The nurse must consider *any* type of communication as beneficial. At the same time, the nurse can indicate acceptance and understanding of the patient's communicative difficulties by asking questions that can be answered within the patient's expressive mode and ability. For example, if the patient's responses are limited to yes–no verbalizations, questions that require exposition, such as "Tell me why you do not feel well," are inappropriate. Questions, such as "Does your head hurt?" and "Do you want a pain pill?" are appropriate.

If the patient's expressive difficulties are caused by motor weakness problems (Chapter 14), a few guidelines can greatly enhance the overall intelligibility of the speech. The nurse must remember that transmission of speech involves four interactive processes: respiration, phonation, articulation, and resonation (Darley et al., 1975). Disruption of any of these processes results in reduced intelligibility. The speech–language pathologist can help by suggesting specific exercises that facilitate stronger and more purposeful interaction of the processes. Generally, the patient with dysarthria should be encouraged to reduce his or her rate of speech, attempt to become cognitively attuned to muscle mobility and patterning, and shorten length of utterance per breath so that speech can be produced clearly with decreased need for repetition. The patient should be taught how significant decreases in overall intelligibility can be minimized by prevention of fatigue.

Realizing that verbal communication involves a complex sequence of linguistic and physical activities alerts the neuroscience nurse to the fact that difficulties in expression can occur and will worsen if not carefully monitored and modified. Frustrations on the part of the patient, family, and medical staff can be reduced effectively if proper evaluation and therapeutic intervention strategies can be implemented in a timely fashion.

Case Study 2

John, a 39-year-old male, suffered a left temporal frontal cerebrovascular accident (CVA). He was admitted to the acute stroke care unit and evaluated by the full rehabilitative team. On physical examination, he was able to demonstrate adequate sensory and motor capabilities and was able to ambulate independently. The patient was able to feed himself and was placed on a regular diet. The primary neurologic deficit noted was his inability to make personal needs known to the nursing staff because of severe word-finding difficulties.

The speech–language pathologist was consulted and diagnosed the communicative disorder as anomic aphasia, characterized primarily by the inability to produce independently the names of objects, body parts, or pictures without significant cueing. The speech–language pathologist's comprehensive evaluation determined that association cues and descriptive cues resulted in increased word-finding ability. A therapy program was initiated, therefore, with the goal of increasing word retrieval skills through multimodal cueing. Nurses were provided with a checklist of important words, such as bathroom and water, that the patient needed to communicate basic functional needs. A common set of cues was established and reviewed by all participating staff and family members. Through consistent cueing strategies and modification of the environment by providing the patient with a writing board and picture word card, the patient was able to make his personal needs known in most contexts of his medical stay. Frustration on the part of all individuals decreased significantly as a result of this functional therapeutic intervention.

☐ **Impaired Verbal Communication Related to Expressive Aphasia**

The ability to express oneself verbally is a complex process and often is impaired in patients with cerebral injury (Carpenito, 1983). The key indicator of John's diagnosis was severe difficulty finding words. Frustration results from the inability to express one's needs. The goals for the nurse caring for the patient with impairment in expressing himself or herself is to create an optimal communication system and to encourage the patient to express himself or herself using the system established.

Specific interventions are as follows:

- *Identify methods by which communication of basic needs can be performed.* As stated earlier, many alternatives can be tried to assure that communication can occur, such as pad and pencil, alphabet list, flash cards. In addition to these methods, the nurse can use gestures and verbal cueing to assist the patient.
- *Reduce client frustration.* The nurse should observe the patient for signs of frustration and address the problems of frustration with the patient. Helping the patient to understand the problem will allow him or her some insight into the frustration being experienced. Patience of the caregiver and the patient is needed. Maintaining a calm, positive attitude will help to reassure the patient and allow for the time needed to communicate. The ability to anticipate patient needs will certainly decrease frustration.
- *Promote continuity of care.* Another means of assuring that patient needs are met is to maintain a specific plan for communication. Writing the method of communication being used will permit caregivers to meet the patient's needs. Incorporating specific measures to reduce confusion over communication and the need for the patient to have to ask for everything will ensure continuity and reduce frustration.

Outcome criteria are that the patient will (1) be able to communicate that needs are being met, (2) follow an established plan for communication, and (3) demonstrate improved ability to express self.

AUGMENTATIVE COMMUNICATION SYSTEMS

Augmentative communication systems refers to any assistive device that enhances functional communication by increasing either comprehension or expression capabilities. The *goal* of any augmentative communication system is to match the current communicative needs of an individual with the functioning of a specific augmentative device (Lubinski, 1981). The interdisciplinary team, with major input from the patient's nurse to the speech–

language pathologist, provides a comprehensive evaluation of a patient's communicative situation.

Questions relating to evaluation or potential use of augmentative communicative devices include the following: What is the present communicative need? How long will the patient require the communicative aid? What potential benefits and risks are present with the preferred communicative aid? What is the potential for acceptance of the device as it pertains to the patient, the family, and the neuroscience nurse? Are there sufficient financial resources for obtaining an expensive piece of equipment? Would a handmade, less-expensive version be more appropriate? Have the patient's physical and cognitive abilities been evaluated?

The answers to these questions should focus on the patient's motor ability, sensory function, mode of mobility, complexity of operation, and comprehension abilities (Mast, 1983). Once questions about the patient's abilities and problems are answered, consideration of various types of augmentative communication systems is necessary.

Types of Augmentative Devices
Research and development of augmentative communication systems is a fast-growing, complex specialty. Because most devices are extremely individualized and because any attempt to provide a comprehensive list of available devices would rapidly become obsolete, only general information is provided here. Consultation with the speech–language pathologist is recommended for more patient-specific augmentative device information.

Generally, augmentative systems can be divided into nonmechanical and mechanical systems, each of which can provide specific or general help to the patient.

Nonmechanical
A communication chart is a commonly used nonmechanical augmentative communication device. Usually a notebook with pictures and words, a lapboard with letters or pictures, or a wall chart may serve as a communication chart. The chart encapsulates specific words or concepts that tend to depict an entire activity that is useful or necessary to the patient. The nurse must ensure that only a *limited* number of purposeful items are used; cluttered communication charts often result in significant confusion and frustration. The patient usually begins with only a few items, practices using them to communicate basic needs, and gradually adds more items as he or she becomes more adept in using the charts. The simplicity or complexity of the completed communication chart will depend on the motor control, manual dexterity, visual abilities, mode of mobility, method of message indication, type and number of required messages, and the amount of time available to make the patient's needs known (Mast, 1983). To keep the communication chart useful for long periods of time, the nurse may wish to preserve it by covering it with clear plastic or hanging it on the wall when not used. Most situations would require the chart to encompass orientation information, yes–no–uncertain response blocks, and listings of basic needs.

Mechanical
Mechanical versions of communication charts are available and may be useful for patients who will need to use them for extended periods of time. These systems usually require preprogramming before patient usage. Power sources, including AC line and battery power, generally adapt to available services; batteries must be recharged or replaced on a regular basis. Mechanical communication charts are not recommended for patients who will not require them for extended time periods because of cost of purchase, service, and operation.

The letter clock has letters of the alphabet located in place of the numbers on a clock face. Using a switch mechanism, the patient rotates a bar similar to an hour hand around the face and stops it when the desired letter is reached. Once the letter has been identified, the patient reactivates the system to locate the next letter.

Sophisticated, computerized augmentative communication systems are available that

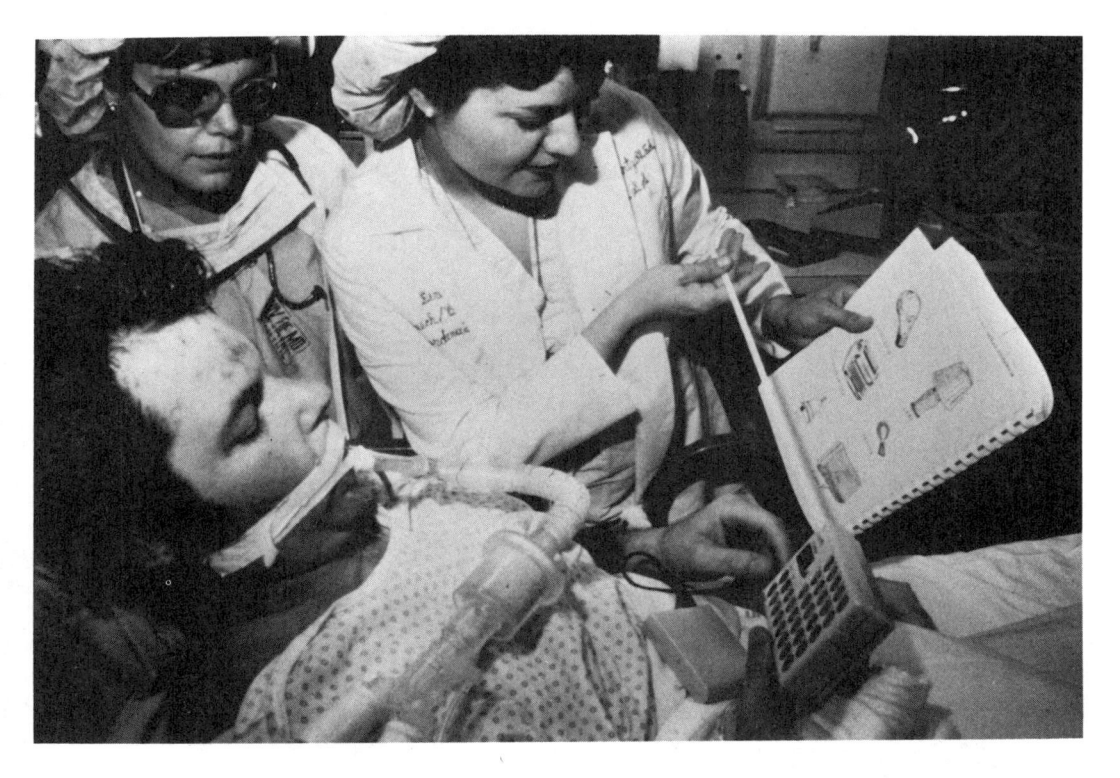

Figure 15–1. An intubated patient regains his ability to communicate by using a small typewriter-like device with a printout record.

can be programmed to produce either visual–graphic or auditory messages. The user simply pushes a button or tab to respond to a message. Printers are available for permanent recordings. Miniature typewriter-like devices are used for spelling and printing messages (Fig. 15–1). Adequate fine-motor coordination skills are needed for a person to use such systems effectively.

Personal home computers have adaptations for the nonverbal patient's use in communication. Patients with high cervical spinal cord injuries can use brow switches, pneumatic devices, and similar methods to control a scanner that produces messages (Fig. 15–2). Many hospital staff members can provide instruction and practice, with the result that the patient's behavior will be enhanced by his or her increased ability to indicate basic personal needs. Programs are available that provide activities dealing with memory, abstraction, reasoning, and judgment for the patient demonstrating cognitive–linguistic disturbances.

The artificial larynx is another type of mechanical device used for nonverbal patients. Although traditionally recommended for use by laryngectomized patients, it has been shown to be effective with a patient who has an endotracheal tube. The artificial larynx mechanism lends itself to patient maneuverability. A vibratory wave is transmitted through the neck wall into the oral cavity, which simulates laryngeal vibration. When the oral musculature is moved freely and precisely, the artificially produced voice is transformed into purposeful speech. The patient must be able to follow commands consistently, capable of manipulating articulators

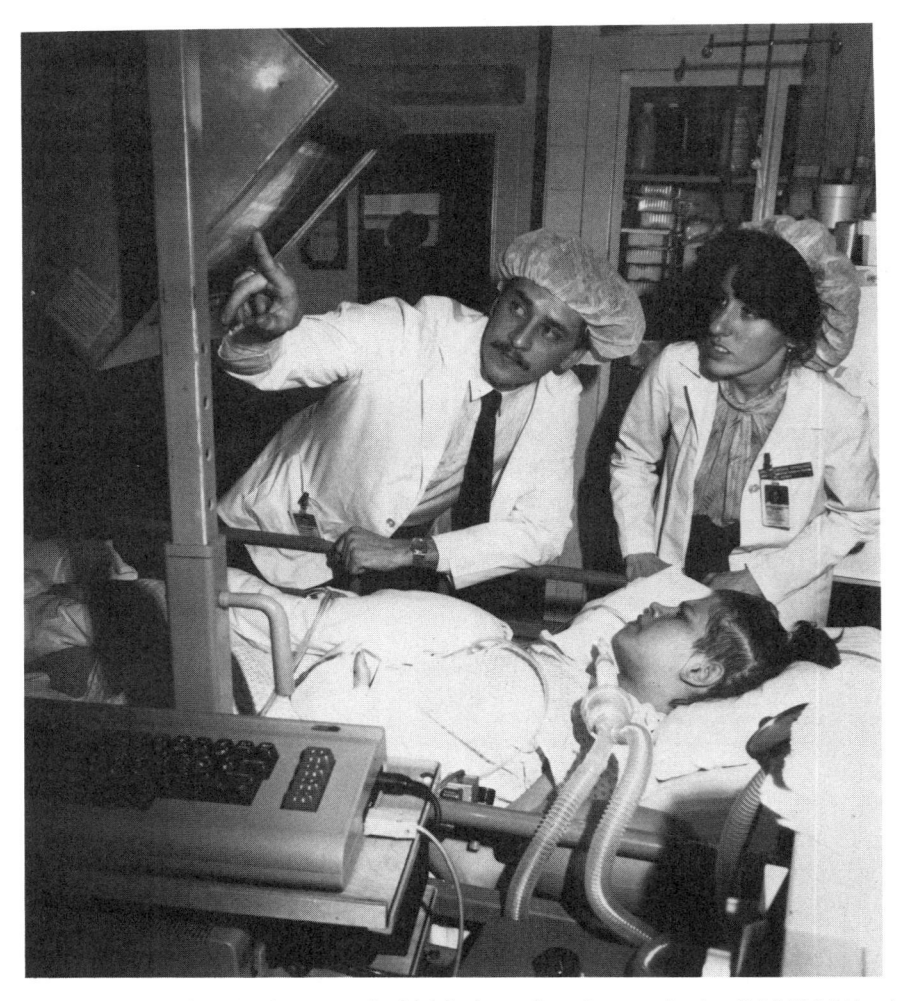

Figure 15–2. A head-injured patient uses the Mobile Acute Care Communication Aid (MACCA) to indicate his basic needs to the rehabilitation staff. The communication system uses input from a single pneumatic switch to select letters, words, or phrases from arrays that are continually scanned on the videoscreen.

with good mobility, and willing to accept the artificial sound of the voice so produced. If the patient cannot hold the apparatus because of weak or nonfunctional upper extremities, the nurse may assist by positioning and holding it.

Because many patients on a neurosurgical unit have significant hearing difficulties, a short, general discussion of the precautions and problems frequently encountered with hearing aids is appropriate here. More detailed information can be obtained from the certified audiologist. Parks and Shanks (1983) suggest the following precautions:

1. Do not expose the aid to excessive heat.

2. Do not allow the aid to get wet. Patients should remove the aid before showering. If the aid gets wet, take the batteries out immediately. Wipe the exterior surface with a dry cloth. Place the aid in a warm (but not hot) place. A hair dryer on a low setting may be used cautiously. Do not place the aid in an oven or microwave oven.
3. Do not use alcohol, acetone, or cleaning fluid on the case.
4. Discard leaking batteries at once.
5. Be sure to remove batteries or open the battery case when the aid is not in use.

Using precautions and good cleaning procedures should extend the functional use of the hearing aid. If, however, the aid does not appear to function properly, Parks and Shanks (1983) suggest the following:

1. If no sound is heard, first check the batteries and be sure to align the positive terminal marking with the appropriate marking in the case. If still no sound is heard, try a new battery.
2. If the aid does not appear to be useful to the patient, make sure that the controls are set according to recommendations outlined by the audiologist. Often the M (microphone) and T (telephone) switch may be set for the wrong listening situation, necessitating adjustment.
3. If feedback occurs, the connections of the ear mold and hearing aid should be examined to locate possible cracks or leaks. If any are found, consult an audiologist to provide the patient with new tubing. Other sources of feedback problems include dirty or clogged ear molds or internal damage to the receiver. A referral to the audiologist is appropriate.

Knowing about and using augmentative communication devices can benefit both patient care and service delivery. The nurse should refer a patient to a speech–language pathologist whenever functional communication of personal needs is limited because of physical, environmental, or physiologic problems.

SUMMARY

Because the neuroscience nurse has significant contact with the daily routine of the patient with acquired neurologic impairment, the nurse is viewed as an integral part of the interdisciplinary team approach to patient care. It is not uncommon for the neuroscience nurse to be confronted with significant needs from the patient. He or she often becomes a spokesperson to and from the communicatively impaired patient. Knowing, understanding, and implementing the functional framework of detailed behavioral observation, informal assessment, and practical intervention strategies for the patient with communicative or cognitive–linguistic deficits will greatly enhance patient communication effectiveness, education, and satisfaction.

REFERENCES

Arnst, D. J., & Purvis, G. O. (1977). Hearing impairment: Basic information for nurses. In S. J. Shanks (Ed.), *Nursing and the management of adult communication disorders*. San Diego: College-Hill Press.

Boone, D. R. (1977). *The voice and voice therapy*. Englewood Cliffs, NJ: Prentice-Hall.

Boss, B. J. (1984). Dysphasia, dyspraxia, and dysarthria: distinguishing features, part II. *Journal of Neurosurgical Nursing, 16*, 211.

Broida, H. (1979). *Communication breakdown of brain-injured adults*. San Diego: College-Hill Press.

Brookshire, R. H. (1978). *An introduction to aphasia* (2nd ed.). Minneapolis: BRK Publishers.

Carpenito, L. J. (1983). *Nursing diagnosis: Application to clinical practice*. Philadelphia: Lippincott.

Christo, S. (1978). A nursing approach to adult aphasia. *Canadian Journal of Nursing, 11*, 34.

Darley, F., Aronson, A., & Brown, J. (1975). *Motor speech disorders*. Philadelphia: Saunders.

Enderby, P. (1980). A nurse's guide to managing the patient with speech handicap following a stroke or head injury. *Nursing Times, 76*, 2114.

Gruen, A. K. (1982). *The effect of presentation rate on the auditory comprehension of adult aphasics*. Unpublished Masters thesis, University of Arizona: Tucson.

Hagen, C. (1984). Language disorders in head trauma. In A. Holland (Ed.), *Language disorders in adults—Recent advances*. San Diego: College-Hill Press.

Hooper, C. R., & Dunkle, R. E. (1984). *The other aphasic person*. Rockville, MD: Aspen.

Lasky, E., Weidner, W., & Johnson, J. (1976). Influence of linguistic complexity rate of presentation, and interphase pause time on auditory-verbal comprehension of adult aphasic patients. *Brain and Language, 3,* 386.

Linebaugh, C. W. (1984). Mild aphasia. In A. Holland (Ed.), *Language disorders in adults—Recent advances*. San Diego: College-Hill Press.

Louis, M. R., & Povse, S. M. (1980). Aphasia and endurance: Considerations in the assessment and care of the stroke patient. *Nursing Clinics of North America, 15,* 265.

Lubinski, R. (1981). Environmental language intervention. In R. Chapey (Ed.), *Language intervention strategies in adult aphasia*. Baltimore: Williams & Wilkins.

Mast, D. L. (1983). Selecting and implementing augmentative communication systems for adults. In S. J. Shanks (Ed.), *Nursing and the management of adult communication disorders*. San Diego: College-Hill Press.

Norman, S., & Baratz, R. (1979). Understanding aphasia. *American Journal of Nursing, 79,* 2135.

Ozuna, J. (1984). Alterations in mentation: Nursing assessment and intervention. *Journal of Neurosurgical Nursing, 17,* 66.

Parks, J. E., & Shanks, J. C. (1983). The nurse and voice disorders. In S. J. Shanks (Ed.), *Nursing and the management of adult communication disorders*. San Diego: College-Hill Press.

Ryan, W. J. (1982). *The nurse and the communicatively impaired adult*. New York: Springer.

Schuell, H. (1953). Aphasic difficulties understanding spoken language, Neurology, 3, 176.

Serbin, S. J., & Sommers, R. K. (1984). *Aphasia and associated problems—A family guide*. Kent, OH: Blaca Enterprises.

Weinhouse, S. (1981). Speaking to the needs of your aphasic patient. *Nursing, 11,* 34.

SECTION 4. AFFILIATIVE RELATIONSHIPS PHENOMENA

16

Affiliative Relationships: An Overview

Catherine Ecock Connelly

Neurologic problems often precipitate major changes in patients' lifestyles, roles, and ability to function independently. Families and significant friends of neurologic patients are struggling to cope with the crises and grieving processes associated with neurologic disabilities. Empathetic reactions of loved ones may provide support to patients; at other times, families may be so overwhelmed emotionally that they become barriers to care. Understanding the nature of affiliative relationships enables nurses to help families or significant friends to mobilize their own support systems throughout the various crises related to the illness. Such understanding enables the nurse to evaluate the impact of family and significant friend responses on the patient's responses to illness and enables the nurse to diagnose situations in which the whole family becomes the client for care.

Affiliative relationships are conceptualized as social systems comprised of significant, patterned, meaningful relationships that are characterized by emotional commitment, intimacy, stability, and continuity. This chapter discusses the various forms of affiliative relationships in our society and the ways in which human needs are met through affiliative relationships. A framework for the assessment of affiliative relationships is presented.

NATURE OF AFFILIATIVE RELATIONSHIPS

Two basic assumptions underlie the analysis of affiliative relationships. The first assumption is that individuals meet their needs for supportive interpersonal relationships in many forms apart from traditional family structure (Stein, 1977). The significance of these relationships is not necessarily dictated by the biologic or legal status of the relationship.

The second assumption proposes that the major theoretical frameworks developed to study family relationships are applicable also in assessing other forms of affiliative relationships. This view recognizes that the human needs for love, sharing, and communication are the basis for affiliative relationships of all types. Fulfillment of such needs distinguishes affiliative relationships from more casual ones. Fulfillment of these basic needs operates as a dynamic process in family relationships (Spanier, 1981) but is not limited to formalized families. These processes operate in other significant relationships as well (Lindsey, 1981).

Consistent with these two assumptions, Naisbitt (1982) calls for a "new definition" of the family. The inclusion of long-standing voluntary relationships in this new definition will lead to "new family models" (Naisbitt, 1982). Trends that characterize the American family are reduced fertility rates, single households, dual career and dual earner couples, high divorce rates, second marriages, cohabitation, single parents, and househusbands (Yankelovich, 1981). Nine of ten Americans eventually marry, and 80% of divorced people remarry. The increase of 41% in the number of cohabiting couples indicates that the search for intimate relationships is a major force in American life (Spanier, 1981). Scanzoni (1983) proposed that a fresh concept of family has the potential for making it a richer institution capable of balancing the interests of society with those of individuals. Howard (1978) concluded that whether the connections are those of choice or chance, the effort people make to create relationships resembling families is one of the most enduring habits of the human race.

FORMS OF AFFILIATIVE RELATIONSHIPS

Affiliative relationships can be categorized as either legal and biologic or achieved and nonbiologic. An examination of the various forms of affiliative relationships within each category demonstrates the diverse kinds of relationships developed by people to meet their needs for intimacy and relatedness.

Legal and Biologic Families

Legal and biologic families include marital couples, nuclear families, extended families, and the family of origin. The marriage of a couple without children, whether by choice or not, is the *childless dyadic marriage* (Kuhn & Janosik, 1980). This may be a temporary stage in the marital relationship for a short or prolonged period of time or may persist throughout the life of the marriage.

The *married childbearing family* includes the marital couple and their biologic or adopted children or both, even when the children are no longer living in the parental home. This is classified as the family of procreation for the spouses (Heffron & Wolff, 1984). This form, frequently called the traditional family, is viewed as having a developmental history based on the age of the oldest child (Duvall, 1977). The life cycle of the childbearing family is conceptualized in eight stages: (1) the married couple, (2) the childbearing family, (3) the family with preschool aged children, (4) the family with school aged children, (5) the family with teenage children, (6) the family whose children are involved in launching a career, (7) middle-aged parents, and (8) the family whose parents are aged. Duvall (1977) theorized that each family developmental stage requires the accomplishment of stage-appropriate tasks that characterize the function of the family during that stage.

The *single-parent family* consists of one parent and his or her biologic or adopted children or both (Heffron & Wolff, 1984). Single-parent families are a result of separation, divorce, widowhood, or childbearing or adoption outside of marriage. The life cycle approach proposed by Duvall (1977) for analyzing the childbearing family is also applicable to understanding single-parent families because of its focus on tasks related to parenting.

The *extended family* includes the nuclear family and other biologically related family members. These may include grandparents, siblings, or other people biologically related to one of the spouses. The extended family sharing the same residence was much more common in the past than it is at present (Heffron & Wolff, 1984). In this age of geographic mobility, extended families tend to be scattered and less intensively involved with one another on a regular day-to-day basis.

The *family of origin* refers to the parental family of an individual (Heffron & Wolff, 1984). The maintenance of intense relationships and the role the family of origin plays in the life of an adult vary from individual to individual. For single adults, particularly those who recently have moved away from their nuclear families, the family of origin often remains the primary source of emotional support and relatedness.

Achieved, Nonbiologic Families

Achieved, nonbiologic families are referred to by Lindsey (1981) as *chosen families*. They exhibit qualities of kinship characterized by love, commitment, and continuity. Chosen or achieved families include those involving cohabitation and those comprising friends as family. The term *cohabitation* implies a sexual relationship, which can be either heterosexual or homosexual in nature. Common law marriages can be included in this category, although it should be noted that, in some states, the law recognizes common law marriages as legal relationships (Heffron & Wolff, 1984).

Lindsey (1981) categorizes *friends as family* as honorary kin, workplace family, and chosen family. Individuals in achieved or chosen families may share the same household, but shared residency is not necessary for achieved or chosen families. Lindsey (1981) described *honorary kin* as people who, because of their intimacy and emotional ties to the biologic family, become absorbed into and are considered a part of the preexisting family structure. They frequently are chosen by the parents often from among their friends and fill roles similar to those of grandparents, aunts, uncles, siblings, or children. Honorary kin are integrated into the family system, and the close relationship continues despite changes and relocation of various family members. They often have played an important role in families in poverty, suggesting that the practical support they provide often precedes and leads to the development of strong emotional ties. *Fictive kin*, as they are sometimes called, are an integral part of the life of the family and share in major events.

The *workplace family* develops among people who spend most of their daily time together for extended periods, frequently stretching into years, sharing a common task or goal. Lindsey (1981) observed that the bonds that develop among people who share common commitment and goals in a workplace often can be as intense and enriching as those of the biologic family.

Lindsey (1981) characterized chosen family as relationships woven into the fabric of a person's well-being and deeply emotionally significant despite separations of time and distance. Friends are chosen as family not always because the biologic family is not available or satisfying needs for bonding and emotional support but often to expand and extend these meaningful relationships. For many single people, especially those separated by time and distance from their families of origin, chosen families are the source of the deep and enduring emotional support characterized by primary affiliative relationships.

The characteristic of permanence is the essence of affiliative relationships. Such permanence is established through the commitment of members, which is based on strong emotional attachment. Kinship involves love, commitment and continuity, and stability amid change through shared experiences regardless of whether the relationship is based on biologic, legal, achieved, or chosen foundations (Lindsey, 1981). We will see, by exploring and analyzing the elements of and human needs met through affiliative relationships, that these relationships are at the core of the human experience. As such, they set the tone for the life experience of the individual. Any major change in life experience, such as disabling neurologic illness, reverberates throughout the entire affiliative network.

Characteristics of Healthy Biologic or Achieved Families

Howard (1978), based on her study of families, summarized 10 "earmarks common to blood or achieved families" that portray system dynamics and bonding in affiliative relationships. *First*, affiliative or family systems have a leader, chief, or founder who is central to the system. Howard observed that although some blood families go for generations without such a prime mover, clans of all kinds need such a figure. She observed also that achieved or chosen families may include several such figures at the same time. *Second*, affiliative systems include a member who assumes the role of communicator, thus ensuring that other system members are kept informed and up to date. The family communicator is the member who keeps albums and scrapbooks to record the family history.

Third, all members in affiliative systems have extrafamilial concerns and relationships. Their relationships within the system, however, provide essential emotional support and are of greater significance. *Fourth*, members seek close relationships, encourage and support one another, and tend to be hospitable. "Good families" suggests Howard (1978) seek to share their relationships and welcome others into their fold. *Fifth*, affiliative systems deal with the "direness" or the crises of their members. The crises and disasters encountered in life are as much a part of the family's concern as are good fortune and triumphs.

Sixth, rituals are an important part of affiliative relationships. Not only do fixed rituals unite a family and deepen the bonds each time they are enacted, but also members of families tend to create their own unique rituals to reflect their history and relationships. *Seventh*, members in affiliative relationships are affectionate toward one another. Families establish their own style of expressing their affection. These expressions range from effusive to restrained; the gestures, whatever their form, however, have a shared meaning for all.

Eighth, affiliative systems share a "hearth" or special place for the members. Whether it is the homestead of an extended family or the office of a workplace family, it is a gathering place for the members that is special. *Ninth*, members in affiliative relationships develop a sense of posterity and a connection with the past. This is the sense of time and history that expresses the cohesive bonds. *Tenth*, Howard (1978) observed, good biologic or achieved families honor their elders. She observed that there are more grandparents and elderly today as the life span is lengthened and noted the mutual support and special contributions they can make to younger generations.

These characteristics suggest several ways in which nurses can plan to use knowledge of affiliative relationships to enhance care. The "communicator" and "prime mover" can be identified and used as a primary source of information and communication. Family rituals can be ascertained and incorporated into care, particularly during lengthy rehabilitation. An institution-based "hearth" or gathering place can be provided to help the biologic or chosen family coalesce during crises.

GOALS OF AFFILIATIVE RELATIONSHIPS

Whether they are implicit or explicit, all affiliative relationships have goals. Goals of affiliative or family systems are broadly classified as biologic, psychologic, economic, and social (Miller, 1980). The broad classification of goals is foundational to understanding the specific goals established in an affiliative system at any point in time. Goals in affiliative systems are not static, nor are they established in isolation by the members of an affiliative system. The priority given to any of the broad scope of goals and the establishment of specific goals are influenced by a number of factors, including the developmental stage of the family or affiliative system, the environment, resources available to the members, societal needs and mores, and specific circumstances and events in the lives of the members of the affiliative system (Duval, 1977; Miller, 1980).

An example of the relationship between goals in affiliative systems is apparent in the childbearing family. The biologic goals of the family in this stage are focused on ensuring the birth and nurturance of healthy children.

The biologic goals of members of affiliative systems in their middle years, however, might be adapting and coping with the physical changes accompanying middle age. Families in poverty need to place a higher priority and concern on economic goals to provide basic necessities. An affluent family easily satisfying biologic goals can focus on psychologic and social goals. In the event of illness in a family member, this family can redirect its focus to biologic goals.

Goals and the priority ascribed to them by individual members of an affiliative system are sometimes in conflict, thus causing disruption within the system. This can occur when adopted goals do not incorporate the needs of one or more members. For example, a family of school aged children continues to prioritize biologic goals at the expense of social goals that accompany that developmental stage. Goals in affiliative relationships can conflict when individuals set different priorities for the goals. An example is a situation in which one member seeks psychologic and social goals through a lifestyle that diverts monetary resources to the point of interference with the economic goals of other members.

Members of affiliative systems need to take the needs of the individual members as well as those of the system as a whole into consideration when establishing and pursuing its goals. Conflict and disruption arise when affiliative systems are unwilling or unable to negotiate and blend the individual and system goals. The goals of affiliative systems as they develop and evolve over time, whether conscious or unconscious, serve to support the steady state of the system and set the tone for function and interaction within the system.

Human Needs Met Through Affiliative Relationships

A hierarchy of human needs was proposed by Maslow (1970), including physiologic, safety and security, love and belonging, self-esteem, and self-actualization. Marston and Chambers (1980), in their proposed eclectic framework for understanding family systems, built on Maslow's hierarchy of human needs. Three core human needs were identified in this framework. These core needs are viewed as behavioral motivators and include the concepts of existence, relatedness, and growth (Marston & Chambers, 1980). The Marston and Chambers conceptualization asserts that existence needs encompass material and physiologic needs, safety, security, stability, dependency, protection, freedom from fear, anxiety, and chaos, and a formal structure providing law, order, and limits. Relatedness needs in this framework include emotional gratification, personal happiness, companionship, and support, whereas growth needs include the need for personal growth and self-actualization (Marston & Chambers, 1980). Both the Maslow (1970) and Marston and Chambers (1980) models predict that individuals are free to pursue higher-level needs when more basic ones are satisfied. Marston and Chambers (1980) described three resource dimensions that are the domains within which core needs are met in family systems: time, the sequential and developmental dimension of the family life cycle; territory, the bounded and unbounded distance-regulating dimension in which family interaction takes place; and technology, the family's ability to use resources and energy to meet their needs.

Although individuals are enabled and supported in meeting the whole range of human needs in affiliative or family systems, some independent adults appear able to meet their existence and growth needs in relative isolation. We all can think of examples of people who seem to satisfy their needs who are not apparently involved in affiliative relationships. Affiliative relationships, whatever their form, however, seem to facilitate and enhance the satisfaction of basic human needs. The unique dimension that relatedness makes to the quality of human life suggests that, indeed, these aspects are significant motivators in establishing and maintaining affiliative relationships. A summary of the satisfaction and personal fulfillment attributed to family and affiliative relations in the literature underscores the importance ascribed to various relatedness needs by experts in the field. The list includes love and intimacy (Brain, 1976; Dyer, 1979; Lindsey, 1981), personal happiness (Dyer, 1979), emotional gratification and support (Dyer, 1979; Scanzoni, 1983; Spanier, 1981), complementarity and companionship (Dyer, 1979), connectedness, continuity, commitment, and solidarity (Howard, 1978; Lindsey, 1981; Parsons, 1965; Scanzoni, 1983), and psychologic validation of identity (Brain, 1976). The importance of these aspects of affiliative relationships reflects the bonds that cement these relationships even when more basic needs for existence are threatened. It is the fulfillment and enrichment of relatedness that enable affiliative systems to survive in the face of physical deprivation, illness, or even the death of one of the members.

ISSUES IN ASSESSING AFFILIATIVE SYSTEMS

The multiplicity of factors and variables having an impact on affiliative systems makes assessment of these relationships a complex task. Theoretical frameworks provide an organizing frame of reference that specifies those aspects that are relevant to a particular problem (Fawcett, 1984). The purpose of theoretical frameworks used to study the family is to guide observation and assessment for interpreting and understanding families and other types of affiliative relationships. It also provides a sound basis for assessment and intervention with families and affiliative systems. Janosik and Miller (1979) concluded that theoretical frameworks to study families are an attempt to produce order from the disorder of family life and to describe the commonalities of all families while recognizing the uniqueness and individuality of each.

The general systems framework that is used extensively to study the family is useful because it is applicable to individuals, all forms of affiliative and family relationships, and society. It also incorporates environmental influences. Other frameworks, although not as broad in scope because of the detail in which they examine various aspects of family life, provide useful insight in assessing affiliative relationships. Various family frameworks developed to understand and explain the dynamics of family life differ from one another in the way they define the family and the factors and variables that influence family relationships. Different frameworks suggest different foci for analyzing and assessing the factors and variables operating in family systems. These frameworks are likewise applicable to other forms of affiliative relationships, that is, chosen or achieved families. Since there is no one framework that explains all the aspects of the dynamics of the family, nurses need to understand the major frameworks and select aspects from each to guide their assessment of affiliative systems (Janosik & Miller, 1979; Marston & Chambers, 1980). The following descriptions of the major theoretical approaches to study the family provide an overview of their focus, assumptions, and implications for assessing affiliative relationships.

MAJOR THEORETICAL FRAMEWORKS

Institutional Framework

The institutional approach applies a sociologic and anthropologic framework to the study of families. This approach views the family as the primary or basic social institution and focuses on comparing family institutions through time and in different societies (Dyer, 1979). It is based on the following assumptions: (1) institutions develop in response to individual and social needs, (2) they are necessary for social control, (3) they are overlapping and interrelated and undergo change as a result of change in one or more institutions, and (4) family forms are culturally determined and have their origin in their historical antecedents (Koenig & Bayer, 1981).

Family assessment in the institutional framework focuses on family patterns. It emphasizes changes and variations in those patterns and a comparison of family patterns with those of other social institutions. The institutional approach to assessment provides a broad, overall view of families in society. This approach does not, however, focus on individual family units in any depth and, therefore, does not provide a framework for understanding individual families or assessing their problems (Friedman, 1981; Logan, 1978).

Structural–Functional Framework
The structural–functional approach to family analysis also is primarily a sociologic framework. In this approach, the family is viewed as a social system that functions to meet the basic needs of individuals and society. This framework replaces the institutional approach and examines the structure or makeup of the family at a given point in time (Dyer, 1979). It emphasizes the function or operations needed to meet the individual needs of its members and those of society (Logan, 1978). The major concepts of the structural–functional approach are based on the following assumptions: (1) certain functional requirements must be met for society to survive, (2) the family is one of the functional subsystems that meets these requirements, (3) the family as a social system has functional requirements that parallel society, and (4) the individual family is a small group possessing the basic characteristics of all small groups (McIntyre, 1981).

Assessment in the structural–functional framework examines the various roles that individual family members fulfill. It focuses on the interaction and interdependence of family members seen as necessary for internal family and societal stability (Heffron & Wolff, 1984). The concepts of nuclear and extended family, instrumental roles (economic and decision making), and expressive roles (socioemotional function) are factors to be examined in the structural–functional framework (Logan, 1978). The tendency to view adherence to "normal" family structure, function, and roles suggests to some critics that this approach tends to be static (Dyer, 1979; Heffron & Wolff, 1984; Logan, 1978).

Psychoanalytic Framework
The psychoanalytic framework looks at the role of the family in terms of its impact on the development of the personality of the child. This framework is based on Freudian theory initially developed to explain neurotic behavior resulting from pathologic early childhood experiences. The psychoanalytic approach is further based on Freud's topographic description (1943) of the personality, specifying three levels of awareness: the conscious, the preconscious, and the unconscious. The structural divisions of the mind are further delineated as the id, the ego, and the superego. The family is viewed as the natural group that disciplines the biologic instincts of the child (Logan, 1978). Three premises are foundational to the psychoanalytic approach to the study of families (Janosik & Miller, 1979). First, there is a collective psychologic life of the family shared and created by each member. Second, attitudes and feelings are transmitted from generation to generation, resulting in continuity in the emotional life of the family. Third, ambivalence and conflict are inherent in family life, resulting from bonding, caring, and involvement.

Family assessment within a psychoanalytic framework focuses primarily on the individual family and its influence on psychic development of the members. Social and environmental factors are not considered crucial in the psychoanalytic framework (Janosik & Miller, 1979). This framework focuses on individual's transference, the displacement of emotional response and investment from an earlier relationship to a current one. It is based further on the assumption that emotional and psychic history, especially the earliest experiences, are operant in motivating present behavior (Phipps, 1980). The psychoanalytic approach has been used extensively in the past to study marital and parent–child relationships. Its failure, however, to attend to environmental and social factors, emphasis on individual behavior as biologically determined, and lack of empirical validation has decreased the acceptance of it by many (Bayer, 1981).

Interactional Framework

The family is viewed in the interactional framework as a social group in which members interact in patterned ways (Dyer, 1979). The interactional framework is a social–psychologic approach often called symbolic interaction (Schvanevelt, 1981). Symbolic interaction refers to socialization processes in which people act in response to individual and environmental events. Specific responses arise from the meaning ascribed to the events and reflect past experiences (Janosik & Miller, 1979). The individual is viewed as both actor and observer, with the self-concept developing as a result of consensually validated relationships with significant and generalized others. The self-concept thus enables the individual to choose roles that can be enacted with others, thus learning complementarity of roles. Because of its focus on roles, some writers call this approach role theory (Schvanevelt, 1981). The assumptions on which the interactional framework is based include (1) humans live in a symbolic as well as physical environment, (2) humans are stimulated by and stimulate others through symbols, (3) humans learn meanings to symbols through interaction with others, and (4) roles are guided and directed by the related meaning of clusters of symbols (Schvanevelt, 1981).

Family assessment from an interactional perspective focuses on the ways families relate as interacting personalities. Specific aspects included in the assessment are internal dynamics, family roles, status, decision making, communication, and coping patterns (Friedman, 1981). The interactional framework assesses the internal processes in families by observing overt behavior to which symbolic meaning is ascribed as family members enact complementary roles. The interactional approach has been criticized because it fails to take biologic, structural, and environmental factors into account (Schvanevelt, 1981).

Situational Framework

The situational framework is closely related to the interactional framework. This approach, however, focuses on family interaction in special kinds of situations (Dyer, 1979). Proponents of the situational approach accept that the family is a unity of interaction but emphasize the family as a social situation (Rollings, 1981). Behavior is seen as adjustive to and a function of the situation, and family behavior is a function of the family situation (Rollings, 1981). Individuals respond to situations in terms of the objective conditions in which they exist, the influence of preexisting attitudes, and their definition of the situation in terms of conditions and consciousness of their attitudes (Rollings, 1981). The situational framework is based on the assumption that social situations exist as objective, separate entities resulting from social, physical, and cultural factors. Social situations are changing constantly and are modified as they change. Human behavior is a function of and adjustment to the situation (Rollings, 1981).

Assessment of families in a situational framework involves observation of family behavior in certain situations, with the expectation that repeated observations will reveal patterns of family interaction (Rollings, 1981). The situational approach to family assessment examines the behavior patterns of a family when confronted with a specific situation, such as the birth of the first child. Observation at this time serves as an indicator of patterns of coping behavior.

Developmental Framework

The developmental approach to family analysis views the family as a unit of interacting personalities with a life cycle and related developmental tasks that evolve over time (Duvall, 1977). Duvall conceptualized an eight-stage life cycle of the family that parallels Erickson's developmental model. Developmental tasks emerge in each life cycle stage from physical maturation, cultural pressures and expectations, and individual internal aspirations and values (Duvall, 1977). The developmental framework is based on the assumption that the family is defined as a nuclear conjugal unit. Success in accomplishing each developmental task is accompanied by a mastery that facilitates function in successive developmental levels. Tasks are goals, not jobs, and each family member has a unique age-role expectation in reciprocity with the other members of the family (Rowe, 1981).

Assessment in the developmental framework looks at the family in a chronologic perspective and examines the extent to which family function, roles, and tasks change over time (Janosik & Miller, 1979). It is concerned with the way family function and interaction patterns support the accomplishment of the appropriate life cycle tasks.

Communication Framework

The communication framework asserts that regardless of the situation or the content, family patterns of communication remain the same. Observation of these patterns, therefore, is the source of information for understanding the family (Phipps, 1980). The communication framework is based on the assumptions that all behavior is meaningful and that the verbal and nonverbal communication within a family reflects the interaction patterns of that family (Logan, 1978). Communication is viewed as multifaceted, including content, context, and affect. It is defined on two levels, the denotative level, or the literal content, and the connotative level, which qualifies the content, expresses the degree of intimacy, conflict, and power (Phipps, 1980). Satir (1967) stressed the concept of metacommunication, the "message about a message." Three components of communication incorporated in metacommunication are (1) syntactics, or the information transmitted by the communication, (2) semantics, the meaning of the communication, and (3) pragmatics, the behavioral aspects, including the context. The communication framework views the family as an ongoing interactional framework with implicit and explicit rules about the kinds of messages that are acceptable to that system.

Assessment in the communication framework examines communication patterns as an indicator of the underlying dynamics and rules they express. Communication patterns are seen also as a reflection of the relationships within the family system, its environment, and the suprasystem. The communication framework focuses on discrepancies between verbal and nonverbal behavior, the denotive and connotative level of messages, and the metacommunication.

This overview of the major theoretical frameworks used to study the family highlights the issues and concepts found to influence family relationships. Some of the family frameworks overlap and share concepts and hypotheses, yet each has its own focus and priority for explaining the way various factors influence families and their functions. They provide different dimensions for assessing affiliative relationships. Although some frameworks clearly limit their focus to biologic, legal family relationships, all deal with concepts applicable to all forms of affiliative relationships.

ASSESSING AFFILIATIVE RELATIONSHIPS

Since no one theoretical framework has been demonstrated to explain and describe all the relevant issues related to affiliative relationships, nurses in their practice need to incorporate and integrate the different aspects from the existing conceptualizations in assessing affiliative relationships. The general systems framework provides a broad framework in which to organize an electic approach to assessment of affiliative relationships.

General systems theory provides a framework for analyzing and understanding the elements constituting social systems, including affiliative systems. General systems theory was deveoped by Von Bertalanffy (1968) and gained wide acceptance as a framework for organizing and explaining relationships and interactions among elements or parts of a whole. The components of a system that are relevant in assessing affiliative systems include structure, boundaries, function, tension, processes, and equilibrium (Heffron, 1984; Kuhn & Janosik, 1980).

TABLE 16-1. FRAMEWORK FOR AFFILIATIVE RELATIONSHIP ASSESSMENT.

Structure

Form: What is the form of the affiliative system? Who are the members who comprise the system?

Cultural background: What is the cultural orientation of the affiliative system, and how does it relate to the predominant cultural environment of the suprasystem of which it is a part?

Developmental stage: What are the developmental stages of the individual members of the affiliative system, and how do they relate and shape the developmental stage of the affiliative system?

Educational background: What is the educational background of the members, and how does it influence the affiliative system?

Boundaries

Environmental factors: What are the internal and external environments of the affiliative system, incuding the physical, social, political, and psychologic factors? To what extent and in what ways do the affiliative system and its members relate to their environment?

Function

Roles: What are the various roles of the members of the affiliative system, and how do these roles fulfill the needs of the individual members and those of the system? How are roles ascribed, achieved, evolved, and changed?

Rules: What are the implicit and explicit rules under which the affiliative system operates? How do they influence system function?

Tension–Processes

Input, throughput, output, and feedback: What are the communication and interaction patterns within the affiliative system and between the system and the members with other systems and suprasystems? How do these patterns influence relationships and function of the affiliative system?

Equilibrium

Goals: What are the explicit and implicit goals of the affiliative system and those of the individual members? What are the power issues in establishing goals and equilibrium? How do the goals express the values, existence, relatedness, and growth needs of the members?

Coping patterns: What are the coping patterns for dealing with the exigencies of everyday life as well as crises that disrupt the equilibrium?

The structure of a system refers to the parts that comprise the system as a whole and the organization and pattern of the relationship among those parts. Describing the structure of an affiliative system would involve identifying the individuals involved and their relationships with each other.

The boundary of the system is the margin separating it from suprasystems and other systems. The boundaries define who participates in the system. Boundaries may be rigid, with members of the affiliative system relating almost exclusively to each other. Conversely, an affiliative system may have loose boundaries, with relatively few emotional ties to one another (Miller, 1980).

The function of a system refers to the processes required to achieve its apparent objectives. The function of an affiliative system is influenced by communication patterns, the environment, and available resources (Kuhn & Janosik, 1980). Communication, a key element in the function of a social system, is categorized as affective and instrumental. Affective communication expresses the emotional aspects of relationships within the system, whereas information is exchanged through instrumental communication (Parsons & Bales, 1955).

The environment encompasses the physical, social, and emotional conditions in which the system operates. It includes the proximate environment and extends to the social and cultural environment of the suprasystem of which it is a part (Heffron, 1984). The resources available to the affiliative system are part of the environment. These resources are both emotional and material and influence the extent and ease with which the system achieves its goals.

Tension refers to the energy in the system that is needed to adjust to the demands of the environment. *Input* is the process by which energy, matter, and information are introduced into the system from the environment. *Throughput* is the process by which the energy is transformed and used. *Feedback* is the process by which the system monitors and regulates its response to internal and external stimuli.

Equilibrium is the dynamic steady-state maintained by living systems. Family and affiliative systems maintain a steady-state that reflects and supports the needs of the members. Factors and events, internal or external to the system, that threaten to disrupt the steady-state are resisted by members of the system.

Assessment of affiliative relationships that uses the general systems framework encompasses evaluation of structure, boundaries, function, tension processes, and equilibrium: Specific factors that might be assessed are shown in Table 16–1.

SUMMARY

Individuals meet their need for affiliation and relatedness in a variety of forms of relationships. Recognition of the importance and influence of these relationships in the lives of individuals is essential in assessing the needs of neurologic patients and clients. A general systems approach provides a framework for assessing affiliative relationships and supports the integration of concepts and issues from the major theoretical family frameworks.

REFERENCES

Bayer, A. E. (1981). The psychoanalytic frame of reference in family study. In F. I. Nye & F. M. Bernado (Eds.), *Emerging conceptual frameworks in family analysis* (2nd ed.) (p. 152). New York: Praeger.

Brain, R. (1976). *Friends and lovers*. New York: Basic Books.

Duvall, E. (1977). *Marriage and family development* (5th ed.). Philadelphia: Lippincott.

Dyer, E. D. (1979). *The American family: Variety and change*. New York: McGraw-Hill.

Fawcett, J. (1984). *Analysis and evaluation of conceptual models of nursing*. Philadephia: Davis.

Freud, S. (1943). *A general introduction to psychoanalysis*. Garden City: Garden City Publishing Co.

Friedman, M.N. (1981). *Family nursing. Theory and assessment*. New York: Appleton-Century-Crofts.

Heffron, P. B. (1984). General systems and adaptation. In J. M. Flynn & P. B. Heffron (Eds.), *Nursing: From concept to practice* (p. 9). Bowie, MD: Brady.

Heffron, P. B., & Wolff, E. M. (1984). The family as a system. In J. M. Flynn & P. B. Heffron (Eds.), *Nursing: From concept to practice* (p. 593). Bowie, MD: Brady.

Howard, J. (1978). *Families*. New York: Simon & Schuster.

Janosik, E. H., & Miller, J. R. (1979). Theories of family development. In D. P. Hymovich & M.U. Bernard (Eds.), *Family health care* (2nd ed.) (Vol. 1, p. 3). New York: McGraw-Hill.

Koenig, D. J., & Bayer, A. E. (1981). The institutional frame of reference in family study. In F. I. Nye & F. M. Bernado (Eds.), *Emerging conceptual frameworks in family analysis.* (2nd ed.) (p. 78). New York: Praeger.

Kuhn, K., & Janosik, E. H. (1980). Establishment of a family system. In J. R. Miller & E. H. Janosik (Eds.), *Family-focused care* (p. 147). New York: McGraw-Hill.

Lindsey, K. (1981). *Friends as family*. Boston: Beacon Press.

Logan, B. B. (1978). The nurse and family: Dominant themes and perspectives in the literature. In K. A. Knafl & H. K. Grace (Eds.), *Families across the lifecycle: Studies in nursing* (p. 3). Boston: Little, Brown.

Marston, M. V., & Chambers, B. M. (1980). Development of family conceptual frameworks. In

J. R. Miller & E. H. Janosik (Eds.), *Family-focused care* (p. 416). New York: McGraw-Hill.

Maslow, A. (1970). *Motivation and personality.* New York: Harper & Row.

McIntyre, J. (1981). The structural-functional approach to family study. In F. I. Nye & F. M. Bernado (Eds.), *Emerging conceptual frameworks in family analysis* (2nd ed.) (p. 52). New York: Praeger.

Miller, J. R. (1980). The family as a system. In J. R. Miller & E. H. Janosik (Eds.), *Family-focused care* (p. 3), New York: McGraw-Hill.

Naisbitt, J. (1982). *Megatrends.* New York: Warner Books.

Parsons, T. (1965). The normal American family. In S. M. Farber, P. Mustacchi, & R. H. L. Wilson (Eds.), *Man and civilization: The family's search for suvival* (p. 31). New York: McGraw-Hill.

Parsons, T., & Bales, R. (1955). *Family socialization and interaction.* Glencoe: Free Press.

Phipps, L. B. (1980). Theoretical frameworks applicable to family care. In J. R. Miller & E. H. Janosik (Eds.), *Family-focused care* (p. 33). New York: McGraw-Hill.

Rollings, E. M. (1981). A conceptual framework for studying the family: The situational approach. In F. I. Nye & F. M. Bernado (Eds.), *Emerging conceptual frameworks in family analysis* (2nd ed.) (p. 130). New York: Praeger.

Rowe, G. P. (1981). The developmental conceptual framework to the study of the family. In F. I. Nye & F. M. Bernado (Eds.), *Emerging conceptual frameworks in family analyses* (2nd ed.) (p. 198). New York: Praeger.

Satir, V. (1967). *Conjoint family therapy.* Palo Alto: Science and Behavior Books.

Scanzoni, J. (1983). *Shaping tomorrow's family: Theory and policy for the 21st century.* Beverly Hills: Sage Publications.

Schvanevelt, J. D. (1981). The interactional framework in the study of the family. In F. I. Nye & F. M. Bernado (Eds.), *Emerging conceptual frameworks in family analysis* (2nd ed.), (p. 97). New York: Praeger.

Spanier, G. B. (1981). The changing profile of the American family. *The Journal of Family Practice, 13*(1), 61.

Stein, P. J. (1977). Singlehood: An alternative to marriage. In P. J. Stein, J. Richman, & N. Hannon (Eds.), *The family: Functions, conflicts and symbols.* Reading, MA: Addison-Wesley.

Von Bertalanffy, L. (1968). General systems theory. A critical review. In W. Buckley (Ed.), *Research for the behavioral scientist.* Chicago: Aldine.

Yankelovich, D. (1981). *New rules: Searching for self-fulfillment in a world turned upside down.* New York: Random House.

BIBLIOGRAPHY

Cain, A. (1980). Assessment of Family structure. In J. R. Miller & E. H. Janosik (Eds.), *Family-focused care* (p. 132). New York: McGraw-Hill.

Chinn, R. (1980). The utility of systems models and developmental models for practitioners. In J. P. Riehl & C. Roy (Eds.), *Conceptual models for nursing practice* (2nd ed.) (p. 21). New York: Appleton-Century-Crofts.

Hazzard, M. E. (1971) An overview of systems theory. *Nursing Clinics of North America, 6*(3), 383.

Von Bertalanffy, L. (1967). *Robots, men and minds.* New York: George Braziller.

17

Alterations in Affiliative Relationships

Susan A. Sutcliffe

The family is a basic societal unit. The sense of cohesiveness that develops among its members is the characteristic that distinguishes the family from other small groups. The diagnosis of neurologic dysfunction requiring hospitalization threatens the family unit and can culminate in a situational crisis if the family perceives these two events as stressful. The situation is sudden and unexpected, taxes the person's immediate resources and ability to cope, or demands a change in behavior. The unique aspects of neurologic disease compound the crisis that patients and families face. Central nervous system dysfunction typically is associated with both acute and chronic problems. The management of these problems requires extensive and expensive time-consuming care, yet many families have limited financial resources. The physical and cognitive dysfunction resulting from central nervous system disease often demands drastic lifestyle changes.

IMPACT OF NEUROLOGIC DISORDERS ON AFFILIATIVE RELATIONSHIPS

Mothers of brain-injured patients frequently report personal reactions of frustration, irritability, anger, and guilt. Caretakers of this patient population also report being threatened with physical abuse or subjected to verbal abuse. These patients often undergo significant personality changes, exhibit inappropriate social behaviors, and have physical disabilities. This leads to feelings of exhaustion in family members and subsequent social isolation. Friends no longer want to visit. Frequently, spouses lose any sexual outlets they previously had. It becomes difficult to travel with patients. Vacation plans may change drastically. The public may be embarrassed by the socially inappropriate person. Families feel that they have no time for leisure activities because of the demands on the caretaker. These lifestyle changes often encompass relationship changes as the marriage moves from one of partnership to a relationship involving dependency and supervision. Children may have a difficult time understanding what has happened to their parent. They feel neglected and insecure. Many families report feeling depressed and overwhelmed for years after the initial injury.

The illness or injury of one family member reverberates throughout the entire family system and threatens the integrity not only of the patient but also of the family. In the last decade, there has been increasing attention to the family in both nursing practice and research, as evidenced in the nursing literature. Several authors have investigated the needs of families of critically ill patients (Daley, 1984; Dracup & Breu, 1978). These researchers identified multiple needs expressed by family members who are experiencing the crisis of critical illness and hospitalization. Several authors did a rank order of the significance of these needs to family members. There was variation among the different study populations regarding need significance. This finding illustrates the importance of conducting a family assessment for each patient in order to develop an individualized plan of care.

Other authors have focused their investigations on the unique needs of families with a member with neurologic illness. Mauss-Clum and Ryan (1981) and Lezak (1978) conducted investigations that revealed common adjustment problems faced by families and their head-injured members. The investigators found that a crisis occurred immediately after brain injury and then at intervals throughout the recovery process. During the early phases, families expressed a lack of information about the patient's prognosis and feelings of being overwhelmed and helpless. Yet, as nurses, we know that the variability and the effect of injury and recovery rates prevent us from giving definitive information for months or even years. Later during the recovery process, families began to acknowledge chronic physical and cognitive deficits. It is at this point that they begin to realize that things will never be the same as they once were. The cost of hospitalization and rehabilitation after brain injury are formidable. Many families experience grave financial burdens, since many of the head-injured population are males who traditionally managed the financial affairs of the family. This often leaves the females feeling incapable and overburdened with managing the finances.

Stroker (1983) conducted a descriptive study to gain insight into how the illness of a patient with cerebrovascular accident (CVA) affects the feelings and perceptions of significant others. In her sample of 11, males had more negative attitudes toward the client regarding commitment and financial problems than did females. Stroker also noted that males seem to have a greater difficulty with their new roles and responsibilities.

Mathis (1984) investigated the needs of family members of critically ill patients with and without acute brain injury. Her findings point out the need for individualized care planning for family members of critically ill patients, since there was much variability in her sample as to whether a need was rated as slightly important, important, or very important.

Families experiencing central nervous system dysfunction confront financial difficulties, radical changes in family roles, and an uncertain future. There is no question that central nervous system dysfunction can have a devasting impact on the family. Families need nurses' help in dealing with the anger and guilt, grief and loss, change in roles, communication problems with the patient, and learning how to maintain family functioning.

HUMAN RESPONSES TO ALTERED AFFILIATIVE RELATIONSHIPS

A variety of needs may be expressed by family members who are experiencing the crisis of critical illness and hospitalization. Empirical data indicate that there is wide variation in the significance of these needs to family members. It is important, therefore, that the nurse conduct a *family assessment* in order to develop an individualized plan of care. Family should be considered in the broadest sense of those who are important to the patient, regardless of whether they constitute a legal or achieved family (Chapter 16). An important component of the nursing admission process is the assessment of the patient's family or other significant affiliation systems. Baseline data are collected about the structure and function of the family. Data are collected regarding family roles, communication and decision making patterns, and resources. The nurse must diagnose the family's perception of the illness and hospitalization and evaluate existing coping behaviors. This initial assessment is used as a baseline for determining the impact of the patient's situation over time. It is helpful to identify family members who will visit, preferred visiting times, the names and ages of household members, and names of members outside the household.

There are four areas to assess regarding family structure and function. It is important to identify the *major roles held by the patient* and any plans the family has for assuming those roles while the patient is ill. Second, the family should describe their *usual communication patterns*. *Decision-making patterns* is the third area, including which members play a major role, who participates, and whether the extended family or others outside the family are consulted. *Economic and human resources* are the fourth area of assessment. The family should identify sources of income and insurance and existing or anticipated economic problems. A description of human resources, such as friends and community groups, is useful in evaluating the effectiveness of existing situational supports.

The family assessment also encompasses the *impact of the illness* on the patient and family. Data are collected about the family's perception of the illness, hospitalization, and prognosis. *Family coping ability* should be described in detail. It is important to list any problems identified by family members themselves. The data collected from the family assessment are used in conjunction with objective and subjective findings about the patient to make nursing diagnoses and develop the plan of care.

The impact of hospitalization and neurologic dysfunction on the family is illustrated by the following case.

Case Study 1

Mr. U, a 45-year-old male, was admitted to the neurosurgical service with a 3-week history of memory loss, difficulty concentrating, and occasional difficulty with speech. A computerized tomography (CT) scan of the head revealed a frontal temporal mass. A craniotomy was scheduled for excision of a glioma.

Mr. U had married his second wife 2 years previously. They each had children by their previous marriages. Two sons were away from home attending college at the time of Mr. U's hospitalization. Mr. U owned and directed the operation of a 3,000-acre farm. His symptoms became evident when he was unable to direct the operation in his usual efficient manner. Mrs. U contributed several hours of her time to volunteer efforts. This couple assumed the traditional husband and wife roles within the family.

The couple had a small circle of friends whom they saw on a social basis. Mr. U was financially secure but extremely concerned about the daily operations of the farm during his absence. Mrs. U was unable to direct the business because of a lack of knowledge and experience.

During the weeks preceding hospitalization, Mr. U used denial followed by knowledge and information seeking as his two major coping behaviors. There were no extended family members who were identified as situational supports.

There are seven nursing diagnoses that describe the alterations in relationships and related human responses Mr. U and his family experienced as a result of his medical diagnosis of glioma and the subsequent hospitalization and surgical intervention required.

Nursing Diagnoses for the Individual

☐ **Anxiety Related to Diagnosis (Brain Tumor), Uncertainty of Prognosis, and Inability to Fill Normal Family Roles**

In Mr. U's situation, this diagnosis was manifested by frequent questions and statements of concern about the operation of his farm. Anxiety is defined as a psychologic response to excess energy. The *defining characteristic* for the diagnosis is a vague, diffuse feeling of dread, uneasiness or general discomfort that results when there is a real or imagined threat to oneself.

Anxiety can be divided into two categories—state and trait. Mr. U was experiencing state anxiety, since he was responding to a situation confronting him at the present time. State anxiety can be altered by intervention. Trait anxiety is defined as stable individual differences in anxiety proneness. This is a tendency of an individual to respond to situations perceived as threatening with an elevation in state anxiety level.

There are two *patient outcomes* expected for this nursing diagnosis: Mr. U and Mrs. U will express less anxiety using the rank order scale of 1 to 5, with 5 being very anxious, in 24 hours; Mr. and Mrs. U will be able to recall key points explained by the nursing staff.

The following *nursing interventions* may be effective in reducing state anxiety levels.

1. Provide brief, accurate answers to questions.
2. Arrange for the intensive care unit (ICU) staff to visit before transfer to explain the equipment in the ICU environment. The ICU nurse should identify equipment and tubes that will be used on the patient, explaining where in the body it is used, how much it will hurt, why it is needed, and when it will be removed.
3. Use words and phrases with which the family is familiar.
4. Keep the family focused on the present.
5. Keep the family informed of changes in condition, medical and nursing plan of care, and so on.
6. Provide support and realistic reassurance.
7. Encourage the family to express feelings.
8. Orient the family to unit, visiting hours, phone numbers, and so on.
9. Assure the family that the best possible care is being provided.
10. Explore sources of concern.
11. Maintain consistency in care, via the Kardex and continuity in caregivers.

☐ Loss of Sense of Control in the Hospital Environment Related to Neurologic Dysfunction

Mr. U's verbal expressions of feelings of helplessness and powerlessness constitute the *defining characteristics* of this diagnosis. Desirable patient and family *outcomes* may include the patient's and family's ability to make decisions about care within 48 hours and their ability to participate in developing the nursing care plan within 24 to 72 hours after admission. *Nursing interventions* that will assist the family in achieving these outcomes include:

1. Encourage questions.
2. Provide factual information to the patient and family.
3. Write the nursing care plan at the bedside.
4. Provide opportunities for decision making related to care.
5. Explain what will happen, when, and why so the family can predict the environment to some degree.
6. Encourage the patient to continue making family decisions that he or she was involved in before surgery.
7. Establish short-term goals to monitor progress.
8. Discuss the progress the patient is making on a regular basis.

Nursing Diagnoses for the Family

☐ Potential for Ineffective Family Coping Related to Limited Situational Support

The immediate period after diagnosis and surgical intervention may be a time of crisis for family members. The family experiences intense feelings of shock, disbelief, denial, repression, and suppression. Other feelings exhibited may include withdrawal, helplessness, depression, or anger. Family members will attempt to preserve and protect the integrity of the family as a system. The coping behaviors they select may be functional or dysfunctional. When confronted with a highly stressful anxious environment, the family will automatically react with behaviors they have used in the past. These behaviors may or may not be effective in helping them to cope with their present situation. Effective nursing interventions are directed at two *patient outcomes* related to this nursing diagnosis.

1. The family should be able to demonstrate the use of two coping behaviors within 48 hours of intervention.
2. Families should be able to describe the emotional responses of others faced with a similar potential crisis situation.

Two specific *intervention* strategies for assisting families to achieve these outcomes are family support groups and family network intervention.

Family Support Groups. Family support groups are defined simply as structured groups for assisting families to deal with their problems. Winterhalter et al. (1985) have established family support groups for families experiencing central nervous system dysfunction. These authors see the purpose of family support groups as providing emotional support. Group facilitators take steps to decrease family members' anxieties and facilitate sharing of concerns, stressors, and coping. The support group also gives the family members an opportunity to communicate with the health team, although the focus of a group is not for information sharing. Family support groups do not replace individual support systems, but complement them.

The need for family support groups may be expressed by either family members or nursing staff. It takes only one sincerely interested nurse to initiate the development of a family support group. In the developing stages, the nurse needs to anticipate road blocks early: identify those people that will stand in the way and seek them out; talk about the idea, solicit suggestions, and make people feel included in the planning stages. Provide information to the staff about family support groups and get them excited and involved.

It is important to investigate what resources are available for group facilitators. A facilitator can either make or break a group. Ideally, facilitators should have experience in group dynamics and expertise in the specialty of neuroscience nursing so that they have the knowledge base necessary to clarify information and questions that may be raised during group sessions. Consistency in group facilitators from session to session is important, although it is important to identify backups.

Winterhalter et al. (1985) made several suggestions about logistics of actually conducting sessions. They highly recommend identifying a room to be used consistently for the sessions, preferably located in proximity to the patient population and providing for the comfort and privacy of those attending. It is a challenge to schedule support session times to avoid competing with visiting hours or meals, and at a time when family members are available in the hospital. The best advertisement for the support sessions comes from personal invitations by the primary nurse to the family members through pamphlets or from other family members that have attended sessions. During the family support group sessions, a facilitator should individually welcome each family member to the group. Introductory comments should define the parameters of the session, including the length of the session and the purpose of the session as providing an opportunity for family members to share feelings. It is important that the families understand that support sessions are treated confidentially.

Throughout the sessions, the facilitator maintains control of the group and keeps the group focused on feelings and subsequent problems with coping. A major role of the facilitator is that of listening. There are two techniques a facilitator can use to encourage group members to verbalize. The facilitator can act as a barometer to measure silence. It may be useful to share common feelings expressed by previous support groups to break the silence. Such statements as "If I were you I'd feel . . . ." may give the family members the permission they need to express any negative feelings. The facilitator should identify common themes being expressed by family members and emphasize the fact that these feelings are not unusual. Some of the common themes identified in family support groups are the need to relive the incident, the unpredictability of the prognosis, the subsequent anger, guilt, grief, and loss, and the devastating impact on family functioning. Families find it difficult to cope with the change in roles and to maintain communication with the patient.

The facilitator should help family members explore coping strategies. The existing strategies useful to family members should be supported and reinforced by the leader. If necessary, the leader can encourage and suggest alternative strategies. It is important to make sure the family realizes it is permissable to take care of themselves during the crisis period. At the end of a session, the facilitator should summarize the major themes expressed during the session and reinforce the importance of the family members' feelings. Encouragement should be given for the family members to take care of themselves in order that they can provide support to each other. The group should close with an invitation for the families to return to subsequent sessions.

There are several *outcomes* expected from participation in family support groups. There is usually an extraordinary comradery that develops among family members who participate. Many families have talked about the fact that they were helped to realize it was important to take care of themselves. The group provides the family with an opportunity to acknowledge the normalcy of their feelings and concerns. Many come away feeling like they have new or refined coping strategies for a crisis. Family members are able to acknowledge the importance of their own feelings and roles during the patient's illness.

Social Network Intervention. Social network intervention is a documented approach to organize and strengthen a family's support system systematically. Speck (1973) defines "network effect" as a type of kinship formed when people share an experience. Network effect is easily witnessed in ICU and hospital waiting rooms. Speck (1973) and Rueveni (1979) define the network as gathering immediate and extended family, friends, and acquaintances together for group problem-solving sessions. This group interaction creates a feeling of responsibility for the family's success.

Rogers and Kreutzer (1984) implemented network intervention strategy at Medical College of Virginia. These authors combined individuals with expertise in mental health–neuropsychology with the nursing staff to work together and initiate family network intervention in that institution. To begin, the nurse and other program resources initiated contact with the family. The purpose of this contact was to identify and discuss family needs. Family members were asked to identify possible participants in their network. Subsequent networking sessions mobilized this group of people to identify and anticipate problems, generate solutions, and provide the human resources to implement the solutions generated.

Rogers and Kreutzer (1984) suggested arranging at least three network sessions during the initial phase of recovery. The primary focus of the initial meeting is to structure the network by building on the strength of preexisting relationships. Nurses can use this session to educate participants about the effects of the neurologic dysfunction and potential outcomes. This information is used as a basis for helping family members to identify a list of potential problems and suggest possible solutions. The session is brought to closure by helping the family to formulate goals. Each participant should leave the session knowing his or her responsibilities for providing strength and support.

Rogers and Kreutzer (1984) suggest that the second and third sessions should be used to discuss progress being made toward the initial goals. As new problems are identified, new goals should be formulated and additional responsibilities should be assigned to members of the network as appropriate. The authors concluded from their experience that networks are effective in sharing the burden of increased responsibility after head trauma. Suggestions from these authors are to arrange network sessions before potential crises in the recovery phases and to anticipate the logistical problems in scheduling meetings for the members of the network.

Specific nursing interventions that may be effective in helping family members achieve the identified outcomes for this diagnosis include:

1. Denial: Carefully remind the family of the reality of the situation without taking away their denial defense.
2. Anger: Help the family focus on the real cause of the anger. Validate the fact that many family members in similar situations feel angry. Reassure them that this is a normal feeling.
3. Remorse: Remind the family of the reality of the situation.
4. Guilt: Encourage the family to leave the hospital to fulfill other obligations.
5. Reassure the family that the feelings they are experiencing are normal.
6. Provide frequent opportunities for ventilation of feelings.
7. Evaluate the effectiveness of existing coping mechanisms.
8. Assist the family in identifying and using effective coping behaviors.
9. Reinforce the strengths of the family and mobilize support systems. Suggest participation in family support groups or implement family network intervention.
10. Talk with the family away from the bedside at least once a shift to find out how they are doing and provide information about the patient.
11. Provide for continuity in caregivers as much as possible.
12. Help the family gain an intellectual understanding of the crisis by providing information about events.
13. Consult available resources as appropriate, including clinical nurse specialist, chaplain, and regional or national support groups and organizations.

☐ Disruption of Normal Family Roles Related to Physical Separation

The defining characteristic for the diagnosis is the family's verbal confirmation of change in roles. Again, there are two *patient outcomes* that will assist the nurse in identifying the effectiveness of her intervention: The family will identify who will assume the patient's normal roles in his absence, and the family will state how they would like to participate in the patient's care throughout hospitalization. Specific *nursing interventions* include:

1. Explain the options for participating: Observe, provide comfort and support, give physical care.
2. Check with the family each day to reconfirm their desires for participating.
3. Demonstrate how to give physical care if appropriate.
4. Recognize the family's contribution to the patient's care with positive feedback.
5. Help the family identify the patient's normal roles, what needs to be done (some are critical, others can be left undone), and who can take over these roles temporarily.
6. Identify the decisions that families must make and discuss all their options with them.
7. Arrange for flexible visiting hours.

☐ Potential for Emotional and Touch Deprivation Related to Physical Separation

One *outcome* expected in response to effective nursing interventions for this diagnosis is family members' ability to discuss their feelings with each other. In addition, the family is able to continue their usual patterns of physical touch. *Nursing interventions* to achieve these outcomes are as follows:

1. Encourage the family to continue their usual patterns of physical touch.
2. Show families how to touch the patient without interfering with the equipment if they desire to be caregivers.
3. Encourage the family to discuss their feelings with each other.

4. Encourage conversation about home events, family, and community news.
5. Provide privacy for family interaction if appropriate.
6. Have the family bring items in from home.
7. Encourage children to visit.

☐ **Knowledge Deficit Regarding Neurologic Dysfunction**

Family questions indicating lack of knowledge constitute the *defining characteristic* for this diagnosis. Desired *outcomes* are that the family can define the neurologic dysfunction in simple terms within 72 hours and that the family can outline the medical and nursing plan of care within 48 hours. Nursing *interventions* to assist the family in reaching these outcomes include:

1. Answer the family's questions honestly.
2. Provide specific facts about the patient's prognosis.
3. Arrange for discussion time between physicians and family and assist the family in asking questions.
4. Give clear, understandable explanations about symptoms, equipment, etc.
5. Inform the family daily about the patient's condition.
6. Call the family at home about changes in condition, transfer plans, etc.
7. Describe exactly what is being done for the patient and why.

Nursing Diagnosis for the Community

☐ **Potential for Ineffective Coping Postdischarge—Related to Family Knowledge Deficit About Community Resources**

Family statements of concern are the *defining characteristics* of this diagnosis. As coordinator of the patient's discharge plan, the nurse is in an excellent position to ensure that families benefit from all available community resources. The effectiveness of nursing *interventions* could be measured by the family's ability to list three resources available in the community. A second outcome of the nursing intervention is that the family should make phone contact with one community resource at least 3 days before discharge. In order to assist the family in achieving these *outcomes*, the nurse may:

1. Maintain a list of national and regional specialty associations relevant to neurologic dysfunction.
2. Explain the purpose of those associations that the family could use for support.
3. Provide contact information for those associations in which the family expresses interest.
4. Describe available resources in the local community.
5. Initiate interdepartmental and interagency referrals from which the family and patient may benefit.
6. Encourage the family to take full advantage of local, regional, and national resources.

SUMMARY

Families and other significant affiliative systems are as affected by neurologic illness as the primary patient. Assessment of the family or other affiliative group is an important part of neuroscience nursing care and may lead to several family diagnoses. Support groups, network intervention, and individual teaching are appropriate family and significant other interventions.

REFERENCES

Daley, L. (1984). The perceived immediate needs of families with relatives in the intensive care setting. *Heart and Lung*, 13 (3), 231.

Dracup, K., & Breu, C. (1978). Using research findings to meet the needs of grieving spouses. *Nursing Research*, 27, 212.

Lezak, M.D. (1978). Living with the characterologically altered brain injured patient. *Journal of Clinical Psychology*, 39, 592.

Mathis, M. (1984). Personal needs of family members of critically ill patients with and without acute brain injury. *Journal of Neurosurgical Nursing, 16* (1), 36.

Mauss-Clum, N., & Ryan, M. (1981). Brain injury and the family. *Journal of Neurosurgical Nursing, 13* (4) 165.

Rogers, P.M., & Kreutzer, J.S. (1984). Family crises following head injury: A network intervention strategy. *Journal of Neurosurgical Nursing, 16* (6), 343.

Rueveni, U. (1979). *Networking families in crisis.* New York: Human Sciences Press.

Speck, R.V. (1973). *Family networks.* New York: Pantheon Books.

Stroker, R. (1983). Impact of disability on families of stroke clients. *Journal of Neurosurgical Nursing, 15* (6), 360.

Winterhalter, M., Richmond, T. & Metcalf, J. (1985). Support groups for families of acute neurological patients. Presentation at Neuro Conference By The Sea, Norfolk, Virginia, September 1985.

BIBLIOGRAPHY

Beglinger, J.E. (1983). Coping tasks in critical care. *Dimensions of Critical Care Nursing, 2* (2), 80.

Bouman, C. (1984). Identifying priority concerns of families of ICU patients. *Dimensions of Critical Care Nursing, 3* (5), 313.

Gillings, C.R. (1981). Nursing intervention with the family of the critically ill patient. *Critical Care Nurse, 1* (6), 27.

Hall-Johnson, S.H. (1986). Ten ways to help the family of a critically ill patient. *Nursing '86,* January, 50.

Warmbrod, L.L. (1983). Supporting families of critically ill patients. *Critical Care Nurse, 3* (5), 49.

Wilson, L. (1982). How to develop a support group for families of open heart surgery patients. *Dimensions of Critical Care Nursing, 1* (2), 108.

SECTION 5. MOBILITY PHENOMENA

18

Human Mobility: An Overview

Linda C. Hodges and Christine Callihan

The ability to move freely is basic to the essence of humanity. Through movement, we express feelings and emotions, carry out work activities basic to life support, and reflect our ability to think as we act on decisions made. Not all of mobility is voluntary; for example, vital life processes associated with movement are regulated through the autonomic nervous system as we take in food, eliminate waste, and engage in acts of procreation. To be human, to be alive, implies constant movement both within the internal environment of the self and in the external environment surrounding us.

The inability to move has a great impact on the concept of self; for example, 50 patients with chronic spinal pain that resulted in limited mobility had scores below normal on the Tennessee Self-Concept Scale, physical self subscale, at initial testing before a chronic pain program. After a treatment program, which included increasing mobility, self-concept scores at discharge and follow-up were not significantly different from the normative population (Beckman et al., 1985).

Altered body image as related to the sexual self can be a major problem when immobility is present. Since movement is an integral part of sexual expression in all human beings, those with restricted movement or hypermobility must be assessed to determine the effect altered mobility has on current and previous styles of physical participation during sex. The nurse must be able to counsel the client in alternative techniques and the use of supportive devices to enhance sexuality (Hodges, 1977, 1978; Weinberg, 1982).

The relationship between movement and the ability to conduct activities inherent in a chosen occupation is well exemplified in all disorders leading to immobility. The inability to pursue an occupation for which one is trained can greatly reduce a person's standard of living and force retraining in a less desirable and economically rewarding career.

The ability to put thought into action is associated with mobility. Indeed, educational theorists have defined learning as a change in behavior (Tyler, 1949). Since behavior occurs through movement, a smile, a frown, movement toward or away from an object or a person gives the observer information about the individual's cognitive processes, values, and emotions. In conditions that retard or inhibit normal movement, such as those producing bradykinesia or dyskinesia, the patient's intellectual ability may be judged by observers as less than adequate. People in the individual's environment may respond inappropriately to the less mobile person and thus compound the associated problems of poor self-concept and low self-esteem.

Adequate functioning of the autonomic nervous system is basic to vital life support systems. Disruption of movement associated with such automatic life processes as heartbeat and blood pressure rise and fall creates life-threatening situations.

Movement is the means by which we humans interact with our environment. For people to be mobile, three essential elements must be present: (1) the ability to move (an intact neuromuscular system or compensated movement), (2) the motivation to move, and (3) a free nonrestrictive environment in which to move.

ABILITY TO MOVE

If normal movement is to occur, the person must have an intact voluntary and autonomic neuromuscular system. In the absence of these, voluntary movements can occur through assistive devices, such as wheelchairs, canes, and walkers, and involuntary movements, such as breathing, can be aided by machines, such as the respirator.

Neuroanatomy and Neurophysiology of Movement

The anatomic elements necessary for the generation of normal movement include the muscles themselves, their afferent and efferent innervations, and the segmental spinal cord connections made by these peripheral nerve fibers. Within the spinal cord, descending motor tracts carry information from higher components of the motor system to influence activity at the spinal segmental level. The higher central nervous system elements in the motor systems include the cerebral cortex, certain brainstem nuclei, the basal ganglia, and the cerebellum (Barr & Keirnan, 1983). Dysfunction in any one of these elements can produce alterations in movement or mobility.

The organization of the neuronal elements involved in human mobility gives rise to the terms suprasegmental and segmental motor neurons, also referred to as upper and lower motor neurons, respectively. The motor neurons of the brainstem cranial nerves and of the ventral horns of the spinal cord are referred to as segmental motor neurons. These neurons directly innervate skeletal muscles and are essential for muscle contraction. The segmental motor neurons receive and integrate activity impinging on them from sensory fibers, local interneurons, and descending and ascending spinal cord tracts. For this reason, the segmental motor neuron is also called the *final common pathway*.

The segmental motor neuron is essential for any muscle movement, and the suprasegmental motor neuron is essential for voluntary movement. Suprasegmental motor neurons give rise to the descending pathways that influence the segmental motor neurons. Many of the suprasegmental motor neurons originate in the primary motor cortex of the cerebrum, whereas others originate within the brainstem. The activity within these suprasegmental motor neurons is influenced and modified by the basal ganglia and the cerebellum (Landau & O'Leary, 1983).

Skeletal Muscle

The basic element in human mobility is muscle contraction. Skeletal muscle is composed of individual muscle fibers or cells. A muscle fiber is made up largely of myofibrils that contain the filamentous contractile proteins, actin and myosin, as well as the regulatory proteins, troponin and tropomyosin. In striated muscle, actin and myosin are highly organized into sarcomeres, the functional units of contraction (Nagy & Samaha, 1984). When stimulated to contract, the actin filaments slide past the myosin filaments and thus cause shortening of the sarcomere and muscle contraction.

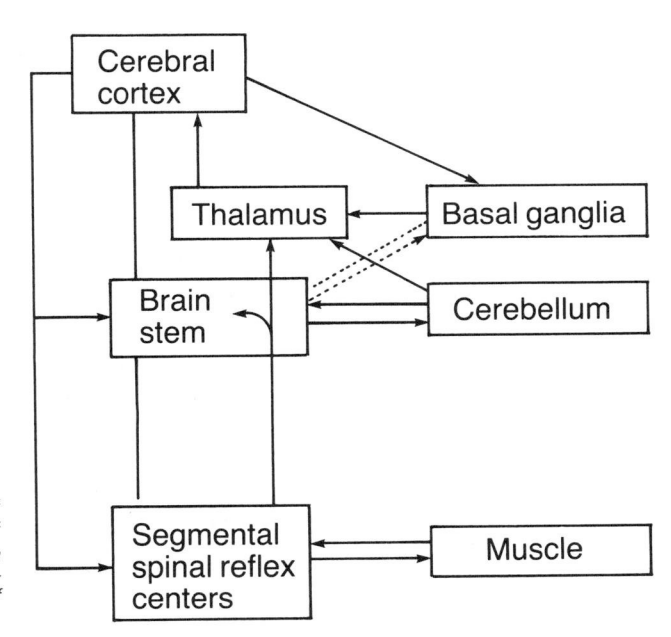

Fig. 18–1. Schematic diagram of the relationship of components of the motor systems. *(Redrawn from H. Patton et al. [Eds.]. [1977]. Introduction to basic neurology. Courtesy of W.B. Saunders Company.)*

The interaction between actin and myosin filaments is accomplished by formation of crossbridges between the two types of proteins. Structurally, these crossbridges are part of the myosin filaments and will interact spontaneously with binding sites on the actin molecules if allowed to do so. This interaction, combined with splitting of adenosine triphosphate (ATP), results in either the movement of actin past myosin and muscle shortening or crossbridge formation with generation of muscle tension rather than shortening. The presence of the regulatory proteins, troponin and tropomyosin, normally prevents crossbridge formation and muscle contraction. The inhibitory effects of the regulatory proteins are removed, however, when the concentration of free calcium around the sarcomeres increases. Conversely, a decrease in the calcium concentration around the sarcomeres causes muscle relaxation (Bullock et al., 1984).

The key to muscle contraction, therefore, is an increase in free intracellular calcium. In skeletal muscle fibers, free calcium concentration in the cytoplasm normally is very low, but the calcium concentration dramatically increases and becomes sufficient to allow contraction in response to motor neuron excitation of the muscle fiber's membrane. In resting muscle, most of the calcium is stored in a specialized form of smooth endoplasmic reticulum, the sarcoplasmic reticulum. When an electrical impulse is generated on the surface of the muscle fiber's membrane, the wave of excitation spreads across the surface of the fiber and penetrates into the interior of the cell via a system of transverse or T-tubules. The T-tubules bring the wave of excitation near to the sarcoplasmic reticulum, which then triggers the release of stored calcium into the cytoplasm, causing contraction (Fig. 18–1). This entire process is called excitation–contraction coupling. Active transport systems pump the calcium out of the cytoplasm back into the sarcoplasmic reticulum, and contraction ceases (Nagy & Samaha, 1984).

Diseases that affect the structural and functional integrity of muscle fibers, such as the muscular dystrophies, congenital myopathies, and inflammatory muscle diseases, can

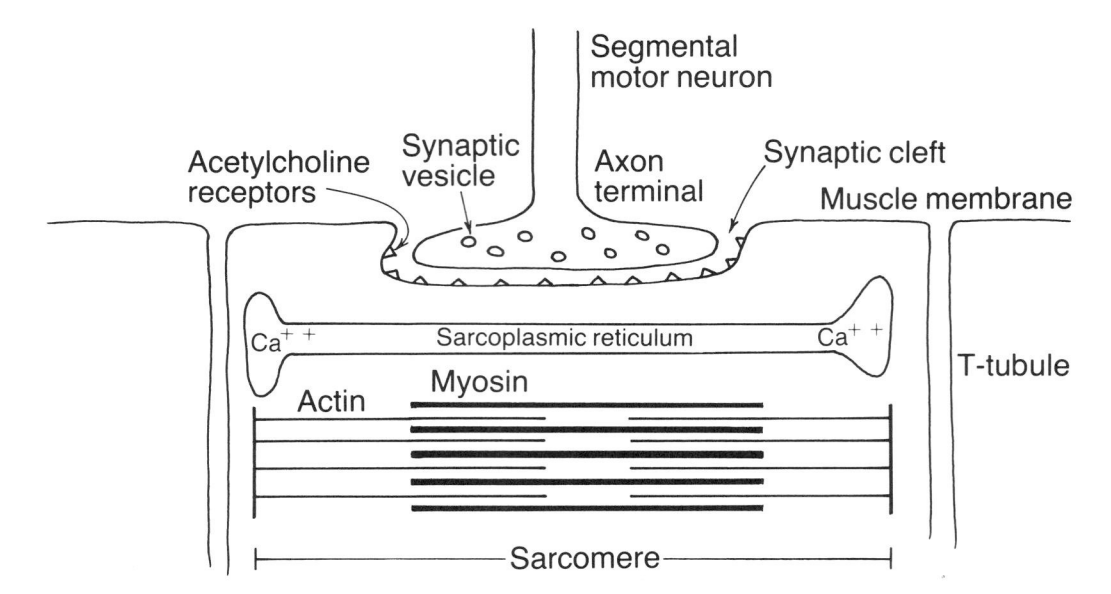

Fig. 18–2. Diagram of the elements involved in neuromuscular transmission. An action potential on the segmental motor neuron causes release of acetylcholine from synaptic vesicles in the axon terminal. The acetylcholine diffuses across the synaptic cleft and binds to specific receptors on the muscle membrane. The interaction of acetylcholine with its receptors alters muscle membrane ion permeability and ultimately results in an action potential, which invades the muscle fiber via the T-tubule system. Calcium is released from the sarcoplasmic reticulum and binds to receptors on regulatory proteins associated with actin. Contractile proteins, actin and myosin, respond to the change in calcium and interact to produce muscle contraction.

interfere with these muscle mechanisms and produce abnormalities in mobility (Robbins et al., 1984; LiVolsi et al., 1984).

Neuromuscular Junction

The action potential on the muscle membrane triggers muscle fiber contraction and occurs in response to an action potential on the motor neuron that innervates the muscle fiber. The bridging step between these two distinct electrical impulses involves the release of a transmitter at the neuromuscular junction, a process referred to as neuromuscular transmission.

The transmitter at the neuromuscular junction is acetylcholine. Acetylcholine is stored in membrane-bound synaptic vesicles in the axon terminals of the motor neuron. When an action potential invades the nerve terminal, the acetylcholine is released by a calcium-mediated exocytotic process. The acetylcholine diffuses across the synaptic cleft, the space between the axon terminal and muscle membrane, and binds to specific receptors on the muscle membrane (Fig. 18–2). The interaction of acetylcholine with its receptor changes the membrane's permeability to ions. The resulting fluxes of potassium and sodium produce a local depolarization, the endplate potential. This potential brings the muscle fiber to threshold and initiates a muscle action potential that subsequently causes muscle contraction (Penn, 1984).

The effect of acetylcholine at the neuromuscular junction is short-lived. Some of the released transmitter randomly diffuses away from the synaptic cleft, although most of the transmitter is rendered inactive through the action of an enzyme, acetylcholinesterase, which also is found in the synaptic cleft.

Rapid inactivation of acetylcholine is necessary in order to have precise neural control of muscle contraction. If acetylcholine remains in the synaptic cleft, it can repeatedly stimulate the muscle. Such repeated stimulation causes hyperexcitability initially but ultimately causes muscle paralysis.

The neuromuscular junction is a site for the alteration of muscle activity by pharmacologic manipulations, toxins, and disease processes. For example, botulinum toxin causes a decreased fusion of synaptic vesicles with the presynaptic membrane. Thus the amount of transmitter released is diminished, creating muscle weakness and paralysis (Walton, 1981). In myasthenia gravis, there is a deficiency of acetylcholine receptors on the postsynaptic membrane. This deficit is believed to be due to an autoimmune condition that results in antibody-mediated destruction of the receptors. The deficiency of receptors decreases the ability of acetylcholine to depolarize the muscle endplate sufficiently to generate an action potential on the muscle membrane. Consequently, the major clinical feature of myasthenia gravis is muscle weakness. Some organophosphate compounds that are used as insecticides can inhibit acetylcholinesterase irreversibly. The resulting prolonged action of acetylcholine at the endplate membrane produces a depolarizing blockade that also effectively inhibits neuromuscular transmission (Penn, 1984).

Motor Neurons

Each muscle fiber has one neuromuscular junction, usually located near the center of the fiber. An individual motor neuron, however, branches out near its distal end, with each branch forming a neuromuscular junction with a single muscle fiber. When an individual motor neuron is excited, the impulse spreads into the axon terminals, causing all the muscle fibers innervated by that axon to contract. A single motor neuron and all the muscle fibers it innervates is called a *motor unit.*

Skeletal muscles are innervated by alpha motor neurons, which have their cell bodies in the ventral horn of the spinal cord. Such neurons are not spontaneously active but must be brought to threshold by the summation of synaptic inputs converging onto them. These motor neurons receive their input from local sensory fibers, local interneurons, and descending and ascending fibers in the spinal cord. Basically, the alpha, or segmental, motor neurons can be excited either by input originating locally and involving activity within the immediate spinal cord segments or by descending input originating in the brainstem and cortex (Bullock et al., 1984).

Muscle Spindles and Tendon Receptors.
Both proprioceptive and exteroceptive sensory fibers that enter the spinal cord can influence motor neuron activity. Most of the proprioceptive fibers carry information that originates in sensory organs located within the muscle itself. These muscle sensory organs are the muscle spindle fibers and the Golgi tendon organs, and they are found in all voluntary muscles. The muscle spindle fibers, or intrafusal fibers, lie in parallel with the main muscle mass, or extrafusal fibers. The sensory fibers arising from the spindle organs are called Intrafusal a (Ia) afferent fibers, and they are stimulated by stretch. On entering the spinal cord, the afferent fibers make direct connections with the alpha motor neurons supplying the same muscle (Fig. 18–3). This spinal cord connection constitutes the monosynaptic stretch reflex. Stretch of the muscle will stimulate the sensory ending on the muscle spindle and will initiate impulses on the Ia fibers. These afferent impulses directly excite the alpha motor neurons that innervate the muscle fibers. The ultimate consequence of stretch of the muscle, therefore, is reflex contraction of the same muscle. The deep tendon reflexes elicited during a neurologic examination indicate the intactness of these reflex pathways (Bates, 1987).

The Ia afferent fibers branch on entering the spinal cord. In addition to making direct synaptic connections with the alpha motor neurons, collaterals from the Ia fibers synapse onto interneurons that are inhibitory to mus-

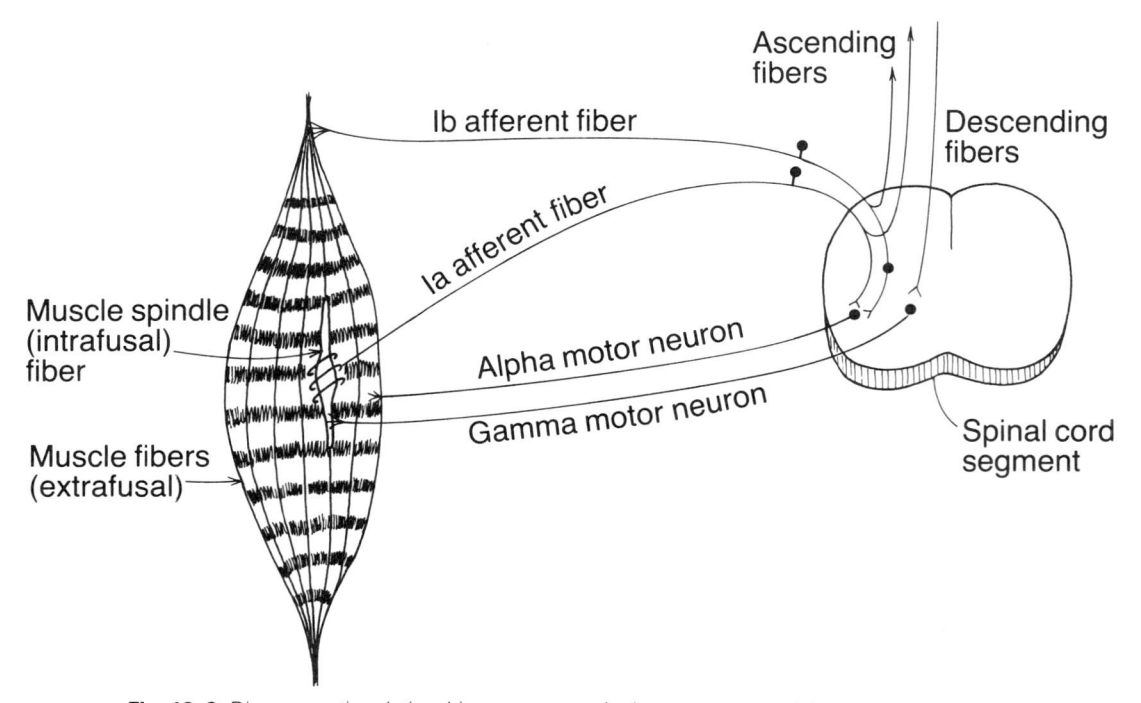

Fig. 18–3. Diagrammatic relationship among muscle, its receptors, and the spinal cord segment.

cles that oppose the contraction. This process is reciprocal inhibition. The Ia collateral fibers also synapse onto interneurons that are excitatory to muscle contraction. Information from Ia afferents is transmitted along ascending pathways to inform higher centers, the brainstem, cerebellum, and cerebral cortex of the length, or contractile state, of the muscles.

Because of the parallel relationship between the extrafusal and infrafusal fibers, it might seem that during muscle contraction the spindle fibers would slacken and be unable to generate important sensory information for movement control. This is not the case, however, because the muscle spindle fibers themselves receive innervation from gamma motor neurons. Motor innervation of the spindle fibers causes them to contract during extrafusal muscle contraction and thereby permit the sensory organs to remain responsive even as the muscle shortens. During the usual course of voluntary contraction, descending commands excite both the alpha and gamma motor neurons to a muscle, causing contraction of both the extrafusal and intrafusal fibers to the muscle. This coactivation of the motor neurons allows sensory input from the muscle during the act of contraction (Guyton, 1981).

The Golgi tendon organs are sensory structures located at the tendon endings of the muscle. The receptors for the afferent fibers originating from the Golgi tendon organs, the Ib afferent fibers, are also stimulated by stretch, but because of their location, muscle contraction increases activity on these sensory structures (Fig. 18–3). These receptors, therefore, respond to the force generated by the muscle as it contracts. The information from the Ib fibers affects neurons locally within the spinal cord and is transmitted along ascending pathways to provide higher centers with important information about the contractile status of the muscles (Guyton,

1981). The information from Ia and Ib fibers is important to the central nervous system in determining if motor commands were carried out appropriately. If the actual signal generated from the muscles does not match the intended motor movement, a correcting signal can be sent out. Thus, a feedback mechanism for the appropriateness of muscle movements exists using these sensory organs in the muscle.

Segmental Spinal Cord Organization

Analysis of the synaptic connections made by muscle afferents onto muscle efferents, either direct or indirect, makes it easy to appreciate how excitation of one pathway can result in the production of a stereotyped movement, that is, a reflex. Other spinal cord reflexes can be initiated by activity generated onto exteroceptive fibers. These latter reflex pathways can be stimulated by pain but also by other sensory stimuli, such as touch and pressure. The principal reflex involving these afferent inputs is the flexor withdrawal reflex. The spinal cord connections in this reflex are far more intricate, involving not only the flexor muscles of the affected limb but also the extensor muscles in the contralateral limb. Noxious stimuli will cause the affected limb to withdraw but the opposite limb to extend. Because this reflex can be initiated by other than noxious stimuli, it is likely that it may be normally elicited during such activities as walking and running, as well as in withdrawal from painful stimuli.

Although local reflex control of spinal motor neurons exists in the human, the nervous system has evolved to the point that descending pathways dominate the expression of these reflexes and, consequently, motor activity. This is demonstrated by the observation that immediately after transection of the cervical spinal cord, all reflex activity within the cord is suppressed, and the patient suffers spinal shock (Landau & O'Leary, 1983). Presumably, descending excitatory input to the spinal cord interneurons is necessary for sufficient stimulation of the alpha motor neurons. In time, however, the cord reflexes reappear and may even be expressed in a hyperactive form.

Spinal Cord Tracts

In addition to the reflex neuronal connections within the spinal cord, the cord provides a vehicle by which information from higher neuronal centers is conveyed to the spinal motor neurons. These descending pathways affect muscle movement either directly by synapsing onto alpha motor neurons or indirectly by synapsing onto interneurons or gamma motor neurons. The descending pathways can be grouped into two categories, the lateral and the medial systems.

Descending in the lateral system are the corticospinal and rubrospinal tracts. Some of the fibers in the corticospinal tract make direct synaptic connection with alpha motor neurons that control the distal musculature. This tract, therefore, is largely concerned with fine independent movements, especially of the fingers and thumbs. The rubrospinal tract is concerned largely with control of the distal musculature. The medial system contains fibers that originate in the vestibular nuclei, the recticular formation, and the tectum. These descending pathways are concerned primarily with controlling neck and trunk muscles and the more proximal muscles of the limbs (Netter, 1983).

Motor Cortex

The corticospinal fibers arise in part from the primary motor cortex, which is located in the frontal lobe anterior to the central sulcus. Direct electrical stimulation of the motor cortex causes discrete muscle movements on the contralateral side of the body. Mapping of the motor cortex in this manner demonstrates the motor homunculus, an image of the body projected on the cortex (Guyton, 1987). The area of the motor cortex devoted to any individual body part is proportional to the degree of cortical influence over that structure rather than to the size of the part. Consequently, the hand has a disproportionately large cortical representation. The leg is represented on the medial surface of the motor cortex, followed by the trunk, arm, and hand. The cortical area controlling the face is located laterally. As mentioned, the cerebral cortex, via its projections in the corticospinal tract, is involved in the control of the distal musculature and is, therefore, involved with those movements that are least automated. It mediates fine hand movements.

The effects of lesions in the primary motor cortex depend specifically on the location and extent of the damage. Primary motor cortex lesions or damage isolated to the corticospinal or pyramidal tract, however, give rise to signs typically associated with suprasegmental (upper motor neuron) lesions. In general, there is a weakness of the involved muscles, loss of skilled movements, and an unwillingness to use the affected limb. The involved muscles initially may demonstrate decreased tone but eventually will become spastic. This hyperexcitability is presumably due to loss of inhibitory inputs that normally originate in the suprasegmental motor neurons to influence the alpha motor neurons. With cortical lesions, there is the appearance of pathologic reflexes, such as the Babinski reflex, which are caused by the increased excitability of the alpha motor neurons (Landau & O'Leary, 1983).

Brainstem Nuclei

The rubrospinal tract originates mainly from the red nucleus in the midbrain. The axons from this nucleus cross the midline immediately, then descend the spinal cord in the posterolateral funiculus just anterior to the lateral corticospinal tract. These axons predominantly influence the motor neurons supplying the distal musculature and synapse on interneurons that facilitate both gamma and alpha motor neurons. The red nucleus itself receives the majority of its input from the cerebral cortex and the cerebellum (Netter, 1983).

Neurons in the brainstem that project to the spinal cord via reticulospinal tracts originate in the pontine and medullary reticular formation. The pontine neurons project via the medial reticulospinal tract and are predominantly facilitory to flexor motor neurons and those neurons innervating proximal and axial muscles. In the medullary reticulospinal system, most of the fibers terminate on interneurons. The exact function of these neurons is not known, but in general they are not concerned with fine, skilled voluntary movements but rather with instinctual reactions and postural adjustments (Netter, 1983).

Basal Ganglia

The basal ganglia are groups of neurons located at the base of the cerebrum, which are organized into pairs of nuclei, the caudate nucleus, the putamen, and the globus pallidus and functionally include the subthalamic nuclei and the substantia nigra. These structures, along with the cerebellum and their various connecting pathways, are generally referred to as the extrapyramidal motor system. The basal ganglia receive their afferent input from the cerebral cortex, the thalamus, and the substantia nigra. The major output from the basal ganglia is to the substantia nigra and to the thalamus and from there to the cerebral cortex and to reticular formation in the brainstem (Barr & Kiernan, 1983).

The connections of the basal ganglia are complex. They do not project directly to the spinal cord; therefore, their influence on motor activity is indirect and the exact function of the basal ganglia is not clearly worked out. Lesions in the basal ganglia give rise to movement disorders, either too much or too little movement, and disturbances in muscle tone. An excess of movement can be called hyperkinesia or dyskinesia. Deficiency of movement can be called bradykinesia, akinesia, or hypokinesia and generally is present in parkinsonism.

Output from the basal ganglia plays an important role in the initiation of movement. The basal ganglia also are important in determining the balance of alpha and gamma motor neuron activity. Consequently, disorders of the basal ganglia may be manifested as inability to initiate movements, excessively slow movements, abnormalities of muscle tone, or tremor. The basal ganglia are necessary for the smooth coordination of voluntary movement as well as for the initiation of voluntary movements, the maintenance of posture and muscle tone, the regulation of postural reflexes, and the conduction of automatic movements (Walton, 1981).

Parkinson's disease provides a good and clinically important example of basal ganglia dysfunction. Parkinson's disease is associated with the degeneration of neurons in the substantia nigra. The substantia nigra is the source of neurons that synthesize the transmitter dopamine. Dopaminergic fibers project to the caudate nucleus and putamen and appear to exert a modulator effect on the level of excitability there. One of the consequences of dopamine depletion in the striatum is that the output from neurons in the globus pallidus occurs tonically rather than physically with movement. This enhanced discharge from the globus pallidus presumably is responsible for symptoms seen in Parkinson's disease, which include rigidity, hypokinesia, and tremor at rest (Fahn, 1984).

Cerebellum

The cerebellum is necessary neither for sensory perception nor for the initiation of movement, but it plays an integral role in motor control. The cerebellum is involved in the timing, duration, and strength of movements and is essential for the fine coordination of movement and the ability to judge distances.

The cerebellum receives afferent information from the vestibular system, from proprioceptors and exteroceptors in the limbs, from the brainstem, and indirectly from the cerebral cortex via relays in the pons. The efferent pathways from the cerebellum project to the brainstem and thalamus and via these areas influence activity in the cerebral cortex and spinal cord (Netter, 1983). Basically, the cerebellum monitors both ongoing afferent information and ongoing information within the motor systems. The cerebellum compares the intended signal with what is actually happening. If the two sets of information do not match, the cerebellum sends a signal to correct the ongoing motor activity and make it appropriate. Lesions in the cerebellum, therefore, produce abnormalities in movement that may be related to interference with vestibular function and cause difficulties with equilibrium and gait, or ataxia. Cerebellar dysfunction also may impair the ability to produce smooth, coordinated movements. With cerebellar damage, there may be decomposition of movement such that muscles act in an isolated rather than a coordinated manner, producing a clumsiness in the motion. The ability to stop movements accurately at the appropriate time can be affected, causing dysmetria. Difficulties with timing and sequencing of movements in cerebellar damage may produce an intention tremor. Also affected by cerebellar damage is the ability to produce rapidly alternating movements, or adiadochokinesia (Lothman and Montgomery, 1984).

Aging and Motor Function

During the aging process, many characteristic changes take place in the motor systems. The elderly often assume a flexed posture and display muscle rigidity, tremor, and a slowness in movements. Disease processes often compound the normal processes of aging, making it difficult to delineate normal from abnormal changes, while adding to the functional motor deficits.

Among the known structural alterations that occur with increasing age are a decrease in brain weight and a decrease in the number of synapses. The neuronal loss is not uniform throughout the central nervous system, and certain areas of the nervous system are involved more frequently in the degenerative changes than other areas. The affected areas commonly include the caudate nucleus, the putamen, the substantia nigra, and the dentate nucleus of the cerebellum (Teravinen & Calne, 1983). The neuronal degeneration in these motor centers presumably contributes to the decline in the motor performance seen in the aged. Among the motor areas affected by aging are those areas also affected in Parkinson's disease. Consequently, some of the motor deficits commonly seen in aging are personified in Parkinsonism. The decline in the number of synapses, along with a decrease in the maximum conduction velocity of peripheral nerves, may contribute to the prolonged reaction time and movement time also characteristic of the elderly. Once again, however, it is difficult to separate the effects of the normal aging process from the effects of physical inactivity.

As more research is carried out on healthy, aged individuals, the effects of normal aging on motor function will be distinguished from the effects of physical inactivity. Identification of the normal process may then open avenues for research into the prevention of degenerative nervous system changes that impair motor functions in the elderly.

Compensated Movement

When an individual has a disruption of the neuromuscular system that results in loss of movement, compensated movement can occur through assistive devices or assistance by others in the environment. According to data from the National Health Survey (1980), 6.5 million people require 8 million assistive devices to increase mobility. The determinants for using these devices should include a comprehensive assessment of the combined neurologic, orthopedic, and functional aspects affecting the body during ambulation. Assistive devices can help improve ambulation by the use of a better gait pattern and stance phase of gait (Rinehart, 1983).

In 1977, over 645,000 people in our society relied on wheelchairs to increase their mobility and functioning. An investment of more than $500 million in wheelchairs was reported in 1983, with the average cost of each chair estimated at approximately $800 (Kohn et al., 1983). Such costs as these require that equipment be adapted as precisely as possible to the person and the environment so that maximum benefit can be realized.

Major considerations in the purchase of assistive devices are the degree of limited movement for which the device will be used, the size and style of the assistive device, and the environment in which the device must be maneuvered. Additional considerations include further growth of the individual, course of the disease, accessibility to repair shops, proximity to rehabilitation or medical facilities, and changes in housing and caretaker arrangements (Kohn et al., 1983).

When the individual is unable to move himself or herself, the nurse or family member may compensate for the lack of movement through a number of activities. To prevent and treat disuse phenomena associated with immobility, people in the disabled individual's environment can participate in (1) body positioning, (2) joint mobility exercises, (3) muscle conditioning exercises, and (4) environmental structuring (Mitchell & Loustau, 1981). The degree and use of specific measures by people in the environment are directly related to the patient's ability and the nature of the immobility phenomenon. These measures are discussed in more detail in Chapters 20 and 21.

ROLE OF MOTIVATION IN MOBILITY

In many cases, the inability of a person to move in a normal fashion can be related to a lack of motivation. The lack of motivation may result from a temporary change in equilibrium, an adaptive response to demands operating in the environment, or the presence of emotional–motivational blocks.

A lack of motivation to move is often associated with psychologic disequilibrium. A common symptom of depression is limited movement, termed psychomotor retardation. Severely depressed people often take to their beds and must be forced to participate in physical activity. Perhaps the classic example of immobility associated with mental disequilibrium is found in people in a catatonic state (Stuart & Sundeen, 1983).

Normal patterns of increased and decreased activity are associated with temporary changes in equilibrium. During periods of minor illness, a decrease in activity is a natural response as the body tries to conserve energy needed for healing. After intense emotional, social, or physical activity, fatigue, our body's signal to rest, decreases our motivation for activity. Activities that conserve energy help to restore our physical bodies and emotional and psychologic reserves. A reduction in movement can bring back a sense of equilibrium with the environment.

Often movement declines as a mechanism of adaptation to environmental changes. When there is a discrepancy in the amount of energy a person has and the demand an environment requires for interaction, the person with limited energy must decrease movement in order to cope. For example, a stroke victim with a weak left side who lives on the second floor may decrease movement in the environment because it is no longer possible to maneuver the stairs without severe fatigue. When an environment is characterized by overwhelming psychologic or social demands, a person usually withdraws. By decreasing physical movement and interaction with others, stress is reduced and energy is restored.

Emotional–motivational blocks in children have been cited as a major cause of poor motor functioning (Stott & Moyes, 1985). In these children, a physical handicap may be the primary reason for poor motor performance. A fear of failure, however, magnifies the effects of the physical handicap. The vicious cycle that follows takes on different forms in accordance with the child's personality. The child who lacks confidence may exhibit a frozen inhibition; the child who is easily distracted has difficulty following instructions and thinking ahead about the steps in a task. The end result in both types of children is a defeatist attitude: "I can't do it." Strategies to help overcome these emotional–motivational blocks are necessary to encourage maximum mobility in a child with a physical handicap.

ENVIRONMENT AND MOBILITY

In some instances, restricted movement can be related to barriers in the environment. A person may have an intact neuromuscular system and the motivation to move about but be faced with an environmental restraint to movement. Examples include the patient in traction, the person with a cast, and those confined to bedrest.

Barriers to movement commonly exist as a component of buildings and structures. In recent years, many of these barriers have come down because of passage of a series of federal laws aimed at enhancing the quality of life for disabled Americans. A major piece of legislation, the Architectual Barrier Bill, was signed into law by President Johnson on August 12, 1968. This law provides full access to any facility wholly or partly financed by federal funds and intended for public use. The law also included buildings to be used for employment or as residences of disabled persons. In 1973, the Rehabilitation Act of 1973 was passed. This law extends to America's disabled all programs, services and benefits that are federally funded. Access to education and job–teaching programs were written into the regulations (DeJong & Lifchez, 1983).

At present, the status of disabled people is somewhat uncertain because of the reluctance on the part of the Reagan administration to enforce laws written to protect the disabled over the last 18 years. The state of the present economy has created some doubt in the minds of taxpayers about the need for an accessible, barrier-free environment. The move to create a barrier-free environment, like many other social programs, has been influenced by retrenchment in federal expenditures.

A barrier-free environment includes the concept of freedom from physical barriers and psychologic barriers. Perhaps one of the greatest barriers to movement is the attitude of others in a person's space. According to Lombama (1980), negative attitudes toward people with disabilities are common throughout all areas of our society. Elliott and Byrd (1982) cited television as one media source that reinforces negative attitudes through misinformation about disabilities and dramatization of negative disabled stereotypes.

Livneh (1982) developed a classification system according to the sources of negative attitudes toward the disabled. He concluded that because of the complexity of factors interacting in the creation of negative attitudes, short-duration interventions aimed at attitude change were futile.

In our efforts to intervene in the environment to create freedom for mobility, political strategies and public education are needed. The attitude of the family, the neighbors, and those in the community must be positive if disabled people with limited mobility are to overcome isolation and find freedom of movement within others' space. Efforts to influence policy at the local, state, and federal level should be viewed as part of nursing intervention in the community if the immobilized are to live in a barrier-free world.

SUMMARY

The ability to move with purpose and freedom within the environment is dependent on an intact neuromuscular system, the presence of assistive aids and people to help when physical limitations are present, a desire to move, and a free nonrestrictive environment. Absence of any of these components can result in disuse syndrome and the resulting consequences of immobility. Since nursing encompasses Nightingale's philosophy of nursing the patient as well as the environment, a comprehensive assessment of each of these components inherent in the concept of mobility is needed if appropriate nursing interventions are to be instituted. Chapter 19 provides a general framework for assessing mobility, Chapter 20 delineates appropriate nursing interventions in the care of people responding to conditions causing acute immobility, and Chapter 21 discusses those who live with chronic immobility as a part of their daily lives.

REFERENCES

Barr, M., & Kiernan, J. (1983). *The human nervous system: An anatomical viewpoint* (4th ed.). Philadelphia: Harper & Row.

Bates, B. (1987). *A guide to physical examination* (4th ed.). Philadelphia: Lippincott.

Beckman, C., Axtell, L., Noland, K., & West, J. (1985). Self-concept: An outcome of a program for spinal pain. *Pain, 22,* 59.

Bullock, J., Boyle, J., Wang, W., & Ajello, R. (1984). *Physiology.* New York: Wiley.

DeJong, G., & Lifchez, R. (1983). Physical disability and public policy. *Scientific American, 248*(6).

Elliott, T.R., & Byrd, E.K. (1982). Media and disability. *Rehabilitation Literature, 43* (11–12), 348.

Fahn, S. (1984). Extrapyramidal system. In E.D. Frohlich (Ed.), *Pathophysiology: Altered regulatory mechanisms in disease* (3rd ed.) (p. 771). Philadelphia: Lippincott.

Guyton, A.C. (1987). *Basic Neuroscience: Anatomy and Physiology.* Philadelphia: Saunders.

Hodges, L. (1977). *Body image and bladder care in cord injured.* Atlanta: Emory University, unpublished thesis.

Hodges, L. (1978). Human sexuality and the spinal cord injured: Role of the clinical nurse specialist. *Journal of Neurosurgical Nursing, 10* (3), 125.

Kohn, J., Enders, S., Preston, J., & Matlock, W. (1983). Provision of assistive equipment for handicapped persons. *Archives of Physical Medicine Rehabilitation, 64,* 378.

Landau, W.M., & O'Leary, J.L. (1983). Disturbances of movement. In R.S. Blacklow (Ed.), *MacBryde's signs and symptoms: Applied pathologic physiology and clinical interpretation* (6th ed.) (p. 669). Philadelphia: Lippincott.

Livneh, H. (1982). On the origins of negative attitudes toward people with disabilities. *Rehabilitation Literature, 43* (11–12), 338.

LiVolsi, V.A., Merino, M.J., Neumann, R.G., & Duray, P.H. (1984). *Pathology.* New York: Wiley.

Lombana, J. (1980). Fostering positive attitudes toward handicapped students: A guidance challenge. *School Counselor, 27* (3), 176.

Lothman, E.W., & Montgomery, E.B. (1984). Control of motor activity by the cerebrum and cerebellum. In E.D. Frohlich (Ed.), *Pathophysiology: Altered regulatory mechanisms in disease* (3rd ed.) (p. 741). Philadelphia: Lippincott.

Mitchell, P., & Loustau, A. (1981). *Concepts basic to nursing*. New York: McGraw-Hill.

Nagy, B., & Samaha, F.J. (1984). Physiology of normal and diseased muscle. In E.D. Frohlich (Ed.). *Pathophysiology: Altered regulatory mechanisms in disease* (p. 805). Philadelphia: Lippincott.

National Health Interview Statistics. (1980). Use of special aids. 1977 Vital and Health Statistics, Series 10, Number 135, U.S. Department of HHS, DHHS, Pub. No. (FHS) 81-1563, October 1980.

Netter, F.H. (1983). In A. Brass & R.V. Single (Eds.), *Nervous system. Part I. Anatomy and physiology*. CIBA.

Penn, A.S. (1984). Neuromuscular junction. In E.D. Frohlich (Ed.), *Pathophysiology: Altered regulatory mechanisms in disease* (3rd ed.) (p. 789). Philadelphia: Lippincott.

Rinehart, M.A. (1983). Considerations for functional training in adults after head injury. *Physical Therapy, 63* (12), 1975.

Robbins, S.L., Cotran, R.S., & Kumar, V. (1984). *Pathologic basis of disease* (3rd ed.). Philadelphia: Saunders.

Stott, D.H., & Moyes, F.A. (1985). Treatment strategies for emotional–motivational blocks to motor functioning in children. *Physical Therapy, 65*(6), 915.

Stuart, B., & Sudeen, S. (1983). *Principles and practice of psychiatric nursing*. St. Louis: Mosby.

Teravinen, H., & Calne, D.B. (1983). Motor system in normal aging and Parkinson's disease. In R. Katzman & R. Terry (Eds.). *The neurology of aging* (p. 85). Philadelphia: Davis.

Tyler, R. (1949). *Basic principles of curriculum and instruction*. Chicago: University of Chicago Press.

Walton, J.N. (1981). Neurology. In L.H. Smith & S.O. Thieu (Eds.), *Pathophysiology: The biological principles of disease* (p. 1265). Philadelphia: Saunders.

Weinberg, J. (1982). Human sexuality and spinal cord injury. *Nursing Clinics of North America, 17* (3), 407.

19

Assessment of Human Mobility

Ann D. Hollerbach

Movement may be defined as a form of voluntary and automatic coordinated skeletal muscle activity that is essential for carrying out the tasks of daily living. It is a highly complex process involving the interaction of man with the environment. The musculoskeletal system provides structure, support, stability, and protection for movement, and the central nervous system provides the necessary neural innervation. The capability for movement is facilitated by the individual's internal motivation and a free, nonrestrictive environment.

Therefore, the physiologic, psychosocial, and environmental components must be considered when assessing mobility (Fig. 19-1). A holistic approach to assessment should be used, including a thorough nursing history, neuromuscular examination related to functional status of mobility, and assessment of the individual's role-related activities.

FUNCTIONAL ASSESSMENT

Lawton (1971) defined functional assessment as "any systematic attempt to measure objectively the level at which a person is function-

Ability to move		Motivation to move
	MOBILITY	
	Free, nonrestrictive environment	

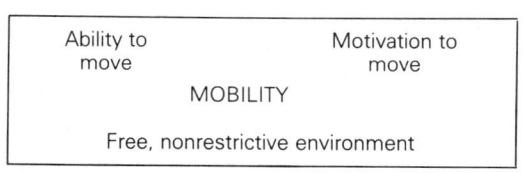

Figure 19-1. Three elements essential for mobility.

ing in any of a variety of areas such as physical health, quality of self-maintenance, quality of role activity, intellectual status, social activity, attitude toward the world and toward self, and emotional status" (p. 466). Sarno et al. (1973) emphasized that the level of the individual's physical function is not a true indicator of the individual's ability to function in life.

Although many instruments have been developed to assess specific mobility functions, a systematic approach to functional assessment of mobility is lacking in the literature. Specific instruments developed for functional assessment in conjunction with the physical examination can be grouped into three categories: (1) *global instruments,* which focus on a comprehensive assessment of an individual's functional status, such as PULSES (Granger & Gresham, 1984) and the Functional Life Scale (FLS) (Sarno et al., 1973), (2) the *activities of daily living (ADL)* scales, such as the Katz Index of ADL (Katz et al., 1963) and the Barthel Index (Mahoney & Barthel, 1965), and (3) *functional profiles*, which enable one to assess a particular disease or condition or to evaluate a single functional parameter, such as the Jebsen Test for Hand Function (Jebsen et al., 1969). The ADL scales are used most frequently to assess mobility functions.

Recently, health care team members have recognized that one problem with developing a comprehensive tool has been a lack of standard terminology and classification for the term disability. In 1967, Townsend (cited in Granger & Gresham, 1984) presented five very distinct meanings for "disability."

1. Anatomical, physiological, or psychological abnormality;
2. A chronic clinical condition altering or interrupting normal physiological or psychological processes;
3. A functional limitation of ordinary activity;
4. A pattern of behavior of a socially deviant kind;
5. A socially defined position or status, usually of inferiority. (p. 7)

Nagi (1965) concluded that the pattern of disabling behavior is influenced in three ways:

1. The effect of the pathologic condition
2. The individual's perception of the situation
3. The perception of the situation by the family, significant others, and health care professionals

Granger (1984) developed a conceptual model (Fig. 19-2) for functional assessment based on the Nagi (1965) and the Wood and Badley (1978) disability models. This model is helpful in sythesizing a framework for assessing the functional status of mobility.

Granger's model (1984) focuses on collecting data to gain a profile of the whole person, including medical status, status in performance of tasks, and fulfillment of social roles, together with knowledge of the individual's level of social supports. This database provides a framework for an orderly review of the needs at the organ, person, and societal levels. These needs are important to the use of skills, the accomplishment of tasks, the fulfillment of social roles, and a satisfactory quality of life.

Functional assessment of the aged is a particular concern for nurses, and Granger's model is applicable for evaluating ADL if expanded to include *instrumental activities*, such as housekeeping, taking medications, transportation, financial management, and care of pets. Thompson and Bowers (1984) have presented an ADL assessment for geriatric clients that is inclusive of many of the instrumental activities. It is a helpful adjunct for identifying needs of the aged (Table 19-1).

The examiner must assess not only the individual's reaction to the impairment or disability but also the effect it has on the individual's performance. Essential components of a functional assessment tool for mobility should include (1) determination of any neuromuscular disabilities, (2) evaluation of independence in self-care and mobility, (3) evaluation of social support, including environmental factors (housing, architectural barriers, and transportation) and financial resources, (4) social interactions and performance of social roles or obligations, psychologic outlook, and coping techniques, family or significant others, and (5) work or educational training.

Mitchell and Irvin (1977) proposed a model for the neurologic assessment that goes beyond the medical model used to identify and diagnose neurologic dysfunction. The instrument is used to assess the functional abilities of the patient in relation to neurologic status. The instrument is directed specifically at the nurse's primary purpose, which is to determine (1) the presence of neurologic dysfunction and (2) the effect that the dysfunction has on the individual's ability to perform

	ORGAN LEVEL	PERSON LEVEL	SOCIETAL LEVEL
CONDITIONS:	PATHOLOGY Anatomic, physiologic, mental, and psychological deficits *determine*	BEHAVIORAL Performance deficits within the physical and social environments *contribute to*	ROLE ASSIGNMENT Environments and societal deficits influenced by norms and societal policy *create*
KEY TERMS:	IMPAIRMENT Organic dysfunction	DISABILITY Difficulty with tasks	HANDICAP Social disadvantage

Limitations in using skills, performing activities, and fulfilling social roles

ANALYSIS:	Selected diagnostic descriptors	Selected performance (behavioral) descriptors	Selected role descriptors

Functional assessment of abilities and activities

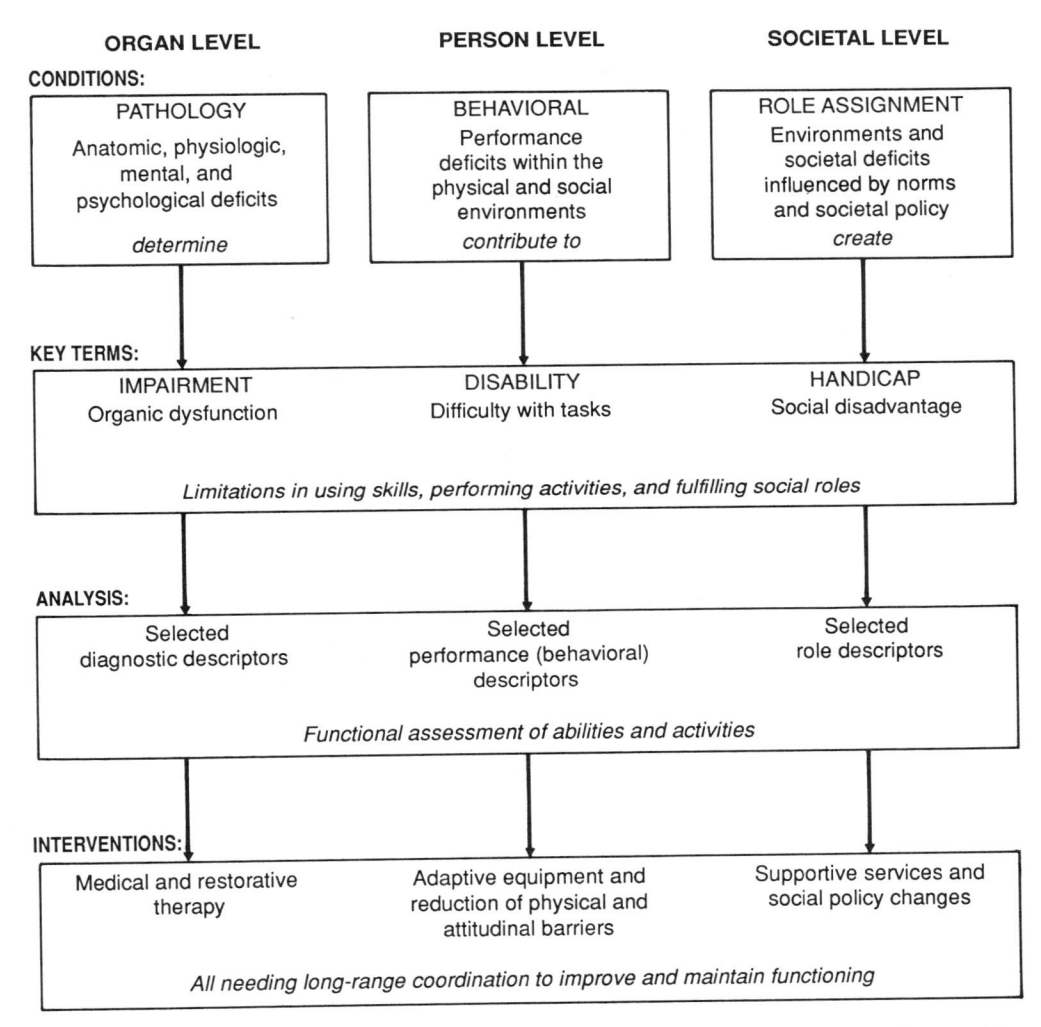

INTERVENTIONS:	Medical and restorative therapy	Adaptive equipment and reduction of physical and attitudinal barriers	Supportive services and social policy changes

All needing long-range coordination to improve and maintain functioning

Figure 19–2. Relationship of functional assessment to the impairment, disability, and handicap model. In the upper half of the diagram, concepts are related horizontally across the three levels of concern: the organ, person, and societal levels. Pathology, manifested as various forms of deficits, determines IMPAIRMENT. DISABILITY is the central person concept, and HANDICAP is the social disadvantage consequent to impairment and disability. The lower half of the figure illustrates functional assessment related to this modified version of Nagi's (1965) and Wood and Badley's (1978) disability models. The most important measure is that of performance related to impairment, disability, and handicap. *(From Granger, 1984.)*

self-care as well as the effect on self-image and safety. The model, as expanded by Mitchell, et al. (1984), consists of six functional categories: (1) consciousness, (2) mentation, (3) movement, (4) sensation, (5) integrated regulation, and (6) coping with disability. This model is used to focus on the basic assessment of movement of the stable, conscious patient. The integrated functions of seeing, speaking, moving, and walking are evaluated fully

TABLE 19–1. ACTIVITIES OF DAILY LIVING (ADL) ASSESSMENT FOR GERIATRIC CLIENTS.

	Yes	No	Comments
A. Self-care			
1. Dressing, undressing, clothing			
a. Keeping clothes in good repair (mending)			
b. Access to clothes			
c. Getting into and out of underwear (bra, girdle, underpants, pantyhose, stockings, garter belt)			
d. Putting on and removing pants			
e. Getting arms in sleeves			
f. Managing zippers, buttons, snaps (especially in back), ties			
g. Putting on socks, shoes, tying laces			
h. Applying prostheses (e.g., glasses, hearing aids)			
2. Grooming and hygiene			
a. Washing, drying, brushing hair			
b. Brushing teeth			
c. Cleaning and putting in dentures			
d. Shaving			
e. Nail care (feet and hands)			
f. Applying makeup			
g. Preparing bath water and testing temperature			
h. Getting into and out of tub, shower			
i. Reaching and cleaning all body parts			
3. Elimination			
a. Position altered for urination or sitting on toilet			
b. Ability to wipe self			
B. Mobility			
1. Difficulty climbing or descending stairs (is bedroom/bathroom on upper level? How many stairs/flights to apartment or house?)			
2. Sitting up, rising from bed			
3. Lowering to or rising from chair			
4. Walking (short and long distances, describe necessity for walking)			

TABLE 19–1. ACTIVITIES OF DAILY LIVING (ADL) ASSESSMENT FOR GERIATRIC CLIENTS. *(Cont.)*

			Yes	No	Comments
	5.	Opening doors			
	6.	Reaching items in cupboards			
	7.	Necessity for lifting (and any difficulty)			
C.	Communication			
	1.	Dialing telephone			
	2.	Reading numbers			
	3.	Hearing over telephone			
	4.	Answering door			
	5.	Immediate access to neighbors, help			
D.	Eating (see nutritional section for details about appetite, weight, food consumption)			
	1.	Access to market			
	2.	Preparing food (opening cans, packages, using stove, reaching dishes, pots, utensils)			
	3.	Handling knife, fork, spoon (cutting meat)			
	4.	Getting food to mouth			
	5.	Chewing, swallowing			
E.	Housekeeping, laundry, house upkeep			
	1.	Making bed			
	2.	Sweeping, mopping floors			
	3.	Dusting			
	4.	Cleaning dishes			
	5.	Cleaning tub, bathroom			
	6.	Picking up clutter (to client's satisfaction)			
	7.	Taking out trash, garbage			
	8.	Use of basement (stairs, cleaning)			
	9.	Laundry facilities (in home or near residence, washtub, clothesline)			
	10.	Yard care (garden, bushes, grass)			
	11.	Other home maintenance concerns (e.g., access to fuse box, storm windows, furnace filters, painting)			

(Continued)

TABLE 19–1. ACTIVITIES OF DAILY LIVING (ADL) ASSESSMENT FOR GERIATRIC CLIENTS. *(Cont.)*

			Yes	No	Comments
F.	Medications				
	1.	Large number of prescriptions			
	2.	Difficulty remembering			
	3.	Able to see labels and directions			
	4.	Medications kept in one area			
G.	Access to community				
	1.	Busline			
	2.	Walking			
	3.	Driving (self or service from others)			
	4.	Church, dry cleaning, drugstore, bank, health care facility, dentist, other community agencies			
H.	Other				
	1.	Caring for spouse/relative/companion			
	2.	Financial management (able to write checks, make payments, cash checks)			
	3.	Care of pet(s)			

Reproduced by permission from J.M. Thompson and A.C. Bowers. Clinical Manual of Health Assessment *(2nd ed.). St. Louis, 1984, The C.V. Mosby Co.*

(Table 19–2). Since the focus of this examination is primarily on the individual's function in relation to self-care, the cranial nerves and motor reflexes are integrated into the functions they serve.

The Mitchell et al. model (1984) does not specifically assess skills and activities, so the Barthel Index, which is a simple index of independence in self-care and mobility, is integrated into the assessment (Mahoney & Barthel, 1965). The Barthel Index (Table 19–3) is a reliable and valid clinical tool for establishing a functional baseline for the patient, monitoring improvement throughout rehabilitation, and identifying the point of maximum benefit therapy. The Barthel Index consists of 10 weighted ADL variables and has a maximum score of 100 for functional competence. The value assigned to each item is determined by the amount of help given in self-care activities and mobility if the person is unable to perform the activity unassisted. The patient's ability to perform independently each activity is scored, and the 10 items are tallied. The index is a beneficial adjunct for periodic assessment of self-care activities, such as feeding, bathing, personal toilet, dressing, bowel and bladder control, and mobility, such as transfers, ambulation, and stair climbing. A major disadvantage to those with a holistic approach to nursing is that the Barthel Index does not include assessment of psychosocial or environmental factors. It has, however, been stressed that the evaluator should recognize

TABLE 19–2. ASSESSMENT OF MOVEMENT.

Functional Category	Anatomic Correlates	Tests
Head		
Seeing (motor aspects)	Oculomotor (III), trochlear (IV), abducens (VI) nerves and brainstem pathways, the cerebellum	Extraocular movements
Eating		
Chewing	Trigeminal (V) and hypoglossal (XII) nerves	Chewing, jaw opening, moving tongue
Swallowing	Glossopharyngeal (IX) and vagal (X) nerves	Swallowing
Expressing	Facial (VII) nerve	Facial movements (eye closing, smile, frown)
Speaking		
Articulating	Facial (VII), glossopharyngeal (IX), vagal (X), and hypoglossal (XII) nerves and the cerebellum	"ma," "la," "ca"
Phonating	Vagal (X) nerve	Vocal sounds "ah," soft palate elevation
The above functions involve 8 of the 12 cranial nerves.		
Body		
Walking	Cortex, basal ganglia, pyramidal and extrapyramidal systems, cerebellum	Observation of gait—arm swing, rhythm, symmetry, coordination
Activities of daily living	As above	Muscle strength testing, assessment of bulk/tone, observation of movement excesses/deficits (involuntary movements, bradykinesia)
Coordination	Cerebellum	Finger–nose, heel–shin, rapid alternating movements, tandem walking, Romberg

From Mitchell et al., 1984.

that these can have an effect on the client's score. Any psychosocial or special requirements should be documented, since they can cause a lower score, for example, bathroom door not wide enough for easy access by wheelchair.

For purposes of this discussion, three essential elements for mobility are required: (1) the ability to move (an intact neuromuscular system or compensated movement), (2) the motivation to move, and (3) a free, nonrestrictive environment in which to move. A workable framework for assessing mobility would include (1) the physical dimensions of mobility (voluntary, involuntary, and compensated) related to functional ability, (2) psychosocial dimension (motivational aspects), and (3) environmental dimensions (assessment of the environment for barriers, assistive devices, and helpers to offer passive movement).

PHYSICAL DIMENSION OF MOBILITY

The assessment should begin by gathering pertinent health history data. Biographical data, such as age, are important parameters, since some neurologic disorders occur most commonly within certain age groups. For example, Parkinson's disease occurs most commonly in people over 40 years of age. Family history is important, since some neurologic disorders may be inherited, and a genogram may be helpful to fully visualize the family history. Other helpful history data regarding

TABLE 19–3. ADAPTATION OF CRITERIA FOR BARTHEL INDEX AS MODIFIED BY THE NEW ENGLAND REHABILITATION HOSPITAL, OCTOBER, 1973.

Index Item	Description of Functional Ability	Score Weight
Feeding	Independent. Able to apply any necessary device. Feeds in reasonable time. Needs help, e.g., for cutting.	10 5
Bathing	Performs without assistance.	5
Personal toilet (grooming)	Washes face, combs hair, brushes teeth, shaves (manages plug if electric razor).	5
Dressing	Independent, ties shoes, fastens fasteners, applies braces. Needs help but does at least half of task within reasonable time.	10 5
Bowel control	No accidents. Able to use enema or suppository if needed. Occasional accidents or needs help with enema or suppository.	10 5
Bladder control	No accidents. Able to care for collecting device if used. Occasional accidents or needs help with device.	10 5
Toilet transfers	Independent with toilet or bedpan. Handles clothes, wipes, flushes or cleans pan. Needs help for balance, handling clothes or toilet paper.	10 5
Chair–bed transfers	Independent, including locks of wheelchair and lifting footrests. Minimum assistance or supervision. Able to sit but needs maximum assistance to transfer.	15 10 5
Ambulation	Independent for 50 yards. May use assistive devices, except for rolling walker. With help for 50 yards. Independent with wheelchair for 50 yards, only if unable to walk.	15 10 5
Stair climbing	Independent. May use assistive devices. Needs help or supervision.	10 5
TOTAL SCORE		

From Granger et al., 1979.

musculoskeletal and neurologic function, available energy, nutritional status, and cardiopulmonary status should be assessed (Table 19–4).

Equipment needed for the examination includes (1) tape measure, (2) goniometer (optional), (3) percussion hammer, (4) Snellen chart or reading material, (5) penlight, (6) cotton swab, and (7) tongue depressor. An overall screening examination of neurologic function can be conducted in approximately 5 minutes if no abnormalities are identified (Table 19–5). This is invaluable in assessing functional abilities as well as dysfunction and its location.

If abnormalities in movement are identified, a thorough mobility assessment is needed. The examination proceeds in a systematic head-to-toe fashion, focusing on the integrated functions of seeing, eating and speaking, moving and walking, activities of daily living, and coordination (Table 19–2).

Seeing

The sensory components of seeing (pupillary response, visual acuity, and visual fields) are described in Chapter 23. For practical reasons, they would be examined at the same time as the motor components.

Extraocular muscle function is tested by examining corneal light reflex, cover–uncover test, and six cardinal fields of gaze. To test the client's corneal light reflex, the examiner stands in front of the client and shines a penlight, held 12 to 15 inches away, between the eyes. The bright dot reflected on the cornea should be located in the same spot on each eye, indicating a symmetrical reflex. If there is an asymmetrical reflex, a muscular imbalance could be the cause of the deviating eye.

TABLE 19–4. HISTORY DATA.

Parameter	Data
Musculoskeletal function	Past or present problems with muscle strength, tone, reflexes, range of motion, motility, muscle control, or physical endurance.
	Perceptual–motor problems: soft signs, such as clumsiness, impaired fine motor coordination, increased or decreased general activity or level of minimal brain dysfunction, hyperkinesis, learning disability
	Activity level
	Aids
	Safety factors related to age or impaired mobility
	Assistance required in activities of daily living
	Description of current muscular impairment or limitation in range of motion
	Current medications that interfere with or enhance muscular functions
	Special needs related to age or impaired functions
Nervous system	Past or current problems with intellectual functions, sensation, movement, or pain
	Past or present problem that was inherited or in other family members
	Communication and speech patterns
	Current medication usage that inhibits or enhances nervous system activities
	Special needs related to age or disease process
Cardiovascular functions	Activity endurance or fatigability
	Medications used that enhance or inhibit cardiovascular functions
Respiratory functions	Past or present respiratory problems
	Shortness of breath (precipitating factors, frequency, measures that relieve symptoms, and effect on ADL)
	Medications used that enhance or inhibit respiratory function
Nutritional patterns	Evaluate adequacy and intake of basic four foods and liquids
	Special needs related to disease or age

Reproduced by permission from B. L. Conway-Rutkowski, Carini and Owen's neurological and neurosurgical nursing (8th ed.). St. Louis, 1982, The C. V. Mosby Co.

The cover–uncover test is used to evaluate the client's ability to maintain parallel gaze, which is essential for binocular vision. The examiner asks the client to gaze at a specific point. The left eye is covered with an opaque card, and the examiner observes the right eye to see if it moves to fixate on the object. If it does move, it was not in straight

TABLE 19–5. SCREENING EXAMINATION OF NEUROLOGIC FUNCTION.[a]

Examination Stimulus	Function or System Tested
Observe gait, symmetry	Motor, cerebellar, position sense
Ask: Why are you here? Has your ability to take care of yourself changed?	Perception, expectations, orientation, self-care change, coping
Read headline, tell meaning, recall later	Seeing, recall, language
Take glass of water, swallow, hand back to examiner (or any act across midline, with three components)	Swallow, right–left orientation, concentration, sensory, coordination
Dress or undress	Motor, sensory, cerebellar
Simultaneously observe language, eye movement	Language, seeing

From Mitchell et al., 1984.
[a] If no abnormality is present, this entire examination can be performed in 5 minutes.

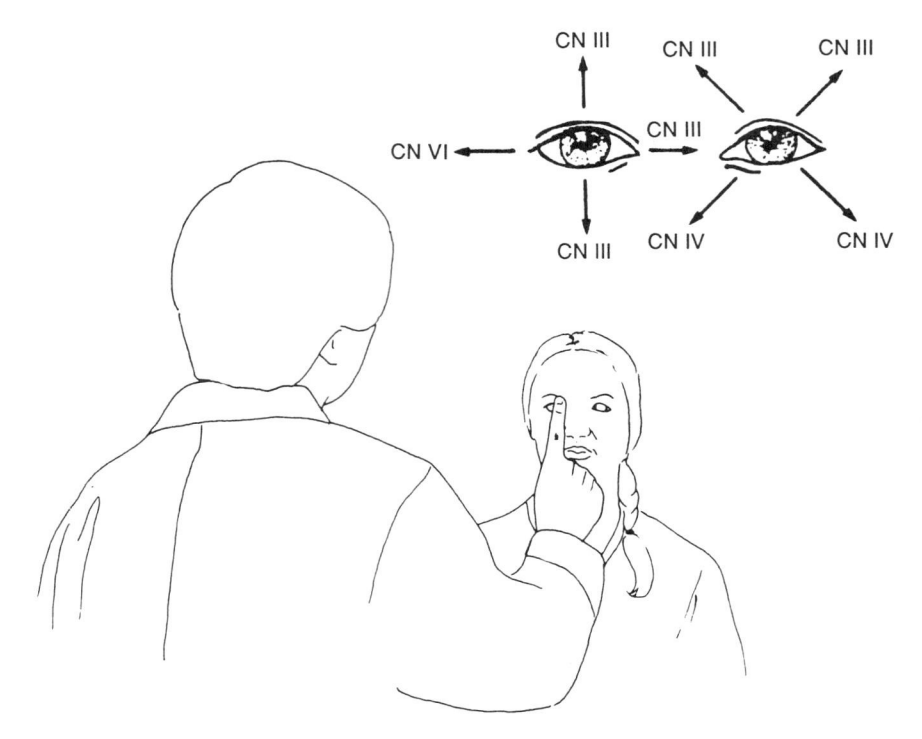

Figure 19–3. Extraocular movements. Arrows show directions in which the examiner's finger should be moved and the cranial nerve innervating that movement. Make an X and a cross across the client's field of vision. (Adapted from Mitchell et al., 1984, p. 42)

alignment. The left eye is then uncovered, and if it jerks into position to again rest on the object, the eye has drifted while resting. This is usually indicative of a muscle imbalance.

The movement of the eyes through the six cardinal fields of gaze is assessed with the examiner being certain to direct the eyes to the extremes of each field (Fig. 19–3). The examiner asks the client to follow with the eyes the tip of a pen or penlight. Nystagmus or abnormal eye movement should be noted.

Eating and Speaking

These integrated functions both require the same intact structures of the peripheral nervous system for normal functioning. For articulation, the facial (VII), glossopharyngeal (IX), vagal (X), and hypoglossal (XII) cranial nerves (CN) and the cerebellum must be intact. For chewing and swallowing, these nerves and the trigeminal nerve (V) must be intact. If a client articulates, chews, and swallows without difficulty, it can be assumed that these nerves are intact. If any difficulties are noted, the various parameters of speech and ingestion must be evaluated to identify the cranial nerve precipitating the dysfunction. Each cranial nerve can be assessed by evaluating the results of various tests.

Cranial Nerve V

The motor component of CN V (trigeminal) serves the muscles of mastication. To test this nerve, the examiner asks the client to clench all teeth, then palpates the masseter and temporal muscles bilaterally, noting symmetry and strength. Absent or weak contractions of the masseter and temporal muscles may indicate a lesion of CN V. Bilateral weakness may result from upper and lower motor neuron involvement. (The absence of teeth obviously complicates interpretation of this test.) To observe symmetry and strength of the pterygoid muscles, the examiner asks the client to open the mouth slightly and press the jaw laterally against the examiner's hand. Any atrophy or deviation of the jaw to one side is rated, and deviation indicates that the muscles of the jaw on the side to which it deviates are stronger than those on the opposite side. Movement will be noted to the opposite side of the paralysis or weakness, not to the paralyzed side.

Cranial Nerve VII
Cranial nerve VII (facial) is the motor component that innervates the facial muscles bilaterally. A sensory component to the taste perception of the anterior two thirds of the tongue also is part of the facial nerve.

To assess the function of CN VII, the examiner should inspect the face for symmetry at rest and during conversation. The client is asked to raise the eyebrows, frown, then close both eyes tightly while the examiner tries to open them. The client then is instructed to show teeth, smile, and puff out the cheeks to assess facial muscle strength, symmetry, or abnormal movements. Muscle weakness may be indicated by drooping of one side of the mouth, flattening of the nasolabial folds, or laxity of the lower eyelid.

Cranial Nerves IX and X
Cranial nerves IX (glossopharyngeal) and X (vagus) are tested clinically as a unit, since they are closely related both anatomically and physiologically and are similar in function. The motor component of CN IX innervates the stylopharyngeus muscle used in swallowing; the sensory fibers innervate the mucous membranes of the pharynx, posterior one third of the tongue, middle ear, and eustachian tube. The motor fibers of CN X innervate the pharynx, larynx, palate, and thoracic and abdominal visceral organs. The sensory fibers of the vagus innervate the heart, lungs, and aortic bodies.

The client is assessed for any hoarseness or nasal speech. The soft palate is inspected for symmetry or any deviation. The client is asked to say "Ah," with the examiner noting if the palate rises symmetrically. Unilateral weakness is indicated by drooping of the palate on the affected side. The palate fails to rise at all if a bilateral lesion of CN X is present. To assess the palatal reflex, the mucous membrane of the soft palate is stroked with a cohton swab, and the side stroked should rise promptly. When the posterior pharyngeal wall is touched with a tongue depressor or cotton swab to elicit the gag reflex, the palate should elevate and the pharyngeal muscles should contract. This reflex may be diminished or absent in some normal people.

Swallowing is assessed by giving the client a glass of water and requesting that the client take a few sips. The examiner observes the swallowing, noting any abnormalities. Ice chips can be used if there is any concern that swallowing may be impaired.

Cranial Nerve XII
Cranial nerve XII (hypoglossal) is responsible for normal tongue movements involved in speech and swallowing. The examiner inspects the tongue for size, symmetry, and fasciculations in its resting state. Then the client is asked to stick out the tongue; it should be midline without deviating to one side and should be devoid of fasciculations. A tongue blade is pressed against one side of the tongue, with the client resisting, to assess muscle strength; then the other side is assessed. Rapid alternating movements, such as moving the tongue rapidly in and out and from side to side, are assessed for symmetry. Diminished or slowed alternating movements may be caused by upper motor neuron disease.

Cranial nerves VII, IX, X, and XII must be intact for speaking. If the individual articulates clearly and without difficulty, the cranial nerves are intact. If an abnormality is noted, a more detailed examination must be performed to determine which sounds are abnormal:

Abnormality	Site
Disrupted labial sounds ("mee, bee")	CN VII
Disrupted lingual sounds ("la")	CN XII
Disrupted gutteral sounds ("ka, ga")	CN IX, X
Hoarseness	CN X
Nasal speech	CN X (Mitchell et al., 1984, p. 45)

If a deficit is noted in any of these sounds, the related cranial nerve should be evaluated (Mitchell et al., 1984).

Moving and Walking

Six areas to observe closely when assessing motor functioning, excluding the face, are (1) posture, (2) muscle coordination, (3) muscle tone, (4) muscle strength, (5) reflexes, and (6) abnormal movements.

The presence and absence of movement, as well as the quality of movement, are always assessed, and motor responses in symmetrical body parts are compared. When interpreting findings, the examiner must consider alterations due to age or unrelated disease or injury.

Posture and Coordination

In assessing gait and posture, the movement of body parts, symmetry of gait, stance, cadence, steadiness of movement, coordination, and type of steps taken if the gait is abnormal must be noted. If it is possible, the client should be observed walking, sitting in a chair, or performing ADL without the client's being aware of the observation. The need for assistive devices should be determined. The client is asked to walk heel-to-toe in a straight line; the ability to do this is impaired in cerebellar disease. The client is requested to walk on the toes, then on the heels.

Coordination is further assessed in the lower extremities by (1) rapid rhythmic alternating movements, such as tapping the examiner's hand with the ball of the foot alternately, and (2) point-to-point testing, in which the client places the foot on the opposite knee and slides it down that shin to the great toe. Note any slowness, hesitation, or awkwardness with both maneuvers.

Muscle Mass, Tone, and Strength

The examiner first inspects muscle mass, comparing symmetrical body parts, and then flexes and extends upper and lower extremities bilaterally to assess tone and resistance to movement. Muscle rigidity or spasticity is noted in increased muscle tone or increased resistance. Decreased resistance denotes decreased muscle tone or flaccidity.

To assess muscle strength of the major muscle groups, the examiner puts them through the normal range of motion, initially against gravity and then against active resistance. The strength of muscles is graded 5 to 0 based on the following standard scale:

Grade	Strength
5	Free range of motion against normal resistance and gravity
4	Full range of motion against moderate resistance and gravity
3	Full range of motion against gravity only
2	Full range of motion with gravity eliminated
1	Slight muscle contraction palpable, but no movement noted
0	No visible or palpable contraction; paralysis of limb

Generally, the person is considered to have a disability if muscle strength is rated below grade 3.

Reflexes

Assessment of reflexes includes both superficial reflexes, graded 0 to 1+ (absent or present), and deep tendon reflexes (DTR), graded 0 to 4+.

Deep tendon reflex grades:

0	Absent
1+	Present but diminished
2+	Normal

TABLE 19–6. SUPERFICIAL REFLEXES.

Reflex	CNS Level	Test and Response
Upper abdominal	Thoracic 7, 8, 9	*Test:* The client lies supine. With the handle end of the reflex hammer, the examiner strokes the skin from the upper abdominal quadrants toward the umbilicus, observing the movement of the umbilicus. *Normal response:* Umbilicus moves up and toward area being stroked. Slight abdominal muscle contraction observable.
Lower abdominal	Thoracic 11, 12	*Test:* The client lies supine. With the handle end of the reflex hammer, the examiner strokes the skin from the lower abdominal quadrants toward the umbilicus, observing the movement of the umbilicus. *Normal response:* Umbilicus moves down and toward area being stroked. Slight abdominal muscle contraction observable.
Cremasteric (males)	Thoracic 12 Lumbar 1,2	*Test:* With the client supine, the examiner strokes the medial side of the upper thigh using the handle end of the reflex hammer. *Normal response:* Contraction of the cremaster muscle, which pulls the scrotal sac upward on the side stroked.
Gluteal	Sacral 3, 4, 5,	*Test:* With the client lying prone, the examiner separates the buttocks and strokes the perianal skin with the handle end of the reflex hammer. *Normal response:* Contraction of the external and anal sphincter muscles.
Plantar	Sacral 1, 2	*Test:* The examiner runs the handle end of the reflex hammer from the heel of the foot up the lateral border of the sole, turning medially and going across the ball of the foot underneath the great toe. *Normal response:* Flexion of the toes. Prior to the age a child walks, the normal response is extension and fanning of the toes.

From Fields & McGinn-Campbell, 1983.

3+ Increased but not necessarily pathologic
4+ Hyperactive with or without clonus present

Superficial reflex grades:

0   Absent
±   Barely present
1+ Normally active

Deep tendon reflexes and superficial reflexes give the examiner information about lower motor neuron function and upper motor neuron function, respectively. The muscle groups that innervate specific reflexes are shown in Tables 19–6 and 19–7.

Deep tendon reflexes are elicited by applying a brisk stimulus with the reflex hammer to a partially stretched tendon, bone, or joint. Superficial reflexes are elicited by stroking the superficial skin surface with a dull object, for example, a tongue depressor. Reflexes should be symmetrical.

After the physical examination, the client's overall motor function should be

TABLE 19–7. DEEP TENDON REFLEXES.

Reflex	Central Nervous System Level	Test and Response
Biceps	Cervical 5, 6 (primarily C5)	*Test:* The examiner places the client's arm over the opposite forearm and holds client's elbow. The client is instructed to relax the arm completely. The examiner places the thumb at the insertion of the biceps tendon superior to the antecubital fossa and taps the thumbnail with the narrow rubber end of the reflex hammer. *Normal response:* Contraction of the biceps muscle, resulting in slight flexion of the forearm at the elbow joint. Normally, the examiner sees or feels a slight jerk of the biceps muscle.
Brachioradialis	Cervical 5, 6 (primarily C6)	*Test:* The examiner supports the client's arm in the same manner used to test the biceps reflex. The styloid process of the radius is located proximal to the wrist. The examiner taps the process with the flat rubber end of the reflex hammer. *Normal response:* Slight flexion of the elbow joint and pronation of the forearm. Slight flexion of the fingers and hand also may occur.
Triceps	Cervical 6, 7, 8 (primarily C7)	*Test:* The examiner supports the client's arm in the same manner used to test the biceps reflex. The examiner taps at the insertion of the triceps tendon superior to the olecranon with the narrow rubber end of the reflex hammer. *Normal response:* Contraction of the triceps muscle, resulting in extension of the arm at the elbow joint.
Patellar	Lumbar 2, 3, 4 (primarily L4)	*Test:* The examiner instructs the client to sit on the edge of the examining table with the legs dangling free, palpates the soft tissue depression on both sides of the patellar tendon, taps the tendon with the flat rubber end of the reflex hammer. *Normal response:* Contraction of the quadriceps muscle, resulting in extension of the leg at the knee joint.
Achilles	Sacral 1, 2 (primarily S1)	*Test:* With the client sitting on the edge of the table with the legs dangling, the examiner dorsiflexes the foot slightly. The insertion of the Achilles tendon is located by palpating the soft tissue depressions on both sides of it. The tendon is then tapped with the flat rubber end of the reflex hammer. *Normal response:* Contraction of the triceps surrae muscle, resulting in plantar flexion of the foot.

From Fields & McGinn-Campbell, 1983.

described quantitatively. The focus is then directed to how the client's impairments are reflected in activities of daily living (ADL).

The nurse must be cognizant of the nursing framework for neuromuscular examination focusing on movement. With this combined framework, the nurse is able to determine nervous system dysfunction, alterations in ADL, safety, self-concept, and coping behaviors. Based on the initial history and the physical examination, specific nursing diagnoses should be stated. Examples of alterations in movement based on the Mitchell et al. model (1984) include the following:

1. Impaired verbal communication related to impaired articulation;
2. Potential for injury related to alteration in the gag and swallowing reflex;
3. Impaired physical mobility related to neuromuscular impairment, intolerance to activity, perceptual or cognitive impairment, or pain and discomfort;
4. Self-care deficit related to neuromuscular impairment, musculoskeletal disorder, or visual disorders;
5. Disturbances in self-concept, body image, self-esteem, role performance, personal identity; and
6. Ineffective individual coping related to situational crises, inadequate support systems, etc. (Doenges & Moorhouse, 1985, p. 11)

PSYCHOSOCIAL DIMENSION

Humans are unique, biopsychosocial beings in constant interaction with the changing environment. To cope with the environment, humans use various mechanisms to maintain homeostasis. The ease of adaptation or ability to cope depends on one's individual characteristics, the influence of others in the environment, and other available resources, such as support systems, finances, and so on.

Since the ability to move about in the environment is so intricately related to all of our activities and perception of self, a functional assessment of mobility would be incomplete without a full understanding of the psychosocial dimension of the individual. Movement not only provides a way for us to express ourselves but also facilitates the attainment of our goals and life pursuits.

Psychosocial aspects, focusing on the motivation to move, are integrated into the overall assessment as follows: (1) self-perception and self-concept patterns, (2) individual strengths and weaknesses, (3) coping patterns, including independency and dependency needs, (4) available support systems, and (5) emotional and social adjustment.

Self-Concept and Self-Perception

Smitherman (1981) states that self-concept is never static. "Throughout life it is continually changing, being altered and expanded to adapt to changes of the self and changes in the environment" (p. 338). She suggests that self-concept consists of three components: (1) the existential self, (2) the physical self, and (3) the psychologic self. The existential self is the most basic of the three components and can be stated as "I exist" or "I am." The physical self correlates with body image and focuses on the "individual's conscious and unconscious beliefs and thoughts about his body—external and internal" (p. 337). This might be stated by the individual as, "I am short" or "I am male." The third component, the psychologic self, focuses on attitudes the individual holds pertaining to self, such as, "I am intelligent" or "I am organized."

People with an alteration in mobility are often confronted with an alteration in self-concept. "The (client's) psychological self may be threatened ('Can I master this?'), his physical self ('Is my body intact?'), or his very existence ('Will I survive?')" (Smitherman, 1981, p. 337). This offers a unique challenge to the nurse to recognize threats to the self-concept and assist the individual to adapt to changes.

Smitherman (1981) also categorized into three areas various events that have the potential for altering one's self-concept. She stated that changes can occur due to altered appearance, functioning, or control. Since each individual attaches special significance to the physical appearance of the self, it is difficult to predict how an individual will respond to a change in body image. Changes can be sudden or chronic, temporary or permanent, visible to others or easily camouflaged. The individual's response to this threat will depend on individual strengths and weaknesses, the meaning attached to appearance, and others' reactions to alteration of appearance. The face, especially the eyes, is usually identified as the most significant aspect of self in relation to physical appearance (Smitherman, 1981).

In addition to altered appearance, events can lead to altered function, which can have an effect on an individual's self-concept. This altered function may be an actual event, or it could be a perceived change. Either way, it will threaten the individual's self-concept and can lead to anxiety, frustration, and decreased self-esteem. The client with Parkinson's disease has an altered appearance, for example, masklike facial expression, akinesia, and loss of posture control. The perception of self, as well as the perception the person believes others hold, can have a profound effect on the self-concept. The person with Parkinson's disease experiences altered function because of difficulty ambulating, change in gait, and tremors. This alteration in mobility may affect the individual's self-concept, leading to a change in the psychologic self.

Information about the client with an alteration in function should include (1) the typical daily schedule in the usual health status and with the current problem, (2) assistance required in ADL, and (3) the effect that illness as a problem has on the pursuit of life goals, ADL, and the ability to support oneself.

Some events may cause the individual to experience altered control of the body, thus creating a threat to the self-concept. In our normal daily routine, we perform many activities without consciously thinking about them. With an illness or mobility problem, the individual focuses energy on the problem and its effect on ADL. This often causes the individual to focus on body changes that can be threatening to the self-concept. Information related to altered control includes (1) ideal versus real roles, (2) the usual methods for coping with stress, (3) the effectiveness of coping techniques, (4) the level of independence in ADL, and (5) priority setting and goals. Alterations in appearance, function, and control can thus occur singly or in any combination. When two alterations occur, it is more problematic for the client. The nurse must be aware of this and assist the client in coping with the changes.

Individual Strengths and Weaknesses

People are motivated by specific goals to meet basic needs and develop to the fullest potential. An understanding of the relationship between basic needs and motivation theory, along with their impact on ADL, is essential to understanding the psychosocial dimension.

Maslow's hierarchy of basic human needs (1970) assists the nurse in identification of the psychologic parameters affecting mobility. This list of basic needs includes physiologic, safety, love, esteem, and self-actualization needs. They usually emerge in that order when lower level needs have been gratified. Gratification of needs has an important role in motivation of the individual.

In limited or absent mobility, the individual is placed in a dependent and somewhat vulnerable position because of reliance on another for such basic physiologic needs as food and water, elimination, activity, and exercise. Mobility can have an effect also on safety and security needs. The person may feel vulnerable and insecure if unable to protect himself or herself from threatening physical and psychologic situations in the environment. Changes in roles and expectations can occur as a result of impaired mobility, leading to an alteration in established patterns of social interaction with family and friends. The role changes often lead to insecurity because the stability of past patterns has been altered. A regression to an infantile state, accompanied by ego regression, may be noted.

Alterations in physical abilities and appearance may lead to fear of rejection by significant others and hinder fulfillment of love and belonging needs. According to Maslow (1970), we all have a need or tendency to flock together or belong to a group. Lack of fulfillment of this need can have a profound effect of self-esteem and self-worth as a result of changes in self-perception, including self-concept and body image. The individual's sense of value and usefulness may be diminished.

Self-actualization needs are dependent on meeting all lower level needs successfully. Since impairment in mobility can hamper achievement of lower level needs, self-actualization may not be achieved. Nursing's goal is to help the individual develop to his or her full potential by assisting in the fulfillment of needs.

Coping Patterns

The concept of human uniqueness is paramount in understanding the impact of neurologic disability or impairment on ADL. Since each person is unique, the psychosocial significance of a mobility problem depends on the characteristics of the individual, the influence of the environment, and the availability of resources (Carlson, 1980).

According to Carlson (1980), to understand the psychosocial significance of a neurologic disorder, the nurse must have knowledge about the neurologic condition and the physical effects resulting from that condition. The nurse must assess the impact of the neurologic condition on the psychologic self—body image, self-esteem, coping—taking into account the individual's social network or environment in relation to the situation.

Some common psychosocial consequences of neurologic conditions that should be considered when dealing with a client with altered mobility include (1) alteration of life patterns, (2) changes in self-perception, (3) visibility of the physical condition, (4) disruption in the method of coping, and (5) impact on significant others (Carlson, 1980, p. 312).

Specific data collection of methods of coping with a disability or alteration in mobility assist in identifying patterns of coping with stressful situations. Mitchell et al. (1984) presented a basic examination for assessing coping behaviors (Table 19–8) that can be completed in an interview or paper and pencil questionnaire. Some helpful parameters to assess coping style that are built into Mitchell et al.'s model include assessment of problems created by the illness or disability, methods for handling the problems, and support from significant others.

TABLE 19–8. BASIC EXAMINATION: COPING WITH DISABILITY.

Self-care competence	Observation: Adaptive aids, deficits
Role competence	History: Effect of disorder
	Observation
Coping	Observation: Congruence of verbalizations, body language
	Body posture, expression
	Adaptive aids
	Interview: Coping style

From Mitchell et al., 1984.

ENVIRONMENTAL DIMENSION

The environment has an impact on the individual's mobility status at various points on the health–illness continuum throughout the life cycle. Stairs may be a problem, for example, for a person with a full-leg cast. Having to maneuver between two levels of a home to carry out ADL will be extremely difficult, as well as exhausting. Even placement of furniture and decorative items, such as throw rugs, can be a safety or environmental hazard for the person trying to maneuver on crutches or with an unsteady gait.

The nurse's responsibility to each client varies greatly depending on the setting of the client and his or her physical and mental capabilities (Mitchell & Loustau, 1981). The client with a recent stroke, for example, will need more assistance to maintain safety than another person who has adapted to the changes created by a disability. Whether the individual is in the hospital or at home will greatly influence the impact the nurse can have. Changes in the hospital are often easier

TABLE 19-9. ENVIRONMENTAL DIMENSIONS.

Physical barriers or obstacles
  Description of home (stairs, layout, conveniences)
  Description of work setting
  Description of neighborhood (proximity, relationships with neighbors, environmental)
  Alterations to improve client health care
Assistive devices
  Rails, ramps, widened doorways
  Crutches, prostheses
Safety factors
  Developmental level
  State of mobility
  Potential hazards
  Sensory deficits
  Use of prosthetic and other supportive devices
Available support systems
  Family and significant others
Sensory stimulation available
Financial resources
  Health insurance
  Effect of health or illness on finances
  Effect of finances on health
Community resources
  Ethnocultural affiliations
  Knowledge of services available
  Transportation

to initiate than in the home, since the nurse is the primary caretaker in the hospital. The nurse must work with the support system in all phases of care and adapt the plan accordingly.

Environmental areas (Table 19–9) that must be integrated in the overall assessment include:

1. Physical barriers or obstacles to mobility (work, living environment, including neighborhood, access to transportation)
2. Assistive devices in the environment (e.g., rails, ramps, widened doorways)
3. Safety factors
4. Available support systems from family unit or significant others
5. Adequate environmental stimulation
6. Financial resources
7. Community resources

When asssessing the external environment for physical barriers or obstacles, the examiner fully assesses the home and work environments to determine if the client has freedom of movement within those settings. Both areas must be described fully regarding layouts, number of floors, if stairs are a problem, and so on. The examiner should assess the client's neighborhood, focusing on location, city versus suburb, relationship with neighbors, and influence from industrial sites.

An assistive device is often the only aid the person needs to be independent and not in need of assistance in ADL. All devices need to be selected for proper fit for the individual and existing environment. Clients should be instructed in proper travel with a wheelchair, how to use crutches correctly, and how to use a prosthesis correctly.

Throughout the life span, safety is a concern. Each developmental level must be considered in terms of expected patterns and variations. As mobility increases with growth and development, the individual is confronted with a variety of hazardous situations. Consider the toddler who has increased opportunities to explore through mobility. Electrical outlets may be a safety problem, since they are now accessible.

Sensory deficits caused by either disease or physiologic changes associated with aging; for example, decreased vision and a less sensitive balance center can have a profound effect on the mobility plan. Sensory stimulation may be inadequate because of primary sensory changes or because mobility is too limited for the disabled individual to join in activities. Such a person is in a socially restricted environment as a result of physical disabilities and living conditions. The aged are the primary group who experience a restricted environment because of their physical or emotional inability to move. People who live in institutions with monotonous environments devoid of sensory stimuli suffer from social limitations. People who are depressed and who choose not to associate with others and people with chronic debilitating conditions are included in this category (Mitchell and Loustau, 1981).

Therapeutically restricted environments are a concern also. A client on a Strykerframe, in Buck's traction, or on bedrest is in an environment that is restricted because of immobility, and sensory stimulation can be greatly decreased. In contrast, in the intensive care unit, an overload of sensory stimuli that are meaningless to the individual may occur and affect psychologic homeostasis (Mitchell and Loustau, 1981).

Other areas to assess include financial resources. Does the client have health insurance or funds adequate to maintain health? Does the recently diagnosed paraplegic or his family have insurance or funds necessary for hospitalization and rehabilitation? Will they be able to sustain its effect without severely damaging the family unit? Even brief illnesses can have a great impact on an individual and family who have a limited income. Insurance may pay the major costs of hospitalization, but the loss of income and child care costs while significant others attend to the client are an added burden and create potential problems.

Knowledge of services available for assistance and affiliation with one's ethnocultural group are important parameters to assess regarding community resources. If the individual lacks knowledge of services, the nurse should guide the individual and family.

One final area to assess is transportation. How does the individual have access to the community—bus, car, walking, or by service of others? This can greatly restrict a person who would otherwise be mobile.

SUMMARY

The ability to move about in the environment is intricately related to one's ability to move, motivation to move, and a free, nonrestrictive environment. Hence, a general framework to assess mobility should be used by the nurse to assess the physical, psychosocial, and environmental dimensions.

REFERENCES

Carlson, C.E. (1980). Psychosocial aspects of neurologic disability. *Nursing Clinics of North America, 6,* 309.

Conway-Rutkowski, B.L. (1982). *Carini & Owens' neurological and neurosurgical nursing.* St. Louis: Mosby.

Doenges, M., & Moorhouse, M. (1985). *Nurses' pocket guide: Nursing diagnoses with interventions.* Philadelphia: Davis.

Fields, W. L., & McGinn-Campbell, K. M. (1983). *Introduction to health assessment.* Reston, VA: Reston Publishing Company.

Granger, C. V. (1984). A conceptual model for functional assessment. In C. V. Granger & G.E. Gresham (Eds.), *Functional assessment in rehabilitation medicine* (p. 14). Baltimore: Williams & Wilkins.

Granger, C. V., Demis, L. S., Peters, N.C., Sherwood, C.C., & Barrett, J. E. (1979). Stroke rehabilitation: Analysis of repeated Barthel index measures. *Archives of Physical Medicine and Rehabilitation, 60,* 14.

Granger, C. V., and Gresham, G. (Eds.) (1984). *Functional assessment in rehabilitation medicine.* Baltimore: Williams & Wilkins.

Jebsen, R. H., Taylor, N., & Trieschmann, R. B. (1969). An objective and standardized test of hand function. *Archives of Physical Medicine and Rehabilitation, 51:*311.

Katz,, S., Ford, A., & Moskowitz, R. (1963). Studies of illness in the aged. The index of ADL. *Journal of the American Medical Association, 185,* 914.

Lawton, M. P. (1971). The functional assessment of elderly people. *Journal of the American Geriatrics Society, 19,* 465.

Mahoney, F., & Barthel, D. (1965). Functional evaluation: The Barthel index. *Maryland State Medical Journal, 14,* 61.

Maslow, A. (1970). *Motivation and personality* (2nd ed.). New York: Harper & Row.

Mitchell, P. H., & Irvin, N. J. (1977). Neurological exam: Assessment for nursing purposes. *Journal of Neurosurgical Nursing, 9*(1), 23.

Mitchell, P. H., & Loustau, A. (1981). *Concepts basic to nursing* (3rd ed.). New York: McGraw-Hill.

Mitchell, P. H., Ozuna, J., Cammermeyer, M., & Woods, N. F. (Eds.). (1984). *Neurological assessment for nursing practice.* Reston, VA: Reston Publishing Company.

Nagi, S. Z. (1965). Some conceptual issues in disability and rehabilitation. In M.B. Sussman (Ed.), *Sociology and rehabilitation*. Columbus: Ohio State University Press.

Sarno, J. E., Sarno, M. T., & Lurta, E. L. (1973). The functional life scale. *Archives of Physical Medicine and Rehabilitation, 54*, 214.

Smitherman, C. (1981). *Nursing actions for health promotion*. Philadelphia: Davis.

Thompson, J.M., & Bowers, A. C. (1984). *Clinical manual of health assessment* (2nd ed.). St. Louis: Mosby.

Wood, P.H.N., & Badley, E.M. (1978). Setting disablement in perspective. *International Rehabilitation Medicine, 1*, 32.

BIBLIOGRAPHY

Bates, B. (1987). *A guide to physical examination* (4th ed.) Philadelphia: Lippincott.

Konikow, N. (1985). Alterations in movement: nursing assessment and implications. *Journal of Neurosurgical Nursing, 17*, 61.

Malasanos, L., Barkauskas, V., Moss, M. & Stoltenberg-Allen, K. (1986). *Health Assessment* (3d ed.). St. Louis: Mosby.

20

Abrupt Alterations in Mobility

Jeanette C. Hartshorn and Mary Gokey

Abrupt changes in mobility can result from a variety of disturbances in the neurologic structures and functions in the systems responsible for normal movement. Diseases and disorders that create these abrupt changes in mobility occur in the brain or spinal cord or in the fiber tracts that connect the higher structures with the segments of the spinal cord that ultimately send the message to move to the muscles themselves. Responses to abrupt loss of function of a part of the motor system can range from hemiplegia to quadriplegia. Although the pathologies that precipitate abrupt loss of movement differ, the disuse syndrome is common to all. In this chapter, acute injury (spinal cord injury and cerebrovascular accidents, CVAs) and their impact on mobility are discussed.

NEUROANATOMIC CORRELATES OF ABRUPT LOSS OF MOBILITY

Impairments in mobility occur as a result of suprasegmental (upper motor neuron) or segmental (lower motor neuron) lesions. A suprasegmental lesion can occur at any level within the brain or spinal cord. A cerebral lesion can be cortical, subcortical, in the internal capsule, or in the brainstem. Spinal cord lesions occur at any segmental level.

Suprasegmental Disruption

Cortical lesions usually involve fewer upper motor neurons because of the wide surface distribution of the fibers (Bannister, 1985). A cortical lesion will, therefore, usually cause a monoplegia or paralysis of the face, with little or no disruption of the adjacent cortex (Bannister, 1985).

Subcortical lesions that occur in the corona radiata involve more fibers because they are closer together than in the cortex. A subcortical lesion causes a greater degree of impairment, usually contralateral hemiplegia or hemiparesis. One limb may be affected more seriously. A lesion of the internal capsule is even more devastating because of the denser distribution of the upper motor neurons. Damage to the internal capsule causes hemiplegia.

Brainstem lesions can cause either hemiplegia or quadriplegia, since the corticospinal tracts lie so close together. Hemiplegia from a brainstem lesion can be differentiated from capsular hemiplegia by associated signs of nearby structures. For example, hemiplegia with involvement of the cranial nerve nuclei would indicate brainstem damage, since the cranial nerves are in close anatomic proximity to the corticospinal tracts. Common characteristics of suprasegmental (upper motor neuron) lesions occur. A group of muscles, rather than an individual muscle, is affected. If any movement is possible, the appropriate functional relationship of the muscle groups, whether agonist, antagonist, synergist, or fixator, remains intact. Paralysis never includes all the muscles on one side of the body, no matter how severe the hemiplegia may be. Bilateral movements, such as of the eyes, jaw, pharynx, larynx, neck, thorax, and abdomen, are little affected if at all because of bilateral cortical innervation of these structures (Adams & Victor, 1985).

Suprasegmental lesions above the pons usually produce deficits that are greater in the arm and hand than in the leg, and muscles of the tongue and lower face are severely affected. Flexor muscles of the arm and extensors of the leg are usually the most severely involved. The muscles exhibit an increased reactivity to a stretch stimulus (Adams & Victor, 1985). The clasp-knife phenomenon can be elicited by quick stretching of the muscle of the affected extremity. Continuous passive extension of the spastic arm can follow a repetitive sequence of moving freely a short distance, stopping abruptly, then continuing its motion of extension. Slow extension of the same arm causes little or no change in muscle tone. Muscle wasting is minimal, in comparison to that with a lower motor neuron lesion. A slight reduction of muscle mass is due to muscle disuse over time.

Segmental Disruption

Disorders that may cause abrupt loss of segmental function include poliomyelitis and spinal cord injury. A segment can be defined as a portion of the brainstem or spinal cord that includes activity from the reflex arc to the individual muscle innervated. When an injury involves a segment, therefore, functions affected include reflex aspects of movement, cranial nerve and muscle stretch reflexes, integration of autonomic nervous system functions, pure motor or sensory functions with respect to the muscle group innervated, and trophic input to the muscles (Nikas et al., 1982).

When a direct injury to the spinal cord occurs, the functional loss experienced depends on the degree of spinal cord damage. Upper and lower extremities are impaired with a lesion above the cervical enlargement. Lower extremities are affected if the lesion is below the cervical enlargement. Because of the varying degrees of spinal shock, however, loss may not correspond directly to the vertebral level, particularly in the thoracolumbar and sacral levels.

There are eight cervical spinal cord segments, which are named for their corresponding vertebrae. When damage occurs to the first two cervical segments, the individual will suffer total quadriplegia and respiratory paralysis. The third, fourth, and fifth cervical segments innervate the diaphragm via the peripheral phrenic nerve. Therefore, segments C3–C5 offer functional control over diaphragmatic excursion. Damage to C3–C4 causes total quadriplegia, a weak diaphragm, and absent intercostal movement. In addition to the diaphragm, C5 also innervates the trapezius muscle along with the spinal accessory nerve (cranial nerve XI [CN XI]), and regulates the individual's ability to shrug a shoulder.

The fifth and sixth cervical segments innervate the deltoid, biceps, brachioradialis, and triceps muscles. This innervation includes the axillary, musculocutaneous, and radial nerves, which allow arm elevation, forearm supination, and neutral forearm flexion. Segmental damage to C5 and C6 causes quadriplegia with retention of gross arm movements. The diaphragm may be impaired initially, but function may return with time. The sixth cervical segment, in conjunction with the seventh and eighth, controls forearm and wrist extension. Specifically, the extensions of carpi radialis and ulnaris muscles are innervated. The seventh and eighth certical segments also control wrist flexion. Damage to C6–C7 causes quadriplegia, with biceps and deltoid function but no triceps function. Damage to C7–C8 causes quadriplegia, with triceps function but no intrinsic hand function.

Grip and finger spreading are controlled by the C8 and T1 segments. The adductor pollicis and dorsal interossei muscles are innervated through these segments as are the peripheral median and ulnar nerves. The first through the twelfth thoracic segments innervate the intercostal, rectus abdominus, and oblique muscles. These segments involve thoracic and lumbocervical peripheral branches and influence respiration through intercostal muscles. In addition, the segments influence the muscles of the trunk.

Damage to the T1–5 produces paraplegia with diaphragmatic breathing and loss of leg, bladder, and bowel function. Arm function is intact, and sensation is present to the nipple line. When there is damage to T6–12, the individual is paraplegic, with no abdominal reflexes at T6 and all abdominal reflexes at T12. Generally, with this level of injury, there is spastic paralysis of the lower limbs. Damage to T12 usually is accompanied by sensation present to the groin area.

The first three lumbar segments control hip flexion through innervation of the iliopsoas muscle and the peripheral femoral nerve. Knee extension is controlled through L2–4. These segments innervate the quadriceps femoris muscle involving the peripheral femoral nerve. The fourth lumbar through the second sacral segment control foot dorsiflexion and knee flexion. This control originates through innervation of the extensor hallucis, digitorium, biceps femoris, and hamstring muscles, including the peripheral deep peroneal and sciatic nerves. Hip flexion, through the gluteus maximus muscle, and plantar flexion, through the gastrocnemius muscle are controlled through L5–S2.

When damage occurs to a segment below the level of L2, the individual may present with mixed sensorimotor loss and bladder, bowel, and sexual loss depending on the nerve roots damaged. Should the conus medullaris be damaged, there is bowel and bladder sphincter dysfunction, lower leg weakness, sacral dermatome hypoesthesia or anesthesia, and back pain. If the cauda equina is involved, there is asymmetric, atrophic, and areflexic paralysis, indicating involvement of the lower motor neurons. Sensory root loss causing decreased sensation in the outer aspect of the legs, ankles, posterior lower limbs, and saddle area will occur. Damage to the cauda equina also causes sphincter dysfunction.

Sacral segments innervate the sphincter muscles through the pudendal peripheral nerves. Damage to sacral segments 1–5 causes loss of bladder, bowel, and sexual function, and some foot displacement may be present. Loss of sensation caused by this type of injury involves the saddle area, scrotum, perineum, penis, anal area, and upper third of the posterior aspect of the thigh.

If the segment is not damaged but cannot receive input from the suprasegmental tracts, such symptoms as spasticity may be seen. Spinal shock is an example of how this type of disruption may occur. *Spinal shock* occurs as early as 30 to 60 minutes after cord injury and involves the complete or nearly complete suppression of all reflex activity below the level of the injury. Tendon reflexes diminish or disappear and temperature control and vasomotor tone are lost. Bladder and bowel paralysis resulting in urinary retention, ileus, and fecal retention also may occur. Spinal shock occurs because of the sudden loss of impulses from the descending pathways, which normally maintain the cord neurons in a ready state of excitability. With the loss of the constant flow of impulses, the resting excitability of the cord is reduced greatly. Occasionally, in a patient with complete cord transection, sacral reflexes may be present immediately after transection. These reflexes show a diminished response, and commonly reflex activity returns after recovery from spinal shock. Without the modulating influence of the central cortex, reflexes are hyperactive. There is a wide variation in the duration of spinal shock, with some resolving in several days and others requiring several months. No specific medical treatment has been identified for spinal shock (Hickey, 1986; Nikas et al, 1982).

PATHOPHYSIOLOGY OF COMMON CONDITIONS PRODUCING ABRUPT IMMOBILITY

Spinal cord injury and cerebrovascular accident (CVA) are two examples of acute disorders that can damage suprasegmental and segmental structures abruptly. These disorders cause disruption of the structures previously discussed and result in partial or complete loss of voluntary movement, involuntary movement, balance, coordination, and postural reflexes.

Pathophysiology of Cerebrovascular Accident

Cerebrovascular accident, or stroke, occurs when acute neuronal and vascular changes in the brain result in ischemia or infarction. Stroke can be classified into two major categories: occlusive and hemorrhagic.

Occlusive disease is caused by an obstruction of the lumen of a vessel, resulting in an *infarction of the brain tissue*. Occlusion may be caused by abnormalities in the vessel wall, such as arteriosclerosis or inflammation. It also can result from red cell deformities, platelet aggregation, increased blood viscosity, dehydration, fever, and hemodynamic changes (Rivera, 1985), which cause thrombosis or embolism. Arteriosclerosis is the most common source of thrombosis. Emboli frequently result from cardiac sources, such as valvular lesions, cardiac arrhythmias, and prosthetic valves. Emboli may originate in extracranial vessels from atherosclerotic plaque. Infarction by embolus frequently progresses to a hemorrhagic stroke. Regional phenomena that occur during infarction include cytotoxic and vasogenic edema and vasomotor paralysis.

Intracranial hemorrhage may occur into the brain substance itself, the subarachnoid space, and the potential spaces below and above the dura. The etiology of hemorrhage can be hypertension, ruptured aneurysm, arteriovenous malformation, trauma, blood dyscrasia, such as leukemia, or brain tumors, or it can be of unknown origin.

After occlusion of a cerebral vessel, damage to autoregulation occurs. Zones of hypoperfusion or hyperperfusion are a result of the degree of autoregulatory damage of the adjacent areas. Hemorrhages appear in the cortex, and ischemic necrosis occurs in the underlying white matter. There is widespread destruction of nerve cells, nerve fibers, and glial tissue (except microglia). Infarction can cause so much swelling that signs of increased intracranial pressure occur (Bannister, 1985). An embolus usually causes vasospasm or cerebral abscess and may be followed by mycotic aneurysm formation (Bannister, 1985). Intracerebral hemorrhage acts as a space-occupying lesion, which compresses surrounding tissue and becomes edematous.

Pathophysiology of Spinal Cord Injury

Acute lesions of the spinal cord affect both the corticospinal tracts (upper motor neuron) and the segmental reflex. Such lesions not only cause a paralysis of voluntary movement, but also a temporary loss of reflexes below the level of the lesion because of spinal shock. After a period of time, this flaccid paralysis will give way to spasticity, with a hyperactivity of tendon reflexes and Babinski's sign. Spasticity is the result of a loss of descending inhibitory input and maintained activity of facilitatory influences (Adams & Victor, 1985).

Several events occur during a spinal cord injury that interfere with voluntary movement. Vascular damage has been identified as a component of spinal cord injury. After injury, a hemorrhagic lesion forms, involving primarily the central gray matter. Chromatolysis, vacuolation, and alterations in cytoplasmic density and stainability are observed. Minimal edematous changes in white matter, more marked in internal than in external layers, have been identified. The mechanical distortion of spinal cord tissue after compression trauma promotes not only intrinsic biochemical changes within the injured cells but also related changes involving extraneural tissues, particularly the blood vessels supplying the cord tissue. Thus, the infiltration by platelets and red cells into the perivascular spaces serves to worsen the intraneural damage normally accompanying the tissue distortion.

After extravasation of the blood elements, polymorphonuclear leukocytes leak into the cord tissue, heralding various degrees of cellular necrosis. Moderately severe impact lesions of this type involve intractions with the myelin sheath, leading to neuronal degeneration in the central gray matter. Within 24 to 48 hours after this type of injury, fibrocytic cells increase substantially. Moderate to severe cavitation of the central gray matter occurs after stabilization of the injury. Distal to the site of trauma, wallerian degeneration or demyelination of the axon sheath occurs. This change is characterized by swelling of the myelinated axon, which then breaks into fragments and finally disappears from the tissue. When the axon regrows in limited circumstances, the glial processes retract, and if synaptic contact is restored between cells, sensorimotor function may return to a degree or completely. The way in which the healing of the injury proceeds is directly influenced by the severity and the site of the injury, by the time elapsed between trauma, and by the observed physiopathologic changes (De La Torre, 1981).

HUMAN RESPONSES TO ACUTE IMMOBILITY

Acute Disuse Phenomena

Acute disuse phenomena occur when mobility is affected by the abrupt loss of functional neurons as a result of a suprasegmental or segmental lesion. Acute disuse phenomena have an impact on all body systems, contributing to multisystem complications. Responses of the cardiovascular, pulmonary, gastrointestinal, and integumentary systems to nervous system injury only serve to compound the deleterious effects of the insult suffered by the patient.

Cardiovascular Effects

As a result of acute immobility, there is an increased workload on the heart. Cardiac output and stroke volume are increased because of the loss of gravity's effect on blood return to the heart. Heart rate increases as a result of cardiac muscle fatigue. Immobility of the lower extremities causes a sluggish venous blood return to the heart. This pooling of blood combined with hypercoagulibility of the blood increases the risk of deep venous thrombosis and pulmonary embolism. In stroke, the risk of deep venous thrombosis in the paralyzed leg is as high as 75%, whereas in the nonparalyzed leg, it is approximately 7% (National Institutes of Health Consensus conference statement, 1986).

Respiratory Effects

With immobility from any cause, there is an increase in the work of breathing, an increase in intraesophageal pressure, and a slight increase in tidal volume. The end result is that more effort is required to expand the lungs and exchange gas. Immobility can be complicated by decreased strength of the muscles of respiration, which leads to decreased chest expansion. The pressure of the bed against the chest decreases expansion, predisposing the person to shallow breathing. Lack of activity decreases the normal stimulus to deep breathing. All of these factors lead to stasis of the normal secretions of the lung, creating a good medium for bacterial growth. When a person is supine, the effects of gravity tend to draw the mucus present in a bronchiole toward the bottom, leaving a dry upper epithelium, which is more vulnerable to bacterial invasion. This can lead to pneumonia. Atelectasis may occur if static secretions become thick and block a bronchiole. If a person is unable to cough, being too weak, unconscious, or in pain, pneumonia is possible.

Patients with high-level cervical cord injury have reduced lung volume and capacity, poor oxygen exchange, and carbon dioxide retention. Each patient demonstrates a variable cough, a progressive decrease in thoracic compliance, and elastic recoil of the lungs because of decreased volume. These people require total respiratory support, at least for a prescribed period of time. The cough reflex is impaired significantly by paralysis of the intercostal and abdominal muscles.

Metabolic Effects

Immobility leads to a multitude of metabolic and digestive changes, including a decrease in basal metabolic rate and oxygen consumption. These decreases reflect a decreased energy requirement of the body.

Negative nitrogen balance may occur with immobility. Normally, anabolism (protein synthesis) is in balance with catabolism (protein breakdown). During immobilization, catabolism increases, as reflected in a marked increase in excretion of urinary nitrogen (urinary nitrogen is a byproduct of protein metabolism). The marked urinary excretion of nitrogen results in a negative nitrogen balance, indicating a depletion of stores for protein synthesis, which is necessary in tissue healing after trauma or surgery.

Immobility may affect the calcium balance adversely. Normally, calcium is released in the process of bone resorption, and the body uses what it needs and excretes the excess. During immobilization, however, calcium is retained in the urine, and since the volume of urine rises only slightly, the calcium concentration is increased. Because the citric acid concentration in the urine does not change, the calcium/citric acid ratio is altered, and the pH of the urine rises, indicating reduced acidity. This combination of factors creates the possibility of calcium precipitation and stone formation (Mitchell & Loustau, 1981).

Elimination Effects

Paralytic ileus may occur with immobility. During the acute stage after spinal cord injury, many patients experience loss of bowel sounds and abnormal distention from the loss of peristaltic movements in the intestines. Peristaltic activities are mediated by the parasympathetic nervous system, and the exact cause of paralytic ileus in these patients generally is attributed to the sudden paralysis and interruption of impulse pathways. Severe gastric dilation from a paralytic ileus can interfere with diaphragmatic functioning. Vomiting can occur, putting the patient at risk for aspiration.

Immobile clients can suffer from alteration in elimination for a number of reasons. One of the most common forms of this alteration is constipation, and several anatomic and physiologic principles explain this. The large bowel musculature has its own neural center within the intestinal wall that responds to distention caused by the fecal contents. Although this type of innervation usually is not greatly affected in stroke or spinal cord patients, the client may suffer from loss of the sensation of fullness in the lower bowel, loss of awareness of bowel evacuation, loss of ability to control the rectal sphincter, and loss of the ability to contract the abdominal muscles and to expel the stool.

Other causes of constipation in the immobile patient include restricted diets that include inadequate amounts of roughage and fluids, insufficient muscle strength to pass stool, and weakened perineal and abdominal muscles as a result of bedrest.

Musculoskeletal Effects

Acute immobility leads to a rapid loss of both muscle strength and muscle mass. As a result of the decrease in muscle strength, the patient experiences a decrease in tolerance for exercise and adapts to the situation by cutting back on activity, which further decreases muscle strength, and the cycle continues.

When muscles and joints are not used to their full capacities, there is a change in metabolic activity that leads to further loss of mobility. Normal mobility depends on the free movement of the joints and muscles and the ability of the loose network of connective (collagen) fibers to stretch to accommodate the full range of motion. When motion is limited, the collagen network becomes dense and rigid, resulting in fibrosis. Muscles become progressively shorter and pull the joints, creating contractures, which can be permanent. Although permanent contractures occur more frequently with paralysis, deformed posture may result from poor positioning during prolonged bedrest.

During immobilization, the bones are not performing their specific functions of weightbearing and motion. This disturbs the balance between bone formation (osteoblastic activity) and bone resorption (osteoclastic activity). Osteoclastic activity increases, and the bone matrix becomes thin and porous, resulting in osteoporosis. Increased osteoclastic activity also degrades collagen fibrils and causes minerals, particularly calcium and phosphorus, to be released and excreted. The osteoporosis of immobilization usually is reversible when the period of immobilization is over, although it can become pathologic with excessive bone and mineral loss.

If a bone that has become porous because of immobility is subjected to weightbearing, a pathologic fracture may result (Mitchell & Loustau, 1981).

Integumentary Effects
A major problem for the immobilized patient is the need to maintain the integrity of the skin. Pressure sores or decubitus ulcers are seen commonly in immobilized people. The lack of muscle tone, voluntary movement, and perception of pain are factors in the development of pressure sores. The most important factor, however, is the lowered tissue resistance to pressure caused by interruption of the vasomotor pathways. Pressure sores involve cutaneous and subcutaneous tissue and occur in areas of the body subjected to unrelieved pressure, such as the back of the head, the sacrum, the heels of the feet, and the trochanters. Skin and subcutaneous tissue die, slough away, and leave areas of ulceration. Cells in these tissues die because sufficient nutrients cannot diffuse from the capillaries to them, and their waste products cannot be carried away. Pressure on the tissues is greater than the hydrostatic pressure in the capillary, and this pressure difference effectively opposes diffusion from the capillaries, leading to tissue ischemia. Prolonged tissue ischemia leads to the production of pressure sores. Pressure sores develop much more rapidly in denervated or paralyzed tissues because of the decrease in trophic factors.

Case Studies
Acute immobility-related nursing diagnoses are examined here through an evaluation of three case studies. These case studies include patients with a cervical spinal cord injury, a CVA, and peripheral nerve injury.

Case Study 1: Cervical Cord Injury
Mr. Jackson, a 21-year-old active duty serviceman, was drinking heavily at a party. He left the party, driving his motorcycle. Shortly after, he remembered that he had forgotten his helmet, but because he was tired, he decided to continue on rather than return for the helmet. While traveling a darkened road, he hit an oncoming vehicle head on and was thrown onto the pavement. He landed squarely on top of his head and immediately lost consciousness. Within 10 minutes, the emergency medical service arrived and transported him to the local trauma center.

On admission, his words were garbled, but he was able to respond to some commands. He had lost sensation from the nipple line down and was experiencing respiratory difficulty. An x-ray examination confirmed the diagnosis of a C4 fracture. After stabilization of the fracture in the trauma center, Mr. Jackson was transferred to the neurologic intensive care unit.

On admission to the unit, Mr. Jackson was found to be unable to move any extremities and was unable to breath. He was placed on a volume ventilator shortly after admission. Mr. Jackson's intercostal muscles were paralyzed, although some diaphragmatic function remained intact. Once his respiratory status was stabilized, it was necessary to begin interventions to stabilize the cervical injury. Cervical tongs were inserted while he was under local anesthesia. Seven pounds of traction were added to stabilize the fracture.

Twelve hours after admission to the neurologic intensive care unit, Mr. Jackson was awake but very frightened. He demonstrated signs of acute anxiety and was unable to recall the events of the accident that caused his injury. Throughout his stay in the neurologic intensive care unit, Mr. Jackson's cardiovascular activity was monitored.

Case Study 2: Cerebrovascular Accident
Mr. F, a 52-year-old father of three children, was admitted to the neurosurgical intermediate intensive care unit, with an admitting diagnosis of a left CVA. He was accompanied by his wife, from whom a history of the present illness and a past medical history were obtained.

Mrs. F stated that her husband had a 20-year history of high blood pressure and blamed this on his job. He was a successful attorney and averaged 10 to 12 hours a day (including most Saturdays and Sundays) at the office. He had been involved in an $18 million law suit for the past year, so "He felt especially pressured." He was 35 pounds overweight and smoked a pack of cigarettes a day. Mr. F had been followed by an internist for his medical care plan. He had taken various medications for his hypertension, with limited success, primarily because "He wouldn't bother to take them as the doctor prescribed." Mr. F had not been able to stop smoking nor lose weight. Mrs. F was distraught, saying, "I'm at my wits' end. I've seen this coming for years."

Mr. F had no history of cardiac disease, neurologic disease, diabetes mellitus, or other major medical problems. He had the usual childhood diseases without complications and had not undergone any surgical procedures. There was a family history of vascular disease. His mother died of a stroke at the age of 76, and his brother survived a myocardial infarction 6 years previously.

Mr. F suffered his first transient ischemic attack (TIA) about 4 months before the hospital admission. He had come home late from the office. While he was sitting and reading the paper, he suddenly experienced right arm weakness and heaviness and felt as if a "curtain covered his left eye." This lasted approximately 1 minute and resolved spontaneously. He had not mentioned this incident to his wife until he experienced the same symptoms twice in 1 day 2 months later. Mrs. F convinced Mr. F to see his internist the following morning.

Mr. F's evaluation for his TIAs revealed a carotid bruit and decreased carotid pulse on the left side. Periorbital directional doppler studies suggested compromise of circulation of the left internal carotid artery. No neurologic deficits were noted, and no evidence of cardiovascular involvement was found. The laboratory results showed his usual hypercholesterolemia. In view of the two recent attacks and the list of risk factors predisposing him to cerebrovascular disease, it was recommended that Mr. F be hospitalized to undergo further evaluation for possible carotid endarterectomy. Mr. F was scheduled for admission to the hospital in 2 weeks and was started on a regimen of aspirin and persantine in conjunction with Hygroton and Lasix for hypertension. Mr. F was unexpectedly detained out of town during the time he was to be hospitalized. "I begged him to reschedule his tests, but he always said he was too busy. Then he woke up this morning with his right side paralyzed and couldn't speak."

The medical evaluation at the time of this admission to the emergency department included a physical examination, 12-lead ECG, chest x-ray, blood work (including complete blood count, clotting profiles, electrolytes, triglycerides, cholesterol, blood urea nitrogen, creatinine, glucose, and uric acid), routine urinalysis, and computerized tomography (CT) scan. The medical diagnosis of left CVA of probable thrombotic origin of the left internal carotid, with emboli to the left middle cerebral artery, was suggested. Mr. F was transferred to the nursing unit with an intravenous catheter, 40% misted oxygen via face tent, and a Foley catheter in place.

On admission to the neurosurgical intermediate intensive care unit, the nursing assessment showed that Mr. F had clear but shallow respirations at 24 breaths per minute. His blood pressure was 170/110, and the apical heart rate was 110. His peripheral pulses were thready and equal. Capillary refill was less than 1 second, and no jugular venous distention or peripheral edema was noted. His skin was slightly diaphoretic and pale but warm to touch. His Foley catheter was draining an adequate amount of clear yellow urine. A thorough neurologic assessment was done. Mr. F was lethargic; he opened his eyes to the examiner's voice, but was unable to respond appropriately to orientation questions. He was able to verbalize "yes" and "no" with difficulty; otherwise his words were unintelligible. Sensory evaluation was deferred because of his aphasia. The motor examination showed marked hemiparesis on the right side. The right upper extremity was assessed to be 1/5, and the right lower extremity was 2/5 on the universal scale. The left side was 5/5 for both upper and lower extremities, and coordination was intact. Asymmetry was noted in Mr. F's face, and on closer examination, weakness was found on the right side when he was asked to puff out his cheeks and smile. When assessing speech, the nurse found consistent articulation errors. Difficulty with lingual and labial sounds were evident. Deviation of the tongue to the right side (the weaker side) was present. Mr. F was uncooperative when he was asked to open his mouth to assess motor function of CN IX and X. Gag reflex testing was deferred. The patient was unable to swallow his own saliva. He was also noted to have a conjugate gaze preference to the left.

Case Study 3: Peripheral Nerve Damage

Mrs. C was a 50-year-old woman who was admitted to the neurology nursing unit with a chief complaint of tingling in her hands and feet and progressive weakness in both legs and arms for the past 2 weeks. She had fallen the day before her admission, which prompted her to consult her family physician. She had suffered an intestinal flu approximately 2 weeks before the onset of these symptoms.

Mrs. C's admission assessment showed a well-developed, well-nourished woman in no apparent distress. She was alert, oriented, pleasant, and relaxed during the interview. Her blood pressure was 110/68, pulse 76, respirations 16 and regular, and temperature 37°C. Her breath sounds were clear, and chest excursion was normal. She denied feeling short of breath. There was no evidence of cardiac abnormalities, and peripheral pulses were equal and strong. Mrs. C denied problems with diet or elimination.

Neurologically, Mr. C's mental status examination was within normal limits. Cranial nerves I through XII were intact. Motor strength was diminished to 4/5 bilaterally in the legs and 5/5 in the arms. Mrs. C complained of some tenderness in her muscles to deep palpation. Proprioception was intact, and vibration was slightly impaired. Heel to shin showed a mild ataxia. Finger to nose and rapid alternating hand movements were performed without deficit. Mrs. C was unable to stand from a sitting position without assistance. She exhibited a wide-base station and gait. Sensation was grossly intact. Deep tendon reflexes were diminished bilaterally. Babinski's reflex was absent. Mrs. C's blood work, ECG, and chest x-ray were within normal limits. Lumbar puncture showed a mild elevation in proteins.

Two days after admission, Mrs. C developed respiratory difficulty and, by that evening, had a flaccid paralysis of her legs and increased weakness of her arms. Sensation remained intact. A lumbar puncture was again performed, which showed a rise in cerebrospinal fluid proteins to 160 mg per 100 ml and 10 lymphocytes. Nerve conduction velocity studies showed a significant slowing. The medical diagnosis of Guillain-Barré syndrome was made based on these findings. Mrs. C was transferred to the intermediate neurologic intensive care unit for observation.

The following day Mrs. C became more dyspneic. Her arterial blood gases showed hypoxemia, a moderate respiratory alkalosis, and a decreased oxygen saturation, and her vital capacity was decreased to 800 cc. She was intubated, and ventilatory support was instituted.

Mrs. C progressed to complete quadriplegia and areflexia by her fifth hospital day. A facial diplegia was present, showing CN VII involvement. Autonomic function was impaired by evidence of urinary incontinence, lability in blood pressure, sinus bradycardia, and profuse diaphoresis.

Nursing Diagnoses Related to the Individual

Patients with acute disruptions in mobility have common nursing diagnoses regardless of the specific cause for the disruption. In this chapter, diagnoses appropriate for the acute phase are discussed. Each of the conditions discussed in this chapter has both acute and chronic components, and in Chapter 21, nursing care for the chronic aspects is discussed.

☐ **Ineffective Breathing Patterns**

Changes in innervation to the muscles of breathing due to the injury and problems specifically caused by immobility make the patient a likely candidate for ineffective breathing patterns, defined as rate, rhythm, or depth of breathing insufficient to support adequate oxygen–carbon dioxide exchange. Whether or not a patient with a spinal cord injury develops respiratory complications is dependent also on the level of injury.

Initial *assessment* of the respiratory function of the immobile patient should include respiratory rate and respiratory excursion. Lung sounds are assessed for the degree of movement of air and the presence of adventitious sounds. Specific respiratory parameters, such as tidal volume and vital capacity, are measured. Arterial blood gases are assessed for levels of oxygen, carbon dioxide, and pH in the blood.

One of the major goals in caring for the immobile client with ineffective breathing patterns is to support ventilation. In addition to the assessment parameters already described, it may be necessary to implement such procedures as suctioning, caring for an artificial airway, and ventilator therapy. A second goal is to prevent respiratory infection or atelectasis. *Interventions* that help in this area include frequent turning, coughing and deep breathing, increasing fluids, and suctioning as necessary. The patient must be monitored for elevations in temperature.

Two types of special beds have been developed to assist in the respiratory care of the immobile patient. The rocking bed is a regular hospital bed attached to a framework with a motor that allows the ends to move alternately up and down. The rocking action takes advantage of gravity; as the head lowers, the abdominal viscera fall lower in the abdominal cavity, allowing the diaphragm to flatten and increase the thoracic space and volume of air inhaled. The patient is taught to inhale as the head rises and to exhale as the head lowers. Both the speed and the degree of tilt of the bed can be adjusted. The speed is set to correspond to the rate of desired respirations; the tilt is adjusted to get the desired tidal air volume. The total rocking arc of most beds is between 40 and 44 degrees.

Another bed with similar characteristics is the kinetic bed. This type of bed provides automated position movement of over a 124 degree range. Because of continuous postural changes, lung secretions are mobilized, allowing for easier expulsion of secretions and better respiratory exchange. In addition to assistance with respiratory care, these beds are useful in preventing other consequences of immobility, such as skin breakdown.

☐ **Impaired Physical Mobility**

Physical mobility is impaired for a number of reasons in the spinal cord injured patient.

Loss of voluntary movement and involuntary movement and the presence of environmental barriers have been discussed. The major characteristic of the immobile person is an inability to move purposefully within the physical environment, including mobility, transfer, ambulation, and locomotion. The degree of impairment of physical mobility is related to the level of injury.

In assessment of the immobile client, it is necessary to check frequently the range of motion of all extremities. Muscle strength and tone can similarly be checked on a routine basis. To test muscle tone, the nurse notes whether rigidity (increased resistance throughout range of motion of the joint), spasticity (increased muscular resistance to brisk movement of the joint), and clonus (oscillation between flexion and extension of the foot when brisk pressure is applied to the sole) are elicited by passive motion. Muscles are palpated for tenderness or spasm.

Muscle strength is tested in several ways. To test the shoulder girdle, the examiner presses on the patient's arms after he or she abducts them to shoulder height. Upper extremities are tested by evaluating biceps, triceps, wrist dorsiflexion, hand grasps, and strength of finger abduction and extension. Lower extremities are tested through the hip flexors, abductors and adductors, knee flexors and extensors, foot dorsiflexion, invertors and evertors. Muscle strength is graded as normal, minimal, moderate, severe weakness, or paralysis.

A major goal in caring for the immobile patient is to prevent complications, such as contractures, through *nursing interventions*. Both active and passive range of motion exercises are needed on a frequent basis. Since the patient is maintained on bedrest, proper positioning is essential. Extremities should be supported at all times. Frequent turning and repositioning of the patient supported may help in maintaining proper alignment. When voluntary muscle contraction is possible, the nurse may assist the patient in performing muscle-conditioning exercises. Setting exercises in which the muscle is contracted as hard as possible for 10 seconds and then released is a type of isometric exercise that may be helpful. Resistive exercises, in which the muscle contracts in pushing or pulling against a stationary object, can be used to help maintain strength.

Associated Diagnoses

A variety of nursing diagnoses occur secondary to the impaired mobility of individuals who have suffered such traumas as stroke, spinal cord injury, and peripheral nerve injury. Although these phenomena are discussed in detail in their corresponding chapters, they are summarized here to emphasize the primary role that mobility plays in all aspects of human response to illness.

☐ Self-Care Deficit

Self-care tasks are performed daily to meet bodily needs and to participate in society. Dependence in this area can impede one's participation in society. Most self-care activities require a significant amount of upper extremity function, which poses obvious problems for patients with cervical cord injury.

The immobile patient with a spinal cord injury can suffer from varying levels of self-care deficit. During *assessment*, inability to move in bed and transfer from bed to chair, difficulty in grasp and grip, and difficulties in using tools and untensils indicate the presence of self-care deficits. Nursing *interventions* are planned to minimize the deficit to the greatest extent possible. The *goal* of nursing care with this diagnosis is to assure that feeding, bathing, dressing, and toileting occur with as much assistance as possible from the patient. It is critical that the patient be involved in his or her own care, maintaining independence for as long as possible.

As the patient nears discharge from the acute care unit, several options for assistance are available. In particular, the occupational therapist can be consulted for assistance in developing new types of utensils that can be used by a patient with a weakened grasp. Occupational therapists can teach the patient ways of dressing despite the restrictions imposed by the injury. This phenomenon is discussed in detail in Chapters 32 and 33.

☐ Alteration in Elimination

Any immobile patient may suffer from problems with *urinary elimination.* Those with spinal cord injury may suffer additional problems due to the flaccidity and areflexicity of the bladder that occur during spinal shock. Depending of the level of injury, control over bladder function may return. Specifically, in upper motor neuron lesions, reflex activity below the cord lesion returns. Chapters 27 and 28 discuss the diagnosis of alteration in urinary elimination. *Bowel elimination* also is impaired with acute spinal cord injury, during the stages of spinal shock as well as chronically. Constipation may occur due to decreased activity. Chapters 27 and 29 discuss concepts of bowel elimination and management of both acute and chronic bowel elimination problems.

☐ Potential Impairment of Skin Integrity

Prevention of pressure sores is a top priority in caring for an immobile client. Skin *assessment* is made at least every eight hours. Generally, one of the first signs of skin breakdown is the presence of reddened areas. Once noted, these areas should be protected immediately. Assessment of the skin should include all areas of the body, with particular attention to the elbows, earlobes, sacrum, and heels of the feet.

Other parameters to assess include the nutritional status of the patient and other medical problems present at the same time. Wound healing is slowed in those suffering from poor nutritional status. These individuals, therefore, are more likely to suffer from pressure sores. Medical diagnoses, such as diabetes mellitus, also may lead to potential problems in skin breakdown. While assessing these parameters, the nurse can build a picture of the risk an individual patient may run for development of pressure sores. Other factors that contribute to the development of ulcers include debilitated conditions, edema, anemia, and trophic skin changes.

There are several *interventions* that are helpful in both the prevention and treatment of pressure sores. The patient should be repositioned to relieve pressure on body parts at least every 2 hours. The skin should be kept clean and dry, particularly in areas prone to the development of pressure sores. Reddened areas are massaged with lotion, and linen should be kept clean, dry, and wrinkle free.

Specific treatment of pressure sores varies from institution to institution. Specialized beds, such as the Clinitron, may be of assistance in keeping the patient off the pressure areas. Other preventive measures, such as sheepskin, air mattresses, egg crate mattresses, and heel and elbow pads are useful. The use of an occlusive plastic film (Op-Site) has gained some popularity over the last few years. This film covers the area, keeps bacteria out, and allows granulation tissue to develop. A number of antibacterial creams have been recommended for different types of pressure sores, and periodic application of heat may be useful in treatment of existing areas of skin breakdown. More severe pressure sores may require surgical debridement and plastic surgery. Research continues in this area, and the nurse should consult the current literature for the lastest information on the problem of pressure sores.

☐ Sexual Dysfunction

Immobile clients may suffer from sexual dysfunction. Those with spinal cord injury probably will have some change in sexual activity related to the level of cord injury. Chapters 30 and 31 discuss sexual dysfunction.

☐ Potential Ineffective Coping

Immobility from any cause leads to multiple problems for an individual. Immobility resulting from spinal cord injury may cause the patient to confront several additional problems. Reactions that can be expected include denial, anger, and depression. Each nurse works with the patient to help in developing methods for dealing with all of the feelings relative to the injury. Studies of the individual's reaction to immobility are based on two major concepts: grief and crisis theory.

Psychologic support of the patient should begin at the time of the injury. As the patient moves through different physical stages, the emotional reactions can vary considerably. For example, in the acute stage of the injury, the patient may be so concerned with holding on to life that there is no opportunity to think about the future in any detail. As he or she becomes more physically stable, the patient may experience some denial of the extent of the injury and eventually some depression. As an understanding develops about the extent of injury and what that means in terms of overall functioning, anger may result. Feelings of inferiority, inadequacy, powerlessness, lack or self-worth, and despair also may occur.

As the patient goes through each of these stages, *nursing interventions* include encouraging expression of feelings. The nurse can learn about the patient's perception of his condition and his expectations. Education at this point will help the patient maintain a realistic view of the future. *Goals* can be set mutually by the nurse and patient so that the patient can achieve and experience the satisfaction that comes with goal attainment. Nurses can do much by repeatedly expressing confidence in the patient's ability to perform successfully, always emphasizing the positive. Working toward maintaining open and honest communication and being sensitive to the patient's need for acceptance are interventions that frequently are successful in working with these patients.

There are times, however, when the nurse is not the best person to help the patient work through these problems. In this situation, the nurse should consider asking for consultation with a clinical nurse specialist in psychiatric nursing or some other health care provider who can establish a relationship with the patient and offer the needed support.

□ Potential for Injury

With limited mobility because of hemiplegia, or hemiparesis, being cared for in unfamiliar surroundings, and visual defects, the patient with an acute disruption in mobility is at risk for injury. Careful *assessment* of visual acuity and visual fields is critical. Room safety, such as placement of the bedside table and accessibility of the call bell or urinal, should be assessed, keeping visual and mobility deficits in mind. Objects should be placed within the visual field. Patients can be taught methods to compensate for visual field cuts. Keeping the bed in the lowest position and keeping the patient oriented to the environment will help to protect the patient from injury.

Nursing Diagnoses Related to the Family and Significant Others

□ Potential for Family Crisis

As the patient works through various stages of anger, depression, and denial, so does the family. There are a multitude of factors that combine to help form the attitudes of the family toward the situation. For example, the family may suffer from guilt, thinking that they may have been able to do something to prevent the accident. The length of time required for hospitalization of the patient may produce an additional strain on the family. Members may disagree about the best decisions to be made on behalf of their family member. For example, once discharge is planned, some would prefer that the patient return to the home setting, whereas others within the same family may ask that the patient be taken to an extended care facility for further rehabilitation.

One of the major goals in dealing with families at this time is to maintain satisfactory family relationships. In *assessing* the family relationship, it is important to accept the family as they are. The approach to the family should be one of determining how they are coping, trying not to impose any personal beliefs. The nurse must assess the family dynamics, coping strategies, knowledge of disease process, and attitudes.

Interventions for the family parallel those for the individual. Initially, it is important to give the family the opportunity to express their feelings. During the early days after the injury, the family may require constant reassurance and explanations. As time progresses, they may feel more trust for the staff and require less explanations. They continue to require a way to express their feelings, however. Support groups for families may assist in this process. Family assessment and interventions are discussed in detail in Chapter 17.

Nursing Diagnoses for the Community

☐ **Potential for Inadequate Community Resources**

Over the past few years, many changes in community resources for the disabled have taken place. Buildings, services, and activities that were off-limits some years ago are now more accessible to the disabled. Yet, more changes are required and should be considered before the patient's discharge.

Perhaps one of the most fundamental issues when the spinal cord injured person is returned to the community is that of role change. Only some spinal cord injured clients will return to their original jobs after the injury. Vocational rehabilitation programs will help some people to return to the community. Generally, vocational rehabilitation programs are funded with federal money and, as such, are always subject to potential decreased funds. Nurses can help in this area by impressing on their legislators the importance of the vocational rehabilitation programs.

Communities may not have the employment opportunities available to help the individual move back into society. Disabled people must have a realistic impression of the types of positions they can fill within the community, and employers must be helped to see the types of jobs within their business that can be filled by disabled people. If a patient is discharged from the health care institution without any thought being given to potential employment opportunities, it is likely that the individual's adjustment to being home will be unsuccessful.

Access throughout the community remains a problem. Although more buildings have been made accessible to those with altered mobility, many buildings continue to be inaccessible. Again, legislative efforts are most likely to influence this situtation. A change in the attitude of society with respect to the worth of disabled people will help in this type of legislative effort.

Implications for the community for the patient who has had a CVA are similar. Stroke ranks third as a cause of death in the United States and is one of the leading causes of disability. Approximately 1.5 million strokes are diagnosed in a year, and at any one time 2.5 million people have suffered strokes in varying degrees. Both U.S. and international data indicate that roughly 70% of stroke victims will survive the first 30 days. Ten percent of those who survive the first month will recover without discernible neurologic deficits. Forty percent have mild residual deficits, another 40% have severe deficits requiring special care, and the remaining 10% require institutional care (Aho et el., 1980; Posner et al., 1984). It is clear that stroke is one of society's leading health problems.

Education of the public is paramount in the prevention of stroke. Information about risk factors, the nature of the disease, prevention, and general care of the stroke patient should be disseminated on an ongoing basis. Education should be available to all age groups, high-risk groups, and the disadvantaged. The general population may be reached through printed material distributed at schools, doctors' waiting rooms, grocery stores, and places of employment. Television, radio programs, and newspapers are effective methods of disseminating information.

Prevention of stroke requires the awareness of health care personnel. Screening programs can identify the population at risk for stroke and refer them to specialists for diagnosis and treatment. Screening programs also can identify people who have warning signs of impending stroke, such as TIAs.

Community resources should be identified and used by patients who have survived the acute stage of stroke. If the patient is at home, resources—such as a visiting nurse, a visiting physician for emergency and follow-up care, a physical therapist, special assistive devices, homemaker or household assistance, and financial assistance—should be available. Public transportation suitable for the handicapped should be easily accessible. Architectural barriers at home and in the community should be eliminated. Whether long-term care is given in the hospital, in ambulatory settings, at home, or in other institutions, emphasis must be placed on rehabilitation and prevention or recurring stroke, which poses an added financial burden on the patient and society.

REFERENCES

Adams, R.B., & Victor, M. (1985). *Principles of neurology* (3rd ed.). New York: McGraw-Hill.

Aho, K., Harmson, P., Hatano, S., Marquardson, J., Smirnov, V.E. & Strasser, T. (1980). Cerebrovascular disease in the community: Results of a WHO collaborative study. *WHO Bulletin, 58*, 113.

Bannister, Sir R. (1985). *Brain's clinical neurology* (6th ed.). London: Oxford University Press.

De La Torre, J.C. (1981). Spinal cord injury review of basic and applied research *Spine, 6*(4); 315.

Hickey, J.V. (1986). *The clinical practice of neurological and neurosurgical nursing.* Philadelphia: Lippincott.

Mitchell, P.H., & Loustau, A. (1981). *Concepts basic to nursing* (3rd ed.). New York: McGraw-Hill, p. 350.

National Institutes of Health. (1986). Prevention of venous thrombosis and pulmonary embolism. NIH Consensus Conference. Journal of the American Medical Association, 256, 744.

Nikas, D. et al. (1982). *Core, curriculum for critical care nursing.* St. Louis: Mosby.

Posner, J.D., Gorman, K.M. & Woldow, A. (1984). Stroke in the elderly: I. Epidemiology. *Journal of the American Geriatric Society, 32*(2), 95.

Rivera, V.M. (1985). Stroke: A guide to differential diagnosis and prevention. *Post Graduate Medicine, 77*(4), 81.

BIBLIOGRAPHY

Adelstein, W., & Watson, P. (1983). Cervical spine injuries. *Journal of Neurosurgical Nursing, 15*(2), 65.

Bracken, M.B., Shepard, M.J., & Webb, S.B. (1981). Psychological response to acute spinal cord injury: An epidemiological study. *Paraplegia, 19*, 271.

Brackett, T.O., Condon, M., Kindelan, K.M., & Bassett, L. (1984). The emotional care of a person with a spinal cord injury. *Journal of the American Medical Association, 252*(6), 793.

Chui, L., & Bhatt, K. (1983). Autonomic dysreflexia. *Rehabilitation Nursing, 8*(2), 16.

Donovan, W.H., & Dwyer, A.P. (1984). An update on the early management of traumatic paraplegia (nonoperative and operative management). *Clinical Orthopedics and Related Research, 189*, 12.

Dudas, S., & Stevens, K.A. (1984). Central cord injury: Implications for nursing. *Journal of Neurosurgical Nursing, 16*(2), 84.

Friedman-Campbell, M., & Hart, C.A. (1984). Theoretical strategies and nursing interventions to promote psychosocial adaptation to spinal cord injuries and disability. *Journal of Neurosurgical Nursing, 16*(6), 335.

Hall, E.D., & Braughler, J.M. (1982). Glucocorticoid mechanisms in acute spinal cord injury: A review and therapeutic rationale. *Surgical Neurology, 18*(5), 320.

Hank, M., & Scott, A. (1983). *Spinal cord injury: An illustrated guide for health care professionals.* New York: Springer.

Hansebout, R.R., Tanner, A., & Romero-Sierra, C. (1984). Current status of spinal cord cooling in the treatment of acute spinal cord injury. *Spine, 9*(5), 508.

Howard, M., & Corbo-Pelaia, S.A. (1982). Psychological after effects of halo traction. *The American Journal of Nursing, 82*(12), 1839.

Kinash, G. (1978). Experiences and nursing needs of spinal cord injured patients. *Journal of Neurosurgical Nursing, 10*(1), 29.

Lagger, L. (1983). Spinal cord injury: Nutritional management. *Journal of Neurosurgical Nursing, 15*(5), 310.

Liebman, M. (1984). *Neuroanatomy made easy and understandable* (2nd ed.) Baltimore: University Park Press.

Stanton, G.M. (1983). Spinal cord injury: Psychological adaptation. *Journal of Neurosurgical Nursing, 15*(5), 306.

Toth, L.L. (1983). Spasticity management in spinal cord injury, *Rehabilitation Nursing, 8*(1), 14.

Tyson, G.W., Rimel, R.W., Winn, H.R., Butler, A.B. & Janes, J.A. (1979). Acute care of the spinal-cord-injured patient. *Critical Care Quarterly, 2*, 45.

21

Chronic Alterations in Mobility

Katharine M. Donohoe, Charlyne Miller, and Brenda Craig

Altered mobility is a common problem for patients with a number of neurologic disorders. The specific pathophysiology may arise from (1) lack of neurotransmitter substances in brain structures (as in Parkinson's disease), (2) altered transmission of electrical signals along motor fibers (as in multiple sclerosis), (3) deficient neurotransmission at the myoneural junction (as in myasthenia gravis), (4) destruction of the anterior horn cell (as in amyotrophic lateral sclerosis) and other portions of the central nervous system (as in stroke or spinal cord injury), or (5) disorders of the muscles themselves (as in the muscular dystrophies). Although the pathophysiology determines the pattern of altered mobility, there are a number of responses to altered mobility that people with chronic changes have in common, including decreased endurance for ordinary activities, potential needs for adaptive mobility aids, potential for social isolation and altered coping ability, and potential for respiratory and nutritional disorders. Chronic disorders that affect mobility make up a large segment of patients requiring prolonged care. Many of these disorders are progressive.

CHRONIC ILLNESS AND MOBILITY

Chronic illness can be defined as a condition that interferes with daily functioning for longer than 3 months in 1 year, causes hospitalization for longer than 1 month a year, or at the time of diagnosis is likely to do so (Hobbs et al., 1984). Severity of illness is much more difficult to measure. Five components suggested to measure the impact of chronic illness in childhood also might be applied to the concerns of adults. These concerns are (1) financial burden (out-of-pocket expenses greater than 10% of family income), (2) restriction of physical development, (3) impaired ability to engage in accustomed and expected activities, (4) significant emotional problems expressed as maladaptive coping strategies, and (5) disruption of family life, as evidenced by increased marital friction and sibling behavior disturbances (Hobbs et al., 1984).

There have been several attempts to describe theories of chronicity and the adjustment process patients and families go through as they cope with chronic illness. Kodadek summarized an application of crisis theory to chronic illness, including three stages of adaptation and resulting tasks that must be addressed (1985). The first phase is the diagnostic or initial stage in which there is a period of disorganization and disequilibrium. The second, or chronic stage, is that of reorganization and can be crucial, because this is when patients and families learn to manage their chronic illness. The third stage, that of resolution, involves accepting the chronicity associated with illness or its terminal nature. The stages described can overlap and change as the nature of the illness changes. The adaptive tasks seen during the chronic phase include the need to learn to (1) function normally, (2) adapt to ongoing change, (3) interact with various health care providers and the health care system in general, (4) manage role shifts, and (5) develop communication channels to prevent isolation (Kodadek, 1985).

Neurologic nurses caring for patients with chronic neurologic problems that impair mobility need a broad understanding of the nursing care measures that these disorders have in common. These patients can be seen in the hospital, outpatient area, or community setting. The importance of early intervention, a rehabilitative focus on abilities, problem solving, adjustment to chronicity, and learning to control one's own life are common themes. It is important for the nurse to have a clear understanding of the natural history of these chronic disorders to be able to set appropriate goals. Patients with chronic neurologic disorders, such as multiple sclerosis, muscular dystrophy, Parkinson's disease, and amyotrophic lateral sclerosis, can have widely different abilities that cannot be predicted from an incomplete or biased knowledge of prognosis. Optimal function for one patient may be to learn to accept the wheelchair for mobility; for another, it may be to avoid dependence on it.

Common Movement Problems in Chronic Neurologic Conditions

Weakness is a common finding in chronic disorders. Disorders such as cerebrovascular accidents and spinal cord injuries usually have an abrupt presentation followed by some marginal improvement and achievement of a static state of deficit. Chronic disorders, such as Parkinson's disease, amyotrophic lateral sclerosis, and the muscular dystrophies, have a more indolent course that can span years. Disorders such as multiple sclerosis and myasthenia gravis often are associated with an abrupt onset of weakness followed by some improvement. *Fatigue* is seen commonly in muscle weakness or caused by overwork of limited available musculature. Fatigue can immobilize a person of normal strength and cardiovascular conditioning. For a patient with chronic immobility, minimal activity can often be a stress that produces muscle weakness and profound fatigue. For patients with myasthenia gravis, Parkinson's disease, and multiple sclerosis, this weakness can be accentuated by nerve or neurotransmitter fatigue. In muscular dystrophy or amyotrophic lateral sclerosis, this can be due to specific muscle weakness or imbalance. *Changes in tone, associated movements, gait,* and *tremor* can alter mobility in patients with Parkinson's disease and Huntington's disease. Immobility resulting from severe muscle weakness and change in muscle tone can result in *contractures* and *atrophy* of the affected muscle group. The effects of *deconditioning* associated with a lack of physical activity may be apparent in a matter of days; the normal individual on bedrest loses strength from baseline levels at a rate of 3% a day. Patients with nerve or muscle pathology are subject to the effects of disuse as well as the intrinsic effects of their disease. The immobilized patient can have weakness of respiratory muscles and muscles of speech and swallowing, as well as altered visual perception. Disorders such as spinal cord injury and multiple sclerosis can be associated with sensory abnormalities that can interfere with perception and comfort. The neurologic disorders associated with chronic immobility may be viewed as affecting the segmental and suprasegmental anatomic structures.

Suprasegmental Disorders

Parkinson's disease, Huntington's disease, and other movement disorders are examples of disorders affecting the extrapyradmidal suprasegmental structures. Cerebrovascular accident, spinal cord injury, and multiple sclerosis are examples of disorders affecting the pyramidal (corticospinal) suprasegmental pathways and that result in chronic alterations in mobility.

Segmental Disorders

Neuromuscular disease and peripheral neuropathies create chronic segmental motor problems. Immobility seen in the patient with neuromuscular disease is characterized by abnormal weakness and fatigability of voluntary muscles. The neuromuscular diseases commonly affect the anatomic area called the *motor unit*, which consists of the anterior horn cells, the motor peripheral nerves, and the muscle fiber innervated. Amyotrophic lateral sclerosis, myasthenia gravis, the muscular dystrophies, and peripheral neuropathies are examples of such diseases. These diseases are discussed in Chapter 5.

HUMAN RESPONSES TO CHRONIC ALTERATIONS IN MOBILITY

The patient with chronic immobility because of muscle weakness or fluctuations in strength will learn to adapt to many changes throughout the lifetime. These changes can range from gradual to abrupt, increasing weakness to improving strength. Coping with limitations in their usual activities can be the most significant problem that faces patients with chronic neurologic disorders. In addition to the problems faced daily by people with chronic mobility alterations, such patients can be acutely immobilized during three situations: (1) during the initial diagnostic period, (2) when a treatment is initiated (such as corticosteroids, immunosuppressants, and temporary drug abstinence), and (3) when a crisis occurs (i.e., respiratory infection, surgery, ventilatory failure). For many patients, these three situations may require hospitalization to resolve. To assess the patient's degree of immobility, the nurse will need to make frequent checks of reliable indicators. The patient may be immobilized both physically and emotionally during crises but function at a near normal level days later. Monitoring vital signs or the patient's subjective perceptions may be of assistance, although in some cases these measures will not allow the nurse (or the newly diagnosed patient) to make reliable judgments about the patient's true functional ability. An experienced patient may be able to describe immobilizing symptoms vividly, but rarely with the sophistication of quantitative objective measures. Quantitative measures a nurse can employ to assess the patient's status are discussed as they relate to the specific nursing diagnosis. A flow sheet (Fig. 21–1) to simplify recording data obtained from patient assessment is very helpful to monitor long-term changes or to signal abrupt deterioration in many chronic neurologic disorders.

Patients should be familiar with the assessment methods used in the hospital and outpatient unit and be encouraged to monitor themselves by keeping a symptom diary that can be useful during telephone calls and outpatient visits.

Nursing Diagnoses Related to Individuals

Nurses may provide care for people with chronic conditions that alter mobility in the community, in outpatient clinics, in long-term care facilities, and in acute care hospitals. The following diagnostic categories frequently have chronic altered physical mobility as the main etiology.

- Potential for injury
- Activity intolerance
- Self-care deficit
- Ineffective breathing patterns
- Inadequate nutrition
- Constipation
- Altered communication
- Altered vision
- Sexual dysfunction

Date: Time	FVC	Count/1 Breath	SW	DBL vision	Arm hang	Med
4:00 PM	2.00 L	20/1 breath	3/5	R lat gaze	30 sec R	Mestinon 60
8:00 PM	1.00 L	9/1 breath	1/5	R lat gaze ptosis bilat	10 sec R	Could not swallow med

A

Date: Time		Worse	Parkinson	Best	Dyskinesias	Worse	Med/dose
	Scale:	0%	−50%	100%	+50%	0	
5:00 PM			−70				Sinemet 20/200
7:30 PM					+15 (Freezing noted)		Sinemet 10/100
10:00 PM			−95		(Mild)		Sinemet 20/200

B

Figure 21-1. Bedside flow sheet for monitoring (A) patients with myasthenia gravis and (B) mobility in patients with Parkinson's disease.

- Discomfort
- Ineffective coping
- Social isolation
- Knowledge deficit
- Home maintenance management
- Alterations in health maintenance

Case studies are used to illustrate several of these diagnoses.

Case Study 1: Chronic Immobility Associated with Parkinson's Disease

Mr. Earl is a 76-year-old man who has had symptoms of parkinsonism for at least 25 years. He was forced into early retirement at age 52 because his parkinsonism interfered with his ability to perform his job as the proprietor of a newsstand. Treatment with levodopa almost completely restored his mobility, although the positive effects were marred by nausea and brief periods of tremor and weakness. Occasionally, he would awaken at night choking on his saliva. These episodes were accompanied by stertorous respirations (labored breathing) that were relieved by walking. In 1974, he switched to Sinemet; this formulation of levodopa eliminated his nausea. With Sinemet, he began to notice slight dyskinesias, periods of (chorealike) extra movements characterized by grimacing, swaying on standing, or, when sitting, a kicking restless leg movement. These movements were not bothersome, and he usually did not notice them unless a family member drew his attention to them. They often accompanied time periods when he felt the most mobile, relaxed, and energetic. After 5 years of treatment with Sinemet, Mr. Earl's dyskinesias began to occur unpredictably throughout the day rather than only after each dose of Sinemet. Attempts to improve mobility by altering the dosing schedule and increasing the amount of Sinemet did not improve mobility and resulted in increased dyskinesias. The dyskinesias on a higher dose were so pronounced that they caused profuse sweating and dehydration. On one occasion, Mr. Earl developed fever and obstipation, which prompted hospitalization. On a lower daily dose of Sinemet, he noticed less relief of symptoms of immobility and continued to have unpredictable periods of freer movement. Swallowing occurred only with effort, even during relatively mobile times. Mr. Earl had lost 10 pounds, to weigh 105 pounds.

Constipation was treated with laxatives, stool softener, suppositories, and enemas. Burning sensations affecting his forearms and the soles of his feet interfered with his ability to be comfortable at night and obtain needed rest. Aching pain in his shoulders and arms was relieved with frequent range of motion exercises day and night. Mrs. Earl was becoming frustrated and overwhelmed with her husband's needs for assistance with all activities; her sciatica was recurring and interfering with her ability to obtain a full night's rest. Mr. and Mrs. Earl could not afford to hire help, nor could they receive reimbursement for Mr. Earl's health care expenses. After several attempts to involve him in day activities for the elderly, several falls, increasing weight loss, and recurring obstipation, Mr. Earl was admitted to the hospital for improvement of his medication regimen under observation and evaluation and treatment of a chronically distended abdomen. Although Mr. Earl has many diagnoses, his case is used to discuss the potential for injury diagnosis.

☐ Potential for Injury

Physical safety is the most basic of human needs. The potential for injury is defined as a state in which the individual is at risk for or has experienced damage to body tissues because of a perceptual or physiologic deficit, a lack of awareness, or maturational age (Carpenito, 1984). Amyotrophic lateral sclerosis, cerebrovascular accident, muscular dystrophy, multiple sclerosis, and many of the chronic motor disorders can cause one's ability to move to be so weakened or disturbed that potential injury is a severe threat. Patients with Parkinson's disease, in particular, have difficulty related to the unpredictability of the degree and timing of response to levodopa therapy. This occurs in patients who have had parkinsonism for several years and have been receiving levodopa therapy usually more than 5 years (Marsden et al., 1982).

These responses may be characterized by extra movements (dyskinesias) or by lack of movement (akinesia or bradykinesia). Dyskinesias place the individual at risk for being thrown off balance or out of chairs. *Off periods* refer to times without satisfactory mobility and may be initiated by gradual or sudden loss of mobility.

Additional problems include a reduced position sense and the slowing of one's ability to correct a loss of balance through movement. This can lead to injury or falls. Reduced sensitivity of the autonomic system can be accentuated by some of the medications used to treat Parkinson's disease, as well as being an independent symptom. Lightheadedness on standing can contribute to loss of balance. Shuffling or short steps of low amplitude associated with parkinsonism are a product of reduced movement and rigidity and can lead to tripping and falls. The patient with footdrop resulting from muscular dystrophy or multiple sclerosis also is in danger of falling without proper intervention. The fatigued or weakened individual, such as the person who suffers from a chronic neurologic disorder, is at risk for injury, since he or she experiences reduced control of movement related to prolonged inactivity.

Defining characteristics include evidence of environmental hazards or lack of knowledge about environmental hazards, a history of accidents, and lack of knowledge about safety precautions. Impaired mobility and sensory deficits contribute to the diagnosis of potential for injury. The activity level may be consciously or unconsciously altered in an effort to compensate for slight but definite changes in mobility and strength affecting safety as well as self-care capabilities.

When attempting to establish the presence of a potential for injury, one examines the client's ability to be aware of the body's position in space and control that position. *Assessment* should include (1) Romberg response, (2) gait, (3) blood pressure and pulse determination for orthostatic changes and autonomic dysfunction, (4) posture, (5) muscle strength, (6) coordination, (7) uncontrolled involuntary movements, and (8) ability to recover position when forcibly displaced. Information obtained from the client should include the number and precipitating factors and times of any injuries or falls. It is important to know if mobility aids are being used properly and successfully. The *expected outcome* for this diagnosis is that the patient be able to maintain maximal independent mobility without physical injury.

Nursing interventions for the person with impaired mobility focus on teaching that person to associate particular symptoms with a potentially injurious situation. Examples of these situations and the precautions that can be taken follow.

Potential for Falls

For lightheadedness or orthostasis, the person should change position slowly; getting up from a resting position to sitting or standing may need to be done over 5 minutes or more. Blocks at the head of the bed may reduce this problem by minimizing the difference between the lying and upright positions by stimulating blood pressure-regulating mechanisms. The marked dyskinesias or freezing that are extremes of on–off fluctuations for the parkinsonian or choreoathetosis for the person with Huntington's disease may necessitate retirement to a chair or bed to prevent loss of balance or injury to the legs or arms from flailing movements. Equipment may need to be padded with sheepskin, foam, or linen to prevent bruising. Frequent repetitive movement can quickly cause a pressure sore where none existed previously, especially at the sacrum, heels, elbows, or ankles. Shuffling steps reduce the size and thus stability of one's base for standing and allow tripping. Leather-soled shoes with low heels are recommended for carpeted areas. Parallel strips of tape about 1 foot apart on the floor provide visual input that paradoxically reduces freezing for the person with parkinsonism.

Mr. Earl required assistance for balance in ambulation most of the time; this was accomplished by having someone walk backward holding onto both of his hands facing him. He was unable to use a walker because of a tendency to fall backward. A sheet restraint tied loosely or a return to bed during dyskinetic periods would help prevent falls. Because of previous problems, when Mr. Earl returned home the public health nurse reviewed the home situation for potential hazards, such as rug placement, grab bars in the bath, the family's plans to cope with falls, and use of appropriate transfer techniques. She noticed that their furniture was comfortable and did not seem to be a barrier, they did not have a gas stove, and their equipment was in good repair. The nurse discussed the correct method of wheelchair use and going up and down ramps safely and reinforced using a seatbelt in the car.

Some homes may require modification, particularly those with bathrooms only on the second floor or steep stairwells that the mobility-impaired patient finds difficult or impossible to climb. The mobility-impaired patient who gets up frequently at night to use the bathroom will need this problem addressed to prevent falls. Ramps, Hoyer lifts, and other home modifications can prevent accidents and injuries to the patient or to the family member who lifts or transfers the patient and should be included in care planning.

The dangers in stair use for the person with reduced mobility are the potential loss of balance backward or forward or inability to complete stair climbing because of weakness. The tendency to fall backward, retropulsion, can be brought out by other situations that challenge position sense, such as reaching or gazing upward, stepping backward when opening a door, sudden movement to avoid injury, or carrying on more than one activity at once. Patients should be cautioned to use additional reference points in space to increase their awareness of position. Examples of common supports are touching furniture or walls when walking, having a back against a wall or leaning into a sink even slightly when standing for long periods.

Potential for Skin Breakdown

The patient with spinal cord injury or multiple sclerosis may have reduced sensory awareness below the level of the lesions that interferes with awareness of ischemic pressure areas. This person must be checked and learn to check himself for areas of skin redness or breakdown periodically. The person with a right hemispheric CVA needs to compensate for input regarding the location and presence of left-sided extremities. These people also need to learn to rethink automatic activities, such as getting out of bed, to include their compromised left side. After they learn which situations can precipitate injury, patients may be more willing to try independent activities with more self-confidence and should continually increase and challenge these skills.

Case Study 2: Immobility Associated with Myasthenia Gravis

Mrs. X was on her way to class; in 2 weeks she would graduate from the community college with an associate degree in nursing with an A average. It did not seem like it had been just 9 years since the birth of her seventh child. She had been only 33 years old and had felt very frightened. Immediately after the uncomplicated birth, the intense fatigue, hoarse voice, and catch in her throat she had experienced over the preceding three months worsened. She was unable to swallow saliva, her eyelids drooped, she saw two of everything, and, worst of all, she could not catch her breath. The next 3 days were a blur, on and off the ventilator, intravenous tubes, infusions, and medications. Pneumonia complicated her hospitalization. A new medicine, edrophonium chloride, finally was used to diagnose a disease she had never heard of, myasthenia gravis. During the years that followed, she had to modify her activities considerably. Mrs. X was not able to climb the two flights of stairs in her home more than once a day and could hold the baby only while sitting down. She was able to rely on her older children to run many errands in the house, such as going up and down stairs and doing the laundry. Managing a home with seven children did not afford her much rest, however, and she frequently had to call on friends and relatives for assistance. Her husband could not cope with the limitations imposed on him by the disease and ultimately abandoned the family. After several years of treatment, which included thymectomy and alternate-day corticosteroids, she was slowly able to resume her usual busy schedule. When her vision and strength stabilized, she resumed driving again. This enabled her to have a great deal more independence. She became involved with the local volunteer ambulance squad and enrolled in nursing school. After 10 years of treatment, she commented, "I know a lot more about nursing now and hope that I can help patients as much as I was helped through those awful years." The diagnosis illustrated by her case is *activity intolerance*.

☐ Activity Intolerance

Activity intolerance can be related to fluctuations in neurotransmitters, failure of neuromuscular transmission, muscle weakness or atrophy due to loss of nerve or muscle fibers, prolonged inactivity, depression, and fear. Patients with myasthenia gravis and multiple sclerosis will occasionally report that heat, particularly hot baths, can increase weakness. The central feature of this diagnosis is that the patient is unable to tolerate an increase in activity.

Defining characteristics include shortness of breath and fatigue after activity, specific patterns of muscle weakness in tested muscle groups, and reports of self-care deficits that may vary throughout the day. Being unable to climb stairs or ambulate for long distances, as well as avoidance of usual activity patterns or exercise is common.

Assessment should include identification of subjective and objective measures of activity tolerance. The patient may describe an inability to perform activities of daily living (ADL) or ambulate independently. The patient should be asked to review daily and weekly activity patterns, including occupation, leisure activity, quiet activity, and exercise programs. Other environmental factors, such as changes in the weather, the number of stairs in the home, and distance traveled walking from work to home, may assist in understanding the baseline activity tolerance. The nurse should record subjective complaints of shortness of breath and objective tests of strength as outlined previously in Chapter 19. Strength and functional ability can vary from hour to hour or consist of a more subtle change in activity pattern in a previously active patient. The activity pattern seen before the onset of illness will influence the nurse's expectations. A young adult who ran or jogged several miles a day will experience different limitations than a less active or aged client. Once the presence of this diagnosis is determined, the *goal* is that the patient will adapt to varying levels of strength in order to pursue a full range of satisfying activities.

Nursing interventions for patients having severely reduced activity tolerance include scheduling activities during periods of maximal strength. This can occur at peak doses of medications, such as levodopa or anticholinesterases, or for some patients in the morning hours when they are fully rested. This may mean a change in the patient's previous activity patterns. Working with the patient to develop a plan for each day can be of assistance. Encouraging the patient to be an executive with a predetermined daily schedule has been suggested (Myasthenia Gravis Foundation, 1979). The patient should plan to incorporate rest periods into both work and leisure activities. This was important to Mrs. X, since she was able to enlist her older children to help supervise the younger children during naps and to do the laundry. In many cases, the patient should double the amount of time he or she would normally expect to prepare for an activity, both to provide a rest period and for unanticipated problems. Asking the patient to rehearse the day also assists in setting realistic goals. A cane or walker provides support; walkers with wheels replacing the front two legs provide support without necessitating picking up the walker (which might put the parkinsonian into retropulsion and cause a fall) and reduces energy requirements for the weakened or fatigued person.

Patients with severe proximal weakness and resultant difficulty in stair climbing will need to consider alternate methods of climbing stairs. These considerations need careful advance planning in patients with progressive disorders who have homes that may become inaccessible as time goes on. Expensive home adaptations need to be considered with this in mind. Stair rails on both walls and wall grips or handles at landings can be helpful. Rails in the shower and bath, as well as bath benches and handheld shower hoses, must be considered. The patient with foot drop that interferes with mobility should be fitted with lightweight plastic short-leg braces, also called ankle–foot orthoses.

When the patient is completely immobilized, which can occur in muscular dystrophy, amyotrophic lateral sclerosis, and spinal cord injury, a range of motion exercises are necessary to maintain joint mobility. Patients with most forms of neuromuscular disease will eventually require a wheelchair to maintain normal activities. There are many new chairs that have features attractive to the patient with a chronic motor disorder. Some are lightweight and have the added feature of being able to assume the standing position or have a motor attached (Fig. 21–2).

For the patient with less variability in symptoms and improving strength, consideration should be given to designing an exercise program. Specific exercise programs that improve flexibility and endurance as well as increase strength have many benefits (Cobble & Maloney, 1985). Most patients avoid exercise because it is perceived as a significant stress. Indeed, many aerobic programs are inappropriate for patients with severe muscle weakness and fatigue. There has been renewed interest in designing individual exercise programs for patients with chronic motor disorders. A successful study of patients with multiple sclerosis demonstrated positive effects on strength, endurance, work, and muscle power using an aquatic fitness program (Gehlson et al., 1984). Before beginning an

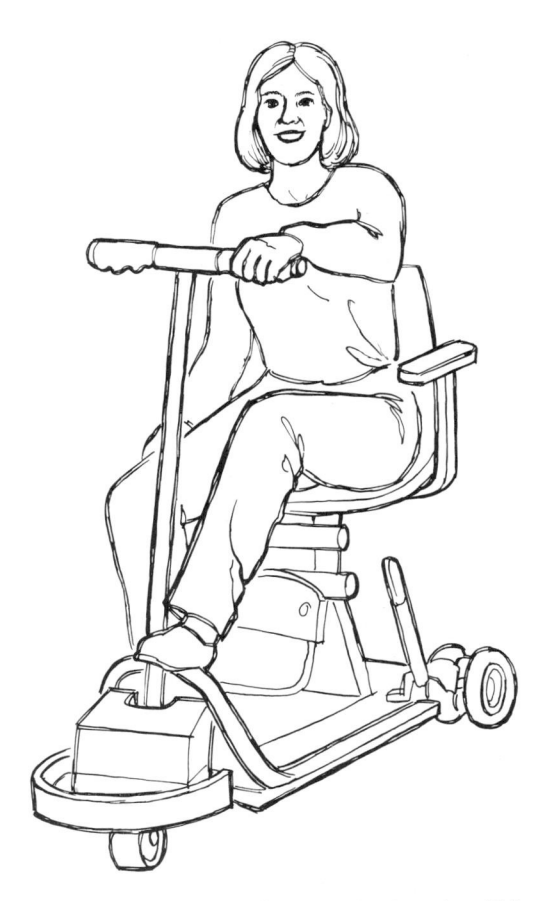

Figure 21-2. A motorized scooter. *(Redrawn from Maloney et al. [1985].)*

exercise program, patients should request the assistance of their health care providers to monitor its effects on their strength and functional ability. Individual exercise prescriptions that address the patient's age, strength, and interests and functional ability can do much to improve the patient's well-being as well as motor strength, flexibility, and endurance.

Transportation and accessibility have been deterrents for wheelchair-bound patients. Several ambulatory patients have reported that participation in a graduated exercise program is possible. In fact, several symptomatic patients with myasthenia gravis and multiple sclerosis have continued exercise programs that include weightlifting, swimming, stationary rowing, and jogging. One patient with myasthenia gravis reported completing a marathon. Many handicapped patients benefit from participation in handicapped sports, such as wheelchair basketball, baseball, bowling, and field hockey. Empiric studies of the benefits of exercise in the patient with chronic motor problems are urgently needed. Until they are completed, each patient needs to be individually considered and carefully monitored. For the extremely weak patient, performing activities of daily living will provide them with all the exercise they need to maintain strength.

Case Study 3: Chronic Immobility Associated with Muscular Dystrophy

Mike was 5 years old when his parents realized that he was not keeping up with his peers. Subsequently, they always felt the worst period in their lives was the time when they were told that he had muscular dystrophy. He has been cared for in a comprehensive multidisciplinary clinic practice since the diagnosis was made at age 6. By age 10, his balance was so precarious that he began to fall frequently. The wheelchair that they formerly dreaded came as a relief. He continued to be able to stand for several hours a day with the assistance of long leg braces and a standing table. His parents wanted him to be treated like any other child, and he enjoyed attending a mainstream school with his older sister. At first, he found it difficult to ask his friends to assist him, especially with toileting. To assist him with this and other problems, a plan was developed each year with the assistance of the clinic staff and school nurse to coordinate transportation between classes, appropriate physical education activities, notetaking, and social activities. He graduated from college with an associate degree in computer science. A work–study program gave him experience as a computer programmer; however, he was not able to find a job when the family moved.

Although always described as quiet, he had many friends. His family was active with the local chapter of the Muscular Dystrophy Association. His mother attended a mothers' group that served to share problems and concerns. They offered such practical advice as how to use assisitive devices, Hoyer lifts, commodes, and wheelchairs. Health care providers from the clinic were often invited guests.

Mike always had trouble getting over upper respiratory infections. At age 19, he had his first severe pneumonia that required hospitalization. He was treated with postural drainage and cupping, using intermittent positive pressure breathing (IPPB) with a bronchodilator before and after the treatment. Broad-spectrum antibiotics and hydration were continued during his 14-day hospital stay. This was a stressful time for Mike. He was secure in his usual home routine and was fearful that the nurses would not understand his needs. Because of his severe contractures, it would often take extended periods of time to position him correctly. Some nurses were patient; others could not understand why he continuously asked for repositioning. He was fearful that he would drop his call bell or that some one would not hear him if he called. He had great difficulty feeding himself while he was in the hospital. The hospital overbed tables were awkward, and unless he was positioned just right he could not feed himself. His forced vital capacity (FVC) was 700 ml during the acute episode and increased to 1 liter several months later. After this episode, he began asking questions about his breathing, and options for future ventilatory support were discussed. *Self-care deficit* and *impaired respiratory function* are the diagnoses discussed in relation to Mike's case.

☐ Self-Care Deficit

Self-care deficit can be related to the severity of muscle weakness and its resultant immobility. This may occur as a static or fluctuating problem in patients with many of the chronic motor disorders, depending on the extent of involvement.

Defining characteristics of self-care deficit include inability to feed or bathe oneself independently and to complete other aspects of hygenic care (care of hair, nails, teeth, skin, make-up application). The patient may manifest difficulty getting on and off the toilet due to proximal muscle weakness. Many patients with severe muscle weakness as seen in muscular dystrophy, spinal cord injury, and amyotrophic lateral sclerosis develop contractures in a specific pattern associated with weakness of specific muscle groups. For patients with multiple sclerosis, cerebrovascular accident, and spinal cord injury, contractures are usually due to severe spasticity and become a significant problem in their management.

Assessment includes physical assessment of the patient's strength and functional ability as well as assessment of daily self-care routines. The *goal* for this diagnosis is to produce an individualized plan of care that would be flexible enough to respond to changes in the patients' abilities and yet promote maximum independence and positive coping.

Nursing interventions may include providing assistance in activities of daily living as the patient directs. The hospital care plan should reflect the patient's home routines as closely as possible to allow the nurse to assess the patient's safety during transfers and the degree of symptom control and to make the patient feel "in charge." For patients with disorders in which fatigue is a factor, such as myasthenia gravis and multiple sclerosis, special considerations must be made. Hospital routines rarely reflect the effort that home activities require. The patient who is not taxed in the hospital or does not participate in care that reflects home requirements may have further difficulties on discharge. While assisting the patient in self-care activities or developing his care plan, the nurse should encourage the fatigued patient not to overextend himself and plan rest periods throughout the day. Discussing how the patient will manage the same activities at home can be accomplished at this time.

For patients with Parkinson's disease, myasthenia gravis, and multiple sclerosis, meals and activities should always be scheduled at periods of peak strength or flexibility. The nurse could use these times to teach the patient to use energy-saving routines, such as dressing and combing the hair while lying down. In addition, for patients with static or more slowly progressive disorders, energy-saving devices, such as a bath bench, handheld shower hose, and easy grip eating utensils, can be suggested for use at home. Special utensils or equipment to maximize use of motor capabilities will save energy, facilitate communication, and allow independence. For patients with severe weakness, positioning may be a key factor in allowing self-feeding. A ballbearing orthosis attached to the wheelchair will allow patients with severe shoulder weakness, yet sufficient biceps, strength to feed themselves (Fig. 21–3).

Other devices, such as wrist splints and built-up utensils, enable the patient with a weakened grip to manage meals independently. An occupational therapist should be consulted to evaluate the patients for these devices. Only in unusual circumstances should the nurse feed the patient with chronic immobility. Feeding oneself may be the only measure of independence such people have, as in Mike's case. For many patients with chronic immobility, bathroom modifications may be necessary. Using a Hoyer lift, raised toilet seat, and wheelchair-accessible shower should be considered. Velcro closures can allow some patients ease in dressing, although they may need the assistance of another if they are pressed by school or employment in the morning. Additional devices or techniques can be obtained from other patients and literature provided by such support groups such as the Myasthenia Gravis Foundation, Amyotrophic Lateral Sclerosis Society, Multiple Sclerosis Society, and Parkinson's Disease Foundation.

☐ Impaired Respiratory Function

The patient with impaired respiratory function has reduced airway clearance or ineffective breathing patterns. These are present in the acutely ill patient with myasthenia gravis but are most frequently seen during the late stages of muscular dystrophy, amyotrophic lateral sclerosis, Parkinson's disease, and Huntington's disease and are often precipitated by respiratory infection. Patients with high cervical (above C3) lesions also contend with ventilatory failure.

Patients with chronic motor disorders rarely have significant blood gas abnormalities on a chronic basis as a *defining characteristic* unless obstructive disease is present. Blood gas abnormalities consistent with alveolar hypoventilation usually follow significant changes in pulmonary function tests or occur only in the presence of respiratory infections. Before the 1960s, many patients with respiratory dysfunction due to neurologic disease died secondary to pulmonary compromise. Crisis seen in patients with myasthenia gravis continues to be associated with upper respiratory infections, significant dysarthria and dysphagia, and aspiration (Grob et al., 1981; Griggs & Donohoe, 1985). Patients with neuromuscular diseases, such as muscular dystrophy, amyotrophic lateral sclerosis, and late stages of multiple sclerosis, have severely reduced objective pulmonary function indicators. Respiratory insufficiency due to a

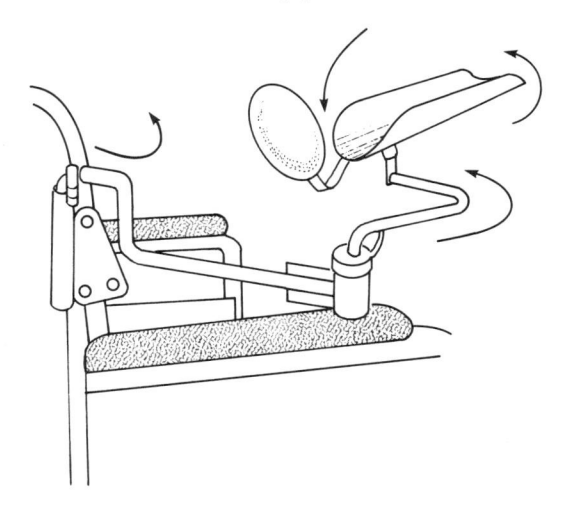

Figure 21–3. Assistive devices: Ballbearing feeder. *(Redrawn from Maloney et al. [1985].)*

decline in pulmonary function is a common cause of death in muscular dystrophy and amyotrophic lateral sclerosis (Griggs et al., 1981). Respiratory compromise was the most frequent cause of death in Huntington's disease patients, according to a survey by Edmonds (1966) and was thought related to dysphagia and aspiration secondary to the involuntary movements affecting swallowing. Studies in patients with parkinsonism have revealed both restrictive and obstructive components to their pulmonary function. Reduced vital capacity and more consistently reduced maximal flow rates were closely correlated with the degree of tremor and rigidity in these patients. The flow rates were postulated to be reduced in relation to the parasympathetic overactivity (Neu et al., 1967).

Assessment should include (1) tests of pulmonary function, particularly FVC, maximum static pressures—maximum expiratory pressure (MEP) and maximum inspiratory pressure (MIP), (2) estimate of counting in one breath, (3) ability to cough and swallow, (4) presence of pharyngeal secretions, (5) subjective sensations of shortness of breath or choking, (6) reduced chest expansion, and (7) presence of adventitious sounds on auscultation. The *goal* for the patient with impaired respiratory function is the maintenance of air passage through the respiratory tract and the exchange of gases between the lungs and the vascular system.

Specific interventions include monitoring activities. Pulmonary function should be tested at frequent intervals. If possible, the nurse should calculate percent predicted FVC, minimum ventilatory volume (MVV), MEP, and MIP for height and age to determine the extent of abnormality. The patient should be monitored while asymptomatic to establish a baseline. With myasthenia gravis, pulmonary function tests and other assessments should be made at intervals to correspond with the anticholinesterase dosage to observe the effects of the medication and determine the lower limit of the patient's strength.

Patients with chronic immobility should be monitored closely because of their ability to change unpredictably and briskly. Patients with muscle weakness rarely show retraction or tachypnea; as their fatigue increases, their muscles become increasingly weak. This may prevent them from asking for assistance or exhibiting the usual signs of pulmonary compromise, such as restlessness and tachypnea.

Nursing intervention also includes patient teaching. The patient should receive instructions on preventing infection, treating it early, and monitoring for signs of respiratory fatigue. The patient should know how to take his or her temperature and take over-the-counter medications to treat cold symptoms, such as antipyretics, decongestants, and cough medicines. Many patients with myasthenia gravis are concerned with the adverse effects of some medications on the neuromuscular junction (this particularly applies to some antibiotics). Sudafed, a commonly used over-the-counter decongestant, usually is suggested because it is very similar to the medication ephedrine, which is used as an adjunctive medication for symptomatic treatment of MG. The patient should be aware of the need to increase fluid consumption to at least 2 liters or more per day during an upper respiratory infection. Patients with chronic motor disorders should receive the pneumonia vaccine (Pneumovax) and a yearly flu shot to prevent pneumonia and influenza.

The patient with poor pulmonary function, that is, anyone with FVC less than 1 liter or less than 10 to 15 ml/kg body weight, may need tracheostomy and ventilatory support after severe respiratory infections or surgery or because of anticipated disease worsening, such as occurs in myasthenia gravis. Appropriate explanations of procedures and sensations to be experienced should be discussed. Many patients recover from these crises to resume their previous activity level; others may not be able to be weaned from ventilatory support. This should be anticipated and discussed well before the acute episode in chronic progressive disorders.

Ventilatory support for patients with chronic motor disorders is not a new phenomenon, yet technology has changed the options for these patients. The poliomyelitis experience of the 1940s and 1950s demonstrated the utility of providing ventilatory support in the hope that the patient would stabilize and improve. The intensive care unit, first described in the literature in 1955, originated from the concept of clustering patients in the polio wards to consolidate those who required highly skilled nursing care (Cadmus, 1980). Today, providing extraordinary means of support has been simplified by the availability of compact portable systems for positive pressure and a renewed interest in the negative pressure devices used in the poliomyelitis era. These devices are being used increasingly in the home with success (Splaingard et al., 1985; Griggs & Donohoe, 1985).

Negative pressure ventilators in use today include the cuirass, wrap-raincoat, and iron lung. The cuirass is a plastic shell that fits over the anterior chest wall and can be molded to conform to a scoliotic curvature. The wrap ventilator, also called the "raincoat," has a metal cage that spans the chest and supports a heavy plastic raincoat-like material away from the body.

The tank or iron lung ventilator can be used to simulate inspiration and promote air exchange. It is very heavy, may require home modifications, and is reported to be in short supply (Curran, 1981). The pneumobelt is another noninvasive device. It has a plastic inflatable bladder that is attached to a corset that fits around the abdomen. It serves as an expiratory assist; with inflation, the abdomen is compressed and the diaphragm is pushed upward. The patient must be sitting to use it comfortably.

Positive pressure devices are the next most frequently used ventilatory support system. They can be used intermittently, such as IPPB treatments, or continuously, with a mouthpiece or tracheostomy. Some patients can use mouth positive pressure comfortably. Most patients with severe respiratory weakness require tracheostomy. The compact portable systems (such as the LP5 and LP6 by the Life Care Corporation and the PPV and Bear system) have been used successfully for home care. Teaching the patient glossopharyngeal breathing to augment vital capacity has been suggested. This procedure requires that the patient take a series of deep breaths without exhaling and has been used by poliomyelitis and spinal cord injury patients successfully to give the patient time off the ventilator (Alexander et al., 1979).

Patients with neuromuscular disease often have pneumonias and retained secretions. Postural drainage and cupping have always been used in conjunction with appropriate antibiotics, hydration, and, if necessary, supplemental oxygen and IPPB. IPPB or other methods provide sighs and hyperexpansion in the patient with hypoventilation due to muscle weakness. The method of postural drainage described in most texts is laborious and time consuming. Few studies have documented its worth on empiric grounds, although it makes sense on practical grounds in patients who cannot produce a sufficient cough, cannot bring up retained secretions, or fatigue rapidly in an effort to do so. Some practitioners and the authors have found that a simpler method is effective and is tolerated better by patients (Lavigne, 1979; Callahan, 1985). It consists of draining the lungs in two positions, with patients lying on their right, then left side, with the hips elevated above the head in the Trendelenburg position (Fig. 21–4). The position is maintained on each side for a minimum of 30 to 45 minutes. The patient should be comfortably positioned to tolerate this time period. Patients with diaphragmatic weakness or severe respiratory insufficiency will need to be on the ventilator during postural drainage and cupping. Other patients will need sighs or IPPB before and after the procedure. Although it takes an hour, the thoroughness of this procedure reduces the necessity of its performance more often than every 4 hours, and it is well-tolerated by patients at home (Callahan, 1985).

Mike and his family successfully learned the postural drainage and cupping procedure

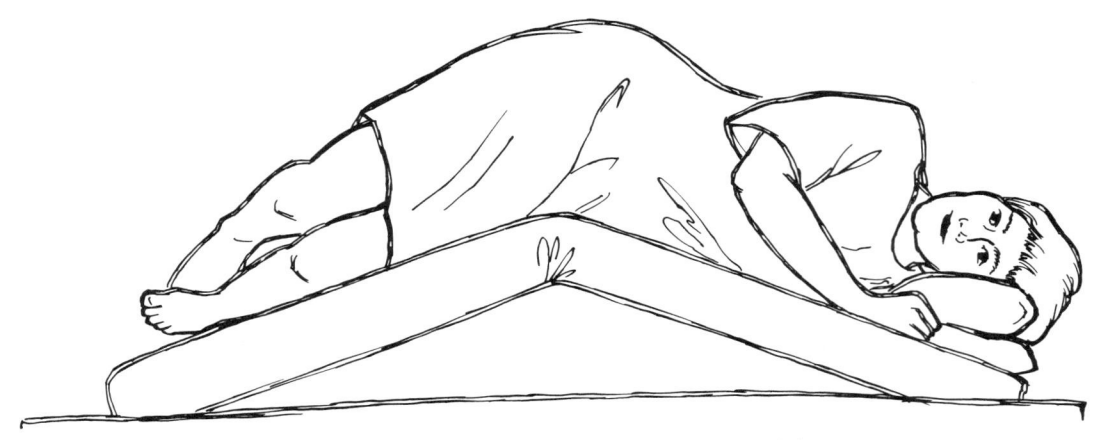

Figure 21–4. Patient in the correct position for postural drainage.

during his first hospitalization for pneumonia and subsequently used it once a day with IPPB to prevent atelectasis and facilitate secretion removal.

Associated Nursing Diagnoses

Chronically altered mobility serves as an etiology for a number of other nursing diagnoses. The relationship of these diagnoses to chronically altered mobility is discussed briefly here.

☐ Inadequate Nutrition Related to Dysphagia

Inadequate nutrition can be related to reduced swallowing and chewing ability, as in the case study of the man with parkinsonism, as well as in other chronic motor disorders. An inability to prepare food can affect the person with weakness or fatigue. Inability to chew and to swallow food is a severely distressing state. Fear of choking or fear of making a mess prevents attempts to eat. Family members or significant others are hesitant to assist the patient because they are afraid of being unable to manage choking episodes effectively. Defining characteristics, assessment, and interventions for this diagnosis are found in Chapter 23.

☐ Constipation Related to Decreased Activity

Constipation is defined as the state in which the individual experiences or is at high risk of experiencing stasis in the large intestine, resulting in hard dry feces and infrequent elimination. All neurologic disorders resulting in chronic immobility place the individual at risk for this problem. Contributing factors to constipation secondary to reduced mobility are outlined in the next paragraph.

As the body's activity level slows, the movement of material through the gastrointestinal track becomes slower also. With slowing, more fluid is extracted from the feces, and it becomes more compact. This process makes elimination even more difficult for the weakened patient. Medications can contribute to the presence of constipation by slowing bowel function further, for example, the anticholinergics used in the treatment of movement disorders. Difficulty in chewing and swallowing can lead to inadequate fluid intake, and reliance on fast, prepared, or pureed foods that have little fiber can lead to constipation. Obesity, which can develop easily in the mobility limited patient, such as the person with muscular dystrophy, can hinder bowel and abdominal muscle function. Hospitalization or the need for assistance with elimination removes privacy.

Irregular patterns may develop because of these factors. In an effort to treat irregularity, laxatives and enemas may be employed; chronically, these make the bowel musculature lazy and contribute further to constipation. "In a society where innumerable approaches to a daily bowel movement are advertised on television and over $200 million are spent annually on laxatives sold over the counter, reeducation is necessary" (Levine, 1985). The older person experiences reduced motility of the gastrointestinal tract related to normal aging. Defining characteristics, assessment, and intervention for this diagnosis are found in Chapter 29.

☐ **Altered Communication Relative to Dysarthria and Dysphonia**

The patient with chronic immobility due to many motor disorders may have poor communication because of dysarthria and dysphonia and limb and hand muscle weakness. Communication is impaired when a tracheostomy is in place. The patient who is quadriplegic secondary to spinal cord injury, multiple sclerosis, muscular dystrophy, or amyotrophic lateral sclerosis, for example, is limited in the ability to communicate verbally or with extremities.

Most patients with chronic neurologic disorders with fatigable weakness, such as myasthenia gravis, Parkinson's disease, or multiple sclerosis, have no difficulty with comprehension. For these patients, dysarthria and dysphonia are evident in prolonged conversation. A patient can be tested for fatigue by being asked to read aloud. Shortness of breath or ineffective breathing patterns will interfere with verbal communication. Assessment and interventions for this diagnosis are found in Chapters 14 and 15.

☐ **Altered Vision Related to Ocular Muscle Weakness**

Altered vision can contribute to immobility or be the result of a chronic immobilizing disorder. Contributing factors include pathophysiologic, situational, and maturational changes. In myasthenia gravis, altered vision can be related to fatigue of ocular muscles at the neuromuscular junction or structural ophthalmologic dysfunction. In Parkinson's disease, reduced ocular accommodation can contribute to blurred vision, and fatigue of the muscles involved in eye movements can interfere with reading or other close work. Slowed eye movements in Huntington's disease can slow receipt of information and increase the effort involved in daily activities, such as driving, reading, and housekeeping.

Defining characteristics of altered vision include difficulty reading, accomplishing ADL, driving, doing fine work with the hands, watching television, movies, or plays, and severe difficulty with spatial orientation secondary to diplopia, ptosis, or other dysfunction of motor ocular structures.

Assessment includes evaluating the patient for signs of ptosis and diplopia and performing tests of visual acuity. The presence of cataracts should be considered when assessing blurred vision. The *goal* is to maximize the patient's visual abilities with supportive devices or to supplement sensory perceptions by using other senses. These methods, hopefully, will reduce the potential for reduced mobility resulting from fear and instability.

Interventions include using lid crutches that support the drooping eyelid or wearing sunglasses to protect the eye from the sun's glare (particularly if the patient is bothered by heat). Diplopia can be relieved by patching one eye. If one eye is covered with a patch, the patient will notice a decrease in depth perception and should be warned that this may impair driving ability. The patient should alternate patches frequently to prevent disuse in the patched eye. The patient who is acutely ill may benefit from having someone read the newspapers and letters aloud. Large print books, talking books, and tape-recorded letters from friends and family can add to the patient's enjoyment. Treatment of cataracts is of great help to patients with diminished activity and is usually recommended when they interfere with functional ability (i.e., driving and reading).

☐ Sexual dysfunction

Sexual dysfunction can be related to fatigue seen with chronic immobility or depression and concerns about self-image. There is no reported physiologic disturbance to impair enjoyment of sexual response in muscular dystrophy, amyotrophic lateral sclerosis, and myasthenia gravis. A physiologic disturbance that impairs the sexual response is seen with spinal cord injury (77% with preserved erection and 10% with preserved ejaculation) (Boller & Frank, 1982) and multiple sclerosis (43% with total or partial impotence after 5½ years of illness) (Vas, 1969). The prevalence and etiology of the dysfunctions are not well understood in Huntington's disease and Parkinson's disease. The improvement in sexual behavior characterized by increased libido and greater coital frequency seen during levodopa therapy (Bowers & VanWoert, 1972) is usually thought to be the result of improved motor activity and affect. Defining characteristics, assessment, and interventions are found in Chapters 30 and 31.

☐ Discomfort

A state in which the patient feels an uncomfortable sensation in response to a noxious stimulus is discomfort. It may be related to a prolonged increase in muscle tone, leading to cramping or uncomfortable dystonias. Maintaining the same position for longer than 1 to 2 hours can cause stiffness of joints and discomfort on movement affecting the joint and muscle. Pressure points are painful because of tissue ischemia. Involuntary movements can lead to repeated trauma to body parts and discomfort. Dysesthesias in Parkinson's disease, spinal cord injury, and multiple sclerosis can become disabling. These may include burning or tingling sensations. Warm or cool temperature intolerances may be present.

The *defining characteristic* is the patient's report of pain or discomfort. For the person with multiple sclerosis or spinal cord injury, the pain may be localized to a referred place. A guarded position, facial expression of pain, or crying and moaning suggest the presence of some discomfort even though the client may not be able to express this problem verbally. Additionally, there may be evidence of autonomic responses to acute pain, such as increased blood pressure, pulse, and respirations, diaphoresis, and dilated pupils.

The *assessment* of discomfort is accomplished by determining any pattern, location, onset, duration, aggravating factors, characteristics, relieving maneuvers, and treatments. The *goal* in any problem characterized by discomfort is to maximize comfort. The nurse does this by correctly determining the cause of the discomfort whenever possible.

Discomfort related to immobility is relieved by the *nursing intervention* of repositioning of limbs or the body, passive range of motion exercises, or such active exercises as walking, swimming, or active range of motion. Movement relieves pressure at bony prominences, especially when massage is applied to the skin over that prominence, and restores circulation. Patients who have not been out of bed for prolonged periods need to be introduced gradually to periods in one position. Water pillows, Gelfoam mattresses, foam rubber pads, or cushions reduce pressure over prominences and potential discomfort. Muscle spasms and cramping are relieved by range of motion exercises. Dysesthesias in Parkinson's disease are thought to be more bothersome in the more immobile patient. If activity can be increased, there may be at least partial relief of this problem.

☐ Potential for Ineffective Coping

Unfortunately for many patients and families with chronic disorders, early diagnosis is the exception and not the rule. This is the most overwhelmingly stressful period of many patients' experience (Sampson & Cosley, 1983; Latham et al., 1983). Changes in body image and self-concept and fluctuations in strength and functional ability make coping a difficult task. Skills developed during the early stages of illness assist the patient to cope with subsequent stages of illness (Moos & Schaefer, 1984).

Defining characteristics include reduced and increased verbalization and inability to make decisions. The presence of confused roles, inability to relinquish control, or inability to meet basic needs can be a cue to inadequate coping.

Assessment should include the patient's previous experiences with illness, particularly how he or she made decisions and coped with adversity in the past. This could also include changes in lifestyle or problems unrelated to health. Asking the patient to discuss previous accomplishments and future plans will assist the nurse in fostering the patient's coping abilities. Rapidity of change is an important factor in the patient's ability to cope. Timing in life cycle can be a significant variable to the different concerns at each stage. The *goal* is to promote coping skills that improve the patient's ability to function.

Interventions include supplying accurate information in a way that clarifies the patient's understanding of his or her illness. During the initial diagnostic phase, education should be designed so that it is not an overwhelming process. The nurse should draw on the patient's past experience and coping ability to provide complete information in small, easily digestable segments. Adequate time should be allowed for patient discussion and clarification. Helping the patient to cope with chronic illness is not something that can be done in one appointment. The patient should feel that he has easy access to his health care provider via frequent appointments or telephone conversations to clarify questions. Praise regarding positive problem-solving ability and achieving realistic goals should be liberally distributed. Rehearsals of how the patient will deal with crises or changes in performance often help the patient to structure his responses in an appropriate way. All life cycle concerns should be addressed at some point, including information about childbearing, marriage, occupational choice, and leisure activities. The patient should know how these concerns will interact in the face of fatigue and changes in strength and mobility.

The nurse should be aware of factors that influence coping ability, such as age, sex, temperament, intelligence, the presence of chronic adversity, and the proximity of social relationships and support. The patient should be encouraged to participate actively in his or her care to have more control over the illness, particularly while hospitalized. In addition to friends and family, another source of support is a peer group. Discussing how one feels with others who have been through similar situations is perceived as being very useful. There are support groups under the auspices of the Multiple Sclerosis Society, Parkinson's Disease Associations, Myasthenia Gravis Foundation, and Independent Living Centers in many areas. Many patients and families learn that their responses to crises are not always unique and are comforted to know that others live through this period in their lives and progress to achieve their goals (Latham et al., 1983).

☐ Social Isolation

Social isolation defines a state in which the person has a need or desire for contact with others but is unable to make that contact. The loss of function of one or more extremities, of verbal skills, or of sensory contact can contribute to social isolation and cause immobility. In multiple sclerosis, loss of bladder control may be a devastating experience, resulting in an altered self-image and social isolation (Ahearn & Schwetz, 1985). In a study of 169 people with Parkinson's disease Singer (1974) noted "premature social aging" when compared to age-matched well controls. This process was characterized by isolation from interpersonal contacts. People with Parkinson's disease were less likely to be working, to participate in household management, or to enjoy a circle of close friends. With illness and disability come loss of income, job, and previous lifestyle. The patient usually becomes dependent on others for some part of socialization. Inability to maintain contact with others can lead to depression and reduced motivation to improve one's situation in other ways (Hyman, 1972).

The *defining characteristics* of this state include expressed feelings of abandonment, underactivity, or uselessness. Irritability may be present and accompanied by other signs of depression. In time, anxiety about going out socially when the opportunity is available may interfere with efforts to treat this problem.

Assessment should include a determination of the frequency and level of social interaction that the patient experienced before the illness or its worsening. When this information is compared with the patient's current social activities, the nurse is alerted to the person at risk for problems and learns those activities the patient may return to most easily. It is important to know if the patient perceives himself or herself as needing more socialization. Evidence of inability to make decisions, irritability, anxiety, failure to interact with others nearby, a change in eating or sleeping habits, and a change from a previous state of good health can signal depression as a consequence of social isolation. The *goal* for this diagnosis is the maintenance of sufficient contact with others despite immobility.

Nursing interventions should include supporting the patient in maintaining the premorbid lifestyle, if possible, including occupation, hobbies, and other forms of social interaction. One's occupation is an important source of socialization as well as recognition. If the patient cannot continue in his or her occupation, it is important to do some anticipatory planning about activities that may occupy time productively during a period of disability. Workshops, day care centers, day programs, exercise programs, and volunteer work are some of the options available to the disabled. Assuming a greater percentage of household responsibilities also promotes self-esteem. The opportunities available often can be increased immensely with the addition of transportation; the mobility impaired may be taught to drive or use special equipment. In one city, volunteers have been organized to visit people in the community weekly who are socially isolated (Compeer; Rochester, NY). Independent living centers teach the handicapped to live on their own or find housing that offers the degree of support necessary so that they may live alone. Such housing can vary; among the options are apartments with emergency call systems, living with a supportive family as a boarder, or living in group homes.

If the patient requires assistance and further education to maintain mobility and overcome environmental barriers, admission to a rehabilitation facility can prove beneficial. As Osberg et al. stated, "Our disabled patients are handicapped only to the extent that we are unable to provide them with enhanced personal abilities, diminished environmental demands, and suitable interface devices to operate or manipulate their environment" (1983, p. 191). The rehabilitation mileu often is an excellent experience for patients who view their illness in terms of deficits; it gives them a chance to concentrate on their strengths. Many rehabilitation facilities offer weekend and evening outings that serve to maintain the patient's links to the real world and keep the treatment program oriented to reality (Osberg et al., 1983).

When anxiety secondary to depression or fear of becoming isolated occurs, the patient needs a supportive individual to help him initiate social activities. At these times, the professional may have more influence than a close family member.

☐ Knowledge Deficit

Knowledge deficit can be seen during any stage of the disease process, particularly following diagnosis. The patient will need to learn about his illness and perhaps new psychomotor skills.

Defining characteristics of this diagnosis include verbal report of difficulty and the patient's expression of inaccurate information. Lack of compliance with desired or prescribed treatments and the presence of anxiety are important factors to assess.

Initially, the nurse should *assess* the patient's knowledge of his or her illness. This includes any previous knowledge of the disorder as well as problems encountered during experiences with the health system in the past. The *goal* is to provide the patient with complete information to allow him to independently manage the problems of immobility resulting from illness.

The patient should be encouraged to learn at his or her own pace. The nurse should take into account the situational and developmental needs as well as anxiety levels. *Interventions* should include a complete discussion of pathophysiology and etiology of the current understanding of the disorder and its effect on functional ability. The patient should know measures that improve and limit strength; for example, the patient with myasthenia gravis should know that rest and timing of anticholinesterases will improve strength and that some medications, such as aminoglycoside antibiotics, beta blockers, and others, will increase weakness (Argov & Mastaglia, 1979). The patient should be encouraged to consult with his specialist before initiation of any new medication. The patient should wear a Medic Alert tag for identification if unable to communicate. Patients should receive thorough instructions about their medications and how these influence their symptoms. Patients receiving corticosteroids or immunosuppressives should understand how these influence pathophysiology and the side effects associated with their use.

Patients feel overwhelmed by the amount of information they will learn. Having contact with other patients or participating in a support group can be a great benefit to a patient. During these initial stages of therapy, the nurse should test the patient's knowledge and not rely solely on head shakes as a measure of understanding. Many patients with chronic disorders are motivated learners and often scour the literature in an attempt to master their illness. For those who ask few questions and appear to deny their illness, the nurse must judge if this is a typical response pattern for that patient or if this coping mechanism is getting in the way of care. For some patients, denial is a comfortable mechanism, particularly when the illness is threatening and the consequences are overwhelming.

☐ Home Maintenance Management Deficit

Home maintenance management can be a potential problem in a patient with chronic immobility and can require that a patient radically change previous patterns. During crisis, many families alter their responsibilities, but when the crisis is over, patients may be burdened with responsibilities they are no longer able to handle.

Defining characteristics include the expression of difficulty by individual family members in accomplishing all activities related to home maintenance. The expectations can be altered significantly by the developmental stage of the family. The spouse or parent will display evidence of anxiety or lack of understanding about the patient's illness or will avoid contact with the care providers. They may show signs of overtaxing the patient with trivial concerns.

The nurse should *assess* the patient's ability to manage self-care activities, occupational concerns, exercise, financial management, home repairs, meal preparation, and leisure activities. The nurse should determine who usually performs these activities and who the patient expects to perform them if he or she needs help. The *goal* is to maintain family functioning during change and fluctuations in the patient's abilities.

Interventions are dependent on the developmental stage and family constellation and their status. The nurse should discuss how the patient might organize the day and accomplish daily needs. For the patient with severe impairment in mobility, supports, such as Meals on Wheels, public health nurses, home health aides, or even private housekeepers, can be employed as a short-term solution. Patients with long-term disorders require extensive home care planning. Financial counseling should be provided, particularly regarding occupational choice, disability concerns, tax planning, and health insurance. Family meetings should begin shortly after hospital admission and should include all members of the multidisciplinary team.

Further information is contained in self-help books, such as those published by the Multiple Sclerosis Society, Amyotropic Lateral Sclerosis Society, the Myasthenia Gravis Foundation, and other related associations. Encouraging the patient to use telephone and mail order shopping and grocery delivery services can be important. Seeking support from family members is necessary. The nurse can assist the patient in learning negotiation strategies to accomplish tasks and to distribute them according to the family member's interests and desires. The patient and family should renegotiate responsibilities at frequent intervals to account for changes in the patient's abilities. The patient should be encouraged to organize himself or herself and the surroundings to prevent wasting energy, such as going up and down stairs. Simple tips, such as sitting on a high stool instead of standing while working in the kitchen and using a portable shopping cart to carry heavy items in the store and to and from the house, can save energy expenditure. A motorized three-wheeled scooter can serve the patient with limited strength on long shopping trips (Fig. 21-2). Patients have considerable difficulty allowing others to complete tasks that they know they could do better than their helper. The nurse should allow patients to express these feelings and let them know that this is a normal reaction.

☐ Health Maintenance

Problems with health maintenance can be seen in the patient with problems of immobility resulting from acute and chronic illnesses when the patient considers his disabilities to be overwhelming. The patient may express inadequate knowledge of preventive health behaviors.

Defining characteristics include noticeably poor oral and body hygiene, obesity, sleep disturbances, poor exercise habits, and visual and hearing problems. Patients who are frequent users of the emergency department or those who lack a consistent source of health care also are at risk for this problem. Those who have frequent minor illnesses related to their immobility that evolve into illnesses requiring hospitalization, such as a cold leading to pneumonia or an injury leading to infection, are experiencing difficulty with health maintenance. Patients with multiple health care providers may be confused about who should provide their care.

Assessment measures include recording who the patient identifies as the usual source of health care and how frequently he or she uses that source. The patient should be asked about his or her knowledge of health and health care practices, particularly problems consistent with age and developmental level. Contributing factors include knowledge deficit about health care practices, previous negative experiences with health care providers, and lack of financial means or transportation to continue to use one's chosen health care source. The perception that the primary illness is the only impediment to happiness fosters delay of return to previous health practices and reflects a lack of acceptance of the problem. Some patients may have differing beliefs and cultural systems that cause them to reject accepted health care practices. The *goal* is to prevent further health care problems and assist the patient in optimizing health.

Interventions include clarifying the roles of the patient's primary and specialty care providers, including nursing's role, and the services unique to each. The nurse should praise the patient for attempting to improve his or her health via diet and exercise plans, dental visits, and ophthalmologic examinations. All women should know preventive health care practices, such as breast self-examination and the importance of Papanicolaou smears. Men should be taught the technique of testicular examination. Detailed health maintenance plans are outlined in many sources (Frame & Carlson, 1975;

Breslow & Somers, 1977). The nurse should consult these sources to develop an appropriate plan of care related to developmental level and age. Patients with chronic motor disorders can be at risk for cancer and other chronic diseases because of such risk factors as family history, smoking, and diet and, for patients with myasthenia gravis and multiple sclerosis, immunosuppressive therapy.

Nursing Diagnoses for the Family and Significant Others

☐ Alteration in Family Processes and Potential for Ineffective Coping

Ineffective family coping can occur during the initial diagnostic period or during any changes experienced during the patient's course of illness. These problems can be related directly or indirectly to the patient's immobility. There are many reactions to the diagnosis of a chronic disorder. Families have been known to react initially to the diagnosis of myasthenia gravis with relief, taking comfort that there was a specific cause and that medicine would control the problem (Sampson & Cosley, 1983). Other families have more difficulty adjusting and are unprepared to cope with the unknown future. Problems may arise when family or significant others deny the reality of the disease. Initially, family members may be angry because the patient has few noticeable signs of weakness or because the illness carries with it the likelihood of other family members being similarly affected, as in Huntington's disease and some of the muscular dystrophies. Mothers who are presumed carriers of Duchenne muscular dystrophy can suffer from guilt and severe stress from within and outside the family. In addition, the patient may not be able to communicate with family members, thus leaving the patient to believe that his or her concerns are ignored or of secondary importance. Defining characteristics, family assessment, and intervention are discussed in Chapter 17.

☐ Knowledge Deficit

Although many families report that they have heard of chronic disorders such as multiple sclerosis, muscular dystrophy, amyotrophic lateral sclerosis, and Parkinson's disease, before their family member was diagnosed few know the ramifications of the disorders. *Defining characterisics* of this diagnosis include the family's expressed lack of knowledge, misconceptions, or lack of support.

The nurse will need to *assess* the family's level of understanding as well as knowledge of the therapeutic regimen and potential genetic implications for such disorders as muscular dystrophy and Huntington's disease. The family may have misconceptions about the limitations imposed by the disease and its treatment. Contributing factors are language and cultural differences and interpersonal problems, such as anxiety, depression, denial, and lack of motivation. The *goal* for this diagnosis is to provide the family with sufficient information to allow them to support the patient throughout his illness.

Interventions can include developing an educational plan for the family that parallels that of the patient. The patient's feelings should be consulted, and, if possible, the patient should be present during all educational family meetings. Many patients like to assist the nurse when educational plans are discussed. This can be a good time to verify the patient's knowledge base. The various foundations have patient and family pamphlets to reinforce teaching plans about medications, symptom control, disease process, and management. Families should have a clear idea of how to handle problems, particularly emergencies. Many would benefit from instructions about cardiopulmonary resuscitation and should know emergency phone numbers. The educational process should not be confined to the initital hospital admission. The family should be encouraged to voice their questions and have a clear idea of when to ask for assistance.

Nondirective genetic counseling should be scheduled initially as part of the educational program for those families affected by diseases with an inheritable pattern, such as the muscular dystophies, Huntington's disease, spinal muscular atrophies, Wilson's disease, the dystonias, and Tourette's syndrome. For some families, tests to determine if a person carries the gene for an illness are available with varying degrees of certainty, for example, Wilson's disease and some forms of muscular dystrophy. This topic is usually a complex one to discuss with those who are uninformed and requires repetition over several sessions and written materials for reference and review at home.

Nursing Diagnoses for the Community

☐ Knowledge Deficit

The patient with chronic neurologic disorders that affect mobility will have to deal with constant change and adjustment throughout the lifetime. For example, the patient with muscular dystrophy may be able to accomplish normal tasks of living one day and be immobilized the next. Immobility is seen as a threat to independence. Today's society values independence, strength, and athletic and competitive ability, all of which are affected in chronic motor disorders.

Since many patients cite that their most stressful period is during the initial diagnostic process, improving public recognition of these diseases may facilitate early diagnosis. Reducing the obscurity of the disease may decrease the fear and anxiety that a chronic neurologic diagnosis carries. Although it is the purpose of nonprofit organizations, such as the Huntington's Disease Society of America, Parkinson's disease associations, the Myasthenia Gravis Foundation, and Muscular Dystrophy Association to increase public and professional awareness of the disease, they cannot do this alone. As nurses, we must continue to educate all health care providers, as well as patients and families. Nurses should encourage positive public attitudes toward the handicapped by looking beyond the wheelchair and focusing on the patient's strengths, not his handicaps. Nurses should become more active in lay organizations that advocate for the handicapped.

The Myasthenia Gravis (MG) Foundation recently formed a National Nursing Advisory Board to coordinate educational efforts for patients and professionals. They have planned a scholarship program to further nursing research on the care of the patient with MG, as well as developing educational programs and pamphlets. In other foundations, such as the Multiple Sclerosis Society and Parkinson's Disease Foundation, nurses are involved actively in patient programs and educational activities.

☐ Barriers to Mobility

There are innumerable physical and social barriers to mobility for patients with chronic immobilizing disorders. These barriers are most easily appreciated for the wheelchair-bound person. In recent years, the efforts of groups of disabled and their advocates have led to legislation or contingencies linking accessibility to facilities with continued funding. Ramps, wide doorways, and low curbs have been added to building codes. Much more needs to be done but the process of change is slow. Barriers to mobility are associated with society's appreciation of the person behind the disability and a history of isolating those who are different from the accepted norm. The effects of the social isolation would be to limit the person that the handicapped individual could become.

Care for the person with chronic immobility is costly. Expenses related to medications, special equipment, nursing assistance for daily care needs, and transportation, including specially equipped vans and ramps, often are not covered by insurance. For the vast majority of people, disability means minimal income. The state offices of vocational rehabilitation offer a skills evaluation, training, or schooling scholarships and generally facilitate the reentrance of the disabled into the job market.

Further research is necessary to clarify the most efficient and effective way of counseling patients with chronic disorders. Coping with a disease that is progressive and chronic, lasting many years, is different from coping with an illness in which the deficit is static. The age dimension needs to be explored as well. Patients who develop a chronic disease in childhood and adolescence have different developmental needs and require different coping strategies than those who are affected by illnesses with onset in middle age. Younger patients can be more severely affected (Singer, 1974).

□ Insufficient Community Resources

There are many needs that the community must address in the case of patients with chronic motor disorders and immobility. One of the most important is who will pay for the chronic care necessary to maintain the quality of life for these patients. The problem of transportation and personal attendants must be overcome to allow these patients to become useful and productive members of the community. In many cases, rehabilitation can make these patients independent. These services must be accessible and supported by the community at large. Many families need respite care to allow them to continue to support their family member.

The development of exercise programs would allow patients to participate in activities outside their homes, to make gradual improvements in strength, and to reduce disuse atrophy. Patients with muscle weakness and fatigue have been excluded from many exercise programs because of their disability or lack of access to many facilities. The success of cardiac rehabilitation and exercise programs for cerebral palsy, Parkinson's disease, and multiple sclerosis lend support to the notion that the chronically ill population should not be overlooked for rehabilitation.

Society must change its values to include the needs of those who are less independent. A renewing of the focus of one's life activities to include community support projects does not apply just to nurses. In the years to come, attendance to community needs should become an expectation and not an exception for all citizens. The work of established health organizations and coalitions of these groups is necessary to lobby for the rights of the disabled if a change in the government support of the needs of the chronically ill is to be effected. This type of work requires energy above and beyond that necessary just to meet the daily needs of the patient. Many patients and families may not have this energy and expertise and will need to elicit the support of friends, health care providers, and elected officials.

SUMMARY

The problems of those with chronically impaired mobility can affect every area of their functioning. Limitations imposed by their physical disabilities can be significant and may be accompanied by or result in psychosocial limitations in functioning. As a society, it is our responsibility to minimize any limitations within our jurisdiction as expeditiously and in the most cost-effective manner possible. Change in society values may be apparent only in generations to come. It will be facilitated only by the amazingly rapid manner in which knowledge of today's events can be shared around the world.

REFERENCES

Ahearn, J., & Schwetz, K. (1985). Comprehensive supportive therapy in multiple sclerosis. *Seminars in Neurology*, 5 (2), 146.

Alexander, M.A., Johnson, E.W., Petty, J., & Stauch, D. (1979). Mechanical ventilation of patients with late stage Duchenne muscular dystrophy: Management at home. *Archives of Physical Medicine and Rehabilitation*, 60, 289.

Argov, Z., & Mastaglia, F.L. (1979). Disorders of neurotransmission caused by drugs. *New England Journal of Medicine*, 285, 773.

Boller, F., & Frank, E.F. (1982). *Sexual dysfunction in neurologic disorders*. New York: Raven Press.

Bowers, M.B., & VanWoert, M.H. (1972). Sexual behavior during L-dopa treatment of Parkinson's disease. *Medical Aspects of Human Sexuality, 1,* 88.

Breslow, L., & Somers. (1977). The lifetime health-monitoring program. *New England Journal of Medicine, 296* (11), 601.

Cadmus, R. (1980). Intensive care reaches silver anniversary. *Hospitals, 54,* 98.

Callahan, M. (1985). A prudent pulmonary rehabilitation program. *American Journal of Nursing, 85* (12), 1368.

Carpenito, L.J. (1984). *Handbook of nursing diagnosis.* Philadelphia: Lippincott.

Cobble, N.D., & Maloney, F. P. (1985). Effects of exercise in neuromuscular disease. In F. P. Maloney, J. Burks, & S. Ringel (Eds.), *Interdisciplinary management of multiple sclerosis and neuromuscular disease* (p. 228). Philadelphia: Lippincott.

Curran, F.J. (1981). Night ventilation by body respirator for patients in chronic respiratory failure due to late stage Duchenne muscular dystrophy. *Archives of Physical Medicine and Rehabilitation, 62,* 270.

Edmonds, C.E. (1966). Huntington's chorea, dysphagia and death. *Medical Journal of Australia, 2,* 273.

Frame, P.S., & Carlson, S. J. (1975). A critical review of periodic health screening using specific screening criteria. *Journal of Family Practice, 2,* 29, 123, 189, 283.

Gehlson, G.M., Grigsby, S.A., & Winant, D.M. (1984). Effects of aquatic fitness program on muscular strength and endurance in patients with multiple sclerosis. *Physical Therapy, 64* (5), 653.

Griggs, R.C., & Donohoe, K.M. (1985). Emergency management of neuromuscular disease. In R. J. Henning & D. Jackson (Eds.), *Handbook of critical care neurology and neurosurgery* (p. 251). New York: Praeger.

Griggs, R.C., Donohoe, K.M., Utell, M.J., Goldblatt, D., & Moxley, R.T. (1981). Evaluation of pulmonary function in neuromuscular disease. *Archives of Neurology, 38,* 9.

Grob, D., Brunner, N.C., & Namba, T. (1981). The natural course of myasthenia gravis and effect of therapeutic measures. *Annals of the New York Academy of Sciences, 377,* 652.

Hobbs, N., Perrin, J.M., Ireys, H.T., Moynihan, L.C., & Shayne, M.W. (1984). Chronically ill children in America. *Rehabilitation Literature, 45*(7-8), 206.

Hyman, M. (1972). Sociopsychological obstacles to L-dopa therapy that may limit effectiveness in parkinsonism. *Journal of the American Geriatrics Society, 20,* 200.

Kodadek, S.M. (1985). Working with the chronically ill. *Nurse Practitioner, 10* (3), 45.

Latham, E.E., Bresnan, M.J., & Sollee, N.L. (1983). Psychosocial issues in raising a child with Duchenne muscular dystrophy: A parent group ethnography. In L. Charash, S.G. Wolfe, A.H. Kutscher, R.E. Lovelace, & M.S. Hale (Eds.), *Psychosocial issues of muscular dystrophy and allied diseases* (p. 221). Springfield, IL: Thomas.

Lavigne, J. (1979). Respiratory care in neuromuscular disease. *Nursing Clinics of North America, 14,* 110.

Levine, J.S. (1985). Bowel dysfunction in multiple sclerosis. In F.P. Maloney, J.S. Burks, & S. Ringel (Eds.), *Interdisciplinary rehabilitation of multiple sclerosis and neuromuscular disorders* (p. 62). Philadelphia: Lippincott.

Maloney, F.P., Burks, J.S. & Ringel, S. (Eds). (1985). *Interdisciplinary rehabilitation of multiple sclerosis and neuromuscular disorders* (pp. 271, 383). Philadelphia: J.B. Lippincott.

Marsden, C.D., Parkes, J.D., & Quinn, N. (1982). Fluctuations of disability in Parkinson's disease—Clinical aspects. In C.D. Marsden & C. Fahn (Eds.), *Movement disorders* (p. 96). London: Butterworths.

Moos, R., & Schaefer J. (1984). The crisis of physical illness: An overview and conceptual approach. In R. Moos (Ed.), *Coping with physical illness: New perspectives* (p. 3). New York: Plenum.

Myasthenia Gravis Foundation. (1979). *Patient to patient memo.* New York: Author.

Neu, H. C., Connolly, J.P., Schwestley, F.W., Lodwig, H.A., & Brody, A. W. (1967). Obstructive respiratory dysfunction in parkinsonian patients. *American Review of Respiratory Diseases, 95,* 33.

Osberg, S., Corcoran, P.J., Dejong, G., & Ostruff, E. (1983). Environmental barriers and the neurologically impaired patient. *Seminars in Neurology, 3,* (4), 180.

Sampson, R., & Cosley, S. (1983). Physical, emotional, social, and family interactions in childhood myasthenia gravis. In L.I. Charash, S.G. Wolfe, A.H. Kutscher, R.E. Lovelace, & M.S. Hale (Eds.), *Psychosocial aspects of muscular dystrophy and allied diseases* (p. 183). Springfield, IL: Thomas.

Singer, E. (1974). Premature social aging: The social-psychological consequences of a chronic illness. *Social Science and Medicine, 8,* 143.

Splaingard, M.L., Frates, R.C., Jefferson, L.S., Rosen, C.L., & Harrison, G. (1985). Home negative pressure ventilation: Report of 20 years of experience in patients with neuromuscular disease. *Archives of Physical Medicine and Rehabilitation, 66,* 239.

Vas, C.J. (1969). Sexual impotence and some autonomic disturbances in men with multiple sclerosis. *Acta Neurologica Scandinavica, 45,* 166.

BIBLIOGRAPHY

Carlson, C. (1980). Psychosocial aspects of neurologic disability. *Nursing Clinics of North America, 15,* (2), 309.

Donohoe, K.M. (1979). Overview of neuromuscular disease. *Nursing Clinics of North America, 14,* 96.

Duvoisin, R. (1984). *Parkinson's disease: A guide for patient and family.* New York: Raven Press.

Goldblatt, D. (1984). Decisions about life support in amyotrophic lateral sclerosis. *Seminars in Neurology, 4,* (1), 104.

Kess, R. (1984). Suddenly in crisis: Unpredictable myasthenia. *American Journal of Nursing, 84* (8), 994.

Rose, N.L. (1985). Nutrition for patients with neuromuscular disorders. In F.P. Maloney, J. Burks, & S. Ringel (Eds.), *Interdisciplinary management of multiple sclerosis and neuromuscular diseases* (p. 341). Philadelphia: Lippincott.

Scheinberg, L. (1983). *Multiple sclerosis: A guide for patients and their families.* New York: Raven Press.

Stern, G., & Lees, A. (1982). *Parkinson's disease: The facts.* Oxford: Oxford University Press.

22

Swallowing Dysfunction in Patients with Altered Mobility

Roberta Schwartz-Cowley and Andrew K. Gruen*

Swallowing dysfunctions are common in patients who demonstrate acquired neurologic deficits. Various sources indicate that swallowing problems can be associated with the disease process, such as cerebrovascular accidents (CVA), Parkinson's disease, Huntington's disease, amyotrophic lateral sclerosis, encephalitis, meningitis, anoxia, demyelinating disease, head trauma, brainstem tumors or trauma, metabolic myopathy, carcinomas, and hypopharyngeal and esophageal webs. Swallowing difficulties have been reported as associated complications after implants and surgical interventions in the oropharyngeal and esophageal areas.

It would appear that swallowing disorders are routinely assessed and treated appropriately in progressive medical settings, although Zimmerman and Oder (1981) suggest that many exceptions can be found in acutely ill patients. They suggest that patients often are left undiagnosed and untreated because of a general lack of understanding of dysphagia and its effects on normal feeding and nutritional support of patients.

The careful evaluation and treatment of neurologically based swallowing disorders requires a consistent interdisciplinary team approach. In many facilities, the dysphagia team is lead by the swallowing therapist (who is often the speech language pathologist [Logemann, 1983]), with input from the patient's physician, nurse, dietitican, and radiologist. The input from occupational therapists also is essential to the team in terms of adaptive equipment needs.

NORMAL SWALLOWING

Before effective evaluation and therapy procedures can be applied to the patient with a swallowing disorder, the neuroscience nurse should review the normal process of swallowing. A brief physiologic review of the process of swallowing follows.

Leopold and Kagel (1983) suggest an *anticipatory phase* to the swallowing process. This phase includes the decisions made by an individual before feeding. Considerations in-

---

*The authors acknowledge the contribution of Connie A. Walleck, who provided nursing diagnosis examples.

clude amount, type, form, and rate of feeding and swallowing. More traditional viewpoints of the feeding process begin at the *oral preparatory phase*, the point where a piece of food is bitten or chewed by use of the teeth, tongue, cheeks, and lips. The bolus is formed by mixing the food particles with saliva. The lips close to form a seal that prevents the bolus from escaping. When chewing is completed, the tip of the tongue rises to the hard palate, and the bolus is thrust to the posterior portion of the pharynx by action of the cheeks and tongue. The tongue acts as a barrier to prevent the bolus from returning to the anterior oral cavity.

Blonsky et al. (1975) report transit time from the oral stage to pharyngeal stage of swallowing to be approximately 1 second. Reflexive action takes over as the bolus becomes involved in the *phyaryngeal stage*. Respiration temporarily stops, and the larynx receives protection by upward and forward movement caused by muscle contraction and covering by the epiglottis, which folds down over the laryngeal area. The hyoid bone displaces upward and posteriorly. The bolus, which has been displaced to the posterior pharyngeal area, stimulates pharyngeal sphincter peristalsis. Sequential contractions and relaxations of the sphincter muscles propel the bolus down the pharynx, around the epiglottis, which is folded over the laryngeal area, and down to the cricopharyngeal segment. Transit time is approximately 1 second (Blonsky et al., 1975).

The *esophageal phase* begins when the cricopharyngeal segment relaxes and the bolus moves into the esophagus. Through the process of peristalsis (and to a lesser extent, gravity), the bolus is transferred through the esophagus and through the gastroesophageal sphincter into the stomach. Mandelstam and Leiber (1970) suggest transit times of 8 to 20 seconds. The interested reader should review the works of Logemann (1983), Dobie (1978), Aliza (1983), Rouecke (1980), and Donner et al. (1985) for more comprehensive information about neural and physiologic aspects of normal swallowing.

The successful swallowing process depends on a rapid sequence of finely tuned muscle movements in voluntary and reflexive control mechanisms. Disorders or disruptions can be found in any phase of swallowing and can significantly affect the patient's ability to take food orally and maintain adequate nutrition. It is essential that the neuroscience nurse carefully monitor the patient's ability to feed and swallow. Clear documentation of behaviors observed, a referral for a complete bedside and radiographic evaluation, and implementation of reasonable effective management programs are necessary to assure a functional feeding program for the patient.

BEHAVIORAL MANIFESTATIONS OF DIFFICULT SWALLOWING

The neuroscience nurse charged with overseeing patient care may observe several behaviors that would suggest the need for a swallowing evaluation protocol. The nurse might observe the patient choking on food, or the patient may do better (or worse) with liquid consistencies than a soft diet. The patient might not swallow food when it is placed in the mouth or may appear to lack enough attention to follow through in the feeding process. This could be an associated characteristic of a cognitive–linguistic disorder. Excessive drooling, especially unilaterally, might be observed. Several hours after meal time, the nurse performing the routine oral hygiene procedures may find food pocketed on one side of the patient's mouth.

A patient who is being tube-fed may appear to be swallowing his or her own secretions, which might suggest adequate oral manipulation and, thus, feeding potential. Questionable secretions resembling thick liquid (such as milkshakes) on the patient's tray may be expelled from a tracheostomy tube. The patient might complain of a sensation of food becoming stuck in the throat. Any of these observations suggest referral to the facility's dysphagia team. If there is no such team, the speech–language pathologist can evaluate or make appropriate recommendations concerning swallowing assessments and treatment protocols.

Assessment

A nurse's concern about the patient's ability to swallow food warrants referral to specific individuals on the dysphagia team. An orthodontist or dentist may be asked to evaluate the patient's teeth or dentures to determine the best possible oral preparation situation for chewing food. If laryngeal aspiration is suspected, referrals for cineradiography or video fluoroscopy can be made to the otolaryngologist, radiologist, or speech–language pathologist. It is beneficial to evalute the actual swallowing process from both a radiographic and a behavioral standpoint. Information obtained from these evaluations is used to establish therapeutic goals. Information from the radiographic studies will include comments on bolus propulsion and bolus transfer in the pharyngeal area and around the epiglottis to the cricoesophageal sphincter into the stomach. Radiographic studies can be replayed frame by frame to outline the sequence of swallow and to delineate any difficulties, peculiar findings, and significant problems, such as laryngeal penetration, laryngeal aspiration, and regurgitation from the esophagus or into the nasal passageway.

The behavioral assessment completed by the speech–language pathologist begins with a focus on comments from the patient's history. Evaluation and comments are made of respiratory status, head–trunk control, and dentition considerations. A comprehensive oral mechanism evaluation of the structure and function of various components of the oral cavity, including both sensation and motor functions, is completed. The patient's ability to communicate basic needs and follow commands is assessed.

The speech–language pathologist conducts a complete swallowing examination to evaluate various consistencies, textures, and temperatures of food. The patient's responses, including comments about oral preparation, bolus, manipulation, swallow, and laryngeal excursion, are recorded and analyzed. Cervical auscultation procedures further classify the patient's performance. Many swallowing centers use evaluative procedures similar to those used at the Shock Trauma Center and Montebello Rehabilitation Hospital of the Maryland Institute for Emergency Medical Services Systems in Baltimore, Maryland. Appendix 22-1 is the Diagnostic Summary of Swallowing Functions form used there.

Various types of swallowing disorders can be identified through comprehensive formalized bedside and radiographic evaluations of the swallowing mechanism and process. A brief notation of disorders associated with the oral preparatory, pharyngeal, and esophageal phases of swallowing is warranted. Oral phase difficulties can arise from the presence of structural abnormalities, such as developmental disorders, trauma-induced injuries, or surgical removal. Patients may not be able to close their lips completely or use tongue movements effectively because of weakness or paralysis of muscles or inflammation. Incoordination of oral musculature movements results in leakage of the bolus out of the oral cavity. Lack of selective attention, perceptual deficits, confusion, and errors in judgment and insight result in possible functional disturbances in oral preparation.

Many problems are noted during the pharyngeal phase of swallowing, including delayed or absent swallow reflexes, structural abnormalities, such as noted previously, or pharyngeal webs, interference of normal swallow as a result of inflammation or accessory sphincter action (although this may help in certain situations), or inadequate weak pharyngeal peristalsis. Patients who have poor control of velopharyngeal closure, such as that induced by progressive neurologic disease processes, may have nasal regurgitation.

Although many swallowing teams do not evaluate or monitor esophageal problems, a comprehensive assessment can disclose such problems as esophageal spasms, immobility, or structural abnormalities. Disorders in coordination of bolus movement through the cricopharyngeal and gastroesophageal segments can pose problems in effective transfer and regurgitation. Radiographic studies are necessary for objective determination of esophageal disorders.

Results of the swallowing evaluation are discussed with the patient, the family, physician, therapy team, and neuroscience nurse. Recommendations about diet consistency, problem foods, supervision of feeding, assistive devices for feeding, the effects of fatigue, and the times for best swallowing activity are provided. For some patients, oral intake of food may not be recommended because of significant physical risks posed by limited structural, physiologic, or mental abilities. Because the neuroscience nurse becomes a key individual in the patient's successful oral intake of food during the neurologic unit course, it is impressive for the nurse to understand basic treatment goals, environmental modifications, and feeding procedures.

Treatment Guidelines

Manipulating environmental controls can influence greatly the success of the swallowing procedure for patients with dysphagia who are candidates for oral feeding. The atmosphere should be calm, quiet, and free from distraction (Aliza, 1983). Other patients, staff, and visitors should be requested to leave or to remain quiet during the feeding process. Although the patient should be as comfortable as possible, proper positioning is extremely important and should not be compromised for the sake of comfort. Ideally, the patient should be in a chair at an angle of 90 degrees, with hips flexed and head bent slightly forward (Logemann, 1983; Rouecke, 1980). If the patient is taking tube feedings, the doctor may order cessation of tube feedings for 1 to 2 hours before oral feeding to help stimulate an appetite. The nurse should clean or freshen the patient's mouth to maximize the taste for the foods presented.

Several feeding assistive devices are available to help the patient with oral dysphagia. These include a push spoon, squeeze bottle syringe, baby spoon, straw, nose-cut glass, and styrofoam cup. Occupational therapists can offer other helpful suggestions specific to the patient's needs.

The patient should be instructed to move the food around the oral cavity with the tongue if possible. Initially, only small amounts of food (generally one-quarter to one-half teaspoon) should be given. Swallow retraining has the initial goal of process, not nutrition. Augmentative feedings, such as nasogastric tube feeding, should not be discontinued until the patient can demonstate the ability to take enough food orally to sustain nutritional requirements.

The patient should be given ample time for the eating process. Family members are encouraged to aid nurses in the time-consuming feeding process. Such family involvement helps also to clarify teaching plans and provide a more natural social environment for eating.

In patients with *chronic* alterations in mobility, the *goal* for the patient with inadequate nutritional status is to provide caloric intake that will meet the need for growth, daily energy expenditure, and weight gain. The *goal* for the overweight patient is to structure the caloric requirements to meet growth and energy needs, in addition to providing an organized pattern of weight loss in the context of the patient's exercise ability.

Interventions include planning meals that coincide with chewing and swallowing ability and reflect caloric requirements. Patients taking medications that would facilitate swallowing (levodopa, anticholinesterases) should schedule meals 1 hour after medication to coincide with the drug's peak effectiveness. The patient may want to avoid talking before or during meals. For patients with fatigable muscle weakness, such as myasthenia gravis and multiple sclerosis, many of the same muscles that are used for speech are used for swallowing, and they are likely to fatigue with repeated activity (Kess, 1984). For the person with a movement disorder, performing two tasks at once interferes with the smooth accomplishment of either. In a patient with severe swallowing difficulty, such high-calorie snacks as puddings, eggnogs, and milkshakes may be used as supplements. A prospective study of weight loss in Huntington's disease reveals that female patients, who have diets higher in fat, lose proportionately less weight than male patients (Shoulson et al, 1984). The overweight patient must be careful not to increase the total caloric intake with such supplements. Patients with problems of chronic immobility on weight loss diets will need to restrict their caloric consumption severely: Diets with as few as 500 calories per day may be required for weight loss in patients who are immobile and in wheelchairs. Such patients should work out a diet plan with a dietitian or nurse that will meet the need for weight loss in the context of their swallowing ability. Patients with myasthenia gravis occasionally report that cold foods are easier to swallow than hot foods. Patients taking corticosteroids should know which foods are rich in potassium and calcium, since depletion of these electrolytes occurs frequently with this treatment.

Case Study 1

Dale, a 23-year-old male, was admitted to a regional tauma center with a diagnosis of severe closed head trauma. The initial Glasgow Coma Score was 4/15. Predominant computerized tomography (CT) findings included significant diffuse cerebral edema and an acute left temporal–parietal epidural hematoma, which was repaired quickly. Because of the low level of response, a tracheostomy was completed 4 days postonset with moist room air. A nasogastric tube was inserted, and the patient received 50% to 75% strength tube feeding on a continuous basis. Behavioral rating was completed 7 days postonset. A Rancho Los Amigos Level of Cognitive Functioning Scale was used to determine level III behaviors.

Characteristics included inconsistent reactions to stimulation provided by the examiner. The patient inconsistently followed simple commands such as "point to floor." These responses were delayed (5 to 10 seconds). Dale was unable to communicate his basic needs to the nursing staff. Responses were more consistent and exemplified higher levels of response when his girlfriend of 5 years gave the commands.

A referral to the speech–language pathologist for a swallowing evaluation was initiated because the patient appeared able to manage his secretions well without drooling. The bedside evaluation indicated impaired head and neck control, necessitating propping pillows and Posey restraint to position him in a Gerichair. Cognitive–linguistic deficits included short selective attention span, inconsistent axial commands, remarkable decrease in gestural expression of personal needs, and nonverbal communication because of tracheostomy.

The oral mechanism examination was not reliable based on inconsistent patient response levels. The patient did, however, arouse when cold stimulation was provided to the teeth and buccal cavities. Dale demonstrated tongue and jaw movements spontaneously. The cuffed tracheostomy tube was deflated. Saliva secretions were swallowed without coughing. Results of cervical auscultation were unremarkable pretesting and posttesting. Ice chips, soft potatoes, and a popsicle were used to determine Dale's ability to swallow specific food textures and consistencies.

Results of oral feeding trials included successful oral manipulation through reflexive swallow. No particles remained in the oral cavity. Breath sounds were normal to cervical auscultation, and an increase in overall awareness and cognitive–linguistic performance was noted. Recommendations were to decrease tube feedings 50% and start supervised oral feeds while the patient was in the chair at 90 degrees. A soft diet without thin liquids was ordered. Suggestions about environmental distractions, positioning, and supervised feeding were provided to the primary nurse.

Dale's speech–language pathologist monitored swallowing functions in addition to the cognitive–linguistic remediation program. Twenty-one days postonset, the tracheostomy table was removed. The patient proceeded to a regular diet with liquids and tolerated oral feeding well. A significant positive change in overall cognitive–linguistic performance was noted also.

Nursing Diagnoses

☐ **Potential for Alteration in Nutrition— Less Than Body Requirements**

Swallowing dysfunctions can considerably reduce the patient's nutritional intake (Carpenito, 1983). Adequate nutritional intake is critical to the healing process. The inability to meet metabolic requirements results in loss of weight as well as a decreased ability of the body to grow and repair itself. Assessment of the patient's swallowing ability is the important first step in designing an appropriate nutritional plan for the patient.

Specific interventions include reducing causative and contributing factors if possible. Before beginning feeding, the nurse must assess that the patient is alert and responsive and has a good cough reflex. Suction equipment should be available. The patient should be positioned appropriately, and food must be given in small amounts and of the proper consistency. Following the plan outlined by the speech–language pathologist will assure consistency of feeding. The use of a calorie count with supplemental intravenous or nasogatric nutritional intake can assure an adequate intake.

The *expected outcomes* for the patient are that he or she will experience an increase in the amount and type of nutrients ingested and describe the rationale for the treatment plan initiated.

☐ **Insufficient Airway Clearance**

The patient experiencing a swallowing disorder has a great potential for aspiration, which could lead to upper and lower airway problems. *Assessment* of the cough and gag reflex is critical in every patient to prevent a possible catastrophe. Collaborating with the speech–language pathologist for guidelines on the best way to feed the patient also contribute to safeguarding the patient.

Specific interventions include the following:

1. Positioning the patient to facilitate swallowing by elevating the head of the bed to a 60 to 90 degree position. Avoiding a position that causes the patient to flex the neck or slouch can facilitate swallowing.
2. Allowing the patient adequate time to chew and swallow. Initially, patients undergoing swallowing therapy should be assessed on the quality of swallowing procedure rather than on the quantity consumed.
3. Avoidance of fatigue and drowsiness is necessary, since they can increase the risk of aspiration during eating. Rest periods before eating allow the patient to be alert and responsive during the meal. Using assistive cough techniques and other pulmonary hygiene measures ensures clearing the airway.

Expected outcomes are that the patient will have a clear upper and lower airway on auscultation, have a decreased risk of aspiration, and demonstrate effective coughing techniques. The family can demonstrate the Heimlich maneuver in chronic care.

Although it is the ideal to have all patients feeding either independently or with assistance, the realistic neuroscience nurse will realize that enteral or parenteral means will be required to maintain nutrition for some patients. Oral gastric and nasogastric tubes are frequently used for short-term swallowing problems. Gastrostomy or jejunostomy may be required for long-term nutritional management. Referrals to the gastroenterologist, internist, or surgeon are made when management issues are considered.

SUMMARY

Knowledge of the functional framework of the swallowing process, indications for assessment protocols, and therapeutic management options for the dysphagic patient aid the neuroscience nurse in developing an effective and appropriate nutrition and feeding program.

REFERENCES

Aliza, B.E. (1983). Retraining swallowing after brain injury. In S.J. Shanks (Ed.), *Nursing and the management of adult communication disorders.* San Diego: College-Hill Press.

Blonsky, E., Logemann, J., Boshes, B., & Fisher, H. (1975). Comparision of speech and swallow function in patients with tremor disorders and in normal geriatric patients: A cinefluorographic study. *Journal of Gerontology, 30,* 299.

Carpenito, L.J. (1983). *Nursing diagnosis application to clinical practice.* Philadelphia: Lippincott.

Dobie, R. (1978). Rehabilitation of swallowing disorders. *American Family Physician, 17,* 84.

Donner, M.W., Bosma, J.F., & Robertson, D.L. (1985). Anatomy and physiology of the pharynx. *Gastrointestinal Radiography, 10,* 196.

Kess, R. (1984). Suddenly in crises: Unpredictable myasthenia. *American Journal of Nursing, 84(8),* 994.

Leopold, N.A., & Kagel, M.C. (1983). Swallowing ingestion and dysphagia: A reappraisal. *Archives of Physical Medicine and Rehabilitation, 64,* 371.

Logemann, J.A. (1983). *Evaluation and treatment of swallowing disorders.* San Diego: College-Hill Press.

Rouecke, J.R. (1980). *Dysphagia: An assessment and management program for the adult.* Minneapolis: Sister Kenny Institute.

Mandelstam, P., & Leiber, A. (1970). Cineradiographic evaluation of the esophagus in normal adults. *Gastroenterology, 58,* 32.

Shoulson, I., Miller, C., Welle, S., Panzik, J., Lipinski, B., Plumb, S., & Forbes, C. (1984). Huntington's disease: Body weight and metabolic indices (Abstr.). *Annals of Neurology 16, (1),* 126.

Zimmerman, J.E., & Oder, L.A. (1981). Swallowing dysfunction in acutely ill patients. *Physical Therapy, 61,* 1755.

APPENDIX 22–1. SPEECH–COMMUNICATION DISORDERS PROGRAM.*

Diagnostic Summary of Swallowing Functions

Date of examination: _____
Examiner: _____

I. **IDENTIFYING INFORMATION**
   Date of birth: _____ Date of onset: _____
   Referring physician: _____ Date of admission: _____

II. **MEDICAL INFORMATION**
   Primary diagnosis: _____

   Reason for referral: (Include subjective complaint if applicable) _____

   Current diet order/method of intake: _____

   Respiratory status: _____ normal _____ impaired
   _____ on ventilator comment: _____
   _____ tracheostomy tube: type _____
       _____ cuffed _____ uncuffed; _____ fenestrated _____ unfenestrated;
       If fenestrated, _____ plugged _____ unplugged; duration plugging tolerated: _____
   Duration of oral intubation: (if applicable) _____
   Ability to manage secretions: _____

III. **BODY POSTURE**
   Head/trunk control: _____ normal _____ impaired
   Comment: _____

	Right	**Left**	
Hemiparesis	___	___	Head/neck extended: _____ yes _____ no
Flaccid	___	___	Head/neck contracted: _____ yes _____ no
Spastic	___	___	

IV. **COGNITIVE–LINGUISTIC COMMUNICATIVE STATUS**
   Rancho level (if applicable): _____
   Attending behaviors: _____
   Follows motor commands: _____ consistently _____ inconsistently _____ absent
        oral commands: _____ consistently _____ inconsistently _____ absent
   Comment: _____
   Expression of wants/needs: _____ functional _____ nonfunctional
       Modality of expression: _____ verbal _____ written _____ gestures _____ augmentative
       system: _____

   Speech articulation: _____ precise _____ imprecise
   Comment: _____
   Vocal quality: _____

V. **ORAL MECHANISM EXAMINATION**
   A. Sensation: (Mark boxes with: + = deficit, − = no deficit, 0 = could not assess)
      Indicate R (right) or L (left) for unilateral deficits

---

*This evaluation is used by the Montebello Rehabililtation Hospital of the Maryland Institute for Emergency Medical Services Systems in Baltimore, MD.

(Continued)

	Temperature		Touch		Taste			
Structure	Hot	Cold	Light	Increased pressure	Sweet	Sour	Bitter	Other
Lips								
Tongue ant ⅓								
post ⅔								
Buccal cavity								
Palate								
Velum								

B. Motor (structure/function): Indicate N (normal), A (absent), or I (impaired) for each movement on each side; make reference to range, strength, speed, and coordination of movements under comments, as needed.

Lips: Right   Left
At rest
Pursing
Retraction
Strength (tight closure)
Drooling: ____yes ____no
Rapid movements: ____adequate
                 ____decreased
Comments: _____
_____

Tongue: Right   Left
At rest
Protrusion
Retraction
Lateralization
Elevation
Depression
Strength
Rapid movements: ____adequate
                 ____decreased
Tongue thrust: ____yes ____no
Comments: _____
_____

Jaw: Right   Left
At rest
Closure
Depression
Lateralization
TMJ noises: ____yes ____no
Comments: _____
_____

Hard palate: Right   Left
At rest
Comments: _____

Velum:
At rest
Elevation
    Reflexive (Gag)
    Gag: ____hyperactive ____hypoactive
          ____intact
Volitional ("ah"):
duration in seconds ____
Comments: _____
_____

Larynx:
   Prolong "ah" vocal quality: ____hoarse ____breathy ____harsh other: _____
   Intermittent phonation (ah-ah-ah): _____
   Volitional cough/throat clearing (check all that apply):
     ____normal   ____weak   ____delayed   ____absent
   Reflexive cough/throat clearing:
     ____normal   ____weak   ____delayed   ____absent/not observed
   Ability to vary pitch: ____adequate   ____limited   ____N/A
   Ability to vary loudness: ____adequate   ____limited   ____N/A
   Ability to impound air: ____adequate   ____limited   ____absent

(Continued)

354 II. 5. MOBILITY PHENOMENA

    Dentition: Indicate presence/absence and/or normal dentition and adequacy of alignment: _____
_____

    Primitive reflexes: (check all that apply)
        ____bite reflex   ____sucking   ____rooting (____L ____R)   ____munching
        Other: _____
    Salivary function: ____adequate   ____dry mouth   ____excess saliva

VI. **DEGLUTITION**
    A. Position of patient for evaluation:
        ____bed   ____chair   ____Stryker frame   ____Clinitron bed   ____Other: _____
        Degree of hip flexion: ____0°   ____45°   ____90°   ____Other: _____
        Comments: _____

    B. Consistencies (check all that apply):
       1. Ice chips: Oral preparation: ____adequate   ____impaired:
                        Comment: _____
                        Bolus manipulation: ____adequate   ____impaired:
                        Comment: _____
                        Swallow: ____complete   ____incomplete
                                ____delayed (time: in seconds _____)   ____Repetitive
                                ____mouth emptied   ____food particles remain (location) _____
                        Laryngeal excursion: ____adequate   ____limited   ____absent
                                ____coughing   ____particles exiting trachea
                        Cervical auscultation: postswallow: ____clear   ____wet
                                       postcough: ____clear   ____wet
                        Not assessed _____
       2. Pureed consistency—specify food, temperature:
                        Oral preparation: ____adequate   ____impaired:
                        Comment: _____
                        Bolus manipulation: ____adequate   ____impaired:
                        Comment: _____
                        Swallow: ____complete   ____incomplete
                                ____delayed (time: in seconds _____)   ____Repetitive
                                ____mouth emptied   ____food particles remain (location) _____
                        Laryngeal excursion: ____adequate   ____limited   ____absent
                                ____coughing   ____particles exiting trachea
                        Cervical auscultation: postswallow: ____clear   ____wet
                                       postcough: ____clear   ____wet
                        Not assessed _____
       3. Soft food consistency—specify food, temperature:
                        Oral preparation: ____adequate   ____impaired:
                        Comment: _____
                        Bolus manipulation: ____adequate   ____impaired:
                        Comment: _____
                        Swallow: ____complete   ____incomplete
                                ____delayed (time: in seconds _____)   ____Repetitive
                                ____mouth emptied   ____food particles remain (location) _____
                        Laryngeal excursion: ____adequate   ____limited
                                ____absent   ____coughing
                                ____particles exiting trachea
                        Cervical auscultation: postswallow: ____clear   ____wet
                                     postcough: ____clear   ____wet
                        Not assessed _____

(Continued)

4. Regular food consistency—specify food, termperature:
   Oral preparation: ____adequate ____impaired:
   Comment: _____
   Bolus manipulation: ____adequate ____impaired:
   Comment: _____
   Swallow: ____complete ____incomplete
   ____delayed (time: in seconds _____) ____Repetitive
   ____mouth emptied ____food particles remain (location) _____
   Laryngeal excursion: ____adequate ____limited
   ____absent ____coughing
   ____particles exiting trachea
   Cervical auscultation: postswallow: ____clear ____wet
   postcough: ____clear ____wet
   Not assessed _____

5. Liquids
   a. Thick liquids—specify type, temperature:
      Check all that apply:
      ____cup ____straw
      Lip protrusion: ____adequate ____limited ____absent
      Sucking: ____adequate ____decreased strength
      ____absent
      Swallow: ____complete ____incomplete
      ____delayed (time: in seconds _____)
      ____repetitive ____mouth emptied
      ____particles remain (location): _____
      ____liquid spills from mouth
      Laryngeal excursion: ____adequate ____limited ____absent
      ____coughing ____particles exiting trachea
      Cervical auscultation: postswallow: ____clear ____wet
      postcough: ____clear ____wet
      Not assessed _____
   b. Thin liquids—specify type, temperature:
      ____cup ____straw
      Lip protrusion: ____adequate ____limited ____absent
      Sucking: ____adequate ____decreased strength
      ____absent
      Swallow: ____complete ____incomplete
      ____delayed (time: in seconds _____)
      ____repetitive ____mouth emptied
      ____particles remain (location): _____
      ____liquid spills from mouth
      Laryngeal excursion: ____adequate ____limited ____absent
      ____coughing ____particles exiting trachea
      Cervical auscultation: postswallow: ____clear ____wet
      postcough: ____clear ____wet
      Not assessed _____

6. Postsuctioning Results: ____clear ____food particles
   ____methylene blue ____unable to suction

VII. **Impressions:**
   A. Diagnosis: ____Dysphagia ____R/O Dysphagia
      Comment: _____
   B. Severity: ____mild ____moderate ____severe
   C. Stages of deglutition affected: ____oral ____pharyngeal (____laryngeal) ____esophageal
   D. Consistencies affected: ____pureed ____ground ____soft ____regular ____thick liquids
      ____thin liquids
   E. Comment: _____

(Continued)

F. Functional status:
   _____Dependent: Requires enteral or parenteral techniques to maintain adequate nutrition.
   _____Limited: Intake is primarily oral but requires constant supervision at meals to maintain nutrition and assure safety.
   _____Assisted: Intake is primarily oral but requires some assistance for feeding or a specialized diet.
   _____Independent: Requires no assistance and is able to tolerate safely most regular foods.
G. Prognosis: ____good ____fair ____poor ____guarded
H. Prognostic indicators: Favorable: ____age ____progress/recovery course thus far
   ____date of onset ____severity ____other:_____
   Unfavorable: ____age ____progress/recovery course
   ____date of onset ____severity ____other:_____

VIII. RECOMMENDATIONS

A. Treatment: _____no treatment at this time _____treatment
   _____pending: _____
B. Estimated LOS: Individual therapy for _____ week(s) for _____ units (sessions)
C. Referrals:_____
D. Treatment goals:
   Long-term goals/short-term goals
   1. _____   3. _____
      a. _____   a. _____
      b. _____   b. _____
      c. _____   c. _____
   2. _____
      a. _____
      b. _____
      c. _____
E. Ongoing patient/family education:_____
F. Suggestions to staff/family:
   1. Optimal positioning for feeding:_____

   2. Diet recommendations:
      _____PO intake
      _____PO intake *is not* appropriate
      _____To be fed only by speech pathologist at present time
      Diet: _____

      Foods to be omitted:_____

   3. Supervision required:_____

   4. Instructions to give patient:_____

   5. Others:_____

The above was discussed with the patient and/or family.

_____
Speech–Language Pathologist

If cineradiography study was completed, see following page for results.

(Continued)

Radiographic Dysphagia Assessment

☐ **Supplemental assessment:**

_____cineradiography   _____videofluroscopy

☐ **Summary of results:**

I. **Oral Stage:** _____normal _____impaired. If impaired,
   A. Check consistencies affected: _____thick barium _____thin barium
      _____barium/cookie mixture _____other:_____
   B. View difficulty noted: _____lateral: R L (circle), _____posterior/anterior
   C. Positioning affected: _____supine _____standing _____sitting other:_____
   D. Specific difficulty: _____

II. **Pharyngeal Stage:** _____normal _____impaired. If impaired,
   A. Check consistencies affected: _____thick barium _____thin barium
      _____barium/cookie mixture _____other:_____
   B. View difficulty noted: _____lateral: R L (circle), _____posterior/anterior
   C. Positioning affected: _____supine _____standing _____sitting other:_____
   D. Specific difficulty: _____

III. **Esophageal Stage:** _____normal _____impaired. If impaired,
   A. Check consistencies affected: _____thick barium _____thin barium
      _____barium/cookie mixture _____other:_____
   B. View difficulty noted: _____lateral: R L (circle), _____posterior/anterior
   C. Positioning affected: _____supine _____standing _____sitting other:_____
   D. Specific difficulty: _____

☐ **Recommendations:** (See evaluation in part VIII of Diagnostic Summary of Swallowing Functions.)

_____
Speech–Language Pathologist

SECTION 6. SENSATION PHENOMENA

23

Sensation: An Overview

Judith A. Metcalf

Sensation is an extremely personal concept, influenced by cultural, environmental, and psychologic factors. One might say that significant function and pure survival rely on the ability of the individual to receive, process, and take action on various forms of stimuli—external, from environmental influences, and internal, from within the individual.

From minute to minute, we experience situations within our environments and changes within our bodies by way of specialized sensory systems: vision, hearing, touch, taste, and smell. Each sensory system is architecturally specialized so that it reacts to a particular range of environmental influences.

Sensation may be provocatively pleasant, irritating, or tearfully painful. It may be accentuated, altered, diminished, or even absent. There may be variety in intensity with no direct correlation to the stimulus, especially when the stimulus is of pathologic origin (Purchese, 1977).

Sensation may be viewed with respect to the implications it has for the person, family, and society. There are many neurologic conditions that alter sensory input, processing, or perception and thereby impose severe restrictions on the individual and the way he or she relates to family and society.

Several questions must be kept in mind: How do normal sensations influence, enhance, or interfere with everyday life? How does an alteration in sensation affect daily living? Can one measure the devastation that is created when one of the senses has been impaired? Why do some people adapt to the effects of spinal cord injury better than others? Is it their support systems, professional interest, culture, life experiences? Should we even try to make a judgment about or should we instead heighten our awareness of the fact that alterations in sensory experiences are individual and may have profound implications on the person, family, and society?

PERIPHERAL SOMESTHETIC SENSORY SYSTEM

Receptors
The skin is considered the major source of sensory input to the nervous system and contains a variety of sensory receptors that relay information about the internal and external environ-

TABLE 23-1. TYPES OF MECHANORECEPTORS.

Type	Purpose	Location
Free nerve endings	To detect touch and pressure	Everywhere in the skin
Meissner's corpuscles	Ability to discern spatial characteristics of touch sensation	Glabrous, nonhairy, skin, especially fingertips and lips
Expanded tip tactile receptors	Provide a continuous signal that gives the ability to determine continuous touch of objects against the skin	Skin
Hair end-organs	Detect mainly movement of objects over the surface of the body due to stimulation of nerve fibers that entwine the base of the hair	Skin
Ruffini's end-organs	Alert to heavy continuous touch and pressure signals	Deep tissues and deeper layers of skin
Pacinian corpuscles	Detect tissue vibration, stimulated only by rapid movement	Beneath the skin, deep in tissues of the body

ment. The sensory receptors are specialized for converting various forms of energy in the environment into action potentials in the neurons (Ganong, 1987). The forms of energy converted by the receptors include mechanical (touch, pressure), thermal (degrees of warmth), electromagnetic (light), and chemical (odor, taste, and carbon dioxide content of the blood). Because sensory receptors are highly specialized to respond to one particular form of stimulus, there must be many different types of receptors. The receptors pertinent to this chapter include mechanoreceptors, thermoreceptors, and nocireceptors.

Mechanoreceptors

Mechanoreceptors facilitate the relative determination of positions and rates of movement of the different parts of the body. They are sensitive to touch, pressure, vibration, tickle, and position. There are six types of tactile receptors, as shown in Table 23-1.

Thermoreceptors

Thermoreceptors detect changes in temperature. There are various thermoreceptors throughout the body that function to inform the hypothalamic heat-regulating center of environmental temperature. That information plus the information from central temperature receptors normally stimulate the hypothalamus to activate either heat-gaining or heat-losing mechanisms; for example, when the body attempts to generate heat via shivering or when the body strives for heat containment by peripheral vasoconstriction.

Sensory information on the continuum of burning hot to freezing cold and the degrees of temperature difference are discriminated by at least three types of peripheral sensory receptors: cold receptors, warmth receptors, and pain receptors. Central receptors are specialized neurons in the anterior hypothalamus (Table 23-2).

Nociceptors

Nociceptors are pain receptors that detect damage in the tissue, whether it be physical or chemical.

Fibers

Sensory nerve fibers transmit impulses from the periphery to specific cortical or subcortical areas. Three types of fibers have been described according to fiber diameter, conduction velocity, and physiologic characteristic. Generally, the greater the diameter of the nerve fiber, the greater is its speed of conduction. The larger fibers are concerned with proprioceptive sensation, whereas the smaller fibers are concerned with pain sensation (Ganong, 1987).

TABLE 23–2. TYPES OF THERMORECEPTORS.

Type	Purpose	Location
Cold receptors	Discriminate degrees of temperature difference, cold	Under the skin (there are three to four times as many cold receptors as warmth receptors)
Warmth receptors	Discriminate the degrees of temperature difference, warmth	Under the skin

Pain receptors
  Warmth pain receptors
  Cold pain receptors
	Pain receptors in combination with cold and warmth receptors are responsive to freezing cold and burning hot sensations (Guyton, 1981)	Under the skin

Central receptors	Monitor temperature of blood (core temperature)	Anterior hypothalamus

Large Myelinated Aβ Fibers

Large myelinated Aβ fibers transmit impulses generated via mechanical stimuli: touch and pressure.

Small Myelinated Aδ Fibers

Small myelinated Aδ fibers serve two functions. First, some fibers transmit impulses from nociceptors and mediate fast pain, such as removing a hand from a hot burner. Second, some fibers transmit impulses from mechanoreceptors. These are the fibers that carry temperature, crude touch, and prickling pain sensation.

C Fibers

C fibers are small, unmyelinated fibers and are concerned basically with pain, temperature, itch, and crude touch sensation. A few C fibers also transmit impulses from mechanoreceptors. Over two thirds of all nerve fibers in peripheral nerves are C fibers. The large numbers of C fibers facilitate the transmission of tremendous amounts of information from the surface of the body, even though the velocity of transmission is slow.

Dermatomes

Cutaneous sensation of a specific area of skin supplied by the fibers of any one dorsal root is a dermatome. The cell bodies of the afferent fibers involved are located in the dorsal spinal nerve root ganglia and in the ganglia on cranial nerves (CN) V, VII, IX, and X. Sensory stimuli express toward the cell body from the periphery and continue to the spinal cord. The anatomic distribution represented by the dermatome correlates with a respective spinal cord segment and can be mapped out schematically. Using astute accurate assessment of the cutaneous distribution of various nerve roots, it is possible to localize the site and level of pathologic disturbance.

Spinal Cord

The spinal cord is a cylindrical, flexible structure that is the caudal continuation of the medulla oblongata. It extends distally from the medulla, ending at the level of the first or second lumbar vertebra. The spinal cord travels through the hollow canal in the center of the vertebral column and serves as a communication cable carrying motor information from the brain to the peripheral nervous system and carrying sensory information from the peripheral nervous system back to the brain.

The spinal cord is approximately 45 cm long in the male and 42 cm long in the female and is divided into cervical (C), thoracic (T), lumbar (L), and sacral (S) segments. Two enlargements are present, one in the cervical region C3 to T2, and the other in the lumbar region, corresponding to vertebrae T10 to T12, to receive additional nerves from the upper and lower extremities.

Spinal Nerves

The spinal roots are bundled together to form the 31 pairs of spinal nerves that originate from the spinal cord. Each nerve has an anterior or ventral root and a posterior or dorsal root. The anterior or ventral nerve root consists of efferent motor fibers originating in the ventral and lateral gray columns, having their attachment to the front portion of the spinal cord. They carry motor information from the brain through the cord to various body parts.

The posterior or dorsal nerve root contains afferent sensory fibers from the nerve cells in the spinal ganglion, or dorsal root ganglion, which is an enlargement containing cells in the dorsal root of each nerve. The dorsal nerve roots have their attachment to the back portion of the cord and are responsible for carrying incoming sensory information to the cord, where it is then relayed to the brain.

The groups of spinal nerves are divided into 8 cervical, 12 thoracic, 5 lumbar, 5 sacral, and 1 coccygeal nerve. The lumbosacral nerve roots are collectively called the *cauda equina* because of the resemblance to the tail of a horse.

Gray Matter

The gray matter within the spinal cord is composed of cell bodies clustered in the central area, appearing like a butterfly or an H. White matter is composed of myelinated nerve fibers and surrounds the gray matter. The gray matter has three columns, the anterior, posterior, and the lateral columns. The *anterior column (anterior horn)* is composed of cell bodies of motor neurons that relay motor information from the brain out through the anterior roots. The *posterior column (dorsal horn)* contains sensory relay cells that transmit incoming information received through the posterior root from the body to the brain. The *lateral column (lateral horn)*, also called the *intermediolateral cell column*, extends from T1 through L2 or L3. This column consists of small motor-type cells and gives rise to preganglionic sympathetic fibers.

The gray matter is divided into 10 layers, or laminae, on the basis of cytoarchitecture and organization of neurons. Lamina I is in the most dorsal section of the dorsal horn, and lamina IX is in the most ventral section of the ventral horn. Each lamina extends the full length of the spinal cord. Laminae I–VI are located in the dorsal horns, with lamina I the most superficial and lamina VI the most deep. These laminae are primarily concerned with *afferent sensory input* to the spinal cord. Specifically laminae II and III correspond to the substantia gelatinosa, which receives information from pain and temperature afferents. Lamina VII is located in the intermediate gray area and extends into the anterior horn. It contains the nucleus dorsalis and the intermediolateral gray column. The anterior horn contains lamina VIII, which has neurons that send commissural axons to the opposite side of the cord. Lamina IX is contained within the ventral horn and has motor neurons that send axons into the ventral roots of the spinal nerves and innervate the skeletal muscles. Lamina X surrounds the central column.

White Matter

The white matter in the spinal cord is composed chiefly of myelinated nerve fibers, although there are some unmyelinated fibers as well. The purpose of the white matter is to link different segments of the spinal cord and to connect the spinal cord with the brain. The white matter is organized around longitudinal columns (funiculi)—anterior, posterior, and lateral. Each column consists of fiber tracts, some ascending (sensory) and others descending (motor).

For the purposes of this chapter, only the major ascending tracts are discussed. The *lateral spinothalamic tract* is the main pathway for conveying impulses of pain and temperature, and the *anterior spinothalamic tract* is the pathway for simple touch and pressure. Recent evidence indicates that both the lateral spinothalamic tract and the anterior spinothalamic tract are capable of mediating nociceptive and tactile sensation. The *posterior or dorsal column tract* includes the fasciculus gracilis, fibers from the leg, and fasciculus cuneatus, fibers from the arm. These pathways are responsible for sensations of motion, movement, touch, and pressure. The *ventral spinocerebellar tract* relays information from pain, tactile, and pressure receptors over an extremity, and the *dorsal spinocerebellar tract* provides information relating to individual muscles and joints. Both the ventral and dorsal spinocerebellar tracts are concerned mainly with the lower extremities and provide predominantly proprioceptive information to the cerebellum. The name of each tract is descriptive to indicate the column (funiculus) in which it travels, the location of its cells of origin, and the location of its axon termination.

There are two major ascending systems responsible for conveying somatosensory information to the cerebral cortex. Current literature divides them into the dorsal column, or lemniscal system, which mediates fine tactile and kinesthetic sensation, and the anterolateral system, which conducts impulses for pain and temperature, touch, and deep pressure.

Dorsal Column System. In general, fine touch, pressure, and proprioceptive fibers ascend on the ipsilateral side in the dorsal columns to the medulla, where they synapse in the gracile and cuneate nuclei. The second-order neurons from the gracile and cuneate nuclei cross the midline and ascend on the medial lemniscus to end in the specific sensory relay nuclei of the thalamus, which projects to the somatosensory regions of the cerebral cortex. Dorsal columns transmit messages exclusively from mechanoreceptors, whereas information from the anterolateral system comes from mechanoreceptors, thermoreceptors, and nociceptors. Dorsal column lesions produce ipsilateral impairment of ability (Schmidt, 1978).

Anterolateral System. The fibers mediating temperature and pain, as well as some touch fibers, synapse on the neurons in the dorsal horn. The axons from these neurons cross the midline and ascend on the contralateral side in the anterolateral quadrant of the spinal cord. This pathway ends in the reticular formation of the brainstem and in the thalamus. Anterolateral lesions produce impairment on the contralateral side (Schmidt, 1978).

Fibers from within both the dorsal column (lemniscal system) and the anterolateral system are joined in the brainstem by fibers mediating sensation from the head.

CENTRAL SOMESTHETIC SENSORY SYSTEM

The body has two major sensory systems that influence and organize sensation. Neither is mutually exclusive, and they depend on each other's normal function and relay of impulses for the total delivery of the sensory experience. The first sensory system, the peripheral somesthetic system, has been discussed. The central somesthetic sensory system includes the fiber connections between the peripheral somesthetic sensory system, which communicates with the brainstem (reticular activating system), thalamus, hypothalamus, and parietal lobes (Schmidt, 1978).

Brainstem, Reticular Activating System

The reticular activating system receives information from all the afferent cranial nerves and is thought to participate in a number of sensory influences. Schmidt (1978) lists these as

> (a) The influence the ARAS has on control of consciousness by influence on the activity of cortical neurons; (b) Mediation of the affective emotional effects of sensory stimuli, for example the transmission of afferent pain information to the limbic system; (c) Vegetative regulatory functions with vital reflexes (cardiovascular, respiratory, swallowing, coughing and sneezing reflexes) in which many afferent and efferent systems must be coordinated; (d) Participation in the motor mechanisms for body support and directed movement. (p. 57).

Thalamus

The thalamus has many subdivisions and is a very important sensory center. The thalamus receives afferent communication from the periphery and from all the other sensory modalities, with the exception of the olfactory impulses. Some of the fibers that terminate in the thalamus are those of the lateral spinothalamic tract, which carry sensations of pain and temperature, as well as fibers from the anterior spinothalamic tract responsible for carrying sensations of light touch and pressure. In his work, Peele (1977) states that, "thalamic nuclei may serve as simple relays, as integrative centers for conscious recognition of certain impulses and as integrative and elaborative centers which project the product of their elaboration to the cerebral cortex" (p. 311).

The thalamus serves to integrate sensory impulses, as in the recognition of pain or in the spectrum of temperature or touch variations. The thalamus also makes it possible for a person to realize the degree of contraction in muscles and around joints, allowing for a sense of movement or position. The ability to recognize size, shape, and quality of objects that have contact with touch receptors and to be able to identify a particular point of stimulation are cortical functions that are possible only if thalamic relay functions are intact.

Hypothalamus

The hypothalamus is directly responsible for a variety of vital regulatory functions of the body and is involved with many aspects of emotion and behavior. With the limbic structures, the hypothalamus seems to be responsible for the interpretive nature of sensory sensation, whether pleasant or painful. Communicating pathways exist with all levels of the limbic system.

Stimulation of various regions of the hypothalmus can create an increase in activity that can create the emotions of fear, rage, and increase in sexual drive.

Parietal Lobe

Adams and Victor (1985) state:

The greater part of the parietal lobe functions as a center for integrating somatic sensory with visual and auditory information in constructing an awareness of the body . . . and of its relation to extrapersonal space. Through frontal connections, proprioception and vision are combined for the movement of the body and manipulation of objects and for certain constructional activities, and impairment of these functions implicates the parietal lobe, especially the right (p. 338).

The somesthetic area, the primary sensory projection area, is responsible for the reception of general sensation and is located in the parietal lobe. It receives fibers from thalamic radiations conveying skin, muscle joint, and tendon sense from the opposite side of the body. The primary sensory areas are arranged topographically on the cerebral cortex to mirror image the primary motor area; this is called the sensory homunculus.

Conditions That May Alter Somatic Sensation

There are many neurologic conditions that may have as a common symptom an alteration in sensation. Only those with an actual or potential marked sensory alteration are discussed.

Complete Spinal Cord Injury

When there is a sudden transverse lesion to the spinal cord, all sensory and motor function is lost immediately below the level of the lesion; these functions do not return. Generally, there may be a hyperesthetic area near the upper margin of anesthesia, and loss of pain temperature and touch sensation may begin one or two segments below the level of the lesion.

Incomplete Spinal Cord Injury Syndromes

The most commonly seen incomplete spinal cord injuries are Brown-Séquard syndrome and Central Cord syndrome.

Brown-Séquard syndrome is caused by hemisection of the spinal cord, resulting most commonly from bullet or stab wounds. This syndrome results in ipsilateral motor paralysis, ipsilateral loss of touch, pressure, vibration, and proprioceptive sensation, and contralateral loss of pain and thermal sensation, usually beginning one to two segments below the lesion.

Central cord syndrome occurs when there is damage located specifically in the area of the central spinal cord. Motor ability of the upper extremities is more severely affected than that of the lower extremities, and sensory loss is variable.

Syringomyelia
Syringomyelia (from the Greek *syrinx*, "pipe" or "tube") is a chronic progressive syndrome of the spinal cord associated with an enlarging accumulation of fluid in the spinal cord. Usually, the central canal of the spinal cord enlarges, or tubelike cavities open in the central region of the gray matter. As a result, there is destruction of the gray and white matter that lies adjacent to the central canal. Because pain fibers that cross anterior to the central canal may be interrupted or destroyed, the first symptom often is loss of pain and temperature sensation in the involved dermatomes. Pain may be a symptom, however, and if so, it is usually unilateral and is of a burning, aching quality located in the region of sensory impairment.

The cavitation, or syrinx, may extend into the anterior horn, destroying motor neurons, and result in atrophy and weakness of the segments involved.

Trigeminal Neuralgia
Trigeminal neuralgia (*tic douloureux*) may result from the degeneration or compression of one or all branches of CN V. It is characterized by mild to excruciating facial pain, described by many as the worst possible pain a person could ever suffer. The pain frequently occurs as severe, lightninglike, electric stabs or searing pain and may be accompanied by muscle twitching of the face. The duration is usually short, lasting from a few seconds to minutes, but frequently pains occur in succession so that it seems endless. At times, the pain may be provoked by a slight breeze, brushing of the teeth, or washing the face. The most common trigger points include the nostril, medial cheek, or one lip.

Thalamic Lesions
Thalamic lesions involving the nucleus ventralis posterolateralis of the thalamus can create a decrease or loss of sensation on the contralateral side of the body. The origin of this thalamic lesion is vascular or a tumor. The sensory function most commonly involved is position sense, and deep sensory loss is usually but not always more profound than cutaneous loss. There may be spontaneous and extremely irritating pain on the affected side that may linger and be extremely unpleasant.

Lesions of the Parietal Lobe
The best known anterior parietal lobe syndrome is described by Adams and Victor (1985, p. 126) as Veger-DeJerine syndrome. It is characterized by disturbances of the discriminative sensory abilities on the contralateral side, especially of the face, arm, and leg. Impaired localization of touch and pain stimuli, loss of position sense, elevation of two point threshold, astereognosis, and tactile agnosia, if the lesion is in the dominant hemisphere, are the most prominent findings. Seen frequently with lesions involving the parietal lobe is a sensory inattention or neglect response of body parts on the affected side. Stroke, closed head injury, and tumors may cause parietal lobe lesions.

Herpes Zoster
Herpes zoster (shingles) is an infection by a virus of the primary sensory neurons. Generally, symptoms of fever and malaise precede the pain and vesicle formation over the segmental distribution of the involved roots. Itching, tingling, or burning sensations of the dermatomes often precede the vesicular eruption.

Any dermatome may be involved, but T5–T10 dermatomes appear to be the most common, followed by the craniocervical regions. The pain and dysesthesia frequently linger for weeks, months, or in some cases years, creating difficult problems with pain management.

Causalgia
Causalgia is a condition of constant burning pain, most commonly along the distribution of the median or tibial nerves. Causalgia usually follows traumatic lesions of the peripheral nerves. Symptoms may begin the first few days after injury and may involve trophic changes on the skin, sweating in the affected extremity, and changes in the hair and nails.

Multiple Sclerosis
Multiple sclerosis is one of the most common neurologic diseases in the United States. It is chronic, often progressive, and characterized by destruction of multiple areas of central nervous system myelin. Sensory disturbances are common and depend on the area of sclerotic patch formation in the central nervous system. Sensory disturbance usually is symmetric and involves the trunk and lower extremities more frequently than the upper extremities. Lhermitte's sign is perhaps one of the most common sensory symptoms noted and is frequently described as a lightninglike sensation that radiates down the neck after neck flexion. Other forms of sensory changes experienced include loss of vibratory sense in the distal lower extremities, bandlike sensations about the trunk, tingling paresthesias or numbness of the face in the distribution of the fifth nerve, and pain that is individualized.

SPECIAL SENSES

Hearing
In the United States, hearing loss is one of the most frequent forms of physical disability and involves 10 to 20 million Americans. The potential for suboptimal educational, economic, and psychosocial advantage is a real concern to both the individual and society. Alterations in hearing affect each person and family unit differently. The meaning this disability has is a uniquely personal experience. Hearing levels adequate for one person, situation, or occupation vary. The effect of hearing loss would be different for a carpenter or a photographer than it would be for an anesthesiologist who requires acute hearing to detect life-threatening air emboli (Meyerhoff et al., 1984).

There are both peripheral and central components to the sensation of hearing. The *peripheral components* include the outer, middle, and inner ear as well as the auditory peripheral nerve (CN VIII). The *central auditory system* includes the brainstem cochlear nuclei, superior olive, lateral lemniscus, inferior colliculus, and medial geniculate body. Auditory representation on the cerebral cortex includes a diversity of connections and pathways. The brainstem assumes some responsibility for sound awareness, and the temporal lobe is responsible for the appreciation of sound, pitch, intensity, and discrimination.

Sound stimuli may be movement created by a moving body in some medium—water, air—or it may be the sound, sensation, or sensory experience known only to the mind of the listener that we can relate to our physical and emotional lives. Sound is translated by the brain as music, information, or noise. We can discriminate between sounds, such as footsteps versus horse's hooves, and even tell the direction of movement based on noise. Sound must begin by a mechanical disturbance, such as that caused by the slamming of a door or striking the keys of a piano. The vibrations of the sound cause the formation of waves that radiate in all directions. It is the moving waves that are heard as sound.

> Sound waves are collected by the auricle and pass along the canal to the tympanic membrane. The pars tensa vibrates in response to sound waves, which are then conducted through the malleus and incus to the stapes. The stapes footplate articulates with the oval window and beneath it lies the utricle and saccule surrounded by perilymph. Movement of the stapes footplate causes sound waves to be conducted through the oval window to move the endolymph. This movement stimulates the

delicate hair cells of the cochlea and from these cells impulses pass along fibers of the auditory nerve to reach the auditory cortex in the superior temporal gyrus on both sides of the brain (Pracy et al., 1974, p. 35).

The auditory pathway contains a series of neurons that make synapses at each station of the ascending pathway and may be described as follows. Acoustic stimulation excites fibers of the cochlear nerve that terminate in the cochlear nucleus. The fibers leave the cochlear nucleus via three main tracts, one of which connects with the superior olivary complex. Fibers continue to ascend in the contralateral lemniscus to the inferior colliculus, which sits on the roof of the midbrain. The inferior colliculus gives rise to fiber tracts that terminate in the medial geniculate body, which is in the posterior portion of the thalamus. From here, fibers form the thalamic auditory relay, which connects to the auditory cortex (Karmody 1983; Bradford & Hardy, 1979).

When hearing loss is assessed, hearing specialists attempt to determine the site of damage within the auditory system. Hearing loss is, therefore, generally broken down into three categories that relate to the anatomic areas of involvement. The first is a *conductive hearing loss*, in which there is damage involving the external auditory canal, eardrum, middle ear, or eustachian tube. The second is a *sensorineural hearing loss*, in which there is involvement of the inner ear, the auditory nerve, or both. The third is *central hearing loss*, in which damage to the auditory system lies in the central nervous system between a structure in the medulla oblongata, the auditory nucleus, and the cortex (Sataloff, 1980).

Some nongenetic causes of sensorineural hearing loss in the neurologic realm include (1) trauma resulting from noise, penetrating injuries, or temporal bone fracture, (2) sudden pressure changes, resulting from cerebrospinal fluid or barometric pressure changes, such as flying, diving, coughing, or sneezing, (3) metabolic disturbances resulting from hypothyroidism or adrenopituitary disorders, (4) toxic substances, such as heavy metals, antibiotics (especially the aminoglycosides, which are capable of destroying the hair cells and stria vascularis of the inner ear), and salicylates, (5) space-occupying lesions in the cerebellopontine angle, such as acoustic neuromas and meningiomas, and (6) inflammatory disease, either viral (herpes, cytomegaloviras, or adenovirus III, which may create labyrinthitis, neuronitis, or vasculitis) or bacterial (meningococcal meningitis, which may involve the inner ear) (Meyerhoff et al., 1984).

Vision

Vision is an extremely complex and still not completely understood sensory modality. We begin by discussing the structure and composition of the eye.

The *cornea* forms the anterior one sixth of the eyeball and is responsible for focusing and transmitting light to the interior of the eye. The *sclera* is white, opaque, and tough and is directly continuous with the edge of the cornea. It encircles the eye completely, except where it joins the emerging optic nerve. The donut-shaped structure that gives the eye its color is the *iris*. It surrounds the pupil, which is essentially a hole in the center of the iris. The two muscles in the iris are responsible for changing pupillary size (Havener et al., 1974). The *ciliary body* is in direct continuity with the iris and is adherent to the sclera. The ciliary muscle directly controls the focusing ability of the eye by controlling the size and shape of the lens. The richly vascular layer, the *choroid*, supplies the nutrition of the outer half of the retina. The *retina* perceives light and is the innermost layer of the eye. Each retina contains more than 125 million nerve cells able to see light and many more millions of nerve cells to coordinate and transmit the impulses from the seeing cells to the optic nerve. The two types of visual cells are called *rods* and *cones* and are the light-sensitive part of the retina. The rods are used for vision in dim light; the cones are used for daylight color and vision. The rods and cones are located in the deepest layer of the retina. The retina develops from the central nervous system and, in its component layers of nerve cells and fibers, resembles the architecture of the cerebral cortex (Havener et al., 1974).

The *lens* is just behind the iris and functions to focus light on the retina. The space behind the lens is the *vitreous body*; it is filled with fluid resembling gelatin and occupies two thirds of the volume of the eye. The *anterior chamber* is the space between the iris and cornea, which is filled with a crystal clear fluid formed by the ciliary body called *aqueous*. The posterior chamber is located between the iris and the lens and also is filled with aqueous.

Optic Nerve
The optic nerve emerges from the back of the globe to enter the cranial cavity via the optic canal. Intracranially, the two optic nerves join to form the optic chiasm. Each optic nerve is covered by the meninges. Since the general cranial subarachnoid space is continuous with that surrounding the optic nerve, increase in intracranial pressure is transmitted through the spinal fluid to the optic subarachnoid space, creating swelling of the optic papilla. The total length of the optic nerve is approximately 4 to 5 cm (Peele, 1977).

Extraocular Muscles
There are six extraocular eye muscles in each eye that are responsible for moving the ocular globe. These twelve must work in harmony all the time. They are amazingly coordinated and automatically aim the two eyes at exactly the same point in space. The innervation for these muscles is from CN III, IV, and VI. Dysfunction of ocular movement is described in Chapters 19 and 21.

Visual Pathway
As the fibers leave the optic nerve, approximately one half of them cross to the opposite side. Once past the optic chiasm, these crossed fibers, which originated from the nasal half of the retina of one eye, intermingle with the fibers originating from the temporal half of the retina of the opposite eye. These intermingled fibers form the optic tract.

Fibers from the optic tracts enter a relay station, the *lateral geniculate body*. From here, the fibers disseminate in a fan shape and traverse parts of the temporal and parietal lobes en route to the occipital cortex, the *striate area*. The area from which the retinas receive light impulses is the *visual field*. Mapping of the visual field provides information about the functioning of the retina and the visual pathways.

Disorders of Vision
The eyes are in close concert with the brain and often supply much diagnostic information that may assist in the localization and diagnosis of central nervous system disorders. When there is abnormal function of the anatomic structures that are in close proximity to the eyes and optic pathways, such as those around the optic chiasm, third ventricle, and pituitary gland and internal carotid artery and optic nerve, there will be dysfunction of ocular movement and visual disturbance.

Optic neuritis is a sudden decrease in vision, often accompanied by central vision field defects. Optic neuritis may be attributed to a wide variety of causes, but sudden central monocular visual loss with pain on ocular movement usually is due to demyelinization of optic nerves. Multiple sclerosis appears to be one of the most common causes. *Pituitary tumors* have such a close proximity to the optic chiasm that the visual finding commonly is bitemporal hemianopsia. *Pupillary abnormalities* occur in *Horner's syndrome*, in which the pupil is small, regular, and unilateral, and is associated with a mild ptosis and loss of sweating of the forehead. Horner's syndrome usually is associated with damage or interruption of the sympathetic nerve supply, usually in the neck.

Argyll-Robertson pupils are small, irregular pupils, usually bilateral, with a poor or absent reaction to light but appropriate response to accommodation. This condition usually is associated with neurosyphilis.

Taste

The sense of taste allows one to discriminate and recognize the salt on a potato chip, the bitterness of bitter lemon, the sweet taste of sugar, and the sour taste of acid. The sense of taste, however, usually must depend on the sense of smell to appreciate the complete array of food flavors, such as fruit, meat, and coffee.

The sense of taste arises from the dorsal surface of the tongue, the epiglottis, and at times from the mucous membranes of the cheeks, lips, and larynx. For taste discrimination, the tongue is divided into the mid-dorsal surface, which is insensitive to taste; the tip, which is most aware of sweet and salt stimuli but responds to all taste; the borders of the tongue, which are most sensitive to sour tastes; and the base of the tongue, which is most sensitive to bitter tastes. Taste buds that recognize these flavors are present on the surface of the tongue and number approximately 100,000 in the human adult (Peele, 1977).

There are both peripheral and central taste pathways. The *peripheral pathways* involve the input from CN VII, IX, and X. The geniculate ganglion of CN VII, the superior petrosal ganglion of CN IX, and the nodose ganglion of CN X pass centrally into the medulla, join the tractus solitaris, and synapse in the nucleus solitarius. The central pathways seem to be the secondary solitariothalamic fibers, which travel in company with the medial lemniscus fibers and synapse within the medial portion of the posteromedial ventral thalamic nucleus (Peele, 1977).

The tongue must be moist enough to allow for solution to stimulate the taste buds. If the tongue is very dry, the sense of taste is thus dramatically reduced. The number of taste buds decreases with age, thus creating a loss of full appreciation of flavor. Bell's palsy may create a loss of taste on one side that is annoying but tolerable. Stimulation of Brodman's area 50 has elicited taste sensations. Taste may be altered by local disturbances of the mouth, and alterations in taste do not always indicate pathology of the taste pathways.

Smell

The airway of the nostril provides access to the sensitive nerve endings that are all but hidden high in a compartment at the top of the nasal cavity. This compartment, the olfactory cleft, occupies an area about 2.5 cm within each nostril. The nasal septum separates the two clefts. Most inspired air passes directly to the pharynx and lungs, bypassing the cleft. Some odor particles do escape the air and find their way to the cleft. The nasal chamber of the nostril has an average volume of 17.1 ml. When one chews food, the movement of the palate and throat create small air movements that project odorous material up to the cleft via the nasopharynx, where it can stimulate the sensitive receptors (Geldard, 1972). The surface of the olfactory cleft, the olfactory mucosa, is composed of millions of tiny endings of CN I and an even larger number of supporting cells. The true endings of the olfactory nerve fibers or rods project through the supporting cells to the surface. Tiny cilia arise from the tip of each rod and project into the mucous layer, which bathes the entire surface of thj olfactory epithelium (Geldard, 1972).

An alteration in the sense of smell is not very common. When it does occur, however, there are three major causes. (1) *Trauma* seems to affect the olfactory tract by tearing or shearing of the tiny olfactory nerves or by avulsion of the olfactory tract if a fracture is present. Compression of olfactory tracts after trauma may result from edema or accumulation of blood clots. All may serve to interfere with the sense of smell. (2) *Tumors*, especially meningiomas of the olfactory groove, may alter smell. The presence of frontal lobe or temporal lobe tumors or any swelling around the vicinity of the optic chiasm may affect the olfactory nerve. (3) *Epilepsy* may produce focal sensory seizures characterized by an olfactory sensation described as unpleasant. The seizure focus may be directly related to the area responsible for normal olfactory perception. This could be caused by electrical discharges involving not only the limbic system but also the olfactory bulb and receptor cells (Douek, 1974). Such seizures may generalize to major motor seizures, in which case the sensory seizure may be called an "aura" by the patient.

ASSESSMENT OF THE SOMATIC AND SPECIAL SENSES

Somatic Sensation

When evaluating sensation, it is most important to have the full cooperation of the person being examined; otherwise the findings will be inaccurate. In order to enhance the assessment, the person should be instructed about what to expect. The face, trunk, arms, and legs are most commonly tested. The examiner systematically tests the right and left sides and evaluates the dermatomes, working upward on the body from the impaired to the normal area.

Light Touch

Light touch may be tested with a wisp of cotton, first familiarizing the person with the stimulus by applying it to a normal body part. The person can be asked to say "yes" everytime it is felt. When an area of impairment is discovered, the stimulus should be moved from the point of impairment outward until normal areas are found to map the boundaries of impairment.

Pain

Pain may be tested with the sharp point of a pin. The person should be asked to indicate the degree of sharpness in addition to the feeling of contact or pressure. As in testing for light touch, the examiner should work upward, beginning with the areas of impaired sensation. The skin may be tested using both sharp and dull ends of the pin to have the person differentiate sharp from dull. Both right and left sides of the body should be tested.

Temperature

The perception of temperature at times is difficult to assess accurately. It depends on the temperature of the test object, the duration of the stimulus, and the area over which it is applied. The test object should be large; a flask of hot or cold water or a metal tuning fork may be used. The test object should be tested over a normal area, and the person should be asked if the thermal sensation is less hot or less cold in comparison to the sensation in the normal part.

Position Sense—Passive Movement

To test for position sense, the examiner asks the person to close the eyes; the examiner moves the patient's extremity and has the person describe the position of that extremity. The person may also be asked to hold the arms up and attempt to touch the nose with the index finger. Passive movement may be tested by the examiner's holding one of the fingers or toes firmly and moving it rapidly up or down. The person should be asked to report each movement as being up or down.

Vibration

Vibration and position sense are often lost together. Vibration sense is evaluated by placing a tuning fork over the sternum, fingers, elbow, iliac crest, ankles, and toes. The examiner must be careful that the person is responding to the vibration and not to the pressure of the tuning fork. When the person no longer feels the vibration, the fork is moved quickly to the same point on the corresponding limb. Perceived vibration at this point indicates an abnormality. (Adams & Victor, 1985)

Discriminate Sensory Function

Lesions in the sensory cortex or thalamocortical projections may leave touch, pain, temperature, and vibration sense intact but interfere with higher integrated sensation, such as form, discrimination, and shape. The following tests are higher level tests of discriminating function.

Two-point discrimination is the ability to distinguish two points from one. The two points must be applied simultaneously and without pain.

Number writing or *graphesthesia* can be tested by tracing a number larger than 4 cm on the person's skin and asking him or her to identify it. *Stereognosis*, or ability to detect shape, is tested by placing objects in the patient's hand and asking him or her to identify the object without looking at it.

Special Senses

Hearing

Hearing can be evaluated by determining the person's perception of the whispered or spoken word. The ear not being tested should be blocked when performing this test. The patient is positioned 20 feet away, and a few words are whispered. This provides a quick rough estimate of hearing loss. If a problem is detected, further evaluation is essential.

Weber's test assesses bone conduction. The base of the vibrating tuning fork is placed on the forehead or top of the skull, and the patient is asked if the sound is heard better in one ear or the other. The *Rinne test* involves placing the vibrating tuning fork on the mastoid process until the vibrations are no longer heard, then immediately moving the fork to the external ear canal to determine if sound is still present. Normally, sound should be heard longer via air conduction than by bone conduction.

Vision

Tests for vision include pupillary reaction, visual acuity, visual fields, and extraocular movement. Pupils are tested for size, shape, equality, and reaction to light, as well as for accommodation and the consensual light reaction.

Visual acuity is best tested with the Snellen eye chart. The person is placed 20 feet from the Snellen chart and asked to read the lines of progressively smaller letters until they can no longer be read. Each eye is tested individually. Test line 8 is what the normal eye should be able to read at 20 feet, and such vision is described as 20/20. (The person has read from a distance of 20 feet what a normal eye should be able to read at 20 feet.)

Visual fields are tested by comparing the patient's peripheral vision with that of the examiner by determining when both patient and examiner can see the object. The examiner stands in front of the person and assesses one eye at a time by having the person close one eye while the examiner closes the opposite eye. The examiner asks that the person fix on a point in the midline and brings his or her finger toward the midline in all four planes of vision. The patient indicates when the object comes into vision.

Examination of *extraocular movement* is described in Chapter 19.

Smell

With the eyes closed, the patient should be able to identify such common substances as chocolate, cinnamon, and tobacco.

Taste

Taste is tested by placing a few salt crystals or sugar crystals on the tongue. The person being tested must describe the taste. Perception of taste and smell diminish with age.

SUMMARY

There are many conditions with a wide range of varying degrees of sensory alteration. The impact of these dysfunctions on living are addressed in Chapters 24, 25, and 26.

REFERENCES

Adams, R., & Victor, M. (1985). *Principles of neurology* (3rd ed.). New York: McGraw-Hill.

Bradford, L., & Hardy, W. (1979). *Hearing and hearing impairment.* New York: Grune & Stratton.

Douck, E. (1974). *The sense of smell and its abnormalities.* London: Churchill-Livingstone.

Ganong, W. (1987). *Review of medical physiology* (13th ed.). E. Norwalk, CT: Appleton & Lange.

Geldard, F. (1972). *The human senses* (2nd ed.). New York: Wiley.

Guyton, A. (1987). *Basic neuroscience: Anatomy and physiology.*. Philadelphia: Saunders.

Havener, W., Saunders, W., Keith, C., & Prescott, A. (1974). *Nursing care in eye, ear, nose, throat disorders*. St. Louis: Mosby.

Karmody, C. (1983). *Textbook of otolaryngology*. Philadelphia: Lea & Febiger.

Maguire, G.H. (Ed.). (1985). *Care of the elderly: A health team approach*. Boston: Little, Brown.

Meyerhoff, W., Liston, S., & Anderson, R. (1984). *Diagnosis and management of hearing loss*. Philadelphia: Saunders.

Peele, T. (1977). *The neuroanatomic basis for clinical neurology* (3rd ed.). New York: McGraw-Hill.

Pracy, R., Sieglar, J., & Stell, P. (1974). *Ear, nose and throat*. London: English Universities Press.

Purchese, G. (1977). *Neuromedical and neurosurgical nursing*. London: Bailliere Tindall.

Sataloff, J., Sataloff, R., & Vassallo, L. (1980). *Hearing loss*. Philadelphia: Lippincott.

Schmidt, R. (Ed.). (1978). *Fundamentals of sensory physiology*. New York: Springer-Verlag.

BIBLIOGRAPHY

Carpenter, M. (1985). *Core text of neuroanatomy* (3rd ed.). Baltimore: Williams & Wilkins.

Chusid, J. (1985). *Correlative and functional neuroanatomy* (19th ed.). Los Altos, CA: Lange.

Creutzfeldt, O., Schmidt, R., & Willis, W. (Eds.) (1984). *Sensory–motor integration in the nervous system*. New York: Springer-Verlag.

Mitchell, P., Ozuna, J., Cammermeyer, M., & Woods, N. (1984). *Neurological assessment for nursing practice*. Reston, VA: Reston.

24

Alterations in the Special Senses

Sharon A. Bray

As an open system, each person is in constant interaction with the environment, exchanging matter, energy, and information. "The constant interchange of matter and energy between man and environment is at the basis of man's becoming. It is this interchange that portends the creativity of life" (Rogers, 1970, p. 54). Information from the environment is perceived by five senses: sight, hearing, smell, taste, and touch, which are important mechanisms for data collection, vital to an individual's very existence in an ever-changing complex environment. A person receives, processes, interprets, and responds to information perceived by the senses in a unique way as an individual.

Perception of the information received from the environment forms the basis for a response. Through experience, a degree of stability and predictability is established in this communication pattern. A deficit in one or more of the senses disrupts the individual's sense of predictability and often can bring chaos to the biopsychosocial functioning of that individual.

The impact of an alteration in one of the special senses is profound and dramatic, for it changes the way an individual has previously perceived and responded to the environment. A person's preference for environmental perception often can be inferred by the response to daily environmental input, "I hear you," "I see what you mean," "That feels right to me." The loss of a preferred sense may have greater impact on an individual's ability to interact constructively with the environment than does the loss of another modality. Neurologic disease processes often are responsible for creating alterations in the senses. As neuroscience nurses, each of us works daily with people who have a sudden or progressive alteration in one or more of the special senses.

The neuroscience nurse cares for, supports, and teaches the individual and family to adapt and repattern their communication with each other and their environment. The goals of the neuroscience nurse are to assess the individual's physical, emotional, and behavioral responses to a sensory deficit, formulate nursing diagnoses, and plan interventions with the patient and family directed toward achieving independence and optimal health within the constraints of the illness. The generalist focuses on the individual, family, and health care team while implementing nursing plans and coordinating overall care. The specialist, whose role includes education, clinical practice, consultation, and research, uses expertise in neurologic and neurosurgical clinical practice to serve as a resource to the generalist, intervene as a change agent, and actively participate in the community to facilitate maximal attainment of skills and capabilities of neurologic patients and their families (Davis, 1985). The ability to cope with and adapt to the changes in sight, smell, hearing, taste, and touch can be facilitated by the nurse's interventions with the individual, family, and community.

This chapter discusses the changes in the special senses that occur in the normal aging process and the impact of these changes on the nurse's interventions with the elderly. Conditions and diseases that result in alterations in the special senses are reviewed briefly, and human responses are illustrated, using a case study format.

AGE-RELATED CHANGES IN SENSORY COMPONENTS OF THE NERVOUS SYSTEM

Signs and symptoms of neurologic dysfunction are common in the elderly. According to Drachman and Long (1984), the reasons for the neurologic deterioration in the elderly are a cumulative summation of four factors:

1. Normal neuronal attrition (involution over time)
2. Previous neural damage
3. Decline in neural reserve, or plasticity
4. Specific disease(s) of the nervous system present at the time of evaluation (p. 97)

There are both structural and functional changes in the nervous system as it ages. Structurally, the brain loses weight and, therefore, volume within the fixed cavity of the cranium, giving it a shrunken appearance. There is loss of both gray and white matter (Kemper, 1984). The extracellular compartment volume decreases and cerebral blood flow decreases, providing fewer nutrients to the neurons and, thereby, decreasing the efficiency of the cell functioning (Meyer & Shaw, 1984). Intracellularly, there is the development of neurofibrillary tangles, or intraneuronal fibrillary material in the cytoplasm, which is thought to decrease intracellular transport and thus cause a permanent decline in neuronal functioning (Kemper, 1984). There appears to be a decrease in the efficiency of neurochemical activity in the aged as a result of a decline in the production of some of the neurotransmitters and also an increase in the activity of the enzymes responsible for neurotransmitter degradation (Solkoe & Kosik, 1984). These age-related changes, in combination with changes specific to the organs in the body, create an overall decrease in the functioning of the sensory nervous system. Age-related changes occur at different rates in each individual and are often complicated by a variety of situational, disease-related, and therapeutic aspects, such as nutrition, hypertension, hyperlipidemia, diabetes mellitus, and drugs. It is, therefore, important for the nurse to assess the elderly person's sensory functioning thoroughly and determine the impact that changes have on the ability to perceive and respond to the environment. Table 24–1 illustrates the changes in the sensory functions, commonly experienced symptoms, and some general nursing considerations when working with the elderly.

CONDITIONS THAT MAY CAUSE ALTERATIONS IN SENSORY FUNCTION

Seeing

Visual anatomy is described in Chapter 24. Neurologic disorders that can impair vision along the visual pathway include degeneration of the receptor cells of the retina, lesions of the macula, retina, or optic nerve, pituitary tumors, temporal or occipital lobe lesions, and disruption of blood supply to the

TABLE 24-1. AGE-RELATED CHANGES IN SENSORY FUNCTIONING.

	Sensory Function		
	Vision	Hearing (Presbycusis)	Combined Vestibular, Visual, and Proprioception
Functional changes	Decreased visual acuity, visual fields, color receptivity, pupil size, reactivity to light; opacification of lens	Stiffening and degeneration of auditory ossicles, auditory nerve cell loss.	Decreased balance, coordination, and equilibrium
Common symptoms	Myopia, hyperopia, tunnel vision, decreased color discrimination, impaired vision in dim light or glare	Decreased ability to detect pitch (high frequencies, initially) and to understand spoken words.	Dizziness, disturbances in gait, falls, difficulty walking and turning on uneven surface
Nursing considerations	Orient to environment; consistent location of furniture, personal objects; position objects within field of vision; adequate illumination; side lighting; annual eye examination	Face client when speaking; speak clearly, distinctly without artificial mouth configurations; keep pitch low in louder tones; use short sentences; request one response at a time; hearing aids; annual auditory examination	Encourage awareness of balance; turn slowly, rise gradually from sitting or lying; sit to put on pants, socks, shoes; use bathtub and stair rails

structures along this pathway. Specialized diagnostic techniques that may be helpful in determining the type and location of these disorders include magnetic resonance imaging (MRI) and pattern-shift visual evoked responses (PSVER) (Adams & Victor, 1985). Medical management is specific to the disorder and may include control of intracranial pressure, surgical removal of tumors or lesions, and revascularization.

Hearing and Balance

The ear is a complicated structure concerned not only with the function of hearing but also with balance. Dysfunctions that can occur along the complicated neural pathways of the auditory system are varied, such as damage from excessive noise, ototoxic drugs, and a variety of neurologic disorders: acoustic neuroma, auditory cortex infarcts, pontine lesions, chronic meningitis, or demyelinative plaque (Adams & Victor, 1985). In addition to the physical assessment findings, specialized hearing testing using audiograms and brainstem auditory evoked potentials (BAEP) can be helpful in identifying the location and nature of hearing deficits (Weldon et al., 1983).

Prevention is the best intervention for limiting impairment from ototoxic drugs. Routine assessment of hearing for patients taking ototoxic drugs can provide early indication of this side effect, at which time the drug can be discontinued or the dosage adjusted if the side effect is dose related.

Conductive hearing loss may be improved by use of hearing aids or surgical replacement of one or more of the auditory ossicles. Sensorineural hearing loss is difficult to treat since the source of the dysfunction is the focus of therapy, such as surgical removal of tumors, revascularization, or antibiotic therapy for infections.

The endolymph in the semicircular canals of the vestibular labyrinth moves in response to changes in motion and position of the head. This neurologic information, in conjunction with visual input and impulses from the proprioceptors of the joints and muscles, is integrated to maintain equilibrium, balance, and orientation in space. Dysfunctions of the vestibular system, such as Ménière's disease, trauma, vertebrobasilar ischemia, and vestibular neuronitis, can cause symptoms of vertigo, nystagmus, and unsteadiness. The goal of medical therapy is to treat the underlying disorder or the symptoms of the disorder; examples of therapy include surgery, antihistaminic agents, rest, and mild sedatives (Adams & Victor, 1985).

Smell

The receptor cells of the olfactory sense are bipolar neurons found in the mucous membranes of the upper and posterior parts of the nasal cavity. Olfaction can be diminished (hyposmia) or lost (anosmia) by such common causes as allergies or rhinitis, in which there is swelling or congestion of the nasal mucosa (Adams & Victor, 1985). The sense of smell is dependent on moistened, volatile air particles reaching the receptor cells and can, therefore, be impaired by inability to breathe in deeply through the nose or inadequate moisture of the nasal mucosa (Brown, 1985). Damage to the receptor cells as they converge and pass through the cribriform plate of the ethmoid bone can be severe as a result of head injuries, particularly fractures of the ethmoid bone (Adams & Victor, 1985).

The central processes of the olfactory receptors (cranial nerve I, CN I) and their connections in the brain are complex; therefore, the influence of smell on the biopsychosocial behaviors of an individual are broad. Brown (1985) offers an overview of the anatomic structures and the interrelationships between the olfactory neuronal connections and other structures and functions of the brain. Other etiologies that may affect the olfactory sense along its neural connections include tumors, multiple sclerosis, Parkinson's disease, and trauma (Adams & Victor, 1985). Olfactory hallucinations or an unpleasant smell (cacosmia) can occur as an aura in uncinate seizures. Again, medical therapy is aimed at treating the underlying causative factors if possible.

Taste

The sensory receptors for taste are distributed over the surface of the tongue, with a smaller number over the palate, pharynx, and larynx. The taste receptors perceive only salty, sweet, bitter, and sour sensations. More complex tastes are the combined sensations of taste and smell (Adams & Victor, 1985).

Decreased sense of taste (hypogeusia) or loss of taste (ageusia) may be caused by extreme dryness of the oral mucosa or lesions of the medulla oblongata or may follow influenza-like illnesses. Unilateral lesions of the thalamic region or the parietal lobe have been characterized by contralateral impairment of taste. Taste distortions can occur with some medications, such as antithyroid drugs, chlorambucil, colestyramine, and some anticancer drugs (Adams & Victor, 1985). Treatment of the underlying cause is the basis of medical management.

Touch

Deficits in sensory touch perception can occur as a result of damage to the many structures in the sensory nervous system. Review of the entire sensory nervous system is beyond the scope of this chapter, but deficits can result from pathologies occurring as distal as the sensory nerve receptor or dorsal nerve root and ganglion. Altered touch can occur as a result of spinal cord disorders in which there is damage of the posterior columns, anterolateral spinothalamic tract, and the thalamus. Increased intracranial pressure or lesions affecting the parietal lobe can cause deficits characteristic of damage to the postcentral gyrus. In addition to a thorough history and physical assessment, computerized tomography (CT) scans, MRI, and short-latency somatosensory evoked potentials (SLSEP) can assist the physician in differential diagnosis of disturbances of touch in the sensory nervous system (Adams & Victor, 1985).

Table 24–2 provides an overview of the anatomic structures involved in alterations in touch sensation, examples of causative neurologic disorders, and options for medical management.

HUMAN RESPONSES TO ALTERATION IN SPECIAL SENSES

The neuroscience nurse, in collaboration with the individual and family, develops a realistic, individualized plan for assisting the patient to regain and maintain functions of daily living safely and as independently as possible. Based on the following clinical case, a nursing care plan is developed for individuals with uncompensated sensory deficits and their families.

Case Study 1: Cerebrovascular Accident

Mr. F, 68 years old, was hospitalized with an admitting diagnosis of septal and posterior wall myocardial infarction (MI). His recuperation from the MI was complicated by several episodes of congestive heart failure, for which he was treated with diuretics. Three days after admission, Mr. F developed atrial fibrillation, which was unresponsive to drug therapy. Since the dysrhythmia had a significant impact on his hemodynamic status, it was imperative that he undergo cardioversion, to which he agreed. Twenty-four hours after a successful cardioversion, Mr. F suffered a cerebral embolus.

His patient profile and social history describes Mr. F as a right-handed, 5 ft. 11 in., 260 lb white male from South Carolina. He is married and has four children, all living away from home. His wife, 58 years old, is healthy, a homemaker, with no prior job experience. Mr. F is a machine mechanic, employed by a local garage. He and his family are Baptist and attend church regularly. Mr. F has no hobbies and often spends his leisure time at the local pool hall with his buddies from town. Mr. F has been looking forward to retiring in a few months and has a modest savings account.

His past medical history revealed the usual childhood diseases: measles, mumps, and chickenpox, with no history of rheumatic fever. He has a history of several broken bones, job related and without complications. Mr. F stated that he had been put on a "water pill" and a "heart pill" about 12 years previously, after several months of headaches, when he was diagnosed with hypertension. Mr. F stated that he sometimes forgets to take his medication and does not seek out medical attention often, "unless it's somethin' I can't fix myself." He stated that he has had several episodes of "indigestion" over the past 3 or 4 months. The present episode "didn't go away, and it was more crushing than the other ones," which is why he agreed to let his wife bring him to the hospital. Mr. F stated that he has noticed a decrease in his hearing bilaterally over the last few years; "My wife keeps saying I'm just ignoring her."

Mr. F's medications before admission were furosemide (Lasix), methyldopa (Aldomet), and potassium chloride.

The day Mr. F sustained a cerebral embolus, there was a sudden onset of the following signs and symptoms: agitation, restlessness, and severe sensorimotor deficit of the right side. Although he did not lose consciousness, Mr. F had decreased orientation to time and place and decreased awareness. He was aphasic initially and did not follow movements when they occurred in his right field of vision. Mr. F was incontinent of stool and urine at this time.

Three weeks after the cerebral embolus, Mr. F shows stable cardiac condition, improvement in motor function of his right leg, and minimal improvement in his right arm and face. He continues to exhibit impairment of sensory function over his right leg, arm, and face to light touch, vibration, position, discrimination, and tactile localization. He understands written and spoken words and shows some improvement in speech. He exhibits right homonymous hemianopsia. His inability to communicate with the health care staff, complicated by his sensorineural hearing loss, is extremely frustrating to Mr. F,

TABLE 24-2. UNCOMPENSATED DEFICITS IN TOUCH.

	Examples of Disorders	Medical Management Options
Anatomic structure: Peripheral nervous system		
	Peripheral neuropathies:	
Chronic	Carcinoma and myeloma, amyloidosis	Removing or controlling tumor growth
Acute	Idiopathic polyneuritis, Landry-Guillain-Barré	Corticosteroid therapy, physiotherapy to prevent pressure palsies
Subacute (symmetrical)	Nutritional deficiency states, uremia, drug intoxications	Nutritional supplementation, dialysis in renal failure; discontinuing or decreasing dosage of drugs
Subacute (asymmetrical)	Diabetes mellitus, polyarteritis nodosa	Control of blood sugar, corticosteroid therapy
Others	Genetically determined, trauma, entrapment neuropathies	Immobilization, physical therapy, surgery

	Examples of Disorders	Medical Management Options
Anatomic structure:		
Central nervous system: Cord (complete, posterior column, partial), thalamus, parietal lobe (postcentral cyrus)		
Specifically	Brown-Séquard syndrome of the *partial* cord	See below
Overall	Complications of surgery, trauma, lesions from tumors, infarcts, hemorrhages, or myelitis (as in demyelinative myelitis)	Therapy to treat underlying cause symptomatology: Surgery Immobilization Corticosteroids

and he often turns his head away when staff enter the room. Mr. F's physical therapy program continues to provide improvement in motor function, particularly walking and gross motor movement in the right leg and arm. Mrs. F's visits have decreased in length and frequency and often when she visits, she speaks to Mr. F infrequently and tears well up in her eyes. She has mentioned to the staff that she realizes that Mr. F wants to come home soon but "I just don't know how I can handle it all."

Nursing Diagnoses

☐ **Partial Self-Care Deficit: Feeding, Dressing, Bathing, Related to Sensory Deficits**

Decreased visual acuity can make it difficult for an individual to locate self-care items as well as perform self-care functions. *Defining characteristics* of decreased visual acuity include myopia, hyperopia, blurring, glare, visual loss, and clouding of the lens. Visual field defects, such as homonymous hemianopsia, bitemporal hemianopsia, quadrantinopsia, scotoma, and central field defects, make it difficult for the individual to locate items in the environment. Additional uncompensated sensory deficits that hinder self-care abilities include impaired depth perception, impaired temperature descrimination, impaired ability to determine objects by touch, and impaired ability to determine position of body parts.

The success of the individual in accomplishing self-care activities can be enhanced by the nurse and the family's encouraging the individual's independence in self-care as much as possible while providing adequate time for each activity. Praise and positive reinforcement of the individual's efforts and accomplishments encourage motivation and enhance the individual's seelf-esteem.

As part of *nursing interventions*, the nurse and family should consistently place items of self-care, such as water, soap, towels, clothes, in designated locations while verbally identifying the location of the objects to the individual. They can assist the individual in finding objects by creating clues, such as a bright colored sign over bathing utensils. When meals are served, they should identify the location of food and liquids on the meal tray or table by clock placement, such as, "The coffee is at 2 o'clock, the fork is at 3 o'clock." Depending on the functional limitations of the sensory deficit, the individual may need assistance with cutting food and pouring hot liquids. The individual can be instructed to pour cups and glasses half full to prevent spilling. If the meal tray has disposable containers, the nurse can open the lids only halfway to prevent spilling.

Emphasis on using intact senses for identifying objects can facilitate self-care efforts. The nurse can teach the individual to hold a knife and fork European style while the patient is learning to identify foods by how they feel through the knife and fork. Foods can be differentiated by an intact sense of smell, particularly condiments, such as salt, pepper, catsup, mustard, lemon juice, and mayonnaise. Amounts of salt, pepper, or sugar can be estimated by pouring them over the fingertips.

The nurse can teach patients with peripheral or central visual field defects to scan the environment visually to locate self-care items and food on a tray or table. Self-care articles and food should be placed on the unaffected side of vision.

Individuals with disturbances in touch should be encouraged to use the unaffected side to determine the temperature of food, liquids, and bath water. These people also should be encouraged to use the unaffected side to identify the location and texture of objects, such as towels or clothes. Individuals with loss of touch need to examine their skin daily for bruises, cuts, burns, and pressure areas; they should be taught to monitor the position of body parts while bathing, sitting, lying, or altering their position.

As the nurse works with the individual and family, she can teach the family the extent of the individual's physical limitations, compensatory techniques that facilitate self-care, and the activities that require assistance.

Collaboration with other members of the health care team in teaching and reinforcing the use of compensatory techniques while in the hospital and in the home is essential to promoting the individual's self-care independence.

The *expected outcomes* are that the individual will use compensatory techniques for maximizing functional abilities in performing self-care and will attain an acceptable level of self-care within the functional limitations, requiring minimal or moderate assistance. The family will assist the individual in those self-care efforts he or she is unable to perform.

With Mr. F's improved cardiac status and motor ability, the nurses were successful in encouraging Mr. F to perform more and more of his self-care. It is apparent to the nursing staff, though, that as Mr. F assumes more independence, he also increases his risks of accidents and falls.

☐ Potential for Injury Related to Impaired Vision and Hearing

Impaired vision and impaired hearing can make it difficult for the individual to receive input from the environment, putting him at risk for falls, accidents from moving objects, or something as simple as not hearing a smoke detector alarm in a house fire. Impaired tactile sense also creates risk of injury from falls, burns, cold, and pressure areas. Additional *defining characteristics* that indicate a potential for injury include impaired motor ability, a history of falls or injury, and lack of knowledge of necessary safety precautions.

To prevent injury, the individual with sensory deficits must reestablish familiarity with the environment. Some general environmental principles include orienting the individual to the environment, such as the location of furniture, lights, and light switches, keeping objects in consistent locations, and informing the individual of changes if objects are moved. People with sensory deficits should always be approached on the side of intact senses to reduce the startle effect. It is important for the nurse to instruct the family about the impact of the individual's physical deficits, environmental hazards, and safety precautions, including eliminating throw rugs, toys on the floor, and furniture that may be situated away from room walls. While in the hospital, the individual's bed should always be kept in the lowest position.

Specific *interventions* for safety for individuals with impaired vision include the following procedures. To optimize visual capabilities, the nurse should encourage the use of adequate lighting, including night lights. Incandescent light offers less glare than fluorescent light. Providing side lighting, or lighting in front of objects rather than behind them, also can help to reduce glare. Encouraging the individual to avoid looking directly at bright lights, such as headlights while driving, and to wear sunglasses while outside on bright days can diminish the blinding effects of glare.

The use of color contrast can enhance greatly the visual discrimination of objects for individuals with impaired vision. The family can help alter the home environment to improve safety, using some of the following suggestions: place color strips on the edges of steps; avoid white on walls, countertops, and any working surface; paint doorframes and doorknobs in bright colors; and use contrasting colors for light switches and electric outlet plates.

If the individual has visual field defects, it is important to teach him or her to scan the environment to compensate and identify safety hazards, such as doorframes, furniture, and stairs inside the home, or moving vehicles outside the home.

Specific safety *interventions* for individuals with impaired tactile sense include the following. To prevent burns, a common injury resulting from this impairment, the individual or family can set the thermostat on the hot water heater to provide warm but not extremely hot or scalding water. The individual can be taught to assess the temperature of the bath water with the unaffected extremity or with a bath thermometer. The individual should use thermal insulated mitts when handling pots and pans from the stove or oven and avoid the use of hot water bottles and heating pads. Skin injury can occur without the person realizing the injury, and, therefore, people with tactile deficits should inspect the skin daily for burns, scratches, bruises, cuts, or pressure areas. A common source of undetected injury occurs to the feet; such individuals should wear well-fitting, low-heeled, soft shoes. Monitoring the position of body parts during activities can help to minimize the risk of injury from uncompensated tactile deficits.

As safety interventions for individuals with impaired hearing, the individual and family should be encouraged to have visual signals installed on smoke detectors, phones, and doorbells. While outside the home, scanning the environment can be helpful for those with this sensory deficit.

The *expected outcomes* for this diagnosis are that the individual will not sustain injury from falls, burns, wounds, or pressure sources, and the individual and family will use safety precautions in the home environment.

Difficulty communicating became very frustrating for both the nurses and Mr. F. Implementation of the nursing care plan was hindered by the nurses' attempts to communicate through the normal visual and verbal signals. It became evident that alternative mechanisms for communication had to be developed to facilitate Mr. Fs interactions with his environment.

☐ **Alteration in Verbal Communication Related to Hearing Compounded by Aphasia**

In an increasingly complex age of information, the mechanisms by which people exchange information with their environment also have become more varied and complex. In addition to face-to-face verbal exchange, radio, television, telephones, newspapers, magazines, letters, and computers have become routine means of communication. Impaired hearing is the most common cause of communication difficulties. When it is accompanied by impaired vision, an individual's inability to receive information is compounded by the difficulty experienced in reading and observing lip movement during verbal exchanges.

Neurologic disorders can cause impairments that further inhibit an individual's ability to interact in the environment, such as, motor or expressive aphasia, sensory or receptive aphasia, total or global aphasia, auditory verbal agnosia, visual verbal agnosia, and agraphia.

Establishment of a calm, unhurried environment is a key factor in establishing effective communication with an individual with uncompensated sensory deficit. Active and careful listening is essential to understanding the communication efforts of the individual, while expressing positive regard for him or her. Approaching the individual with sensory deficits on the side of intact senses is a principle that is important in facilitating communication. In the hospital setting, this includes situating the patient's bed in the room with the side of intact senses facing the door.

The nurse initially must determine with the patient an effective alternate form of communication. Some alternative *interventions* include the use of hand signals, pointing to letters on an alphabet board, or using a magic slate. The effectiveness of these methods of communication depends on the form of uncompensated sensory deficit as well as on the dexterity of the patient.

To facilitate communication, it is important to stand facing the individual when speaking. Speaking clearly, in low-pitched tones, can help the individual with hearing impairment understand spoken words. If it is appropriate, address verbal communication to the individual's ear with the best hearing.

To maximize the individual's sensory abilities, annual professional vision and hearing examinations should be performed. Visual aids, such as glasses, magnifying glasses, and hearing aids, may be useful in improving vision and hearing.

With the individual and family, the nurse can determine the need for various resources, such as speech therapists, large-type materials, and talking-books available through the Library of Congress, closed-caption television services, and the Commission for the Blind and Visually Handicapped.

The *expected outcomes* are that the individual will be able to communicate effectively within physical limitations; and the individual and family will use compensatory techniques to enhance communication.

CONSEQUENCES OF SENSORY ALTERATION

Consequences for the Individual

Uncompensated sensory deficits severely alter the individual's established pattern of interaction with people and objects in the environment. Inability to receive stimuli from the environment can elicit fear, anger, anxiety, and frustration. Until an effective alternate method of receiving information is established, the individual may be unable to carry out activities of daily living, as well as normal role responsibilities.

Frustration and fear underlie the individual's desire to limit interaction with people. If alternate forms of communication are not established, social isolation can result.

Nursing interventions can assist the individual in emphasizing intact senses for receiving environmental input. Collaboration with the individual and family is essential in evaluating the effectiveness of compensatory techniques.

Consequences for the Family

Often it is the family who must assume the responsibilities of the roles of an individual with uncompensated sensory deficit. Breadwinner, parent, and homemaker are difficult roles for the family to assume. If the individual is unable to carry out activities of daily living, he or she may assume a childlike role, requiring assistance in eating, dressing, and bathing. The profound changes in the family structure and functioning may stimulate feelings of anger, resentment, and frustration. It is extremely important that the family participate in the planning and implementation of the nursing actions in order that they may learn the necessary techniques for compensation of sensory deficits and subsequently encourage the individual to use them.

Consequences for the Community

Alterations in the senses of vision, hearing, or touch may mean that the individual is no longer capable of performing work responsibilities. New jobs may have to be learned in which responsibilities require use of intact senses. The financial impact and loss of work contributions resulting from uncompensated sensory loss can be significant unless effective rehabilitation is achieved.

UNCOMPENSATED SENSORY DEFICIT: IMPAIRED SMELL AND IMPAIRED TASTE

Deficits in smell and taste are discussed together because they are clinically interdependent and have similar impact on the individual's response to the environment. Two characteristics unique to the sense organs of smell and taste are that their receptor sites are both chemoreceptors and the receptor cells are constantly dying and being replaced, "the only examples of neuronal regeneration in humans" (Adams & Victor, 1985, p. 197).

Compared with vast amounts of research and literature available about deficits in the other special senses, there is a scarcity of information about the impact of impaired smell and taste on an individual's interaction with the environment.

The recognized impact that impairment of these two senses has on the individual is the lack of interest in or enjoyment of food. Just as do the elderly (who have decreased functioning of these sensory receptors), individuals with impaired taste or smell often complain that everything "tastes the same."

Nursing Diagnosis

☐ Alteration in Nutrition: Less Than Body Requirements Related to Altered Taste and Smell

An interview with the individual with impaired smell and taste may reveal the *defining characteristics* of lack of interest or enjoyment in food, often with a subsequent decrease in food intake. There may also be a verbalized decrease in appetite. The individual with impairment in these two senses usually does not seek medical care for this as a primary problem, but the history would indicate a weight loss without other medical cause.

As an initial *intervention*, the nurse can discuss the specific foods that the individual avoids, likes, or dislikes. This will provide a basis for working with a diet plan that will be agreeable to the individual and, therefore, have greater chance of success.

Small, frequent, visually appealing meals may be more enticing to the individual and should be provided in a quiet, nondistracting environment. Adequate time must be made available for eating. Liquid supplements, provided in acceptable flavors, can supply the needed calories between meals. Thorough oral hygiene before and after meals may be helpful in improving the flavor of the food.

The individual and family should be informed about the basic food groups and recommended daily allowances to meet the individual's needs. Teaching the meal preparer of the family and the individual some simple, yet effective methods of enhancing the enjoyment of food can improve the appetite of the individual with altered taste and smell. Some examples of these methods include varying the textures in food selections; using spices, such as mint, cloves, basil, thyme, or lemon juice, to enhance the taste or aroma of foods; adding supplements to routine food preparation to increase the nutritional quality of the meal, for example, adding powdered milk or eggs to sauces, gravies, puddings, or casseroles or adding raisins and nuts to cereals.

The individual can monitor the success of these efforts by maintaining a dietary log with calories to demonstrate adequate intake and monitoring weight gain or loss once a week.

Expected outcomes for this diagnosis are that the individual will increase the quantity and quality of nutritional intake necessary to meet metabolic needs, and the family will support the individual in meeting dietary requirements.

SUMMARY

The neurologic deficits that can impair an individual's ability to perceive input from the environment through the special senses are complex and varied. An impairment in the senses can have a profound impact on the individual's ability to function and communicate with the people and objects in the environment. The neuroscience nurse can assist the individual and the family within the community setting in maximizing independent, safe, and satisfying functioning within the constraints of the illness.

REFERENCES

Adams, R.D., & Victor, M. (1985). *Principles of neurology* (3rd ed.). New York: McGraw-Hill.

Brown, I.A. (1985). The widespread influence of olfaction. *Journal of Neurosurgical Nursing, 17*(5), 273.

Davis, A.E. (1985). Focus on rehabilitation in the acute care setting: The role of the neuroclinical nurse specialist. *Journal of Neurosurgical Nursing, 17*, 244.

Drachman, D.A., & Long, R.R. (1984). Neurological evaluation of the elderly patient. In M.L. Albert (Ed.), *Clinical neurology of aging*. New York: Oxford University Press.

Kemper, T. (1984). Neuroanatomical and neuropathological changes in normal aging and in dementia. In M.L. Albert (Ed.), *Clinical neurology of aging*. New York: Oxford University Press.

Meyer, J.S., & Shaw, T.G. (1984). Cerebral blood flow in aging. In M.L. Albert (Ed.), *Clinical neurology of aging*. New York: Oxford University Press.

Rogers, M.E. (1970). *An introduction to the theoretical basis of nursing*. Philadelphia: Davis.

Solkoe, D., & Kosik, K. (1984). Neurochemical changes with aging. In M.L. Albert (Ed.), *Clinical neurology of aging*. New York: Oxford University Press.

Weldon, P.R., Murray, T.J., & Quine, D.B. (1983). Hearing changes in multiple sclerosis. *Journal of Neurosurgical Nursing, 15*(2), 98.

BIBLIOGRAPHY

Albert, M.L. (1984). *Clinical neurology of aging*. New York: Oxford University Press.

Carpenito, L.J. (1983). *Nursing diagnosis: Application to clinical practice*. Philadelphia: Lippincott.

Hayes, D., & Jerger, J. (1984). Neurotology of aging: The auditory system. In M.S. Albert (Ed.), *Clinical neurology of aging*. New York: Oxford University Press.

Kopac, C.A. (1983). Sensory loss in the aged: The role of the nurse and the family. *Nursing Clinics of North America, 18*, 373.

Sabin, T.D., & Venna, N. (1984). Peripheral nerve disorders in the elderly. In M.L. Albert (Ed.), *Clinical neurology of aging*. New York: Oxford University Press.

Smith, J.F., & Nachazel, D.P. (1980). *Ophthalmologic nursing*. Boston: Little, Brown.

Stewart, C.M. (1982). Age-related changes in the nervous system. *Journal of Neurosurgical Nursing, 14*(2), 69.

Weinberger, M., & Radelet, M.L. (1983). Differential adaptive capacity to hearing impairment. *Journal of Rehabilitation, 49*(4), 64.

25

Alterations in Peripheral Senses

Carol Gohrke Blainey

Coping with alterations in peripheral sensation can be frustrating when the changes are due to both apparent causes (e.g., painful or bizarre sensations with accompanying motor loss), and obscure causes (e.g., aberrant or painful sensations with a lack of demonstrable pathology, or a seeming lack of responsibility for oneself due to lack of sensation). Assisting people to cope with these alterations is a considerable and continuing challenge for nurses.

MANIFESTATIONS OF ALTERATIONS OF PERIPHERAL SENSATION

Terms used to describe alterations of sensation are:

Analgesia	Lack of pain sensation
Hypalgesia	Decreased sensitivity to pain
Hyperalgesia	Increased sensitivity to pain
Anesthesia	Lack of tactile sensation
Hypesthesia	Decreased sensitivity to touch
Hyperesthesia	Increased sensitivity to touch
Paresthesia	Abnormal, tingling sensation
Dysesthesia	Perverted interpretations of sensation, such as burning or tingling in response to tactile or pain stimulation
Neuralgia	Severe paroxysmal pain along the course of a nerve
Causalgia	Burning sensation secondary to peripheral nerve damage (Mitchell et al., 1984, p. 140)

CAUSES OF ALTERED PERIPHERAL SENSATION

The etiology of alterations in peripheral sensation is determined by the underlying disease process; exact manifestations of the alteration vary somewhat with each individual. The major sources of altered peripheral sensation can be categorized into two groups: age-related nerve changes and peripheral nerve pathologies.

Age-Related Changes in the Peripheral Nerves

The increasing numbers of aged patients needing nursing care necessitates that nurses appreciate the peripheral nerve changes attributed to the aging process, aside from any specific pathology.

After age 40, there is a 5% to 8% loss of nerve fibers per decade and a progressive slowing of maximal sensory and motor conduction velocities at a yearly rate of 0.12 to 0.16 meters per second. The number of abnormalities in myelination increases with advancing age. The longer and larger fibers are most affected. Some of the changes, particularly the alteration in myelination, might be due to cumulative effects of trauma or vascular disease or both, although primary degeneration of nerve cells and axons also is taking place (Albert, 1984).

Pathologic Causes of Alteration of Peripheral Sensation

Pathologic etiology of alteration in peripheral sensation can arise from one of several causes. Clements (1984), in listing a differential diagnosis of diabetic polyneuropathy, included the following:

Toxic neuropathies

1. Drugs (e.g., allopurinol, phenytoin, hydralazine)
2. Heavy metals (e.g., arsenic, lead, mercury)
3. Industrial toxins (e.g., acrylamide, carbon tetrachloride, insecticides)
4. Ethanol

Hereditary neuropathies

Infectious neuropathies (e.g., Guillain-Barré syndrome, infectious mononucleosis, syphilis)
Other metabolic neuropathies (e.g., acute intermittent porphyria, hypothyroidism, uremia)
Neoplastic neuropathies (e.g., carcinoma, lymphoma, leukemia)
Structural neuropathies (e.g., spinal cord tumors, syringomyelia, spondylosis) (p. 75).

The remaining etiology of alteration in peripheral sensation is trauma (e.g., spinal cord damage or transection or peripheral nerve damage or transection). When the pathology is trauma or transection of the spinal cord or a peripheral nerve, transmission by the sensory nerve stops at the level of the trauma.

Diabetes mellitus and chronic renal failure are diseases that frequently have peripheral neuropathy as a sequela. Large numbers of people with these diseases may come to nurses for help in managing alterations in peripheral sensation. The following case study illustrates multiple nursing diagnoses that arise in a patient with altered peripheral sensation as a sequela to diabetes mellitus.

Case Study 1

Mrs. Zella H, a 68-year-old woman, came to the diabetes clinic for treatment of a 1½ inch skin ulcer on the plantar surface of her right first metatarsal bone. The ulcer had a firm, thick eschar covering.

Mrs. H had a 20-year history of type II, noninsulin-dependent diabetes mellitus (NIDDM), currently controlled with 22 units of lente insulin once daily at 8 AM. (Many people with NIDDM take insulin daily. These individuals would become symptomatic without the exogenous insulin but would not lapse into ketoacidotic coma without insulin. People with insulin-dependent diabetes mellitus [IDDM] would lapse into ketoacidotic coma without exogenous insulin.) Mrs. H's blood glucose levels, as measured by Chemstix testing, were between 180 and 240 mg/dl. She noted rapid elevation of her blood glucose whenever she ate fresh fruit, particularly pears. She was obese, with body weight of 180 lb and height 5 ft. 3 in. Her blood pressure was 156/88, and heart rate was 77 regular. Mrs. H was sedentary, and her overall muscle strength was weak. Other medications taken were levothyroxine sodium 0.3 mg daily for hypothyroidism and ibuprofen 600 mg, which she took at bedtime for rheumatoid arthritis noted primarily in the left hip.

She lived with her 70-year-old husband, who was in good health. They never had children but had one niece who was close to them, and they thought of her children as their grandchildren. Both Mr. and Mrs. H were retired and shared the tasks of homemaking.

On *assessment*, it was found that the skin on both feet was soft and pliable, with no excessive callus formation. There were no other breaks in the skin and no reddened areas. The toenails were not thickened and were cut straight across. Dorsalis pedis and posterior tibial pulses were present but diminished bilaterally. Mrs. H's feet were evenly pale in color and slightly cool to the touch. She was able to view her own feet and was independent in her own care with the exception of toenail trimming, which was done by her husband. She wore snug but not restrictively fitted support panty hose. Mrs. H never sat with her legs crossed and had never used tobacco in any form.

A neurologic examination was notable for the following abnormalities: inability to distinguish light touch to midcalf level bilaterally, inability to distinguish temperature sensations to midcalf level bilaterally, decreased Achilles tendon reflexes, and diminished vibratory sensations of the toes bilaterally. Although proprioception was normal, Mrs. H stated that when she walked she did not feel "certain" where her feet were, especially when going down stairs. She stated that she felt she was "walking on pillows during the day" and had "burning and tingling pain in her feet at night." Her gait was slow and broad-based. She used a cane in her left hand when her left hip was particularly painful.

Although Mrs. H had several relatives and friends who also had diabetes, including one who had a below-the-knee amputation, she was not alarmed by her ulcer because it "did not hurt." She stated that her only serious concerns and discomforts were the burning and tingling she had in both feet at night and her occasionally painful and stiff left hip.

Nursing diagnoses applicable to Mrs. H included alteration in comfort: pain related to diabetic neuropathy; sleep pattern disturbance related to alteration in comfort; potential for injury related to absent pressure sensation; potential for injury related to loss of vibration and proprioception; impairment of skin integrity related to absent sensation.

Collaborative medical and nursing management had fairly comprehensive results. Blood glucose was closely monitored with Chemstix four times daily, and the insulin dose was adjusted to gain tighter control of the diabetes. The small amount of cloudy yellow drainage that could be expressed from the wound was cultured and revealed *Staphylcoccus*. Mrs. H was started on a 10-day course of tetracycline hydrochloride 250 mg orally four times daily. Then the ulcer was debrided. The pressure distribution on the soles of both feet was analyzed using a process such as the Shurtrak static and dynamic gait analysis (Fig. 25–1). Based on the results of the pressure analysis, individualized pads for Mrs. H's shoes were prepared, and she was fitted with extra-depth shoes. As empirical treatment for the burning, tingling nocturnal pain in her feet, phenytoin sodium 300 mg was instituted. The treatment was effective, but the dose was decreased to 200 mg every even day and 300 mg every odd day because Mrs. H was experiencing the side effect of hypertropy of her gingival tissue, which interfered with the fitting of her dentures.

Nursing *interventions* included instruction in twice daily washing of the feet with mild soap, then soaking in warm water (measured with wrist) for 20 minutes, and, finally, an application of Eucerine cream to the feet; teaching the importance of daily visual examination of her feet; carefully checking shoes each day to detect any objects or loose inner soles inside the shoes; wearing warm stockings at night if her feet are cold; *never* putting feet near any heat source (e.g., heating pad, fireplace).

Mrs. H's sleep pattern returned to her normal cycle of midnight to 6 AM, with arising once during the night to walk to the bathroom to void. She believed the walk to the bath-

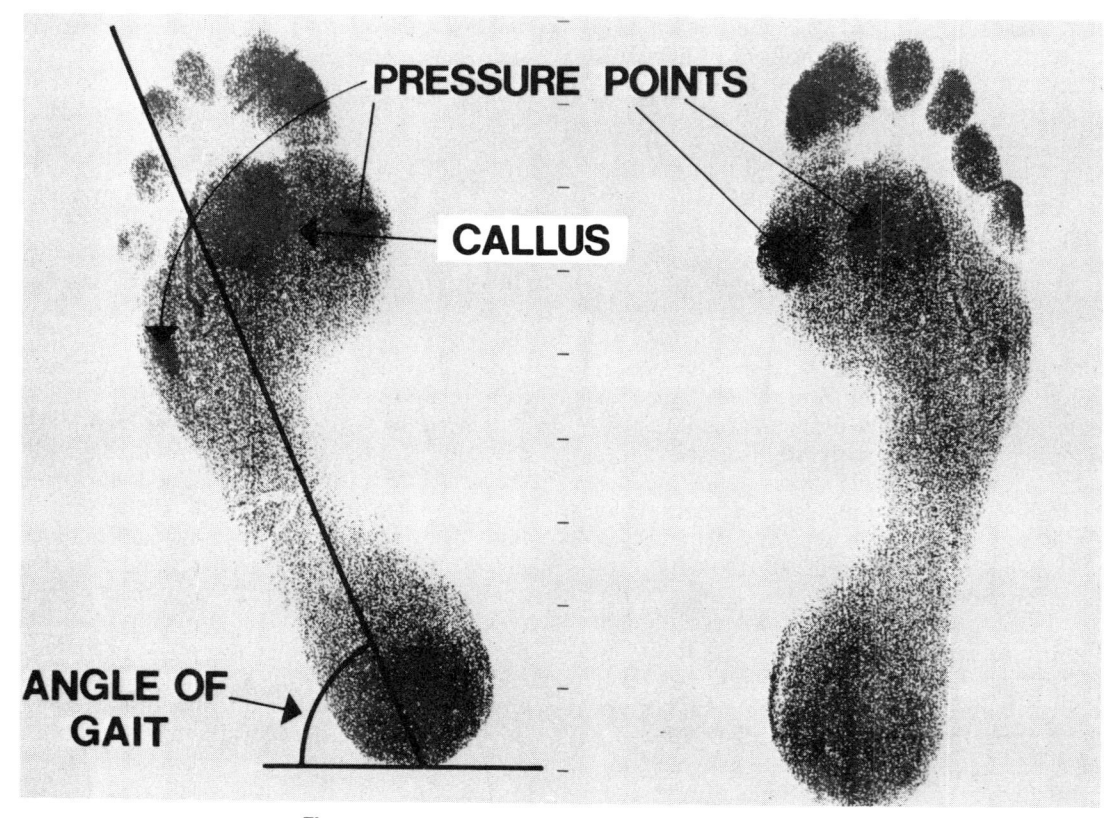

Figure 25-1. Static analysis of pressure points on feet.

room during the night decreased her generalized morning stiffness.

Over a period of 9 months, the metatarsal ulcer slowly filled in from the base, and eventually the skin closed over. The area remained easily damaged; stepping on a small stone directly under the area or prolonged standing would result in a darkening of the skin in that area. A general program of care for her feet, primarily special attention during her every other day bath, was sufficient to keep the area healed. Whenever the area became darkened, she returned to the every day soaking routine.

Mrs. H disliked the extra-depth shoes because she thought they were unattractive. She did wear the shoes, however, and felt they were comfortable. Mrs. H joked about being "vain" at her age and about how she could count on having visitors at her home. She said all she had to do was get her pan for soaking her feet all set up, turn on the television set, put her feet in the water, and the doorbell would ring. Her body weight did not decrease despite her best efforts, but she never gained weight even with her sedentary lifestyle.

The outcome of this case was that Mrs. H's ulcer healed, and she never had another episode of nonhealing trauma to her feet in a 9-year period. Her husband died suddenly of a myocardial infarction, and she moved from the area to be nearer her niece.

HUMAN RESPONSES TO ALTERATION OF PERIPHERAL SENSATION

Nursing diagnoses discussed in this section are those that occur frequently when people have alterations in peripheral sensation.

Nursing Diagnoses for the Individual

☐ Alteration in Comfort—Pain

People who have alterations in peripheral sensation in whom pain is the prominent feature verbalize the quality of sensations in their hands, feet, and legs as numbness, burning, tingling, boring, or hot, shooting stabs. Verbalization of discomfort is often the only *defining characteristic* of existing pain. The sensations are ill-defined, ill-localized, and particularly noted at night. The pain can be complicated by the changing nature of the sensations. There can be a marked discrepancy between the severity of the discomfort and the presence of clinical neurologic abnormalities. This discrepancy and the changing nature of the sensation make adaptation particularly difficult. The discrepancy between severity of discomfort and clinical findings may lead others to convey a sense of confusion or doubt about the individual's suffering. The individual must live with the promise of relief or the threat of increasing severity of discomfort.

There are many *interventions* available to the nurse for assisting these people to adapt to this type of pain. The nurse should take time to establish a strong helping relationship with the person. It is important to have a clear understanding of what is known about the individual's clinical picture, including what is thought to be the cause of the discomfort and if the discomfort is related to continuing tissue damage or is a result of previous tissue damage. Determining the coping style used by the individual in previous stressful situations will help explain current behavior and give guidelines to use in developing interventions.

The person should be encouraged to discuss feeling about the pain: What is the worst part of the pain? What does he or she think the pain means? What might be the outcome of the pain? What relieves the pain? The patient should be encouraged and guided in the use of prescribed drugs such as analgesics and phenytoin sodium. The nurse and patient together should strive for the best possible control of underlying disease (e.g., blood glucose or renal function).

For greater comfort, the nurse should encourage the patient to use a counterirritant before retiring (e.g., soaking feet in warm water, massaging feet) and to wear stockings at night. A cradle placed over the feet to keep the weight of the bed clothes off the feet and legs is often helpful. The nurse can teach the person that the discomfort is due to damaged nerves and is not a signal that further damage is occurring, when this is the case.

The patient can be taught about imagery and the use of imagery as a means of pain control, while being encouraged to keep trying to do things and to be as active as possible. Providing the person with support is important. Schoenhofer (1984) believes that support can be used as a deliberate element of nursing practice. She states that support allows expression and confrontation of dependency and security needs and assures the helpee that he or she can help himself or herself.

Outcome criteria to evaluate the effectiveness of the nursing interventions are that the person will receive validation that pain exists; relate that he or she has a repertory of techniques to decrease painful sensations; and report an increase in comfort and a decrease in painful sensations.

☐ Potential for Injury Related to Diminished or Absent Sensation

The *defining characteristic* of this diagnosis is evidence from the physical examination that there is a loss of touch or pressure sensation. This creates the threat that the individual may incur trauma to the part of the body where sensation is diminished or absent (e.g., feet, legs, buttocks, or hands).

Nursing *interventions* are primarily educational. The person must learn to use his or her eyes or the eyes of others to prevent injury and for early detection of injury. The person should check shoes for foreign objects—tacks that may have come through the soles of the shoes, wrinkles in the insoles, or wrinkles in the stockings. Hours spent walking on small objects or wrinkles can result in trauma that may require considerable effort and time to heal. The individual with a cord transection needs to make similar observations about objects in pockets on which they may bear weight. The person must be taught to do a daily visual examination of areas of the body affected by diminished or absent sensation. If the person cannot make her or his own visual examination because of a vision problem or the location of the affected area, someone else should do the daily visual examination.

The passage of time rather than the presence of discomfort must become the signal to alter position, since pressure and discomfort will not be perceived by these people. Increasing circulation to affected areas that bear weight can be accomplished by a regular program of massage to the areas.

Another nursing intervention is to teach the person to assess bathwater temperature via a thermometer or by using an area of the body that has retained a sense of temperature. These people should not use heating pads on affected areas, and they should not place affected body parts near heaters or fireplaces.

Outcome criteria to evaluate the effectiveness of nursing interventions are that the person will relate a pattern of daily visual examination of parts of the body with diminished or absent sensation and not incur preventable injuries to parts of the body with diminished or absent sensation.

☐ Potential for Injury Related to Loss of Proprioception or Vibration

Defining characteristics of the loss of the sense of proprioception and vibration are that people may trip more easily on uneven ground, fall in the dark, or have difficulty negotiating stairs. They may not be able to safely manage foot controls on an automobile because they cannot detect the location of the pedals quickly.

Interventions in these alterations include liberal use of night lights and rails on walls in appropriate areas in the home. Increasing proprioceptive input from hands can be accomplished by using a cane, and visual input may be improved by teaching the person to watch the feet when moving. Hand controls in place of foot controls may be sufficient to allow such people to drive safely.

Physical therapy may be beneficial in helping people adapt to a loss of proprioception and vibration. Merenstein and Schenkman (1984) suggested that physical therapy goals be directed toward a general reconditioning program to increase range of motion, strength, and endurance. In addition, gait training may be indicated.

To evaluate the effectiveness of nursing interventions in this diagnosis, *outcome criteria* are that the person will report using hands and eyes to determine the location of parts of the body with diminished or absent sensation and not incur preventable injuries to parts of the body with diminished or absent sensation.

☐ Noncompliance

The *defining characteristic* of noncompliance is that the person voluntarily does not follow prescribed care for affected areas of the body. Further evidence for this diagnosis is that these individuals sustain injuries to areas of the body with altered or absent sensation. The lack of care and presence of injuries are related to the person's not ascribing value to the potential for injury or not appreciating that injury has actually occurred in a body part that has no pain sensation.

Other etiologic factors may be involved in noncompliance, such as (1) not believing the care will accomplish anything, (2) feeling that the energy requirement for compliance is too great, and (3) thinking that the financial cost of compliance is beyond the family's means.

The diagnosis of noncompliance is differentiated from knowledge deficit by the fact that the individual with noncompliance can independently describe appropriate care. The person may not value the necessary care, however, primarily because he or she attaches seriousness or importance only to sensations of pain. Alternately, the person may verbalize lack of energy or funds to follow the treatment plan.

Interventions in this diagnosis begin with the nurse establishing a very open relationship with the person. Communication must be clear and open to be effective, particularly in the area of values. If the relationship is such that the person simply responds to the nurse in the way the patient believes is correct or appropriate rather than as an expression of true feelings, nothing will be accomplished. The patient will go on behaving in the same way, and no change will be made. A second step is to verify the person's understanding about potential and actual problems related to the lack of sensation, as well as the person's understanding about the prescribed care for the affected area. Once the knowledge component has been verified, the nurse can begin to determine the individual's beliefs about the usefulness of preventive efforts and treatment. The person may have memories of the experience of relatives or friends with similar conditions and believe that nothing of value can be done to prevent or help. Conversely, the person may believe that the efforts are not necessary because nothing serious will happen.

Appropriate use of anecdotal incidents can be used to impress patients with the seriousness of the problem of lack of sensation and the potential for injury. Anecdotal incidents can be used to illustrate situations in which people have understood intellectually the seriousness of injury yet not behaved in a way that evidenced acceptance of the seriousness.

A 60-year-old man came to the diabetes clinic, and in the course of a routine examination of his feet, the nurse discovered an abrasion, measuring 3 inches by 4 inches, on the dorsal surface of his right foot. He stated that he was aware of the injury and that it had occurred 2 weeks earlier when he wore some old, ill-fitting boots to paint a room in his home. He had first noted the injury when he removed the boots and socks, which had a small amount of blood over the area of the injury. In previous clinic visits with the same nurse, he had been able to verbalize appropriate care for his feet, as well as why the care was important (e.g., lack of sensation and decreased circulation). The nurse was clearly concerned at seeing the abrasion, but the patient quickly reassured her she need not be so concerned because this injury did not and had never hurt. When the nurse explained that the lack of pain was the primary reason the injury had occurred and that was the whole point of the previous discussion, the patient said "Oh, I see what you mean" but still seemed dubious about the need for concern.

Appropriate use of anecdotal incidents is emphasized because some people have been frightened by the anecdotal incidents and subsequently have avoided health care.

Mutually agreed upon contracts to do preventive self-care routines is another technique that can be employed to help the individual become more compliant with the suggested treatment. Support groups are an option that provides the person with opportunities to interact with people who have worked out appropriate methods of coping with similar problems.

Outcome criteria for this diagnosis are that the person will follow prescribed treatment plans with increasing compliance and will not incur preventable injuries.

☐ Body Image Disturbance

Defining characteristics of this diagnosis include description of changed or absent sensation from affected areas of the body (e.g., numbness, walking on pillows, not "knowing" where affected areas of the body are without looking at the area). These people can view but not feel an injury. An objective component of this diagnosis is that the person is unable to do customary activities because of alteration in peripheral sensation.

Nursing *interventions* in this diagnosis revolve around the grieving process. Talking with the person to determine the stage of grieving for lost function begins the process of helping the person cope with an altered body image. Nursing activities are directed toward helping the patient reconstruct the body image. A deliberate examination of lifestyle points out unaltered aspects of life and positive areas of functioning. An exploration of lost function begins the process of designing methods of compensation and alternatives to previous ways of functioning.

Outcome criteria to evaluate the effectiveness of nursing interventions are that the person describes the basis of the altered body image and displays movement toward a reconstruction of body image by carrying out daily living activities with appropriate changes.

☐ Potential Impairment of Skin Integrity

This is certainly a problem for people with alteration of peripheral sensation. Specifics of care for these people has been discussed in the "Potential for Injury" sections in this chapter.

☐ Sleep Pattern Disturbance

People with this nursing diagnosis state that painful sensations in affected areas interrupt their sleep and require them to rise and move or try other methods of distraction. This discomfort results in the *defining characteristics* of fewer total hours of sleep and a break in the continuity of sleep. People feel tired and irritable and lack motivation during the day.

Nursing *interventions* to help people adapt to this changed activity of daily living begin with specifying etiology of the sleep disturbance. Is the disturbance in sleep due to pain, too much sleep during the day, lack of physical activity, hunger, or anxiety? The nurse must identify the individual's pattern of preparation for sleep. Perhaps the person has not developed a useful, repeated pattern that begins the process of sleep; for example, a small snack, a warm bath, mild exercise, or watching television or reading. A review of what is effective in dealing with what may be disturbing the sleep, such as pain, is conducted. Perhaps night sleep would be enhanced by phenytoin taken nightly or by the use of a bed cradle to keep the weight of bed clothes off the feet and legs or some form of counterirritation, such as massage of the feet or a soak of the affected area in warm water. It may be necessary to determine if other times of the day are available for napping if adequate night sleep cannot be managed.

Outcome criteria for these nursing interventions are that the person will describe factors interfering with the usual sleep patterns, describe techniques to induce sleep, and report feeling more rested.

Nursing Diagnosis for the Family and Significant Others

☐ Ineffective Family Coping Related to Role Changes

Manifestations of this diagnosis stem from role shifts made by the ill person that are a result of the discomfort associated with peripheral neuropathy. Pain, sleep disturbance, and loss of mobility may interfere with the person's ability to carry out responsibilities in the family group (e.g., wage earner, homemaker). This shifts responsibilities to other family members and may create anxiety about how the family will manage. *Defining characteristics* are that family members may feel that the person is not trying to help himself or herself because of neglecting to follow the treatment plan. There may be strong feelings in the family of frustration or anxiety about the endlessness or inheritability of the condition.

Nursing *interventions* include interpersonal techniques to get the family verbalizing feelings and perceptions to the nurse, each other, and the family group. The group can be helped to reorganize family responsibilities and to learn how to assist in the care of the affected individual. The nurse can teach and encourage anticipatory coping as the illness progresses. Anticipatory coping involves preparations and adaptive strategies initiated before the occurrences of stresses that are predictable (Hamburg & Inoff, 1983).

Outcome criteria to evaluate the effectiveness of nursing interventions are that the family would report discussions of feelings related to the ill family member and reorganize family responsibilities to incorporate changes in the ill family member.

☐ Knowledge Deficit

Defining characteristics of this diagnosis are evidenced when family members are unable to describe independently the disease process and the affected person's response to the disease. The ill family member may have been able previously to manage the situation alone and may have preferred not to involve the family. Perhaps, the person feels some stigma attached to the primary disease. As the disease progresses and the individual ages, he or she might not be able to manage without family member participation.

Interventions are to determine the family members' knowledge and perceptions about the affected member's disease and responses. The nurse must determine family members' ability and willingness to participate in the affected member's care. Appropriate teaching about the disease and treatment may allay some anxiety in family members who have not been involved previously in the care. For example, family members may believe that the patient intentionally ignores the ulcers on affected areas and may not truly appreciate that the patient does not feel the ulcers and, hence, simply forgets to do the care. The family can then work on a plan to assist the patient to remember to care for affected areas.

Outcome criteria for this diagnosis are that family members independently verbalize an understanding of the disease process and the affected person's response to the disease experience and provide appropriate assistance to the ill family member.

Nursing Diagnoses for the Community

☐ Knowledge Deficit (Stigma)

The *defining characteristic* of this diagnosis is a societal discrimination against people with chronic diseases in the job market or in line for promotions. Employers may believe that people with chronic diseases will not function efficiently at work or may overuse sick leave and abuse health care plans. The environment must be made more usable for people who need aids for mobility, (e.g., liberal use of hand rails, elevators, curb cutouts).

Interventions include nurses' involvement in public education programs that present facts about work attendance and use of health care plans. This can be accomplished by participation in fairs and by contacting major employers. Nurses can participate in public service organizations to encourage adaptations of the environment to be more accommodating to individuals with alterations in mobility.

Outcome criteria to evaluate nurses' participation in public education are community allocation of funds to make the environment more accessible to individuals who need aids for mobility and that more individuals in the community can verbalize correct information about work habits of chronically ill people.

☐ Lack of Emphasis on Health Promotion and Disease Prevention

A *defining characteristic* of this diagnosis is that society at large has erroneous ideas about what causes chronic diseases (e.g., eating too much sugar in childhood causes diabetes mellitus; all diabetes mellitus and renal disease is inheritable and nothing can be done anyway). There is a lack of knowledge about sources of stress and methods of dealing with stress.

Interventions are education about healthy lifestyles and stress reduction techniques. Nurses can participate in public education programs that present accurate information about the etiology of chronic diseases and that through sound self-management people with chronic disease can live productive lives.

NURSING ROLES IN CARING FOR PEOPLE WITH ALTERED SENSATION

The nurse *generalist* can maximize her functioning through the following methods:

1. Increasing his or her awareness of people who may be at risk for alterations in peripheral sensation (e.g., people with diabetes mellitus and renal disease).
2. Directing specific attention to the assessment of the person's current state of peripheral sensation.
3. Having a clear understanding of the disease process and the current treatment program.
4. Conducting a careful evaluation of the person's ability to do self-care and follow the treatment plan.
5. Conducting patient and family teaching when indicated.
6. Initiating contact with a nurse specialist when that becomes necessary.

The neuroscience nurse *specialist* can be effective in the following ways:

1. Being available for participation in the management of complex patient situations in which there are social, physical, and economical extenuating situations.
2. Participating in community education about the nature of neurologic conditions in general and peripheral neuropathies specifically.
3. Participating in educating nurse generalists to teach patients and to be alert to prevent problems that come from lack of sensation.
4. Designing and participating in research projects in related areas to increase knowledge about nursing management of alterations in peripheral sensation.

SUMMARY

Loss or aberration of peripheral sensation can create serious problems in terms of potential for injury, decreased mobility, and pain. Peripheral neuropathies subsequent to a number of systemic diseases are a common source of such altered sensation. Care of people with altered peripheral sensation is as common in general nursing settings as it is in units specializing in neuroscience nursing care.

REFERENCES

Albert, M. (Ed.). (1984). *Clinical neurology of aging*. New York: Oxford University Press.
Clements, R. (1984). Diabetic neuropathy: Diagnosis and treatment. *Clinical Diabetes, 2,* 74.
Hamburg, B.A., & Inoff, G.E. (1983). Coping with predictable crises of diabetes. *Diabetes Care, 6,* 409.
Merenstein, A., & Schenkman, M. (1984). Pernicious anemia: The disease and physical therapy management. *Physical Therapy, 64,* 1076.
Mitchell, P.H., Cammermeyer, M., Ozuna, J., & Woods, N.F. (1984). *Neurological assessment for nursing practice*. Reston, VA: Reston.
Schoenhofer, S.C. (1984). Support as legitimate nursing action. *Nursing Outlook, 32,* 218.

BIBLIOGRAPHY

Carpenito, L.J. (1983). *Nursing diagnosis application to clinical practice*. Philadelphia: Lippincott.
Conway-Rutkowski, B.L. (1982). *Carini and Owens' neurological and neurosurgical nursing* (8th ed.). St. Louis: Mosby.
Green, D.A., Lattimer, S., Ulbrecht, J., & Carroll, P. (1985). Glucose-induced alteration in nerve metabolism: Current perspective on the pathogeneses of diabetic neuropathy and future directions for research and therapy. *Diabetes Care, 8,* 290.
Mitz, M., Benedetto, M., Klingbeil, G., Melvin, J., & Piering, W. (1984). Neuropathy in end-stage renal disease secondary to primary renal disease and diabetes. *Archives of Physical Medicine and Rehabilitation, 65,* 235.

Mooney, V., Gottschalk, F., & Powell, H. (1985). The diabetic foot ulcer: Treating one, preventing the next. *Clinical Diabetes, 3*, 36.

Sabin, T.D., Geschwind, N., & Waxman, S.G. (1978). Patterns of clinical deficits in peripheral nerve disease. In S.G. Waxman (Ed.), *Physiology and pathobiology of axons*. New York: Raven Press.

Schnatz, J. (Ed.). (1982). *Diabetes mellitus: Problems in management*. Menlo Park, CA: Addison-Wesley.

Seidlen, M. (1981). *Practical management of chronic neurologic problems*. New York: Appleton-Century-Crofts.

Snyder, M. (Ed.). (1983). *A guide to neurological and neurosurgical nursing*. New York: Wiley.

26

Pain: Acute and Chronic

Nancy Wells

Pain is one of the symptoms most often managed by health professionals. Common factors influence an individual's responses to pain, but the responses to and, therefore, treatment of acute and chronic pain differ. The purpose of this chapter is to delineate these differences and guide the practitioner in effective nursing management of both acute and chronic pain.

NEUROPHYSIOLOGY OF PAIN

Pain is regarded as primary sensation, with nociceptor stimuli from the periphery transmitted to the central nervous system. This neurophysiologic approach to pain adequately explains acute pain with known pathology but excludes much of chronic pain, where the organic basis and, therefore, the sensory receptor stimulus are unknown or absent. In the instance of chronic pain, the phenomenon is better described as the subjective interpretation of perceived nociceptive input. Several authors argue that pain is a perceptual rather than a sensory experience (Chapman, 1978, p. 178; Fordyce, 1978, p. 53). Perception, in this context, is defined as "the awareness of a noxious sensation, appreciation of negative emotion, and attribution of meaning to the experience" (Chapman & Bonica, 1983, p. 16). This definition eliminates the need for sensory input in the pain experience.

Although pain generally describes a somatic or body experience, the work of Melzack et al. (Melzack & Wall, 1965; Melzack & Casey, 1968; Melzack & Torgerson, 1971; Melzack, 1975) indicates that pain includes sensory, affective, and cognitive dimensions. The most useful clinical definition is a verbal report from the person experiencing pain (McCaffery, 1979; Wolff, 1985).

Gate Control Theory

Current thinking about the psychophysiologic basis of pain was introduced in the gate control theory proposed by Melzack and Wall in 1965. This theory proposes that both peripheral and central nervous systems influence pain. The primary processing area, or gate, is composed of cells in the substantia gelatinosa (SG), located in the dorsal horn of the spinal cord. From the periphery, the balance of large-diameter and small-diameter fibers regulates ascending nociceptive input through the gate. Descending input to the SG originates centrally—from the cerebral cortex, midbrain, and brainstem. Reticular projections to the dorsal horn have an inhibitory effect on cells in the SG. The presence of opiate receptors and high concentration of enkephalins and other neurotransmitters in areas of the thalamus, midbrain, and dorsal horn provide possible mechanisms for descending control of pain.

The multiple ascending and descending projections are shown in Figure 26–1. Nociceptive input ascends the cord via the neospinothalamic (rapid transmission) and paleospinothalamic (slow transmission) tracts. The neospinothalamic tract carries sensory and discriminative information to the thalamus and cerebral cortex. Multiple synapses of the paleospinothalamic tract in the reticular formation and limbic system relate to the affective and motivational dimension of pain. Communication via neurotransmitters from the periaquaductal gray area to the SG is linked to descending modulation (Pert, 1982). Cortical projections also may exert descending control indirectly via the reticular projections and directly via the pyramidal tract. Despite current lack of knowledge about the mechanisms, it is apparent from clinical observation that both affective and cognitive factors greatly influence pain and responses to it.

Persistent pain in the absence of peripheral stimulation is explained by the gate control theory. Degeneration of nerves produces abnormal, high-frequency firing and bursting activity analogous to the neural activity found in epilepsy (Crue et al., 1979). This neural activity occurs without nociception and, in some cases, without peripheral stimulation at all. Continued pain may be caused by (1) overwhelming input from bursting activity into the SG, (2) a lack of or reduced effect of the descending inhibitory system, and (3) memory patterns developed by prolonged, intense nociception (Melzack & Wall, 1982).

DIFFERENTIATION BETWEEN ACUTE AND CHRONIC PAIN

Recognizing the differences between acute and chronic pain is important in providing effective pain management. The most consistent differentiator of acute and chronic pain is temporal, with 6 months duration being the usual dividing point. Both acute and chronic pain may begin with organic pathology, in which pain is a symptom that warns of impending or actual tissue damage. Acute pain is self-limiting; as healing occurs, the pain resolves. Once pain has persisted past the healing phase, it no longer functions as a warning signal. The individual begins to question whether there will be an end to the pain. As the individual moves from the acute to the chronic state, pain becomes a syndrome rather than a symptom.

Acute Pain Responses

The most common sources of acute pain are trauma, planned surgery, and childbirth. Cancer pain, although its duration may be more than 6 months, also is included in the acute pain category because of the self-limiting nature of the disease process. The observable responses to acute pain include physiologic, behavioral, and affective.

Physiologic Responses

Acute, rapid-onset pain produces sympathetic arousal, the "fight or flight" response, which is mediated by the reticular formation. Manifestations include increased heart rate, systolic and diastolic blood pressure, respirations, skeletal muscle tension, and palmar sweating. The person may experience nausea and a dry mouth because of decreased gastrointestinal motility and salivary flow. Typically, the sympathetic nervous system adapts rapidly, making it difficult to rely on these observations to indicate the presence of pain.

Behavioral Responses

There is a set of reflexive responses that follows the onset of nociception. The sequence

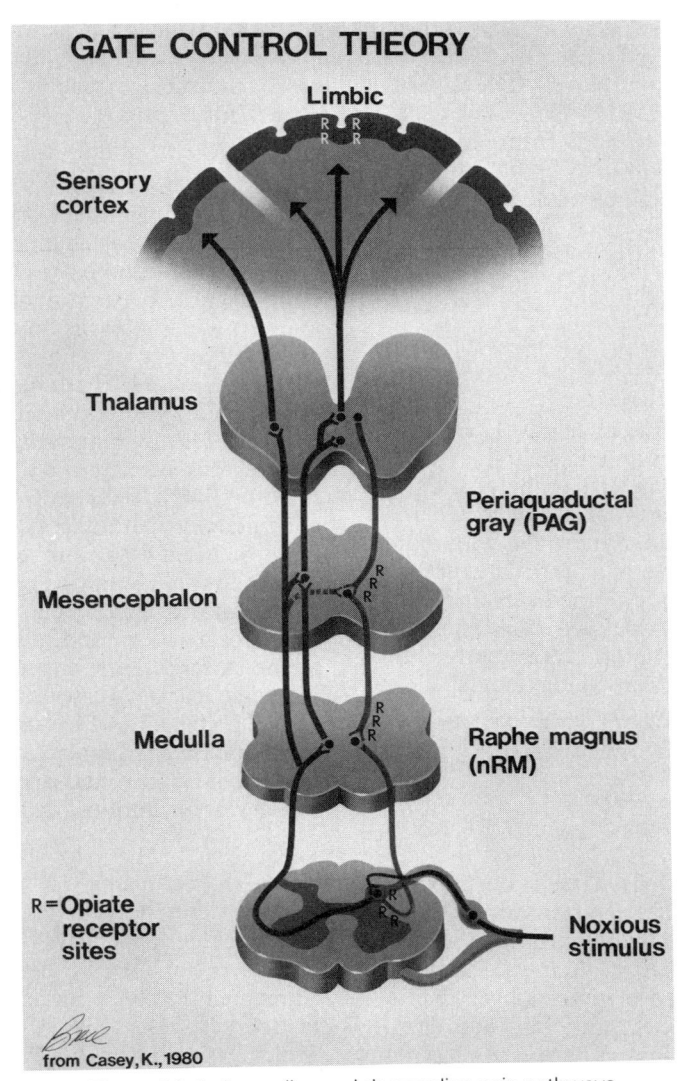

Figure 26–1. Ascending and descending pain pathways.

of events includes sudden withdrawal of the injured part, turning the head to examine the injury, vocalization, and muscle splinting to protect the injured part (Melzack & Wall, 1970).

Affective Responses

Anxiety, like pain, is a subjective experience that produces nonspecific sympathetic arousal. Sources of anxiety associated with acute pain are identified easily: Why does it hurt? Will I have more pain than I can bear? Will this pain affect my future (immediate or long-term)? Acute pain is associated with a transient situational, or state, anxiety that motivates the individual to cope with acute pain. Keefe et al. (1982), describe three important coping behaviors: reducing activity until healing begins, using medications to relieve pain, and seeking medical assistance. At this time, the person relies on medical professionals to diagnose and cure the source of pain. An active cognitive coping style is prevalent (Keefe et al., 1982), using such techniques as distraction and future-oriented planning.

These responses—physiologic, behavioral, and affective—reflect observations of acute pain but bear little resemblance to responses of the individual who is suffering with chronic pain.

Chronic Pain Responses

There are many disease states labeled as chronic pain. Arthritis and migraine headaches, which are characterized by periods of pain with intervals of no pain, are considered recurrent chronic pain. Syndromes with more constant pain, such as postherpetic neuralgia and low back pain, are termed *chronic benign pain* (CBP), which is defined as pain of unknown origin that is not life-threatening. The intensity of the pain complaint cannot be explained by pathology. In the intractable syndrome, the pain is refractory to medical treatment. In contrast to the variable nature of acute pain, clients with chronic pain report a constant and high intensity of pain (Keefe et al., 1982).

The behaviors developed during the acute pain stage continue to be used. Unfortunately, they are no longer appropriate in coping with persistent pain. Activity has been limited over a period of time (longer than 6 months), leading to deconditioning of skeletal muscles, heart, and lungs. The person has not worked or has done so in a limited capacity since the onset of pain. Reliance on pain medications may lead to narcotic and nonnarcotic dependence. The client continues to look for the medical cure, which leads to doctor shopping and potentially engaging in pain games (Sternbach, 1974).

Physiologic Responses

Nonspecific sympathetic arousal is not typically observed in chronic pain. Muscle hyperactivity may be a direct or indirect source of persistent pain, whereas muscle hypoactivity may be a result of decreased activity. In both cases, the muscle tone is abnormal and requires intervention.

Behavioral Responses

From a learning framework, the duration of chronic pain allows changes in behavior patterns to occur in both the client and his or her family. These patterns evolve as the environment provides rewards for behavior or avoidance of negative consequences. Fordyce (1978) has labeled these behaviors, which are determined by environmental consequences, *operants*. The operant nature of behavioral responses has been termed *pain behavior*, defined by Block (1982, p. 52) as "overt indices of a putatively painful condition—all of which are influenced by a number of nonpathological variables." Some pain behavior seeks to communicate pain; facial expressions, posture, vocalization, and guarding alert others to the suffering experienced. Fordyce (1978) includes inappropriate coping behaviors as well. The benefits of having pain behavior include spouse and family attention, spouse and family control, avoidance of social (home and work) responsibilities, and financial gain.

Affective Responses

Many studies have investigated the psychologic profile of clients with chronic pain (Capka, et al., 1979; Gentry et al., 1974). Agreement has been found on a pattern of affective responses, based on the Minnesota Multiphasic Personality Inventory (MMPI), consisting of increased scores on measures of hypochondriasis, depression, and hysteria. It has been suggested that people who develop chronic pain have difficulty expressing emotions. Somatic preoccupation (hypochondriasis) and hysteric denial allow the person to repress unpleasant affect (depression [Sternbach, 1974]; anxiety [Capka et al., 1979]). Although people with chronic pain have multiple personal and interpersonal problems, they commonly insist that with alleviation of their pain all of their problems will be solved (Pilowsky, 1978).

Depression is the affective state most closely related to chronic pain. This reactive or neurotic depression is related to internal conflict or loss (Pinsky, 1979). It is easy to understand how feelings of sadness, hopelessness, and helplessness arise after long-term persistent pain. Losses as a result of pain may be great: loss of function, support systems, and job. Many depressive symptoms are indicative of chronic pain. These include decreased mobility, productive activity, and appetite, loss of libido, a change in sleep pattern, and withdrawal from social activity (Fordyce, 1978; Keefe et al., 1982; Melzack & Wall, 1982; Sternbach, 1974). The chronic pain client's approach to interpersonal relations has been described as hostile and manipulative (Timmermans & Sternbach, 1974). Slow thought and constipation, additional vegetative signs, also are found frequently in chronic pain; these manifestations overlap with the adverse effects of narcotics. As with anxiety and acute pain, the behavioral responses to chronic pain are closely related to those of depression. Chronic anxiety, which is almost as prevalent in chronic pain as depression, also may produce some of these vegetative symptoms (Sternbach, 1974.)

Chronic pain has the potential to disrupt all aspects of life: physical, psychologic, and social. This disruption affects not only the individual suffering from chronic pain but the individual's family as well.

Influencing Factors

In all pain states, there are many factors that influence perception of and response to pain. Factors that influence pain involve the cognitive–evaluative and affective–motivational aspects of pain, which explains the highly variable and individual responses to pain. The sensory–discriminative aspect of pain is relatively stable across individuals with normal sensory capabilities (Melzack & Wall, 1982). Individual factors that influence the severity of pain include attention meaning attached to pain, familial model, culture, personality, and socioeconomic characteristics. *Attention* has long been one of the manipulable factors of pain perception. Attention focused on pain increases the perception of pain. Applying the gate control theory, attention activates descending control mechanisms that either open or close the gate in the substantia gelatinosa.

The response to pain attributed to "heartburn" differs from that of "heart attack," although the location and quality may be similar. This exemplifies the effect *meaning of pain* has on response to pain. The meaning of pain may be influenced, in turn, by familial models and culture. The influence of *familial models* on pain experience arises from social learning theory. Behavior patterns may be learned by observation, that is, vicarious learning. The rewards and punishments for pain behavior are observed easily in the family setting. In recent studies, the influence of family modeling significantly affected complaints of pain in a general population (Edwards, et al., 1985), and was significantly related to chronic pain (Violon & Giurgea, 1984). Craig (1978) suggests that modeling begins in the family context and may be the underlying mechanism for observed cultural differences.

The classic study of cultural differences by Zborowski (1969) suggested that *culture* influences the expression of pain rather that any physiologic or sensory factors. Zborowski found that people from Mediterranean areas (Italians and Jews) were more expressive of pain, whereas Anglo–Saxons (Irish and Old Americans) were stoic. Some of the findings from this study are accepted as generalizations but may not be observed in our culturally mixed American society. The sources of cultural differences in response to pain are not clear, but a learned rather than innate source is suggested (Craig, 1978; Sternbach, 1982; Wolff, 1985).

It is important to recognize that health care providers also carry cultural biases, again based on learning of past familial models. The American medical system operates on an Anglo–Saxon model of illness behavior (Wolff, 1985). Adhering to this model means that clients control their expression of pain and submit to necessary painful procedures without complaint. Health care professionals reward clients who respond in the appropriate manner by giving more credence to their pain complaints (Wolff, 1985) and, it is presumed, by providing faster and more adequate pain relief (McCaffery, 1979).

Research and clinical observation have identified several *personality characteristics* that influence pain responses. Neuroticism, of which the largest component is anxiety, is related to higher levels of reported pain (i.e., lower pain tolerance) in both acute and chronic pain states. Introversion–extroversion, in contrast, is related to willingness to express pain (Sternbach, 1974). This characteristic also may be related to culture (Zborowski, 1969) and social learning.

Socioeconomic factors influence pain responses. Sternbach (1978) describes the chronic pain patient as a member of the working class, engaging in physical labor, with a high school level of education. Physical labor increases the possibility of being injured at work, a common location of initial injury (Carron et al., 1985). Sternbach concludes that a lack of higher education and, hence, formal education in psychology lead to emotional conflicts being expressed in somatic complaints. The medical compensation system, however, particularly in the United States, gives greater support for physical than for psychologic disabilities and treatment (Carron et al., 1985).

Involvement in litigation may be a strong influence on pain, since receiving money for disability can be a potent secondary gain. Sternbach et al. (1973) found the MMPI scores for hypochondriasis, depression, and hysteria to be greater in client's involved in litigation than in those who were not. Carron et al. (1985), in a comparison of low back pain in the United States and New Zealand, found that although clients entered with similar pain intensity and frequency, subjects in the United States had more emotional and behavioral disruptions. These authors proposed that the emotional distress was related to the cumbersome compensation system in the United States.

HUMAN RESPONSES IN ACUTE PAIN

Acute Pain

The *defining characteristics* of acute pain are primarily behavioral responses. Behavioral signs, such as verbalization ("I hurt"), restlessness or agitation, guarding, avoidance of activity, and the physiologic sign of increased muscle tension, indicate the presence of pain. Of these manifestations, verbal report of pain may be the only sign present. Nevertheless, in clients who conform to the stoic model of expression, pain may be denied despite other clinical signs.

Assessment of pain is organized according to the sensory–discriminative, affective, and cognitive dimensions. Responses and influencing factors are initially assessed; ongoing assessment of relevant factors is derived from the initial contact with the client.

The client's self-report of pain is important in obtaining information to evaluate nursing care and in communicating to the client that his or her pain is believed. Several tools are available to assess clinical pain. The PPQRST (*P*rovocation, *P*alliation, *Q*uality, *R*adiation, *S*everity, *T*emporal), a simple, nonresearch-oriented interview guide, is summarized in Table 26–1. The PPQRST provides comprehensive data on the sensory and cognitive dimensions but lacks complete affective information. It is, therefore, necessary to assess affect through observation of behavior and client self-report.

The McGill Pain Questionnaire (MPQ) and Pain Rating Scale (PRS) are two instruments developed for research purposes that may be helpful in clinical assessment. The MPQ is conceptually congruent with the gate control theory and includes rank-ordered verbal descriptors of the three dimensions of pain (Melzack, 1975; Melzack & Torgerson, 1971). In addition, location, influencing factors, and palliative measures are assessed with this instrument. The PRS, developed by Johnson (1972), is useful, since it measures the sensory and affective dimensions of pain. It is comprised of two 10-cm lines and uses numerical descriptors (0 to 10), verbal des-

TABLE 26–1. PPQRST PAIN ASSESSMENT GUIDE.

Key Word	Data Obtained	Dimension
Provocation	Is there an identifiable incident related to the initial onset of pain?	Cognitive
	What provokes the pain? (including activity, affect, environmental stress)	Affective
Palliation	What reduces or relieves the pain? (activity changes, analgesics, assistive devices, medical assistance)	Cognitive
	Exposure to alternative methods? (relaxation, imagery, hypnosis)	Cognitive
Quality	What words are used to describe the pain?	Sensory
Radiation	Where is the location of pain? Is the pain localized or generalized? Does it radiate and, if so, where?	Sensory
Severity	What is the intensity of pain? [on a scale of 0 (no pain) to 10 (worst cognitive pain imaginable)—or using the descriptors, none, mild, moderate, severe]	Sensory Cognitive–evaluative
Temporal	Is there a pattern to the pain? Is the pain constant or intermittent?	Sensory

criptors (none, mild, moderate, severe), or both. One line assesses intensity of pain sensations (sensory dimension), and the other assesses distress (affective dimension) caused by these sensations. Whereas the MPQ is a multifaceted, comprehensive instrument, the PRS is simple to use, and therefore more appropriate for serial measures.

Acute pain typically has an organic basis. Peripheral free nerve endings respond to thermal and mechanical stimuli, and these comprise the initial stimulus for acute pain. *Etiology* may be organized by the anatomic structure(s) affected by pathologic changes. *Medical management,* which is directed at the source as well as palliation of pain, is summarized according to anatomic structure in Table 26–2.

Nursing *intervention* involves application of the nursing process to both the individual and his or her family. Interventions specific to pain and its effects are organized as peripheral and central, following the gate control theory. *Peripheral techniques* alter receptor input entering the SG, whereas *central techniques* alter the affective and cognitive dimensions, thus exerting descending control from the supraspinal structures.

Case Study 1

Grace C is a 51-year-old woman with pain of 3 months duration. The pathologic source of pain is an invasive pelvic tumor. Grace is admitted for pain control. On admission, she displays a tense facial expression, a slightly flexed posture (guarding), and slow, rigid movements. She reports pain in the low back and pelvis only when asked. She denies any familial pain models and, in fact, finds it difficult to remember either of her parents expressing pain. The pain, to Grace, indicates that the tumor is growing and, hence, is anxiety producing.

In assessing the primary complaint, Grace notes that the pain worsens with vigorous activity (e.g., a half-day shopping trip) and when she is tired. Emotions seem to play a part, for when she is feeling low, the pain is at its worst. Rest and the analgesics ordered by her physician (acetaminophen and 60 mg codeine) reduce her pain from 6–7/10 to 4–5/10 on a scale of 0 to 10. She used imagery during chemotherapy but is not using it to control pain. The pain is usually located in her low back, pelvis, and perineum and occasionally radiates to the lower extremities. She rates her present pain at 6/10 and distress at 8/10 on a scale of 0 to 10.

A general systems review reveals an adequately nourished female with lower abdominal and pelvic tenderness. Trunk mobility is decreased; range of motion in extremities is within normal limits. The client reports a re-

TABLE 26-2. ETIOLOGY AND MEDICAL MANAGEMENT OF ACUTE PAIN.

Type of Pain	Anatomic Origin	Medical Management
Myofascial	Muscle and fascia	Activity: mobilization Procedure: local nerve block Pharmacology: muscle relaxants, nonsteroidal anti-inflammatory drugs (NSAIDs) Surgery: none Other: stress management, counterirritation
Rheumatic	Bone, joint, ligament	Activity: mobilization Procedure: deep heat Pharmacology: NSAIDs, corticosteroids Surgery: joint replacement
Neuralgia	Peripheral and dorsal root nerves	Activity: mobilization for peripheral, immobilization for dorsal root (e.g., intervertebral disk) Procedure: local nerve block Surgery: nerve release from entrapment (e.g., diskectomy) Pharmacology: analgesics
Trigeminal neuralgia	Central neuron	Activity: mobilization Procedure: none Pharmacology: antiepileptic (phenytoin, carbamazepine) Surgery: CN V root division (trigeminal neurectomy)
Causalgia	Sympathetic nervous system	Activity: mobilization Procedure: ganglion block Pharmacology: alpha blockers Surgery: sympathectomy
Vascular	Vascular	Pharmacology: vasodilators Surgery: specific to site (e.g., bypass surgeries)

cent decrease in appetite and constipation, which she attributes to the pain and analgesics ordered.

Nursing Diagnoses in Acute Pain

☐ **Alteration in Comfort—Acute Pain**

Client involvement in the planning and use of selected interventions increases the likelihood that the techniques will be effective (Moss & Meyer, 1966). If the client has used methods of pain relief, they become the basis for instruction in additional techniques. The rationale for newly introduced techniques should be explained in understandable terms and in a way that is congruent with the client's pain model (Meichenbaum & Turk, 1976).

Pain relief is related to the expectation the client has for success of the treatment. As an *intervention* for the nurse generalist, approaching the client with a positive *suggestion*, such as, "I think this will relieve your pain," may increase the likelihood that it will work. Giving false reassurances, such as, "After this analgesic you shouldn't feel any pain," may be counterproductive because the client may stop trusting the nurse.

Massage is a common nursing intervention for immobility. The effects include muscle relaxation and, potentially, sedation, both of which provide comfort. Massage may close the gate to nociception because of large-diameter fiber stimulation. It also may reduce a source of nociception by promoting muscle relaxation.

Assessing the client's knowledge and use of imagery provides a basis for instruction as an *intervention* for the nurse specialist. *Imagery* is the use of cognitive activity to produce a therapeutic goal (McCaffery, 1979), in this

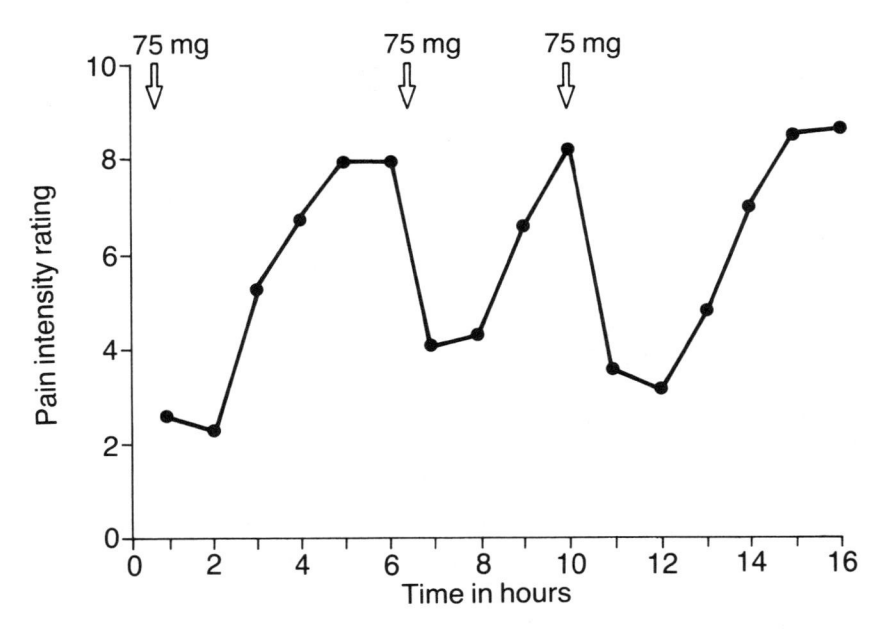

Figure 26–2. Report of pain intensity with variable administration of meperidine 75 mg.

case pain reduction. If Grace had used, for example, diversional, pleasant imagery to cope with the adverse effects of chemotherapy, it would be appropriate to begin with this technique. Relaxation typically precedes imagery. Images to promote muscle relaxation may reduce muscle tension as well as anxiety. Imagery also may be used to transform sensations (sensory transformation) and context and produce disassociation (Turk et al., 1983). Postimagery suggestion, which is similar to posthypnotic suggestion (McCaffery, 1979), may prolong the analgesic effects of imagery. Imagery is considered a benign therapy but should be used with caution in clients with depression and not used in clients with psychotic disorders.

As *outcome criteria* to evaluate nursing intervention, the client will participate in the planning and evaluation of therapeutic modalities used, report increased comfort and decreased pain, report an increased sense of well-being, and use imagery as a self-initiated pain relief measure.

Because of the severity of Grace's pain and the etiology, meperidine (Demerol), 50 to 100 mg intramuscularly every 4 hours as required, is ordered. The principles of analgesic administration are to (1) match analgesic dosage and pain severity, (2) prevent severe pain, and (3) individualize dosage and interval of administration. Parenteral meperidine is indicated for pain of moderate to severe intensity, which Grace experiences (i.e., pain of 5–8/10 on a scale of 0 to 10). From observation, it is apparent that Grace continues to experience pain with activity. A review of analgesic administration reveals that she is receiving meperidine 75 mg at variable intervals ranging from 4 to 8 hours (Fig. 26–2).

It is apparent that Grace is not requesting analgesics to prevent severe pain, or the nursing staff is not offering it on a regular basis. Because of this, the dosage (75 mg) is not sufficient to relieve severe pain. After talking with Grace, the nurse finds that fear of addiction and losing control are preventing her from requesting medications to prevent pain.

☐ Ineffective Coping with Acute Pain Related to Lack of Knowledge

Fear of addiction is a common reason for undertreatment of pain with narcotics. McCaffery (1979) states that tolerance (decreased effectiveness of a drug after repeated administrations) and physical dependence (development of withdrawal symptoms when a repeatedly administered narcotic is abruptly stopped) are involuntary physiologic effects of narcotic administration. In contrast, addiction and drug abuse are voluntary behavior patterns that result in psychologic and social disruption for the individual.

The incidence of addiction is less than 1% in clients with acute pain requiring narcotics (Marks & Sachar, 1973). In clients with progressive cancer pain, such as Grace, comfort is the first priority. Because of the limited nature of pain, addiction should not be an issue. If pain has not been adequately relieved, the client may behave like an addict, that is, crave narcotics; in fact, what they crave is pain relief (McCaffery, 1979). Once the pain has been relieved, the addictive behavior disappears.

The *goal* of treatment for acute pain is pain prevention. If pain is prevented or kept at a manageable level, anxiety is reduced, which in turn reduces the amount of analgesic required. The common practice of *pro re nata* (p.r.n., as needed) administration of analgesics has been criticized recently because the variable intervals between administration produce wide swings in pain intensity that require variable doses of analgesic. Meperidine, the most frequently ordered narcotic, is typically prescribed in doses from 50 to 100 mg at 4-hour intervals, although its mean duration of effectiveness is 3 hours.

Respiratory depression is the most dangerous adverse effect of narcotics. To prevent respiratory depression, assessment of respiratory rate, depth, and character is necessary before administration and at the onset of the first two doses of a narcotic (McCaffery, 1979). Additional adverse effects and potential nursing diagnoses are summarized in Table 26–3.

After discussing the issue of addiction and the need to keep on top of the pain, a mutually agreed upon plan of interventions by the nurse generalist is determined. Meperidine is administered on a regular schedule, every 4 hours, and effectiveness and adverse effects are evaluated over the next several days. Figure 26–2 displays the peaks and valleys of pain intensity that occur with this type of medication schedule.

Evaluation of regular administration reveals that the interval between doses is too long (i.e., pain returns to its initial level before the next dose is due). The interval of meperidine administration is reduced to every 3 hours, which flattens out the pain intensity curve (Fig. 26–3). Because of the moderate pain intensity, the dosage of meperidine may be reduced. Alternatively, meperidine could be replaced by a longer-acting narcotic, for example, morphine.

Regular administration of analgesics seeks to eliminate blood level variability and provide more adequate relief. It also eliminates the need for the client to prove he or she has pain and, therefore, reduces the risk of receiving reinforcement for pain behavior. Although regular administration provides excellent pain control, it allows little control for the individual suffering from pain.

On-demand or self-administered analgesic systems have been developed to allow individual control over pain management. Systems developed for self-control include intravenous, intramuscular, and epidural administration of various narcotics. Research suggests that client-controlled administration decreases the total amount of narcotic used and increases alertness (Stimmel, 1985). These benefits are a result of reduced anxiety from anticipation of pain and enhanced feelings of self-control. The pain intensity curve is relatively flat, which eliminates the need for narcotic adjustment because of variable pain intensities. Tolerance will occur with long-term administration, but since tolerance develops to both the analgesic and the adverse effects of narcotics, increasing dosages of narcotics do not pose any greater danger.

TABLE 26–3. ADVERSE EFFECTS OF NARCOTICS.

Adverse Effect	Mechanism of Action	Nursing Diagnoses
Respiratory depression	Reduced responsiveness of respiratory center to CO_2 levels	Potential for inadequate ventilation
Nausea and vomiting	Stimulation of chemoreceptor trigger zone depresses medullary vomiting center	Potential for fluid and electrolyte imbalance
Orthostatic hypotension	Local effect of peripheral vasodilation	Potential for unsafe ambulation (falling)
Increased intracranial pressure	Cerebral vasodilation	Potential for altered level of consciousness
Constipation	Increased smooth muscle tone and decreased motility	Potential for constipation

The only adverse effect noted is mild sedation. Grace finds this bothersome, in that it limits the amount and type of activity in which she can engage. Most narcotics have similar actions and adverse effects at equianalgesic doses; however, an individual may receive a better response and less adverse effects from one drug than another. One action, therefore, is to discuss with the physician a change in narcotic. Since the client is concerned about losing control, a better alternative is to institute an adjunctive self-management technique, such as analgesic imagery, and reduce the dose of meperidine to 50 mg.

Imagery is used as an *intervention* for the nurse specialist. Grace is instructed to imag-

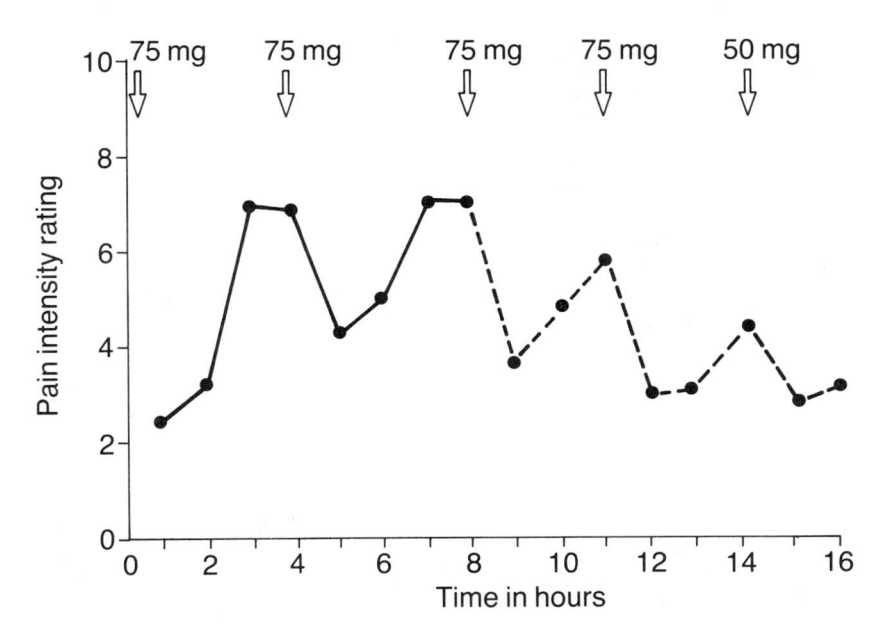

Figure 26–3. Report of pain intensity with regular administration of meperidine 50 to 100 mg. Key: ●———● every 4 hours; ●-----● every 3 hours.

ine the girdle area as numb or warm rather than painful. After achieving this sensory transformation, the nurse suggests that this sensation will remain on termination of the imagery session. In planning, the nurse may suggest the use of imagery on either a regular basis, for example, 2 hours after analgesic administration, or as required. It is important to discuss the preventive use of imagery because it is more effective if used for pain of moderate intensity (Melzack & Wall, 1982).

Outcome criteria to evaluate the effectiveness of nursing interventions are that the client will participate in the planning and evaluation of therapeutic modalities used, report increased comfort and decreased pain, report an increased sense of well-being, and use imagery as a self-initiated pain relief measure.

There are several palliative medical therapies avilable to manage Grace's pain. Injectable narcotics, although effective, may be replaced by an oral or epidural route of administration for home use. In client's with a limited life expectancy, neurolytic blocks or cordotomies may be effective means of pain control. In both procedures, the success rate is approximately 50%, but the pain tends to recur 6 to 12 months after the procedure.

After discussion with Grace and her family, the decision is made to continue to use narcotics to manage her pain. Oral methadone is tried, but the adverse effects of nausea and sedation are distressing to Grace. The next step is to insert a temporary epidural catheter for self-administration. Grace is scheduled for this procedure, to be performed under local anesthesia.

☐ **Anxiety Related to Painful Procedures**

Preparatory information alters responses to the distressful aspects of pain during anxiety-producing procedures. Preparatory information includes temporal, sensory, and coping skill information. Providing the sequence of events and describing some of the equipment, environment, and personnel involved comprises *temporal information*. *Sensory information* includes the sensations that are typically experienced during a procedure. Sensory information reduces the affective dimension of pain, with little effect on the sensory experience (Hartfield et al., 1982; Johnson, & Levanthal, 1974; Padilla et al., 1981), by providing accurate expectations of the sensations experienced (Levanthal & Johnson, 1983). *Coping skills information* instructs the client in activities that will reduce pain or distress during the procedure (e.g., deep breathing and swallowing during nasogastric intubation) or postprocedure to prevent complications and hasten recovery (e.g., turning, deep breathing, and coughing after general anesthesia). There is an additive effect when sensory information and coping skills are combined (Johnson et al., 1978).

Although responses are influenced by individual differences, such as preference for control (Padilla et al., 1981) and level of preoperative fear (Klos et al., 1980), there are no contraindications to providing preparatory information. This intervention is most effective if the level of knowledge is initially assessed, the level of understanding is checked frequently, and information is tailorerd to the client's needs and anxiety level. Methods of pain management are included to reassure the client that he or she will not suffer severe pain and to inform the client of expected behavior.

Providing *temporal and sensory information* is an *intervention* for the nurse generalist. A description of the sequence of events before epidural insertion and the sensations that may be experienced are provided the evening before the procedure.

Specific *coping skills*, such as deep breathing and distraction, can be taught, since they require little concentration and can be reinforced during the procedure with short commands. Deep breathing is a component of relaxation, since taking deep breaths counteracts the rapid, shallow respirations associated with sympathetic arousal. Deep breathing, therefore, has a calming effect that may help the client gain control over his or her responses to pain and reduce anxiety. There are many types of deep breathing exercises that act as distractors, for example "he–who" breathing and counting and breathing (McCaffery, 1979). Distraction redirects attention or awareness from the pain to other environmental stimuli, thus providing a sensory shield (McCaffery, 1979). Many activities, such as counting, singing, listening to music, describing pictures, or engaging in conversation, are distractors that can be used during stressful procedures. Grace was asked to describe several complicated pictures during the procedure.

As *outcome criteria* for the nursing interventions, the client will verbalize temporal and sensory information relevant to the procedure, participate in planning interventions to be used during the procedure, report mild to moderate discomfort during the procedure, and engage in coping skills necessary for recovery from the procedure.

The administration of epidural morphine is successful in controlling Grace's pain with minimal adverse effects. Several days later, she undergoes permanent placement of the catheter, with the end extending through a fistula in the abdomen. This surgical procedure is performed under general anesthesia. Preparatory information, including postoperative coping skills of deep breathing, coughing, and turning, are used to reduce presurgical anxiety and promote postoperative recovery. Grace and her husband are instructed in self-administration and care of the catheter (Regan, 1984).

CONSEQUENCES OF ACUTE PAIN

Consequences for the Individual
Acute pain produces many responses, but the most significant to the individual is suffering. Suffering is defined as "negative affective response generated in higher nervous centers by pain and other emotional situations, such as loss of loved objects, stress, anxiety, or depression" (Loeser, 1980, p. 4). The individual may be asking such questions as, Why is this happening to me? What does it mean? Will I be able to cope? Seeking medical attention is an appropriate response to acute pain, for medical therapies may treat the source of pain and thus eradicate it. Nursing interventions assist the client in controlling the perception of pain through knowledge of pharmacologic and self-initiated techniques. Collaboration with the client is essential in effective management of acute pain.

If pain limits the individual's ability to engage in daily activities, there will be a temporary change in role function and responsbilities. Hospitalization is the most obvious situation in which this occurs; a functioning adult who enters the hospital forfeits most responsibilities to become a patient. This may be a welcome rest for some, but the majority of patients have some difficulty giving up control and fitting into the hospital's structured routine. The client may be unable to meet family responsibilities, which places an added burden on family members.

Consequences for the Family
The family is typically concerned about the client's suffering, related again to the meaning of pain (Is it life-threatening?) and the diagnostic and therapeutic procedures necessary to relieve it. Inability of the client to fulfill his or her family role responsibilities means that the remaining members must do so. Preoccupation with pain and related anxiety may make the client irritable with those closest to him or her, possibly leading to confusion or anger in family members. This, in turn, may produce guilt: How can I be angry when my husband is experiencing such pain? Both the person in pain and the family need to adapt to the temporary changes brought about by pain.

Consequences for the Community
The person with acute pain may be unable temporarily to fulfill work responsibilities. The incidence and impact of acute pain on the community has not been investigated. Since pain is one of the most prevalent symptoms that motivates people to seek medical care, however, the overall consequences for the community presumably are significant.

HUMAN RESPONSES TO CHRONIC PAIN

Nursing Diagnosis in Chronic Pain

☐ Ineffective Coping with Chronic Pain

The *defining characteristics* of ineffective coping with chronic pain are behaviors learned during the acute phase of the process. Activity reduction is related to exercise avoidance, work avoidance, and minimal social participation. There is a continued reliance on medications, leading to overuse of addictive and nonaddictive drugs. This overuse leads to mental cloudiness, disorientation, memory loss, and demands for more medications (Ready et al., 1980). Repeated contact and failure of the health care system to alleviate pain result in manipulative and alienating behavior toward caregivers that carries over to all interpersonal relationships. Depression, and the vegetative signs associated with it, also assist in diagnosing ineffective coping with chronic pain. The result of these behaviors is an inability to meet role demands and responsibilities.

The *assessment* of chronic pain includes the areas identified under acute pain: primary complaint, sensory, affective, and cognitive dimensions. The manifestations of anxiety may be coupled with depressive symptoms. The client may focus totally on physical problems experienced (hypochrondriasis) and deny any other affective or interpersonal difficulties (hysterical denial). Because of the dysfunctional nature of the pain problem, more data are gathered on daily activity, medication use, family relations, social participation, and employment status. Assessment of these areas are included under the relevant nursing diagnosis.

The *etiology* of ineffective coping with chronic pain falls into three categories: personal, psychodynamic, and environmental. Personal etiologies include failure to relate the pain to psychologic as well as physical factors and lack of knowledge of pain management techniques based on psychology. Psychodynamic etiologies include an inability to express feelings and resolve conflicts. Continued pain meets the need for dependency and conflict avoidance. Inability to cope with life stressors is one environmental etiology. Reinforcement of pain behavior is the second environmental etiology. Pathology may be included as a contributing factor in chronic pain, although not as an etiology of ineffective coping. The philosophy held about the etiology of chronic pain guides the approach to treatment.

The most effective treatment of chronic pain is in multidisciplinary pain programs, which have multiplied rapidly over the past 10 years. The objective of most pain programs is to assist the client in developing effective coping mechanisms. If, in the process, pain is alleviated, the client has received a bonus. The emphasis of each program is unique and in part dependent on the philosophic and etiologic orientation of the therapist. For example, programs with a pathologic (or peripheral) focus would result in the use of techniques that interrupt nociception before it reaches the SG. In contrast, a psychodynamic (central) focus would place more emphasis on altering the affective and cognitive responses to pain. Regardless of the focus, all programs combine, to some degree, both peripheral and central approaches.

The physician may orchestrate the therapeutic program, but multiple disciplines are involved. The *goals* of most pain programs include: increasing functional status, reducing pain-related medication use, and increasing use of effective coping mechanisms. These goals, if attained, will produce a better quality of life for the client with chronic pain.

Case Study 2

Paul K, a 32-year-old man, is admitted to an inpatient pain treatment program with a diagnosis of low back pain of myofascial origin. Paul has a tense facial grimace, algetic (painful) gait, and difficulty sitting for more than 5 minutes. His affect is withdrawn, speech is slow and hesitant, and he avoids eye contact. He becomes more animated when discussing his pain and the poor treatment received from health care professionals.

The injury to his low back occurred on a construction site 2 years previously. The initial pain was severe, leading him to seek medical treatment. He underwent many diagnostic tests, which revealed some evidence of a herniated disk. A diskectomy of L4–L5 was performed, which provided relief for 2 months. With the return of pain, Paul began searching for another physician to do the surgery right. A second back surgery to remove the scar tissue provided little relief of his pain. Assistive devices were then tried, and on admission Paul uses a back brace and cane as required. He describes his pain as continuous and severe (8–9/10 on a scale of 0 to 10). Distress is rated at 6/10. The location includes the lumbar area, with dull aching pain radiating down both legs to the knee. He obviously experiences pain when changing position but can stay in one position for only 5 to 10 minutes. He is taking multiple medications, none of which really relieves his pain. The only palliative measure he uses is distraction with television. Paul reports that his wife had used some type of relaxation for childbirth, but he never paid much attention to it. He has not worked since the original injury 2 years ago.

Paul is married, with two school-age children. He expresses guilt about his behavior toward his family, the fact that his wife had to take a full-time job to help with the expenses, and his inability to be a real father for his two sons. Paul attributes these difficulties to his pain and believes things would return to normal if the pain could be relieved. He reports a familial model for pain behavior: his mother suffered from severe migraines that frequently disrupted family life.

On examination, Paul is nourished but pale and reports a 10 lb weight loss over the past year. He complains of a poor appetite and frequent constipation. Difficulty with sleep onset and frequent awakenings are also problems. Physical examination of the back and lower extremities is difficult because of his anticipatory responses (i.e., increased pain behavior) to pain.

☐ Altered Muscle Tension in Lumbar Area Related to Guarding and Anxiety

Muscular hyperactivity commonly is the only physiologic *defining characteristic* noted in clients with chronic pain. It may be directly related to the etiology, as in Paul's case with myofascial pain, or may indirectly increase another source of pain through reflex muscle contraction. There is typically a trigger point, which is a small, tender nodule found in the muscle belly. The primary interventions aim at reducing muscle tension, either peripherally with heat, cold, or transcutaneous nerve stimulation (TENS), or centrally with somatic relaxation.

Application of heat is an *intervention* for the nurse generalist. Heat produces several physiologic changes: increased pain threshold, muscle relaxation, and increased blood flow, all of which may influence pain perception. Heat may be dry, for example, heating pads and hot water bottles, or moist, for example, hydrocolator packs and warm soaks. Trapping the body's own heat with unbreathable materials, for example, plastic, may reduce joint stiffness and pain (Carpenito, 1983; McCaffery, 1979). All applications of heat should be wrapped adequately to prevent burning the skin. Heat should be applied with caution to clients with altered sensation (peripheral vascular disease, paresthesias) and altered ability to communicate (post-CVA, coma, vegetative state). Because of the increased blood flow produced by heat, it is contraindicated in clients with malignancies or a potential for hemorrhage (McCaffery, 1979).

Cold application decreases nerve conduction velocity and, therefore, increases the pain threshold. In addition to promoting muscle relaxation, cold application is particularly useful in pain of inflammatory origin, since it decreases blood flow and edema, thus reducing the inflammatory process. Cold may be dry (icebag, gel pack) or moist (ice-soaked towels). Cold application is indicated for pain of musculoskeletal origin, for example, muscle sprains and strains. Although heat is more commonly used for stiff arthritic joints, cold may be helpful in reducing inflammation and pain and in improving function. Cold also can burn the skin and, therefore, the cold pack should be well covered to prevent injury. Cold is contraindicated in clients with altered sensation, altered ability to communicate, and sensitivity to cold (Raynaud's disease).

Electrical stimulation using TENS or mechanical stimulation using a vibrator are two methods of *counterirritation* that the nurse specialist uses as *interventions*. Following the gate control theory, it is hypothesized that counterirritation closes the gate peripherally by stimulating large-diameter fibers. Because the analgesic effects long outlast the treatment, it is believed to act centrally as well by stimulating descending inhibitory mechanisms. The most effective electrode placement, pulse wave intensity, and frequency are identified by trial and error. An intact nerve supply is needed in the area of electrode placement. Counterirritation may be applied for 10 to 60 minutes at regular intervals but can be used for up to 24 hours a day.

Counterirritation increases muscle relaxation and blood flow (McCaffery, 1979) and, therefore, has added effects in pain accompanied by muscle tension. TENS has been used primarily in the treatment of chronic pain, providing relief in 20% to 30% of clients (Ready et al., 1980). The use of TENS is contraindicated in clients with pacemakers and cardiac arrhythmias. Instruction in the use of counterirritation is imperative if the client is to increase self-control of pain.

Relaxation techniques are most appropriate for clients with muscular hyperactivity. Because of the negative influence of anxiety and the prevalence of anxiety in chronic pain, relaxation may be beneficial for any type of chronic pain state. Relaxation increases susceptibility to the suggestions of comfort (McCaffery, 1979), which is why hypnosis and imagery commonly are preceded by a short relaxation technique.

Relaxation is a common technique used in multifaceted pain programs because it enhances the effects of other pain management techniques and places increased responsibility for pain management on the client. The suggested use of relaxation is 20 to 30 minutes twice a day (Benson, 1975). If used more frequently, withdrawal and psychotic manifestations may occur. Consequently, relaxation is contraindicated in clients who have a history of psychosis and should be used with caution in clients who are depressed (McCaffery, 1979; Snyder, 1984). In clients with cardiovascular disease, tight muscle contraction used in progressive relaxation should be avoided (Snyder, 1984).

Although relaxation is considered a relatively benign procedure, some adverse effects have been noted. Muscle cramps, feelings of suffocation, and increased awareness of pain are effects that may be reduced by altering the technique. Intrusive thoughts, either anxiety provoking or sexually arousing, may occur early in therapy (Bernstein & Borkovec, 1973). The nurse must be aware of these difficulties and openly discuss them with the client. In clients who keep tight control over their feelings, the open awareness suggested may increase feelings of fear, anxiety, or sadness. In this case, the nurse should terminate the exercise and therapeutically listen to the individual.

Paul learns a progressive relaxation technique (Bernstein & Borkovec, 1973), and to provide structure to the program, hydrocolator packs are available every 4 hours and are applied for 20 minutes. Because Paul has some difficulty with back and leg muscle relaxation, a collaborative decision is made to apply the hot pack for 20 minutes before relaxation. The use of heat is effective, and Paul begins to fall asleep during the relaxation exercise. Since Paul has difficulty with sleep onset, he decides to use the relaxation technique in the early afternoon in a sitting position to prevent sleep and at bedtime to promote sleep.

Outcome criteria for this program are that the the client will participate in the development and implementation of a pain management program, report an improved sense of well-being, and demonstrate effective use of heat application and relaxation.

Pain Preoccupation Related to Narrowed Focus of Attention

Preoccupation with pain is a manifestation of somatization (hypochondriasis), which may be inadvertently reinforced by staff. The approach to chronic pain management is focusing on wellness. Therefore, emphasis and, hence, reinforcement are placed on well behaviors, one of which is nonpain-related interpersonal interactions. It is important to *assess* initially the client's pain and convey that the pain is believed. Once this attitude is communicated, the general nursing *intervention* related to chronic pain is selective nonintervention (Yarton, 1979). Ignoring pain behavior and reinforcing well behavior will alter the client's behavior but will not alleviate the pain. This presents a double-edged sword, since nursing responsibility includes early detection of nonpain-related problems, of which pain may be an early symptom.

Pain behavior, which includes verbalization of pain complaints, algetic gait, facial grimaces, and moaning or sighing, are acknowledged but not acted on in nursing *intervention*. Nurse–client interactions are initiated surrounding well behaviors, such as increased activity and the use of alternate self-management techniques. The structure of a pain program and the milieu provide opportunities for the client to engage in these well behaviors.

Program structure is important in setting consistent limits on client behavior, thus avoiding manipulation of staff. Structure may reduce anxiety as it identifies expected client behaviors.

Milieu therapy is defined in the context rather than the content of the therapy (Pinsky & Malyon, 1979). Exposure to pain peers may reduce feelings of isolation and assist individuals in identifying and owning up to dysfunctional or maladaptive behaviors. The health team members function as part of the milieu. Their responsibilities include assisting clients in developing awareness and insight into their responses and working through alternative modes of behavior and showing role model responses to emotions, such as anger, joy, and adaptive interpersonal exchanges.

Paul responds to the milieu by taking an active role in the group. As he gains insight into other client's behavior, he is able to apply these ideas to his own behavior. Paul accepts responsibility for planning and implementing extracurricular activities for the peer group.

Outcome criteria are that the client will participate in nonpain-related group activities and engage in nonpain-related interactions with health professionals.

The three most dysfunctional pain responses are activity reduction, drug abuse, and continued reliance on medical therapies to eliminate pain. Paul completed the Daily Activity Diary (DAD) (Fordyce, 1976), which identifies on an hourly basis the number of minutes spent standing, sitting, and reclining during the week before admission. Paul's activity tolerance is assessed in preparation for physical and occupational therapy. His tolerance for sitting is 10 minutes, standing 25 minutes, and, from the diary, he spends as much as 18 hours a day reclining. The DAD also includes medication use, and the following pattern of medication use is identified: acetaminophen (60 mg codeine) two tablets four to five times daily, diazepam 5 mg three times daily, methocarbamol 250 mg two times daily, and diphenhydramine 50 mg at bedtime.

To provide effective treatment, nursing works interdependently to support and reinforce treatment programs designed to increase activity, reduce medication use, and increase self-management of pain. Table 26–4 presents multidisciplinary management of chronic pain, and Table 26–5 shows specific nursing diagnoses and interventions.

Paul begins an activity program designed by the physiotherapy department, and his tolerance for activity increases as he is weaned from the back brace and cane. Paul successfully completes detoxification with only mild withdrawal symptoms. Because he was skilled in relaxation by the time detoxification began, Paul is able to control his withdrawal symp-

TABLE 26-4. MULTIDISCIPLINARY MANAGEMENT OF CHRONIC PAIN.

	Client Behaviors		
	Activity reduction	*Dependence on addictive medications*	*Reliance on health professionals for pain management*
Goals	Restore muscle tone, strength, and flexibility to increase activity tolerance Decrease or eliminate assistive devices	Eliminate use of medications with minimal withdrawal symptoms Reduce use of nonaddictive medications	Self-management of pain
Management	Replace pain contingent rest with time or activity contingent quotas, increase by 10% each week (Fordyce, 1978; Sternbach, 1982) Increase functional activity Physical education: anatomy and physiology, body mechanics	Time contingent medication schedule, reducing active analgesic by 10% each day (Fordyce, 1978; Sternbach, 1982) Sedative and tranquilizers (hydroxyzine, chlorpromazine) to manage withdrawal symptoms Drug education	Set small, mutually agreed upon goals to increase belief in self-efficacy (Turk et al., 1983.) Review progress frequently and concretely (e.g., flow charts) Explore relationship between thoughts, emotions, and behavior (Turk et al., 1983) Identify maladaptive patterns and plan adaptive alternatives Problem-solving education

toms with relaxation. This success increases his ability to cope with pain.

☐ Ineffective Family Coping Related to Lack of Knowledge

Assessment of the interaction between spouse and client yields information about the possible rewards gained from pain behavior. The spouse may provide rewards for pain behavior that make it difficult for the client to give up his or her symptom. Spouse support may, in contrast, be an important variable in pain reduction and positive mood elevation (Kerns & Turk, 1984). The shift in family roles and the added burden on the spouse may be important in explaining their interactions. The previous (i.e., prepain) pattern of function will indicate the adaptation that has taken place. Flor and Turk (1985) suggest that the development of chronic pain may be a reflection of family function and may, in fact, be a stabilizing force.

The perception of marital satisfaction may significantly differ between client and spouse, with the client denying difficulties that the spouse reports (Maruta, et al., 1981). Maruta et al. (1978, 1981) also report a high incidence of sexual dysfunction in clients with chronic pain. Marital adjustment and sexual satisfaction should be discussed with the client and spouse individually.

Since effective self-management is a goal of treatment for the client, nurse specialist *interventions* involve the spouse as well. If the chronic pain is indicative of family dysfunction, self-mangment techniques may assist in the development of more effective family coping mechanisms. Counseling is recommended as well. Both client and spouse should be instructed in promoting well behaviors, and spouse involvement in techniques to manage pain may be one aspect of this.

If the spouse is providing reinforcement for pain behavior, operant techniques to develop his or her awareness of this process are

Chronic pain (p. 59). New York: S.P. Medical and Scientific Books.
Edwards, P.W., Zeichner, A., Kuczmierczyk, A.R. & Boczkowski, J. (1985). Familial pain model: The relationship between family history of pain and currrent pain experience. *Pain, 21,* 379.
Flor, H., & Turk, D.C. (1985). Chronic illness in an adult family member: Pain as a prototype. In D.C. Turk & R.D. Kerns (Eds.), *Health, illness, and families* (p. 255). New York: Wiley.
Fordyce, W.E. (1976). *Behavioral methods in chronic pain and illness.* St. Louis: Mosby.
Fordyce, W.E. (1978). Learning process in pain. In R. Sternbach (Ed.), *The psychology of pain* (p. 49). New York: Raven.
Gentry, W.D., Shows, W.D., & Thomas, M. (1974). Chronic low back pain: A psychological profile. *Psychosomatics, 15,* 174.
Hartfield, M.T., Cason, C.L., & Cason, G.J. (1982). Effects of information about a threatening procedure on patients' expectations and emotional distress. *Nursing Research, 31,* 202.
Johnson, J.E. (1972). Effects of structuring patients' expectations on their reactions to threatening events. *Nursing Research, 21,* 499.
Johnson, J.E., & Levanthal, H. (1974). Effects of accurate expectations and behavioral instructions on reactions during a noxious medical examination. *Journal of Personality and Social Psychology, 29,* 710.
Johnson, J.E., Rice, V.H., Fuller, S.S., & Endress, M.P. (1978). Sensory information, instruction in a coping strategy, and recovery from surgery. *Research in Nursing and Health, 1,* 4.
Keefe, F.J., Brown, C.J., Scott, D.S., & Ziesat, H. (1982). Behavioral assessment of chronic pain. In F.J. Keefe & J. Blumenthal (Eds.), *Assessment strategies in behavioral medicine* (p. 321). New York: Grune & Stratton.
Kerns, R. D., & Turk, D.C. (1984). Depression and chronic pain: The mediating role of the spouse. *Journal of Marriage and the Family, 46,* 845.
Klos, D., Cummings, K.M., Joyce, J., Graichen, J., & Quigley, A. (1980). A comparison of two methods of delivering presurgical instruction. *Patient Counseling and Health Education, 2,* 6.
Levanthal, H., & Johnson, J.E. (1983). Laboratory and field experimentation: Development of a theory of self-regulation. In P.J. Wooldridge, M.H. Schmitt, J.K. Skipper, & R.C. Leonard (Eds.), *Behavioral science and nursing theory* (p. 189). St. Louis: Mosby.

Loeser, J.D. (1980). A definition of pain. *University of Washington Medicine, 7*(1), 3.
Marks, R.M., & Sachar, E.J. (1973). Undertreatment of medical inpatients with narcotic analgesics. *Annals of Internal Medicine, 78,* 173.
Maruta, T., & Osborne, D. (1978). Sexual activity in chronic pain patients. *Psychosomatics, 19,* 531.
Maruta, T., Osborne, D., Swanson, D.W., & Hallnig, J.M. (1981). Chronic pain patients and spouses. Marital and sexual adjustment. *Mayo Clinic Proceedings, 56,* 307.
McCaffery, M. (1979). *Nursing management of patients in pain* (2nd ed.). Philadelphia: Lippincott.
Meichenbaum, D., & Turk, D. (1976). The cognitive behavioral management of anxiety, anger, and pain. In P.O. Davidson (Ed.), *Behavioral management of anxiety, depression, and pain* (p. 1). New York: Brunner/Mazel.
Melzack, R. (1975). The McGill pain questionnaire: Major properties and scoring methods. *Pain, 1,* 277.
Melzack, R., & Casey, K.L. (1968). Sensory, motivational, and central control determinants of pain: A new conceptual model. In D. Kenshalo (Ed.), *The skin senses* (p. 423). Springfield, IL: Thomas.
Melzack, R., & Torgerson, W.S. (1971). On the language of pain. *Anesthesiology, 34,* 50.
Melzack, R., & Wall, P.D. (1965). Pain mechanisms: A new theory. *Science, 150,* 971.
Melzack, R., & Wall, P.D. (1970). Psychophysiology of pain. *International Anaesthesia Clinics, 8*(1), 3.
Melzack, R. & Wall, P.D. (1982). *The challenge of pain.* New York: Penguin.
Moss, F.T., & Meyer, B. (1966). The effects of nursing interaction upon pain relief in patients. *Nursing Research, 15,* 303.
Padilla, G.V., Grant, M.M., Rains, B.L., Hansen, B.C., Bergstrom, N., Wong, H.L., Hanson, R., & Kubo, W. (1981). Distress reduction and the effects of preparatory teaching films and patient control. *Research in Nursing and Health, 4,* 375.
Pert, A. (1982). Mechanisms of opiate analgesia and the role of endorphins in pain supression. *Advances in Neurology, 33,* 107.
Pilowsky, I. (1978). Psychodynamic aspects of the pain experience. In R. Sternbach (Ed.), *The psychology of pain* (p. 203). New York: Raven.
Pinsky, J.J. (1979). Aspects of the psychology of pain. In B.L. Crue (Ed.), *Chronic pain* (p. 301). New York: S.P. Medical and Scientific Books.
Pinsky, J.J., & Malyon, A.K. (1979). The eclectic nature of psychotherapy in the treatment of

chponic pain syndromes. In B.L. Crue (Ed.), *Chronic pain* (p. 321). New York: S.P. Medical and Scientific Books.

Ready, B., Murphy, T.M., Loeser, J.D., & Fordyce, W.E. (1980). The management of chronic pain. *University of Washington Medicine, 7*(1), 13.

Regan, P. (Ed.). (1984). *Teaching guides for patients with neurological disorders.* Reston, VA: Reston.

Snyder, M. (1984). Progressive relaxation as a nursing intervention. *Advances in Nursing Science, 6*(3), 47.

Sternbach, R.A. (1974). *Pain patients: Traits and treatments.* New York: Academic Press.

Sternbach, R.A. (1978). *The psychology of pain.* New York: Raven.

Sternbach, R.A. (1982). The psychologist's role in the diagnosis and treatment of pain patients. In J. Barber & C. Adrian (Eds.), *Psychological approaches to the management of pain* (p. 3). New York: Brunner/Mazel.

Sternbach, R.A., Wolf, S.R., Murphy, R.W., & Akeson, W.H. (1973). Traits of pain patients: The low-back "loser." *Psychosomatics, 14,* 226.

Stimmel, B. (1985). Pain, analgesia, and addiction: An approach to the pharmacological management of pain. *The Clinical Journal of Pain, 1*(1), 14.

Timmermans, G., & Sternbach, R.A. (1974). Factors of human chronic pain: An analysis of personality and pain reaction variables. *Science, 184,* 806.

Turk, D.C., Meichenbaum, D.H., & Genest, M. (1983). *Pain and behavioral medicine: A cognitive-behavioral perspective.* New York: Guilford Press.

Violon, A., & Giurgea, D. (1984). Familial models for chronic pain. *Pain, 18,* 199.

Wolff, B.B. (1985). Ethnocultural factors influencing pain and illness behavior. *The Clinical Journal of Pain, 1*(1), 23.

Yarton, P. (1979). The role of the nurse on the pain unit. In B. Crue (Ed.), *Chronic pain* (p. 413). New York: S.P. Medical and Scientific Books.

Zborowski, M. (1969). *People in pain.* San Francisco: Jossey-Bass.

SECTION 7. ELIMINATION PHENOMENA

27

Elimination: An Overview

E. Elaine Lloyd, Janet Giroux, and Linda Toth

The elimination of stored waste products in the form of urine and feces is essential to maintaining health. The content varies with the quantity and quality of food and fluids ingested. Elimination during health is affected by physical activity, maintenance of body temperature within 1°F above or below the usual, and the amount of usual life stress experienced. The ability to respond to the cortical signals of the urge to defecate or urinate affects the patterns of elimination (Boroch, 1976).

Bladder elimination, or micturition, involves the *kidneys* with the formation of urine, the *bladder* for storage, the *bladder neck* through which the urine flows after voluntary relaxation, and the *urethra*, which carries the urine out of the body. Disruption of bladder elimination can occur with disease processes in the structures themselves, when neurogenic pathways are interrupted, or when cortical control centers are affected.

Bowel elimination in the form of bowel movements or evacuation of stool involves the *ingestion* and *digestion* of food and fluids, the *small* and *large intestines*, the *anal canal*, and the *rectum*. Voluntary relaxation of the external anal sphincter is under cortical control. The neural pathways include the sacral spinal cord, ascending and descending spinal cord tracts, and spinal nerves. Several key reflexes, such as the gastrocolic reflex, play an important role in defecation. As with bladder elimination, bowel elimination can be disrupted when disease processes invade the structures involved with digestion and storage, when the neural pathways are interrupted, or when cortical control centers are involved.

BLADDER ELIMINATION

Voiding, or micturition, is primarily a spinal reflex that is facilitated and inhibited by higher voluntary centers in the brain (Ganong, 1987). The elimination of urine is the response of the body in regulating the internal environment in relation to water content and requirements, osmotic relationships, and acid–base balance (Crouch, 1965). The organs that make up the urinary system are the kidneys, ureters, bladder, and urethra. Other than the kidneys, which produce urine, the remaining structures are involved primarily in transportation, storage, and elimination.

Anatomy of the Urinary System

The *kidneys* are approximately 11.25 cm in length, 5 to 7.5 cm wide, and 2.5 cm thick. They lie retroperitoneally anterior and lateral to the twelfth thoracic vertebra. The major structures of the kidney are the pelvis, medulla, and cortex. The renal pelvis is the expanded upper end of the ureter and lies within the renal sinus. The medulla is made up of a varying number of renal pyramids. The cortex forms the peripheral layer under the fibrous capsule covering the kidney. The major functions of the kidneys are filtration, reabsorption, and secretion.

The *ureters* are approximately 28 to 35 cm long, arise from the pelvis on the medial side of the kidney extending to the base of the bladder, and are composed of smooth muscle. The ureters enter the bladder through the trigone and travel under the bladder epithelium for several centimeters before opening into the bladder (Crouch, 1965; Guyton, 1987). The mechanism of the ureterovesical junction allows free efflux but prevents any reflux of urine (Tanagho, 1976).

The *bladder* is a hollow muscular organ composed of (1) the body, which is primarily detrusor muscle, (2) the trigone, a small area through which the ureters and urethra pass, and (3) the bladder neck or posterior urethra. The detrusor, posterior urethra, and trigone are smooth muscle.

The *urethra* extends from the bladder to the surface of the body. In females the urethra is approximately 4 cm long. Striated (voluntary) circular muscle, which is under voluntary control, forms the external sphincter of the bladder, where the urethra passes through the urogenital diaphragm. The male urethra is approximately 20 cm long and is divided into three parts; the prostatic, membranous, and cavernous (Crouch, 1965). The prostatic urethra extends from the bladder for approximately 3 cm and passes through the prostate to the pelvic floor. The ejaculatory ducts empty into the urethra on the posterior wall of the prostatic urethra. The membranous urethra is approximately 1 to 2 cm long and passes through the external sphincter to form the cavernous urethra for its remaining length.

Neural Regulation of Micturition

The neurologic control of micturition involves the micturition reflex, sympathetic and parasympathetic nerve supply, and cerebral centers involved in voiding (Fig. 27–1).

Process of Micturition

The bladder fills at an average rate of 1 milliliter per minute. As it fills, intravesicular pressure rises. The micturition reflex is stimulated at a threshold pressure, accompanied by a conscious desire to void. Voiding will occur if there is no voluntary inhibition. In adults, the desire to void is usually felt when the bladder contains 300 to 400 ml of urine. Cystometrographic studies of the bladder demonstrate that as the bladder fills, there is a gradual rise in intravesical pressure from approximately 0 when the bladder is empty to five to 10 cm water with 100 ml of urine. This pressure does not change dramatically until approximately 400 ml is collected. The pressure can then rise to over 400 cm of water because of reflex contractions of the detrusor (Guyton, 1987).

As the bladder fills to 300 to 400 ml of urine, stretch receptors in the bladder wall send sensory impulses through the pelvic nerves to the sacral spinal cord segments. Impulses from the spinal segments return to the bladder through parasympathetic fibers in the pelvic nerves. This initiates reflex contractions of the detrusor, which are self-regenerating: each contraction activates further afferent impulses from the bladder. These bladder contractions send sensory input to the micturition center in the brain, which responds with inhibitory signals to the bladder (Zinner et al., 1976). As the bladder fills, the external sphincter remains contracted. Perkash (1982) describes this as the holding

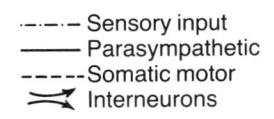

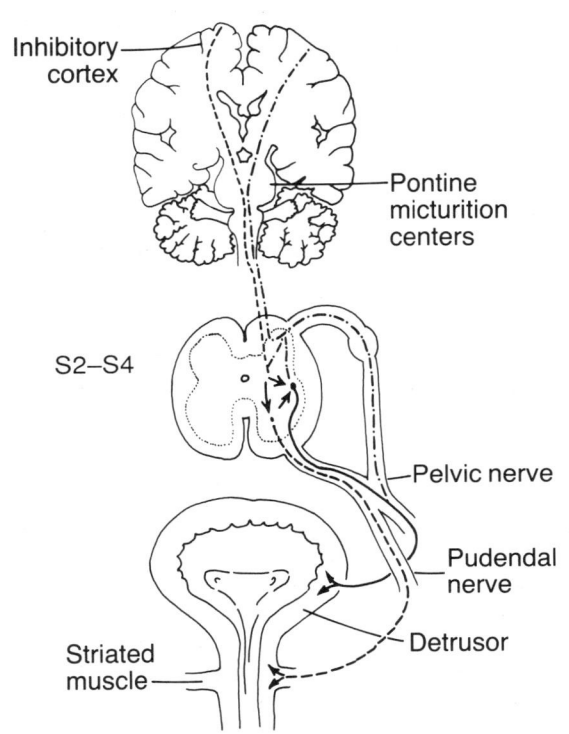

Figure 27–1. Neural regulation of micturition at three levels: cortex, spinal cord, and end-organ. *(Modified from Mitchell et al. [1984]. Neurological assessment for nursing practice.)*

reflex. The voiding process begins with relaxation of the holding reflex and is followed by relaxation of the bladder neck. The opening of the bladder neck is accomplished by immediate contraction of the detrusor, which allows urine to flow from the bladder through the open bladder neck and urethra. The flow of urine usually continues until the bladder is empty but can be stopped voluntarily.

Central Innervation

Both voluntary and involuntary control over the micturition reflex is represented in specific anatomic areas of the brain. The pons contains centers that both facilitate and inhibit the micturition reflex. In addition, there are centers in the medial cerebral cortex that serve voluntary inhibition of the reflex (Guyton, 1987). Afferent impulses for the sensation of the desire to void travel from the S2–S4 spinal cord segments to the pons and cortex via the spinothalamic tracts (Nathan, 1976).

Parasympathetic Nerve Supply

The detrusor muscle is supplied by parasympathetic fibers that originate in the S2–S4 segments of the cord and pass through pelvic splanchnic nerves. Postganglionic fibers travel to the detrusor muscle. Initiating and sustaining bladder contractions during micturition are under parasympathetic control (Perkash, 1982).

Sympathetic Nerve Supply
The sympathetic nerve supply originates in the T11 and L2 segments of the spinal cord and serves to prevent semen from entering the bladder during ejaculation. Sympathetic stimulation functionally closes the bladder neck by stimulating relaxation of the detrusor muscle (Perkash, 1982).

Factors Affecting Micturition
Many variables can affect bladder elimination, such as injury, infection, and disease. These factors can affect the normal structures of the genitourinary system, afferent or efferent neural pathways, or the cortical control centers. Abnormal bladder function due to interruption of the neural pathways is termed *neurogenic bladder*. Several forms of neurogenic bladder are sources of alterations in bladder elimination. These are discussed in Chapter 28.

BOWEL ELIMINATION

Patterns of elimination of stool vary from individual to individual, from once or twice daily to once every 3 days. A neurogenic bowel may result when there are disruptions in the ability to initiate or inhibit bowel evacuation secondary to disease or injury to the brain, spinal cord, or spinal nerves (Sayles, 1981).

Digestion
Food enters the alimentary canal through the mouth and undergoes a series of changes in the process of digestion, absorption of nutrients, and the elimination of waste products. Enzymes and digestive juices assist in the process in the stomach to break down food substances. In the small intestine, complete digestion occurs with the aid of additional enzymes, and it is here that absorption of nutrients occurs. Chyme enters the large bowel, where the absorption of water and electrolytes takes place primarily in the proximal half; the distal half of the colon is concerned with the storage of stool.

The content of stool is inorganic material, undigested plant fibers, bacteria, and water. Variations in diet do not affect stool content greatly because the largest percentage of stool content is of nondietary origin. Even with prolonged starvation, feces will continue to be passed because of the nondietary component. The transit time varies in individuals, but it usually takes 8 to 9 hours for a meal to reach the colon. In 72 hours, approximately 70% of the meal has been evacuated from the colon, and the remaining 30% may take as long as a week to be passed (Ganong, 1987).

Anatomy of the Defecation System
The *colon* is approximately 5 feet, or 100 cm, long and is wider in diameter than the small bowel. Small longitudinal muscular bands called *teniae coli* run the length of the colon. This configuration produces outpouchings along the bowel, called *haustra*. Mucus is secreted by colonic glands, which are short inward projections of the mucosa (Ganong, 1987).

The four major parts of the colon are the ascending, transverse, descending, and sigmoid colon. The hepatic flexure is formed as the ascending colon turns abruptly forward and to the left. The transverse colon turns downward to become the descending colon at the splenic flexure. The descending colon is the narrowest part of the large intestine; it swings in an S curve to midline, forming the sigmoid colon, which gives way to the anal canal and rectum, which terminates with the internal and external anal sphincters. The internal anal sphincter is composed of circular smooth muscle, and the external anal sphincter is composed of striated (voluntary) muscle. The mucosa of the rectum and anal canal is thick and highly vascular (Crouch, 1965). The angulation of the rectum and the spiral folds, or valve of Houston, serve to maintain continence.

Neurogenic Control of Digestion and Defecation

Neural control of digestion and defecation occurs at several levels of the nervous system, similar to the levels of control described in bladder elimination. The defecation reflex involves central voluntary control as well as spinal cord and autonomic reflex control. Several reflexes play a key role in defecation. The *gastrocolic reflex* is initiated by distention of the stomach after a meal. This distention produces contractions of the rectum, accompanied by a desire to defecate (Ganong, 1987). *Mass movements* are several strong peristaltic movements that occur one after another and propel fecal material in the colon. These occur two or three times in 24 hours and often are initiated when some part of the colon becomes overfilled (Guyton, 1987).

The *defecation reflex* produces reflex relaxation of the internal anal sphincter and contraction of the gut wall in response to fecal material in the rectum. The bowel empties if the external anal sphincter is also relaxed. This reflex subsides after several moments and usually will not return for several hours, but it can be initiated by straining (Guyton, 1987).

Process of Defecation

When stool enters the rectum, the stretch response initiates signals that spread through the myenteric plexus. This response initiates reflex peristalic waves in the descending and sigmoid colon. These waves move toward the anus, causing relaxation of the internal anal sphincter. Stimulation of the rectum initiates afferent signals, which are transmitted to the S2, S3, and S4 segments of the spinal cord. Impulses travel to the descending colon, sigmoid, rectum, and anus along parasympathetic nerve fibers, intensifying peristalsis. Stretch receptor impulses also travel from the sacral segments to the brain, where the desire to defecate is perceived.

The spinal cord reflex initiates contraction of the abdominal muscles, inhalation of a deep breath, and closure of the glottis, as well as contraction of the pelvic floor musculature.

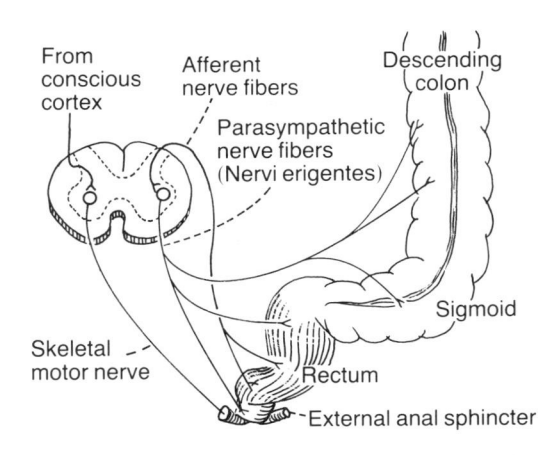

Figure 27–2. Neural regulation of defecation reflex. *(Redrawn from Guyton, 1981.)*

If the external anal sphincter is voluntarily relaxed, defecation will occur. Defecation can be prevented if the timing is not appropriate by maintaining the normal tonic contraction of the sphincter until a more propitious time. These pathways are shown in Figure 27–2 and described in detail below.

The *intramural plexus* of the intestine is composed of two layers of neurons and connecting fibers: the outer is the myenteric plexus or Auerbach's plexus, and the inner is the submucosal or Meissner's plexus. These plexi begin at the esophagus and end at the anus. The primary effects of stimulation of the intramural plexus are increased tone of the gut wall, intensity and rate of the rhythmic contractions, and velocity of conduction of excitatory waves along the gut wall. Coordination of peristalsis also is controlled by this plexus (Guyton, 1987).

Parasympathic Innervation

The vagus nerves innervate the esophagus, stomach, pancreas, part of the small intestine, gallbladder, and the first half of the colon. The sacral parasympathetic supply originates from the S2, S3, and S4 segments of the spinal cord and passes through the nervi erigentes to the distal half of the large intestine, the sigmoid colon, and the rectum. Stimulation of the parasympathetic nervous system increases activity of the intramural plexus, which, in turn, excites the reflexes of the gastrointestinal tract.

Sympathetic Innervation
Sympathetic fibers involved in digestion and defecation originate in the spinal cord between T8 and L3. Postganglionic fibers spread to all parts of the gut. The overall effect of sympathetic nervous system stimulation is inhibitory except when sympathetic stimulation excites contraction of the ileocecal sphincter, the internal anal sphincter, and the muscularis mucosae throughout the entire gastrointestinal tract.

Central Innervation
Afferent impulses travel by way of the spinothalamic tracts to the brain from the S2–S4 segments of the spinal cord, which provide for the sensation underlying the desire to defecate. The pudendal nerve innervates the striated muscle of the external anal sphincter (Ganong, 1987).

Factors Affecting Bowel Elimination
Diet is an important variable in the process of elimination. Certain foods add bulk to the stool, which is needed to provide the stimulus for bowel reflexes to occur. Inadequate fluid intake promotes constipation or infrequent, hard stools. Medication often can cause constipation or diarrhea and needs to be considered when bowel problems are being assessed. Activity and exercise enhance digestion and bowel motility as well as the strength of the Valsalva maneuver, which is necessary to initiate defecation (Benda, 1983). As Staas and DeNault (1973) note, it is difficult to defecate without the ability to sit for any length of time. Severe emotional stress can cause excessive parasympathetic stimulation, with resultant overproduction of mucus in the colon. Such excess mucus can contribute to diarrhea, which contains little or no fecal material (Guyton, 1987). Disease or injury causing neurogenic effects to the bowel are discussed in Chapter 29.

ASSESSMENT OF ELIMINATION STATUS

Assessment of the type and extent of voiding or defecating dysfunction is mandatory as the initial step in the nursing process. Baseline and ongoing assessment direct the nurse in planning individualized programs and preventing complications that could compromise renal or intestinal functions. The following assessment areas can be evaluated simultaneously in a given individual but are separated into bladder and bowel for clarity here.

Neurourologic Assessment
Before appropriate interventions are initiated, the nurse must make a general urologic assessment. This collection of subjective and objective data is essential for formulation of an individualized plan of care. A past and present *voiding history*, noting both volume and frequency of voiding and fluid intake, type of urinary incontinence, and present method of management, is crucial. In addition, any *preexisting urologic symptoms* or complications and a *medical history* should be noted. A 24-hour intake and output record for 3 to 4 days provides baseline data. Measurement of residual urine provides information on bladder capacity.

A *physical assessment* reveals important diagnostic information. The perineal and perianal areas are evaluated for degree of sensation. Can the patient discern bladder fullness, sensation during voiding, or feeling of wetness after voiding? Any anal tone or a positive bulbocavernous reflex would indicate some degree of sacral sparing with an intact reflex arc. Visual inspection of the abdomen would detect any asymmetry or localized swelling. The normal abdomen is symmetrical and soft when palpated. A full bladder can be palpated in the lower abdomen; however, when distended, it can expand to the umbilicus. Palpation of the abdomen should proceed cautiously in an asensory patient. Percussion of the abdomen also can offer information on bladder distention. If dullness rather than a tympanic sound is heard when percussing the suprapubic area, the bladder is probably distended.

When the perineum and genital area are inspected, any anatomic abnormality and evidence of bruising, bleeding, swelling, skin breakdown, or urethral discharge should be noted. For the male patient, the penis and scrotum are examined, and it is noted if he is circumcised, since this may influence the type of urinary management if an external collecting device is used. With females, the labia and location of the urethral meatus are examined and a menstrual history and the date of the last menstrual period are obtained.

Two final general assessment areas are the patient's *physical abilities* and *potential for cooperation*. Evaluation of self-care skills for bladder management must begin early. Physical assessment of upper extremity strength and hand function and any limitations in mobility are necessary before program planning can begin. The ability of the patient to cooperate fully in the bladder management program is crucial to the outcome. Communication problems and decreased mentation, motivation, and receptiveness to learning can all have a negative impact on the goals and success of the program.

Diagnostic Studies

In conjunction with data gathered from the general urologic assessment, the nurse must incorporate findings from medical diagnostic tests describing the functional state of the external urinary sphincter, bladder, ureters, and kidneys. Evaluation and knowledge of laboratory, radiologic, and urodynamic studies will assist in these determinations. The use of these data is essential in formulating an accurate nursing diagnosis and establishing appropriate interventions.

Laboratory tests detailing composition and physical properties of the urine include (1) urinalysis, (2) urine culture, and (3) urine and serum creatinine clearance. In a *urinalysis*, evaluation of certain properties can signal subtle changes occurring in urologic function. The specific gravity (1.010 to 1.025) is an indicator of urinary concentration, and a low reading can herald the development of early loss to tubular reabsorption. Urine pH (4.5 to 7.5) is determined by its hydrogen ion concentration. Normal urine is usually slightly acidic, but infection can cause the urine to become alkaline. Maintaining urine pH levels below 6 may be indicated in people with neurogenic bladders to prevent urinary infection and calculi formation. Evidence of microscopic hematuria could be indicative of trauma, stones, tumor, or acute cystitis. Pyuria greater than five white blood cells per high powered field signifies an inflammatory response, with probable bacteriuria, and urinary casts indicate an inflammatory or renal parenchymal disease.

Urine cultures are necessary to monitor the incidence of bacteriuria, which is a constant threat in patients with urologic dysfunction. A colony count greater than 10^5 per milliliter of urine, along with pyuria, represents significant bacteriuria and usually requires antibiotic treatment (Perkash, 1982). It is important to remember that some patients with neurogenic bladders may not exhibit the classic symptoms of a urinary tract infection because of their neurologic deficit. Therefore, observing the patient for subtle changes, for example, dysreflexia symptoms, increased cloudiness or odor to the urine, general malaise, or a spastic bladder with increased incontinence, can provide clues to the presence of bacteriuria.

Both *urine and serum creatinine* clearance are used to determine the glomerular filtration rate. Serum and 24-hour urine creatinine clearance tests are run simultaneously. Creatinine blood levels are normally 0.6 to 1.2 mg/dl and are generally constant unless renal failure has begun. The 24-hour urine measurement gives the amount of creatinine that can be cleared by the kidney in 1 minute. Normal value is 100 ml/minute.

Initial *radiologic studies*, such as intravenous pyelography (IVP) and voiding cystourethrogram (VCU), assess the anatomic structure of the upper and lower genitourinary tract and delineate any abnormalities. Abnormalities that can be visualized include

(1) calculi, (2) hydronephrosis or chronic pyelonephritis indicating parenchymal damage, and (3) vesicoureteral reflux. Recently, renal scintiradiography with ^{131}I-hippuran has become an important diagnostic tool for assessing actual renal function through calculation of effective renal plasma flow (ERPF) (Tempkin, et al., 1985).

To diagnose the functional state of the neurogenic bladder definitively, *urodynamic evaluation* is mandatory. In general, urodynamic testing encompassess simultaneous measurement of (1) bladder pressure during filling and voiding, (2) urine flow rate during voiding, (3) urethral pressure, and (4) electromyography of the periurethral striated sphincter (Friedland & Perkash, 1983). These measurements assist in identifying (1) sensation of normal bladder filling, (2) bladder pressure response to increased volume, (3) urethral pressure to assess urinary continence and detrusor sphincter dyssynergia, (4) ability of the detrusor muscle to contract, and (5) pelvic floor and external sphincter muscle activity.

Gastrointestinal Assessment

Bowel habits are unique and specific to the individual. The presence of a neurogenic disorder complicates the individual's predisability bowel regimen. A logical, rational, and comprehensive assessment of bowel function must be instituted, therefore, before an effective approach can be planned or a bowel management program can be implemented. Often, bowel programs are instituted without adequate assessment and planning in regard to the unique needs of the individual. A program based on trial and error is discouraging for the individual as well as for the nurse or care provider and is doomed to failure. Successful bowel management must be based on careful evaluation.

Physical Status

Physical status assessment includes evaluation of the neurologic status, abdominal status, mobility, and communication abilities.

Neurologic Status. The etiology of the disability, the current neurologic status, and the location and extent of the lesion are considered in determining the type of bowel dysfunction and, therefore, in planning an appropriate bowel program.

Sensory and motor examination is used to help diagnose the type of neurogenic bowel dysfunction present. *Saddle sensation* is a perianal sensation elicited by response to pinprick or light touch. It indicates intact sensory function at the sacral spinal cord level. The patient should be questioned about ability to sense the urge to defecate. The *bulbocavernous reflex* also indicates intact sacral cord function. The reflex is relayed through the pudendal nerves and is elicited when the glans penis or clitoris is squeezed. The reflex is present when contractions of the bulbocavernous and ischiocavernous muscles are felt, and there is a visible contraction of the external anal sphincter.

The anal reflex or anal "wink" is relayed through somatic pudendal nerves. This reflex consists of a visible contraction of the external anal sphincter in response to pinprick of the adjacent perianal skin.

Abdominal Assessment. Assessment of the abdomen assists in evaluation of elimination dysfunction, particularly in regard to constipation, diarrhea, and paralytic ileus. With the patient in a supine position, the entire abdomen is inspected for contour, symmetry, masses, peristalsis, and pulsation. Auscultation is performed in all four quadrants and the epigastrium, noting the frequency and character of bowel sounds. Bowel sounds may be increased with diarrhea or early intestinal obstruction and are absent in the presence of paralytic ileus. Percussion is useful for identification of air in the stomach or bowel. A tympanic percussion note may be associated with gaseous distention. If distention is suspected, the abdominal girth at the level of the umbilicus should be measured and serial comparisons should be made daily, with the examiner being alert for the absence of flatus. A dull sound on percussion of the descending colon may be due to accumulation of fecal material. Palpation is required to delineate abdominal organs and masses, to elicit areas of tenderness, and to evaluate for signs of constipation.

Activity Level. Physical activity and exercise generally promote peristalsis and bowel activity. If an individual is immobilized because of bedrest, functional limitations, or neurologic or orthopedic instability, bowel motility is slowed, and constipation results. The bowel program, therefore, will progress through different stages as functional abilities progress, making it important to keep in mind the prognosis of the disability. As activity levels increase, musculature and physiologic responses improve. The goals of bowel management progress from initially maintaining peristalsis and preventing obstruction to attaining a predictable bowel routine. Functional ability and muscle strength must be assessed in order to determine (1) the use of accessory muscles in exerting a Valsalva maneuver, (2) sitting tolerance, (3) trunk balance, and (4) ability to transfer to a bowel care chair or toilet. Hand function also must be considered in planning for the level of self-care ability in carrying out a bowel program.

Communication Ability. The ability to recognize and communicate must be evaluated. The aphasic patient may have communication difficulty that interferes with the ability to understand instructions about a bowel routine or to elicit meaningful responses about toileting needs.

History
Concomitant medical history, nutrition history, bowel history, and medication history are all important in determining factors influencing elimination.

Concomitant Medical Conditions. The presence of concurrent or previous medical conditions, such as diverticular disease, bowel surgery, anal fissures or abscesses, hemorrhoids, ulcerative colitis, cancer, diabetes, psychiatric history, or depression, and the effects of the aging process must be assessed for any relationship to the current elimination problem.

Nutrition History. Diet assessment includes meal patterns and routines and food preferences, with consideration of cultural influences on diet, fluid intake, and type of food that caused an alteration in the normal bowel patterns before the disability. Foods that promoted regular evacuation or upset the individual's bowel routine previously will likely have similar effects after the onset of neurologic dysfunction. In addition, mechanical problems, such as teeth in poor repair or ill-fitting dentures, may cause mastication problems and the avoidance of foods that would otherwise be encouraged to promote an adequate bowel regimen.

Neurologic deficits that affect facial and tongue sensation or interfere with the swallowing process may compromise an adequate diet. Roughage may be particularly deficient, causing further digestion and evacuation problems. Tube feedings may increase the frequency of evacuations or cause stools of loose consistency, further complicating a regular bowel routine. Disorders that create dependence on others for feeding may interfere with food and fluid intake. Functional limitations of the upper extremities and positional restrictions may decrease the food and fluid intake.

The examiner must assess the fluid intake to determine if it is adequate to prevent constipation. Water is reabsorbed into the systemic circulation from the stool in the proximal colon. If fluid intake is inadequate, hard, dry stool will result. A fluid intake of 2,000 to 3,000 ml/day is recommended to maintain a stool of soft, yet formed consistency. One must also consider the type of bladder management program the individual is on. Fluids may be restricted during an intermittent catheterization program, and planning for the bowel program must take this into account.

Bowel History. Previous bowel habits, including the history of any gastrointestinal disorders, must be reviewed with the patient. Bowel habits that were healthful and workable previously should be continued insofar as possible. In particular, frequency and time of day when evacuation usually occurs should be noted. Specific methods previously used to stimulate defecation, such as warm beverages or certain foods, should be determined. Problems encountered in the past, such as constipation, diarrhea, or incontinence, precipitating factors, and how these problems were dealt with should be included in the data collection. It must be kept in mind that such terms as "diarrhea" or "constipation" have different meanings to different people. It is, therefore, important to ascertain specifically the individual's interpretation. A history of laxative or enema usage or taking of medications that have a constipating effect should be explored.

One must assess how the bowel pattern has changed since the onset of the present illness or disability. Is incontinence due to an alteration of the defecation process secondary to the neurologic lesion, a communication problem, functional limitations, or environmental factors? The presence of a fecal impaction, paralytic ileus, or an obstruction must also be determined. The person's ability to differentiate between the presence of stool or gas, as well as the ability to hold the stool after feeling the urge to defecate, needs to be assessed.

Description of the character of the stool will aid in planning an appropriate bowel management program. A normal stool is softly formed and has a composition of 75% water and 25% solid materials (Zejdlik, 1983). It should be noted if the stool is hard or dry and difficult to pass or loose and watery, with spontaneous evacuation occurring between planned intervals. The presence of frank blood in the stool or dark, tarry stools warrant further investigation.

Medication History. Medications that affect elimination may cause either constipation or diarrhea. Anticholinergics, antihypertensive agents, analgesics, tranquilizers, anticonvulsants, and certain antacids containing calcium or aluminum may have a constipating effect. Antibiotics may deplete the bowel of normal flora and can contribute to diarrhea. Habitual use of laxatives or enemas can cause atony of the rectal musculature, which results in decreased awareness of rectal sensation. Decreased appreciation of the urge to defecate can cause further constipation.

Diagnostic Tests

In the presence of abdominal tenderness, distention, or increased or absent bowel sounds, an abdominal x-ray will help to rule out bowel obstruction. The condition of the intestinal pathways and the extent and location of intestinal distention will be revealed.

Barium enema and proctosigmoidoscopy are performed when an acute change in bowel habits has occurred that is inconsistent with changes expected secondary to the neurologic dysfunction or when there is blood in the stool. The purpose of these tests is to help rule out other organic causes, such as cancer of the colon, ulcerative colitis, or diverticulitis.

Chemical and microscopic examination will determine the presence of occult blood or the actual composition of the stool. If diarrhea persists and cannot be explained as a result of antibiotic therapy, fecal impaction, or dietary factors, a gram stain, stool culture, or test for ova and parasites is useful to determine the source of an intestinal infection.

REFERENCES

Benda, S. (Ed.). (1983). *Spinal cord injury. Nursing education-suggested content.* Chicago: American Spinal Injury Foundation.

Boroch, R.M. (1976). *Elements of rehabilitation in nursing. An introduction.* St. Louis: Mosby.

Crouch, J.E. (1965). *Functional human anatomy.* Philadelphia: Lea & Febiger.

Friedland, G. W., & Perkash, I. (1983). Neuromuscular dysfunction of the bladder and urethra. *Seminars in Roentgenology, 18,* 255.

Ganong, W. F. (1987). *Review of medical physiology* (13th ed.). E. Norwalk, CT, Appleton & Lange.

Guyton, A.C. (1987). *Basic neuroscience: Anatomy and physiology*. Philadelphia: Saunders.

Guyton, A.C. (1981). *Textbook of medical physiology* (6th ed). Philadelphia: Saunders.

Nathan, P.D. (1976). The central nervous connections of the bladder. In D.I. Williams & G.D. Chisholm (Eds.), *Scientific foundations of urology: Vol. II. Urogenital tract, oncology and urological armamentarium* (p. 51). Chicago: Year Book.

Perkash, I. (1982). Management of neurogenic dysfunction of the bladder and bowel. In F.J. Kottke, G.K. Stillwell, & J.F. Lehman (Eds.). *Krusen's handbook of physical medicine and rehabilitation* (3rd ed) (p. 724). Philadelphia: Saunders.

Sayles, S.M. (Ed.). (1981). *Rehabilitation nursing: Concepts and practice—A core curriculum*. Evanston, IL: Rehabilitation Nursing Institute.

Staas, W.E. Jr., & DeNault, P.M. (1973). Bowel control. *American Family Physician 7*(1), 90.

Tanagho, E.A. (1976). The ureterovesical junction: Anatomy and physiology. In D.I. Williams & G.D. Chisholm (Eds.), *Scientific foundations of urology: Vol. II. Urogenital tract, oncology and urological armamentarium* (p. 23). Chicago: Year Book.

Tempkin, A., Sullivan, G., Paldi, J., & Perkash, F. (1985). Radioisotope renography in spinal cord injury. *Journal of Urology 133*, 228.

Zejdlik, C.P. (1983). *Management of spinal cord injury*. Belmont, MA: Wadsworth.

Zinner, N.R., Ritter, R.C., & Sterling, A.M. (1976). The mechanism of micturition. In D.I. Williams & G.D. Chisholm (Eds.), *Scientific foundations of urology: Vol. II Urogenital tract, oncology and the urological armamentarium* (p. 39). Chicago: Year Book.

28

Alterations in Bladder Elimination

Janet Giroux

A variety of neurologic disorders can cause bladder dysfunction and impair urinary elimination. "Neurologic dysfunction of the bladder can result whenever a lesion or trauma compromises the function of the higher voiding centers in the brain, the ascending and descending pathways in the spinal cord, the S2–S4 of the spinal cord, or the micturition reflex arc" (Johnson, 1980, p. 294). The result is failure in the micturition process that affects either the storage or emptying capability of the bladder. The location and extent of the trauma or injury have a direct effect on the type and degree of neurogenic dysfunction.

The nursing diagnosis "alteration in patterns of urinary elimination" (Kim et al., 1984) is too broad to guide nursing management in patients with neurogenic bladder dysfunction. Specific retraining techniques are required for each type of elimination dysfunction. The key to effective nursing management, therefore, is to understand the type of neurogenic mechanism involved and establish a plan that enables the patient to achieve and maintain an acceptable urinary elimination pattern. This understanding can be best achieved by thinking of the types of neurogenic bladder as etiologies for the broad categories of altered urinary pattern.

HUMAN RESPONSES TO NEUROGENIC BLADDER DYSFUNCTION

Neurogenic bladder dysfunction has been classified into five major types based on the response or action of the bladder rather than on the location of the lesion (Lapides, 1970): *uninhibited, reflex, autonomous, motor paralytic,* and *sensory paralytic.* Although the majority of voiding dysfunctions can be placed into these general categories, mixed lesions can occur. For each type of bladder dysfunction, use of the nursing process is indicated to make a nursing diagnosis and plan appropriate interventions. General assessment techniques are described in Chapter 27. This chapter describes each type of bladder dysfunction and illustrates assessment and intervention strategies that assist the neuroscience nurse in managing specific alterations in bladder elimination. Table 28–1 depicts elements of the nursing process in relation to Lapides' categories of bladder dysfunction.

TABLE 28–1. SUMMARY OF NEUROGENIC BLADDER DYSFUNCTION AND MANAGEMENT TECHNIQUES.

Pathophysiology	Symptoms	Physical Findings	Bladder Retraining Methods	Adjuvant Medications
Uninhibited Neurogenic Bladder[a]: Defect in corticoregulatory pathways	Urinary frequency, urgency, and uninhibited contractions	Sensation intact, Bulbocavernous reflex normal	Timed voiding schedule	Anticholinergics to decrease uninhibited contractions
Reflex Neurogenic Bladder: Lesion above S2–S4 segments	Involuntary reflex voiding	Sensation absent, Bulbocavernous reflex hyperactive	Stimulation of reflex voiding through suprapubic tapping	Alpha adrenergic blockers to decrease urethral resistance
Autonomous Neurogenic Bladder: Lesion involves S2–S4 segments	Varies from constant urinary dribbling to overflow incontinence	Sensation absent Bulbocavernous reflex absent	Stimulation of voiding through Credé-Valsalva maneuver	Alpha adrenergics to increase urethral resistance
Motor Paralytic Neurogenic Bladder: Lesion involves anterior horn cells and anterior roots of segments S2–S4	Ability to perceive bladder fullness but unable to initiate voiding May strain to void	Sensation intact Bulbocavernous reflex variable	Stimulation of voiding through Credé-Valsalva maneuver	Cholinergics useful in partial motor paralysis only, ineffective in complete motor lesions
Sensory Paralytic Neurogenic Bladder: Lesion involves dorsal horn cells or dorsal roots of S2–S4 segments	Inability to perceive bladder fullness but can initiate voiding May have overflow incontinence if chronically overdistended	Sensation intact Bulbocavernous reflex diminished or absent	Timed voiding schedule	Cholinergics to increase detrusor contractions

[a]Types of neurogenic bladders as delineated by Lapides 1970.
Adapted from Johnson, 1980.

Nursing Diagnoses

☐ **Urinary Frequency, Urgency, or Hesitancy Related to Uninhibited Neurogenic Bladder**

The primary cause of the uninhibited neurogenic bladder is a defect in the corticoregulatory pathways, leading to a disruption of the inhibitory efferent impulses from the higher brain centers (Fig. 28–1). Involvement of these pathways that control inhibition results in frequent, uninhibited bladder contractions that can decrease bladder capacity. The lesion may be present at the cortical origin of the tract and be produced by a cerebrovascular accident (CVA) or brain tumor that affects the medial cortex. In the spinal cord, the pathways transmitting inhibitory impulses to the bladder may be involved by tumor, trauma, or a demyelinating disease, such as multiple sclerosis (MS). *Defining characteristics* include urinary frequency, urgency, and hesitancy. A routine neurourologic assessment, as outlined in Chapter 27, would give the nurse data to begin formulating a nursing diagnosis and

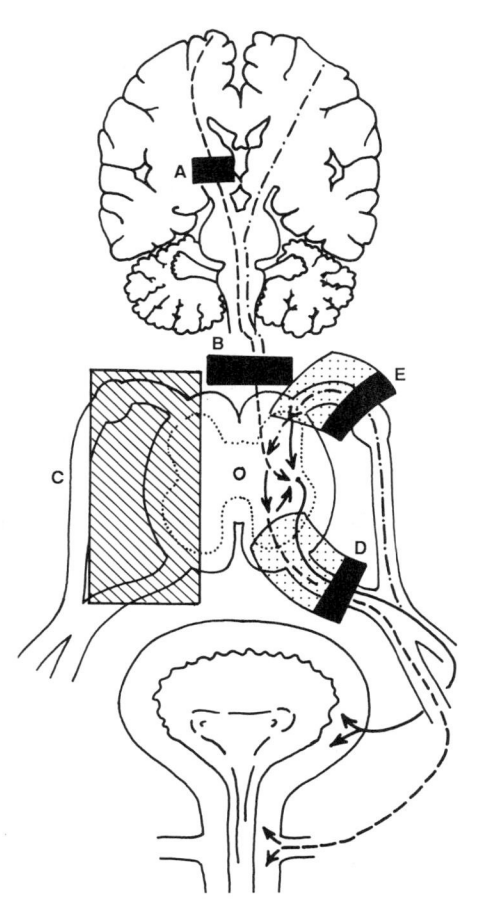

Fig. 28–1. Types of bladder dysfunction related to level of lesion in nervous system. Sensory input is indicated by the •———• key. Lesions at point A or anywhere along the corticobulbar spinal tract produce uninhibited neurogenic bladder. Lesions that transect the spinal cord above the sacral level (B) produce reflex neurogenic bladder. Autonomous neurogenic bladder is produced by lesions that involve both limbs of the spinal reflex arc (C), whereas motor paralytic neurogenic bladder occurs with lesions of the motor cells or efferents (D). Sensory paralytic neurogenic bladder occurs when sensory efferents from the bladder, dorsal horn cells, or sensory tracts to the brain are impaired (E).

subsequent interventions. On examination, bladder sensation is usually intact, and the bulbocavernous reflex is normal. The cystometrogram will show uninhibited detrusor contractions with a decreased bladder capacity.

Once the defining characteristics and alteration have been identified, *nursing intervention* can begin. The primary *goal* is to decrease or eliminate episodes of incontinence. A schedule of frequent timed toileting, based on the patient's bladder capacity and voiding pattern, would be appropriate to maintain low intravesical volumes and reduce bladder hyperactivity. A moderate fluid restriction, especially at night, might help control enuresis. Anticholinergic medications, such as propantheline bromide, may be recommended to decrease the number of uninhibited detrusor contractions and to enlarge the bladder capacity (Wein, 1979). The nurse, however, must be cognizant of the fact that this drug may cause partial or complete urinary retention and may be contraindicated in the elderly patient.

Case Study 1

Mr. S is a 40-year-old male admitted with exacerbation of his multiple sclerosis (MS). Mr. S has been experiencing more episodes of urinary frequency and urgency, with incontinence and occasional hesitancy. The cystometrogram shows uninhibited detrusor contraction at 100 ml. On examination, Mr. S has a normal bulbocavernous reflex and intact bladder sensation. From this information, the nurse knows the reflex arc is intact, since stimulated voiding is possible. Nursing interventions include instituting intake and output records and planning a timed toileting schedule based on Mr. S's bladder capacity and voiding pattern. For Mr. S to achieve an effective voiding technique, stimulation of trigger areas to induce reflex voiding is begun. For Mr. S, manual percussion or tapping of the suprapubic region facilitates maximum voiding. An every 3 hour voiding schedule is necessary initially to avoid incontinence.

To decrease urinary hesitancy, Mr. S is taught such methods as running water from the tap and relaxation techniques. Pharmacologic management includes a trial of propantheline bromide to reduce bladder contractility and increase bladder capacity. As Mr. S's bladder capacity increases, an every 4 to 5 hour voiding schedule becomes sufficient. Additional important teaching areas would include (1) potential side effects of propantheline; (2) monitoring urinary output; (3) adhering to a timed voiding schedule; and (4) limiting fluids after dinner if nocturia is a problem.

☐ Incomplete Involuntary Bladder Emptying Related to Reflex Neurogenic Bladder

Lesions or trauma to the spinal cord above the S2–S4 segments may cause this reflex neurogenic bladder, which results from complete disruption of the motor and sensory tracts (Fig. 28–1). Other neurologic causes include MS, meningitis, and spinal tumors. Since the micturition or reflex arc remains intact, voiding is reflexive in nature but involuntary. Clinically, the patient has no perception of bladder filling or sensation, residual urine is usually increased, and voluntary voiding is not possible. A hyperactive bulbocavernous reflex is elicited. Cystometry reveals uninhibited bladder contractions that may occur at any volume. Combined cystometry and electromyography discloses two basic patterns of bladder and sphincter activity: the coordinated and the uncoordinated. The coordinated bladder and sphincter illustrate reflex bladder contraction and simultaneous relaxation of the periurethral muscles, thereby allowing low pressure emptying. Uncoordinated bladder and sphincter, which is generally the rule (Koff et al., 1979), is known as detrusor sphincter dyssynergia (DSD). During detrusor contraction, the periurethral muscles also contract. This contraction causes increased resistance to outflow and results in high intravesical pressure, high residual urine, and poor emptying.

The *desired outcome* for a patient with a reflex neurogenic bladder is to achieve a catheter-free, reflex voiding state with a urinary residual under 100 ml. In the initial phase of *retraining*, intermittent catheterization (IC) is an appropriate method to effect adequate bladder emptying while avoiding the problems of overdistention or vesicoureteral reflux. A bladder retraining program would emphasize regular bladder emptying. The nurse and the patient work together to discover the most appropriate triggering mechanism to stimulate reflex voiding. Recently, transrectal sonography, as a diagnostic and teaching tool, has shown that suprapubic tapping is the most effective way to trigger and empty reflex bladders (Perkash & Friedland, 1984).

Based on the results of urodynamic testing, pharmacologic manipulation might be necessary to promote effective voiding. For a weakened detrusor muscle that cannot override a stronger external urethral sphincter, a cholinergic medication, such as bethanechol chloride, can be useful (Perkash, 1982). It should be noted, however, that this drug is contraindicated in patients with urinary outlet obstruction or patients with spastic bladders. In the case of increased urethral resistance and evidence of dyssynergia, alpha adrenergic blockers, such as prazosin, can reduce bladder neck and sphincter spasticity. If the patient does not respond to medical management, a transurethral sphincterotomy may become necessary (Perkash, 1978). This procedure surgically reduces bladder neck and periurethral striated sphincter resistance and permits more adequate emptying. In some cases, however, this may result in some degree of incontinence, loss of erectile ability, or retrograde ejaculation. It is essential that the physician inform the patient of these possibilities before a surgical decision is made.

Once a balanced bladder state and reflex voiding are achieved through either bladder retraining, medication, surgery, or a combination of these, an external method of urinary collection usually is required. For the male patient, this does not usually present a problem, since there are many types of external catheter devices from which to choose. For the female, however, there is not an acceptable external collection device at present, and a sphincterotomy is not a viable choice. Remaining choices are limited to continued intermittent catheterization, an indwelling catheter, or incontinence pads. Generally, incontinence pads or garments should be used with discretion in all females, especially asensory patients, because of the potential risk of skin breakdown.

Case Study 2
Mr. M is a 20-year-old C6 to C7 quadriplegic recently injured in a diving accident. On admission, he has an indwelling catheter for bladder management. An intermittent catheterization program every 4 hours is instituted. Twenty-four hour intake and output recordings are started, with fluids restricted to 100 ml per hour. After resolution of the spinal shock phase, some reflex bladder activity is observed. The nurse stimulates triggered voiding before each intermittent catheterization by suprapubic tapping. Because his level of injury precludes fine hand movement, Mr. M is taught to use the ulnar surface of his hand to initiate suprapubic tapping when he is in an upright position. With increased spontaneous and stimulated voiding, Mr. M's catheterizations are reduced in frequency to every 6 hours and then to every 8 hours.

Residual urines, however, remain greater than 250 ml, and Mr. M occasionally displays signs of autonomic dysreflexia, that is, sweating above his level of injury, headache, and rise in blood pressure. Nursing interventions use knowledge of the signs and symptoms of dysreflexia, causes, and appropriate actions. During an episode of dysreflexia, the nurse would elevate the head of Mr. M's bed, monitor his blood pressure and pulse, and check for the source of the stimuli. In the case of urologic involvement, the bladder must be assessed for overdistention caused by kinked or plugged catheters, full drainage bags, or a full bladder. After manual stimulation produces no bladder emptying, the nurse catheterizes Mr. M, with resolution of the dysreflexic symptoms. The physiology of autonomic dysreflexia is discussed in Chapter 29.

Mr. M's cystometrogram shows evidence of DSD from a pattern of uncoordinated bladder and sphincter activity. This may have contributed to Mr. M's continued episodes of dysreflexia. Left untreated, DSD could eventually lead to vesicoureteral reflux and kidney damage. A trial of prazosin, an alpha adrenergic blocker, is begun, but Mr. M's residual urines remain high, and occasional dysreflexic symptoms persist. After weighing all the facts, Mr. M decided on a sphincterotomy to eliminate bladder neck and urethral obstruction. Postoperatively, Mr. M is instructed on the importance of regular, timed reflex bladder triggering. Since Mr. M has limited hand and finger function, a self-adhesive external catheter is recommended. This allows Mr. M to maintain maximum self-care skills and increase his independence.

Additional areas of instruction would focus on (1) daily inspection of penile skin for cuts or abrasions, (2) daily perineal hygiene and condom change to reduce risks of bladder infection, (3) signs and symptoms of urinary infection, (4) importance of fluid intake (2,500 to 3,000 ml/day) including fluids that help to acidify the urine, and (5) daily cleaning of the urinary drainage bags with a disinfectant solution.

☐ **Urinary Retention and Overflow Incontinence Related to Autonomous Neurogenic Bladder**

In the autonomous neurogenic bladder, the reflex arc (S2–S4) is lost, affecting both the motor and sensory components (Fig. 28–1). Damage to the conus medullaris or cauda equina will eliminate all reflex bladder activity. Etiologic factors include (1) traumatic or nontraumatic spinal cord lesions, (2) spinal shock after acute spinal cord transection, (3) infection, and (4) surgical procedures (abdominoperineal resection). The patient cannot perceive bladder distention and is not able to initiate voiding voluntarily. Because of this loss of bladder and sphincter tone, urinary retention, accompanied by high residual urines, leads to overflow incontinence. A history of straining to void and an absent bulbocavernous reflex would assist in the diagnosis of an autonomous or areflexic bladder. The cystometrogram reveals no detrusor contractions, complete or partial denervation of the periurethral striated muscles, and a variable bladder capacity.

Nursing interventions should be directed toward preventing an overdistended bladder by reducing residual urines and managing incontinence. Primary to effective management is institution of a voiding schedule to empty the bladder regularly when a capacity of approximately 350 ml is reached. In the completely denervated bladder, voiding can be accomplished with the use of Credé and Valsalva maneuvers. The Credé maneuver involves external manual pressure applied over the bladder to force urine out. The Valsalva maneuver can be used in conjunction with the Credé maneuver to increase intraabdominial pressure. If feasible, the patient should be taught abdominal strengthening exercises. Normally, this type of bladder is unresponsive to drug therapy. In some patients, however, urinary incontinence between timed bladder emptyings may be controlled by increasing urethral resistance with an alpha adrenergic drug (Wein, 1979). If incomplete voiding cannot be overcome with these methods, intermittent catheterization usually becomes the treatment of choice.

Case Study 3

Ms. A is a 45-year-old female who has developed urinary retention and overflow incontinence after acute transverse myelitis. After urodynamic studies, Ms. A is diagnosed as having an autonomous bladder with complete motor and sensory loss. Intermittent catheterization (IC) is initially started every 4 hours in efforts to keep residual urines under 350 ml. Fluid intake is limited to 100 ml/hour to avoid bladder overdistention, and intake and output records are monitored. As stimulated voiding volumes increase and residual urines remain consistently below 100 ml, Ms. A's intermittent catheterizations are discontinued. A normal sitting position is encouraged to facilitate voiding, and a program to strengthen abdominal muscles is begun. In order to maintain a bladder capacity of approximately 350 ml, the nurse works with Ms. A to determine her voiding schedule by correlating fluid intake with predicted urinary output.

Even though the bladder program is successful in the hospital, Ms. A elects to manage her elimination disorder with an indwelling catheter. Mrs. A feels that her hectic work and travel schedule would not afford her the opportunity to adhere to a rigid bladder emptying schedule. The nurse instructs Ms. A on insertion and care techniques of an indwelling catheter, as well as proper positioning and taping to reduce urethral damage. Other predischarge information includes (1) the risk of catheter-associated ascending bacteriuria, (2) signs and symptoms of urinary infection, (3) fluid intake of at least 3,000 ml/day, (4) daily perineal hygiene and drainage bag care, and (5) catheter management for sexual activity.

☐ **Urinary Retention with Intact Sensation Related to Motor Paralytic Bladder**

Damage to the anterior horn cells or anterior roots of the S2–S4 segments is the cause of motor paralytic bladder (Fig. 28–1). Even though motor function is lost, bladder and perineal sensations remain intact. The patient senses bladder fullness but is not able to initiate voiding. Spinal cord injury, poliomyelitis, Guillain-Barré syndrome, and tumor are some causative factors. The patient may be unable to void except when straining or may have painful bladder distension in the acute stage or overflow incontinence. Cystometric findings are similar to those found in the autonomous bladder except that there is normal exteroceptive and proprioceptive sensation.

Preventing bladder overdistention in the acute phase, either through urethral catheter or intermittent catheterization, is essential. During the rehabilitative phase, the nurse should implement similar techniques for bladder retraining, for example, Credé–Valsalva maneuvers and abdominal strengthening exercises, as are used with autonomous bladders. With motor paralytic bladder, however, the patient has the advantage of bladder sensation and can more readily assess when emptying is necessary. Intermittent catheterization may be a management option if acceptable residual urines are not achieved.

Case Study 4

Mr. C, a 60-year-old male, developed a motor paralytic bladder as a result of Guillain-Barré syndrome. Initially, his bladder elimination was managed by an indwelling urethral catheter to prevent overdistention. The urologic workup revealed a complete motor paralysis of the bladder, and Mr. C chose intermittent catheterization management rather than the use of the Credé–Valsalva maneuver. An every 4 hour intermittent catheterization schedule is begun to assess the amount of residual urine. Mr. C is instructed to become aware of any bladder filling sensations that will assist in regulating his voiding schedule. After evaluation of intake and output records and residual urines, Mr. C's intermittent catheterizations are decreased to every 6 hours. This timing schedule allows for residual urines of under 400 ml without any leakage between catheterizations. A 12 or 14 French straight catheter should be used to minimize urethral trauma due to repeated catheterizations.

Important aspects to stress during bladder retraining include adhering to a catheterization schedule to prevent overdistention, limiting fluids to 2,000 ml to decrease episodes of incontinence, and maintaining sterility during the catheterization procedure. When Mr. C is ready for discharge, changing the intermittent catheterization to a clean procedure would be appropriate.

☐ Difficulty Initiating Urination or Urinary Retention Related to Sensory Paralytic Bladder

Any disease process that interrupts the sensory limb of the lower reflex arc or the long afferent tracts to the brain may result in a sensory paralytic bladder (Fig. 28–1). Perception of bladder fullness is lost, but the patient has voluntary control over voiding. This motor function, however, may be severely compromised if the bladder has become atonic from prolonged periods of overdistention. A sensory paralytic bladder is most often seen in peripheral neuropathy secondary to diabetes mellitis, tabes dorsalis, or pernicious anemia. The onset may be insidious at first, with complaints of difficulty in starting a stream, decrease in size and force of stream, and infrequent voiding pattern. Yet as lack of sensation progresses, overdistention from retained urine causes development of atonicity and decompensation of the bladder musculature.

On examination, *defining characteristics* are a palpable bladder, diminished or absent perineal sensation, and variable bulbocavernous reflex. The cystometrogram will demonstrate no uninhibited detrusor contractions, with an increased bladder capacity.

After testing and *assessment, nursing interventions* are based on degree of bladder contractility. If the bladder has not decompensated from persistent high urine residuals, a planned voiding schedule would be the essential part of the bladder retraining program. The patient should be instructed to void every 2 to 3 hours instead of waiting for a sensation of bladder fullness. A nighttime voiding schedule is important to prevent overdistention. If bladder decompensation has already occurred, a trial of bethanechol chloride might be beneficial. The cholinergic effect of this drug strengthens the contractility of the bladder muscle to produce more effective bladder emptying. The nurse must be aware of the potential gastrointestinal side effects of this drug. Such side effects might require reduction in dosage or discontinuation of use. If bladder retraining through frequent voiding, with or without adjuvant medication, fails, intermittent catheterization becomes necessary.

Case Study 5

Mrs. R is a 55-year-old diabetic who has progressively developed peripheral neuropathy. She has noticed a decrease in perineal sensation with periods of incontinence, especially during exertion. Mrs. R also complains of an infrequent voiding schedule. Urodynamic studies show an enlarged bladder with an increased amount of residual urine. Mrs. R is responsive to a bethanecol chloride test and is given this cholinergic agent to improve her voiding. The nurse plans a timed 24-hour voiding schedule with Mrs. R. By limiting fluids after dinner, a voiding schedule that would allow maximum sleeping time but not compromise her bladder becomes possible. Mrs. R is catheterized after voiding to check for residual urine. These catheterizations are discontinued when urines of <100 ml are demonstrated. Since diabetes can increase the risk of developing bladder infections, the nurse instructs Mrs. R about the signs and symptoms of bacteriuria. Other predischarge teaching areas include (1) fluid intake of at least 2,000 ml/day, (2) daily perineal hygiene, and (3) the potential side effects of bethanechol chloride.

Psychosocial Concerns
Any alteration in urinary elimination is a natural source of concern for an individual. It may signify a loss of control over a very private bodily function and lower self-esteem. Disruption of daily routine and lifestyle, as well as work and family dynamics, can occur. Coping with these alterations and achieving acceptable forms of bladder elimination are of prime importance to the patient. To attain success, a bladder reconditioning program must be individualized, taking into consideration the patient's psychosocial, vocational, and physical needs. Personal preference is also a factor that cannot be overlooked.

The outcome of a bladder retraining program depends on a realistic plan and maximizing involvement of the patient and family. The nurse has a unique role in coordination of the patient's bladder rehabilitation program, incorporating essential components from all the disciplines involved in the team. By assessing the patient's total needs and including clinical and diagnostic findings, the nurse is able to assist the patient in a healthy adaptation to the genitourinary disorder. Within the realm of the team's therapeutic program, the knowledgeable and skilled nurse can help the patient choose the type of urinary drainage most suitable and plan a mutually workable regimen. It is important to remember that these adjustments, made initially in a hospital setting, must be adaptable to the patient's home and community environment. Anticipating these changes will benefit discharge planning and ensure a realistic management regimen for the patient.

Urinary Complications
Two primary goals in urologic rehabilitation are prevention of life-threatening complications and preservation of renal function. These goals should be ever present as the nurse assesses, formulates a diagnosis, plans interventions, and evaluates the patient with a urologic dysfunction. Because of the basic inability of the neurogenic bladder to empty effectively, these patients are prone to recurrent urinary tract infection, calculi formation, and overdistention. The nurse must be alert to the clinical signs of *urinary infection* and monitor urine cultures. Patient education would include (1) fluid intake of 2,500 to 3,000 ml/day, (2) observation of urine for change in color or odor and presence of sediment, (3) change in voiding pattern due to irritable infected bladder, (4) checking and maintenance of an acid pH, and (5) proper personal hygiene and appliance care. Since retained urine is usually the causative factor in overdistention and bacteriuria, providing effective drainage is essential (O'Flynn, 1978).

Another more subtle complication is *detrusor sphincter dyssynergia* (DSD). This incoordination of bladder and sphincter can cause bladder outlet obstruction and ineffective bladder emptying. If not diagnosed and recognized early, DSD will result in vesicoureteral reflux and, ultimately, parenchymal damage (Perkash, 1982). If pharmacologic management by alpha adrenergic blockers (e.g., prazosin) or other voiding techniques are not adequate, transurethral resection of the bladder neck and external sphincter may become necessary in male patients.

Untreated DSD may be the causative factor in autonomic dysreflexia. This syndrome usually affects spinal cord injured patients with neurologic lesions above the micturition reflex arc, specifically T7 and above. Stimulation of the sympathetic nervous system, usually from a distended bladder or bowel, leads to altered hemodynamics and a rise in arterial pressure. Normal vasodilation cannot occur because efferent impulses from the vasmotor center cannot be conducted beyond the level of the cord lesion. If not relieved, this continued vasoconstriction could precipitate severe hypertension, renal damage, or stroke. Knowledge of precipitating causes, symptoms, and appropriate nursing interventions are important aspects in the care of these patients.

Alternate Methods of Bladder Management

Part of the success in adjusting to any alteration in urinary elimination is allowing patient preference in choice of management regimen. Appropriate options should, of course, be presented, but the final choice is with the patient. If feasible, catheter-free methods are preferred to reduce the risk of catheter-associated morbidity, but this may not be practical in all patients. A female patient who continues to be incontinent despite medication, manipulation, and intermittent catheterization may have no other option but to use an indwelling catheter. Other methods include suprapubic cystostomy and ileal loop diversion. The risks and long-term management problems should be thoroughly reviewed with the patient before a final decision is made. Even for those male patients deciding on external urine collecting devices, a complete nursing evaluation is required to assure proper fit without leakage and skin irritation. During the initial trial period, the penis should be checked daily for signs of skin irritation from skin adhesives or from the condom itself. In some males, particularly those who are obese or elderly, retraction of the penis might cause a problem when wearing an external condom. Different styles and adhesive combinations should be tried to maximize holding ability before deciding that a method of drainage is a failure. The newer self-adhesive external catheters have shown promise in some males with retraction difficulties. Regardless of which urinary option is chosen, a teaching program that includes patient and family return demonstrations is vital as a prerequisite to discharge.

Helping the patient cope and adjust to a voiding dysfunction is fundamental in the scope of nursing practice. Through theory-based practice, the neuroscience nurse can play a vital role in coordinating a comprehensive management program focused on alterations in bladder elimination.

REFERENCES

Johnson, J.H. (1980). Rehabilitation aspects of neurologic bladder dysfunction. *Nursing Clinics of North America, 15*(2), 293.

Kim, M.J., McFarland, G., & McLane, A. (1984). *Classification of nursing diagnoses.* St. Louis: Mosby.

Koff, S.A., Diokno, A.C., & Lapides, J. (1979). Neurogenic bladder dysfunction. *American Family Physician, 19,* 100.

Lapides, J. (1970). Neuromuscular vesical and ureteral dysfunction. In M.F. Campbell and J.H. Harrison (Eds.), *Urology* (3rd ed.) (p. 1343). Philadelphia: Saunders.

O'Flynn, J.D. (1978). Early and late management of the neuropathic bladder in spinal cord injury patients. *Journal of Urology, 120,* 726.

Perkash, I. (1978). Intermittent catheterization failure and an approach to bladder rehabilitation in spinal cord injury patients. *Archives of Physical Medicine and Rehabilitation, 59,* 9.

Perkash, I. (1982). Management of neurogenic dysfunction of the bladder and bowel. In F.J. Kottle, G.K. Stillwell, & J.F. Legman (Eds.), *Krusen's handbook of physical medicine and rehabilitation* (3rd ed.) (p. 724). Philadelphia: Saunders.

Perkash, I., & Friedland, G.W. (1984). Using transrectal sonography to teach patients with spinal cord injuries to retrain their bladders. *Radiology, 152,* 228.

Wein, A.J. (1979). Pharmacologic approaches to the management of neurogenic bladder dysfunction. *JCE Urology, 18,* 17.

BIBLIOGRAPHY

Friedland, G.W., Perkash, I. (1983). Neuromuscular dysfunction of the bladder and urethra. *Seminars in Roentgenology, 18,* 255.

Martin, N., Holt, N.B., & Hicks, D. (Eds.). (1981). *Comprehensive rehabilitation nursing.* New York: McGraw-Hill.

Nursing skillbook. Coping with neurological problems proficiently. (1979). Horsham, NJ: Intermed Communication.

Rudy, E.B. (1984). *Advanced neurological and neurosurgical nursing.* St. Louis: Mosby.

Vogt, G., Miller, M., & Esluer, M. (1985). *Mosby's manual of neurological care.* St. Louis: Mosby.

Wein, A.J. (1981). Classification of neurogenic voiding dysfunction. *Journal of Urology, 125,* 605.

Zejdlik, C.P. (1983). Maintaining urinary function. *Management of spinal cord injury* (p. 269). Monterey, CA: Wadsworth Health Services Division.

29

Alterations in Bowel Elimination

Linda L. Toth

Patterns of normal bowel elimination may be altered as a result of neurologic disorders, such as a cerebrovascular accident (CVA), a spinal cord lesion, multiple sclerosis, diabetes, or poliomyelitis. Such disorders may directly compromise bowel function or voluntary control of defecation, and, thereby, affect the pattern of elimination. An interruption of the nerve pathways between the brain, the spinal cord, and the gastrointestinal system results in impaired bowel control as a result of loss of cerebral awareness and the ability to inhibit defecation, loss of anal sphincter control, or loss of anal sphincter sensation. The term *neurogenic bowel* is used to describe the dysfunction that occurs as a result of this interruption in the neural pathways. The location and extent of the lesion determines what type of neurogenic bowel is present. Assessment of bowel function and of defecation patterns was presented in Chapter 27.

HUMAN RESPONSES TO NEUROGENIC BOWEL DYSFUNCTION

Neurogenic bowel may be defined as a bowel dysfunction that occurs as a result of an interruption of the neural pathways that supply the rectum, external sphincter, and accessory muscles for defecation and that results in an inability to inhibit or initiate evacuation. Five classifications of neurogenic bowel dysfunction, based on the location of the neural lesion, are discussed; unhibited, reflex, autonomous, motor paralytic, and sensory paralytic. These categories, their neural correlates, related disease states, and associated signs and symptoms are shown in Table 29–1.

Uninhibited Bowel (Cortical and Subcortical Lesions)

Central nervous system lesions that occur at the cortical and subcortical level are associated with cerebrovascular accidents (CVA), multiple sclerosis (MS), head injuries, and brain tumors. This type of lesion results in an *uninhibited bowel*. Because the lesion is above the level of the spinal cord, the sacral reflex arc and perianal sensation are intact, but cerebral inhibitory or facilitory interpretation of sensory impulses to defecate is interrupted.

As the rectum is distended with feces, the spinal sacral reflex initiates defecation. In the presence of a cortical lesion, awareness of

TABLE 29-1. LEVELS OF NEURAXIAL DYSFUNCTION AFFECTING DEFECATION.

Bowel Function	Level in Neuraxis	Possible Etiology	Upper Motor Neuron Lesion	Lower Motor Neuron Lesion	Sensory Loss	Saddle Sensation	Bulbo-cavernous Reflex	Fecal Incontinence
Uninhibited neurogenic	Cortical and subcortical	CVA, MS, brain tumor, brain trauma	+	0	0	Normal	Normal or increased	Present—associated with sudden urge
Reflex neurogenic	Spinal cord above conus medullaris	Trauma, tumor, vascular disease, MS, syringomyelia, pernicious anemia	+	0	+	Diminished or absent	Increased	Present—occurs without warning or during mass reflex
Autonomous neurogenic	Conus medullaris or cauda equina	Spina bifida, trauma, tumor, intervertebral disk	0	+	+	Diminished or absent	0	Present—may be continuous or may occur during stress
Motor paralytic	Anterior horn cells or S2, S3, S4 roots (ventral)	Poliomyelitis, intervertebral disk, trauma, tumor	0	+	0	Normal	0	Rare, except in widespread disease
Sensory paralytic	S2, S3, S4 roots (dorsal), cells of origin or dorsal horns of spinal cord	Diabetes mellitus, tabes dorsalis	0	0	+	Diminished or absent	Normal, decreased or absent	Rare, except in advanced stages

From Staas & DeNault, 1973.

sensory input from a distended rectum and urge to defecate are diminished, and there is decreased voluntary control of the external anal sphincter. A sense of urgency and involuntary elimination or incontinence occur because the sacral reflex acts alone without inhibition from higher cerebral centers.

☐ **Urgency or Bowel Incontinence Related to Uninhibited Neurogenic Bowel**

In uninhibited neurogenic bowel, there is no sensory loss, bowel sensations are not impaired, saddle sensation is normal, the bulbocavernous reflex is intact or increased, and fecal incontinence associated with a sudden urge is present.

Nursing interventions focus on establishment of a habit pattern of elimination. The individual with a cerebral lesion may have difficulty integrating stimuli and a decreased attention span and may be easily distracted and have speech and language deficits. Therefore, the program must be geared toward a basic routine that the individual can master.

During the acute stage of recovery from a cerebral hemorrhage as well as in the presence of hypertension or cardiovascular disease, the importance of preventing straining during evacuation is stressed. At this stage, immobility, lack of diet roughage, or sedation contributes to constipation. Maintaining an accurate elimination record assists in monitoring the evacuation pattern. Stool softeners or occasional mild laxatives may be necessary to prevent constipation, although their use should be temporary and replaced with a high fiber diet and adequate fluids when the individual's condition permits.

Rectal suppositories may be used initially to establish a habit time by intensifying rectal sensation and increasing awareness of the urge to defecate. Glycerin suppositories act by irritating the rectal mucosa. The resulting increase in mucus secretion lubricates the feces. Such suppositories are generally effective in stimulating planned defecation in the uninhibited bowel. Frequency of use is based on preexisting bowel habits, if they are healthful, as well as present needs (see the section "Principles of Bowel Management" in this chapter for suppository administration procedures). As the individual demonstrates an awareness of the urge to defecate, a consistent pattern of adequate evacuation is established and the occurrence of incontinence between planned evacuation has subsided, the routine use of suppositories should be discontinued (Martin et al., 1981).

As the individual's condition stabilizes and physical activity and functional ability increase, the emphasis is on establishment of a persistent, predictable elimination routine. The bowel retraining program at this point should include consistent timing, taking advantage of the gastrocolic reflex, a diet high in fiber with adequate fluid intake, and encouragement of physical activity.

Goals for this diagnosis are compliance with a comprehensive and consistent program and absence of constipation and incontinence.

Case Study 1

Mrs. C, a 63-year-old right-handed woman came to the emergency room with left-sided weakness and slurred speech. The symptoms had progressed since their onset the previous morning shortly after she arose from bed. Findings included left hemiparesis with diminished position sense and stereogenesis of the left hand, left homonymous hemianopsia, and Babinski reflex on the left. A diagnosis of a right CVA secondary to thrombosis of the right middle cerebral artery was made. Mrs. C had a history of untreated transient ischemic attacks (TIA) persisting for the past 2 to 3 months. She had been treated for hypertension.

Mrs. C was admitted to the neurologic unit. Her nursing care plan, which focused on immediate as well as long-term physical, functional, and psychosocial needs, included the nursing diagnosis: potential constipation and fecal impaction, an altered bowel elimination pattern exhibited by a person with a cerebral lesion. Expected outcomes included the establishment of a habit pattern of elimination in which a persistent and consistent approach was used in order to encourage Mrs. C to focus attention on elimination.

During the acute recovery stages, Mrs. C's nursing care focused on maintenance of normal body functions. The bowel management program, in particular, was directed toward prevention of constipation and fecal impaction. A comprehensive nursing assessment included investigation of previous bowel habits, nutrition, and diet history. She had been accustomed to a daily evacuation in the morning. Her present neurologic and physical status was reviewed. Saddle sensation and bulbocavernous reflex were intact. The gag reflex was intact. She was initially on bedrest. After 48 hours, it was determined that there was no further neurologic deficit, and nutrition advanced from intravenous to a regular diet as tolerated. The left-sided hemiparesis persisted. When solid foods were tolerated, Mrs. C. was encouraged to feed herself while sitting in a high Fowler's position. She was encouraged to place food in the right side of the mouth because of left lower facial muscle weakness involving the mouth and cheek.

At this point, Mrs. C's bowel program consisted of 30 ml of milk of magnesia at bedtime followed by a glycerin suppository in the morning after breakfast to coincide with the gastrocolic reflex and previous patterns. An elimination record was started. Her stool was soft and firm, negating the need for a stool softener. She had a sense of urgency just previous to defecation, resulting in incontinence. The occurrence of incontinence was embarrassing for Mrs. C and discouraging for her husband. Emotional support, understanding, and explanations were provided. Initially, bowel care was performed in bed in a side lying position (see section "Principles of Bowel Management" for positioning techniques and suppository administration procedure). Privacy was insured, and a relaxed atmosphere was established. She was instructed not to bear down for defecation.

Within the first week poststroke, Mrs. C tolerated her diet well. Increased fiber was then added to her diet. She was taking fluids well without restriction. When bathroom privileges were allowed, toileting was done on a commode chair in the bathroom. She required assistance with transfer activities, and a safety belt was used on the commode chair. Feet were supported on a footstool to encourage a squat-like position. Abdominal massage was used to facilitate defecation.

Bowel management goals soon advanced to establishment of a planned "habit time" elimination routine. As Mrs. C's therapy program progressed, ambulation and functional abilities increased. The bowel record showed that Mrs. C was having daily adequate bowel movements after suppository administration, without spontaneous stools between elimination times. Suppository use was discontinued, and Mrs. C started using the toilet for evacuation. A schedule of toileting daily immediately after breakfast was maintained. Milk of magnesia at bedtime was later replaced with prune juice. At the time of hospital discharge, a bowel care routine of prune juice at bedtime and toileting after breakfast had proved workable for Mrs. C. A habit routine of elimination had been attained.

Neurogenic Bowel Patterns with Spinal Cord Lesions

Spinal cord lesions can result in two patterns of neurogenic bowel dysfunction: reflex neurogenic bowel and autonomous neurogenic bowel.

☐ **Potential Fecal Impaction or Incontinence Related to Reflex Neurogenic Bowel**

Central nervous system lesions that occur above the conus medullaris, specifically the S2, S3, and S4 spinal cord segments, result in a *reflex neurogenic bowel*. These lesions occur secondary to spinal cord trauma, spinal tumors, a vascular insult, or a disease process, such as MS or syringomyelia. The presence of a spinal cord lesion at this level causes an interruption of ascending sensory signals between the sacral reflex center (S2–S4) and the brain, resulting in an inability to feel the urge to defecate. Descending motor signals are interrupted, resulting in loss of voluntary control over the external anal sphincter. The external anal sphincter maintains its normal closed resting state or may be spastic. Because the spinal cord lesion is above the conus medullaris, the S2, S3, and S4 nerve segments that govern defecation are intact. It is, therefore, possible to develop a stimulus–response type of evacuation that capitalizes on the intact spinal reflex arc. Fecal incontinence is present but occurs infrequently, since the external anal sphincter remains in a contracted state due to parasympathetic innervation through the sacral segments of the spinal cord (Martin et al., 1981).

Spinal cord lesions that occur above the conus medullaris result in a reflex (automatic) bowel. *Defining characteristics* include absent cerebral awareness and voluntary control. Saddle sensation is diminished or absent, and the bulbocavernous reflex is of increased intensity. Fecal incontinence, if present, occurs without warning or as part of a mass reflex.

Management of the reflex bowel focuses on stimulation of the intact sacral reflex arc to move stool through the rectum for the *primary goal* of planned and predictable elimination. A structured bowel management program is developed to ensure adequate emptying and prevent incontinence.

During the acute stages after spinal cord injury, the focus of *nursing interventions* is on prevention of gastrointestinal complications and control of incontinence. Gastrointestinal complications include *paralytic ileus* and *stress ulcers*.

Initially following spinal cord injury, there is a state of spinal cord shock that may result in a loss of gastrointestial activity for as long as 2 to 3 days (Perkash, 1982). Absence of intestinal peristalsis results in loss of bowel sounds and abdominal distention. Frequent assessment for signs of distention and presence of bowel sounds is crucial during the acute stage. Progressive abdominal distention can cause vomiting, with possible aspiration, or may interfere with diaphragmatic excursion, resulting in respiratory distress. Food and oral fluids are withheld. Nasogastric tubes for drainage, intravenous fluids, and intermittent use of rectal tubes are helpful in preventing complications secondary to paralytic ileus. Rectal tubes should not be left in place continuously because there is danger of ischemia to the rectal mucosa from constant pressure.

When bowel sounds return and flatus is passed, the patient may progress from fluids to a light and then a full diet. A manual rectal examination and evacuation of any stool is performed daily.

During the acute period, the patient is prone to the development of gastric mucosal hemorrhages and *stress ulceration* in the stomach or duodenum. The occurrence of stress ulcers is generally within the first 4 weeks of injury and can result in hemorrhage (Kewalramani, 1979). Stress ulcers are thought to be caused by increased levels of catecholamines and steroids after injury. Acute ulceration is more frequent in spinal cord injury patients who have undergone surgery in the acute phase or who have had multiple injuries (Rudy, 1984). Patients with a previous history of gastric or duodenal ulceration are particularly susceptible to recurrence (Perkash, 1982). Drugs such as cimetidine or antacids are useful in the prevention of stress ulcers. Emesis, gastric drainage, and stool should be guaiac tested for the presence of blood.

Bowel Retraining. Initially, a comprehensive nursing assessment includes stool elimination patterns, previous bowel habits, present neurologic and physical status, functional levels, diet, and lifestyle. A consistent and workable time for evacuation is determined. Either a morning or evening schedule, after breakfast or the evening meal, is planned to coincide with the gastrocolic reflex. For the reflex bowel, generally an every other day program for evacuation is satisfactory. Certain individuals can maintain an every third day plan; longer than 3 days without evacuation predisposes to an impaction.

Diet should be high in fiber and fluids adequate to maintain a soft, formed stool. If bulk is inadequate, a methylcellulose product may be used, although dietary fiber is preferred. Laxative and stool softener use is avoided. Positioning progresses from recumbent to commode or toilet when functional ability permits. Bedpans are not used with spinal cord injured persons because of the potential for injury related to sensory impairment (see section "Principles of Bowel Management" in this chapter).

The individual is encouraged to participate actively in the bowel program at this time. Patients and families, as well as attendant if needed, must learn all aspects of bowel management. If the individual has adequate hand and finger function, he or she will assume the responsibility of independent bowel care before return home. If hand function for gloving and digital stimulation is lacking, a digital stimulator may be appropriate. For high cervical level quadriplegics with very limited hand and finger ability, attendant care is necessary for elimination.

Bowel Stimulation Techniques. When sacral reflex activity returns, the reflex bowel is managed by a stimulus–response type of bowel program. This involves the use of suppository or digital stimulation technique to empty the lower bowel of stool adequately. The eventual goal is to use digital stimulation alone to elicit reflex elimination.

At the preplanned time, the lower rectum is examined with a gloved, well-lubricatied finger. If stool is present, it is digitally removed. A suppository is inserted to stimulate reflex peristalsis and the movement of stool into the lower rectal vault (see section "Principles of Bowel Management" for suppository administration procedure). Facilitatory techniques, such as the Valsalva maneuver, forward bends, push-ups, and abdominal massage, should be used. If no evacuation has occurred within 15 to 30 minutes, digital stimulation is attempted. Digital stimulation may be used from the onset of bowel training as the primary stimulation method. If it is effective, it can be used alone without the adjunct use of suppositories.

Digital stimulation techniques: A gloved, well-lubricated finger is inserted into the rectum approximately $1^{1}/_{2}$ inches and pointed posteriorly to avoid pushing against the bladder. The finger is then rotated in a gentle circular motion to stimulate peristalsis and trigger the defecation reflex. Stimulation is continued for 30 seconds or longer until the internal sphincter relaxes. Stimulation is stopped if severe spasms of the anal sphincter occur or if symptoms of autonomic dysreflexia appear. The Valsalva maneuver and techniques to increase intra-abdominal pressure are helpful. The procedure should be repeated every 10 minutes three or four times until adequate evacuation has taken place.

Autonomic Dysreflexia. After the spinal shock phase, individuals who have a spinal cord injury at or above the T7 level are at potential risk of a complication called *autonomic dysreflexia*, also known as hyperreflexia. This exaggerated autonomic response is a medical emergency and can result in convulsions, CVA, respiratory arrest, or myocardial failure if untreated.

This mass reflex syndrome is set into action when afferent impulses ascend the spinal cord, most often due to an overdistended bladder or bowel. When the impulses reach the level of the spinal cord lesion, they are interrupted, resulting in sympathetic hyperactive outflow. This hyperactivity is thought to cause an exaggerated outpouring of norepinephrine from adrenergic nerve endings in the blood vessels and internal sphincter smooth muscle. The outflow stimulates arteriolar spasm, vasoconstriction below the level of cord injury, and subsequent hypertension (Wurster & Randall, 1975). The hypertension is noted by carotid sinus baroreceptors and is transmitted to the vasomotor center of the medulla and on to the sinoatrial node of the heart. Bradycardia results as a compensatory mechanism meant to decrease hyptertension. Blood vessels above the level of cord injury dilate, but vasoconstriction persists below the lesion. As a result, the hypertension persists. Hypertension can be critically severe as blood pressure continues to mount to dangerously high levels.

Symptoms of dysreflexia can be precipitated by an overdistended bowel because of fecal impaction or an overdistended rectum and can occur during routine bowel evacuation. Nursing staff, patient, family, and home attendants must be knowledgeable about the causes, symptoms, and treatment of dysreflexia in order to prevent its occurrence or progression to a medical emergency. Constipation and fecal impaction need to be avoided. People with spinal cord injury who have a history of dysreflexia as well as those at risk must be identified. The patient should wear a Medic Alert bracelet or carry a card explaining dysreflexia and recommended treatment.

Symptoms indicative of autonomic dysreflexia include elevated blood pressure (for many individuals with spinal cord injury, a normal blood pressure may be 90/60—in this case, 150/90 is considered elevated and may be indicative of autonomic dysreflexia); severe, pounding headache secondary to hypertension; bradycardia; profuse sweating, goose bumps, and redness of the skin above the level of the lesion; nasal congestion; blurred vision; and extreme nervousness and apprehension.

If dysreflexia occurs during bowel elimination or if an overdistended bowel is suspected as the cause of dysreflexic symptoms, the following *nursing intervention* should be implemented immediately. The patient should be in a sitting position to induce orthostatic hypotension, thus lowering the blood pressure. Blood pressure and pulse are monitored every 3 to 5 minutes. If the symptoms occur during bowel care, the procedure must be stopped until symptoms subside. (Continued rectal stimulation can cause progression of symptoms.) A topical anesthetic ointment is inserted into the rectum, and after 5 to 10 minutes, gentle manual evacuation of feces is resumed. Vital signs must be monitored during the procedure, and the examiner must be alert to recurrence of dysreflexic symptoms. If symptoms persist, the physician must be consulted. Administration of ganglionic blocking agents occasionally may be indicated.

☐ Constipation and Overflow Incontinence Related to Autonomous Neurogenic Bowel

Central nervous system lesions that occur at the sacral segments (S2–S4) or cauda equina result in *autonomous* bowel function. An *areflexic* or *flaccid* bowel is exhibited. These lesions occur as a result of trauma, spinal bifida, tumor, or intervertebral disk disease. The presence of a spinal cord lesion at this level destroys the sacral reflex center, with loss of the defecation reflex. A flaccid paralysis, including loss of anal tone, results. As with reflex bowel function, there is an interruption of sensory and motor pathways to the brain, resulting in an absence of cerebral control of elimination. The individual is unaware of the urge to defecate, and voluntary control of the external anal sphincter is lost.

Spinal cord lesions that occur at the level of the conus medullaris are of an areflexic (autonomous) type. *Defining characteristics* include absence of cerebral awareness and control. Saddle sensation is diminished to absent, and the bulbocavernous reflex is absent. Because the lesion involves S2, S3, and S4, the activity of the sacral reflex arc is destroyed. Signals are not transmitted to or from the bowel, and reflex (stimulus–response) emptying of the bowel is not possible. Even though the intrinsic contractile responses of the colon remain, peristalsis movements are ineffective without the influence of the sacral reflex arc. The result is a sluggish bowel causing retention of stool, with oozing of stool through the relaxed anal sphincter. Incontinence is especially prevalent when the consistency of stool is too soft.

Nursing interventions for the areflexic bowel focus on keeping the rectum free of stool and maintaining a stool of firm but not hard consistency. A diet high in fiber assists in maintaining a firm stool. Foods or fluids that tend to make the stool too soft must be avoided. Stool that is too hard will be difficult to evacuate. The primary goal of a daily bowel program is to keep the rectum free of stool, thereby preventing incontinence.

Fundamentals of bowel care, discussed under "Reflex Neurogenic Bowel," including acute care, nursing assessment, consistent timing on either a morning or evening schedule, positioning, physical activity, and emotional support and education, also must be part of the bowel management program of the individual with areflexic bowel. Bowel retraining for areflexic bowel, however, differs in its purpose. Absence of the sacral reflex arc results in a flaccid anal sphincter. Incontinence may occur if the rectal vault is not emptied on a regular daily schedule. Techniques used to trigger a stimulus–response reflex, such as digital stimulation or suppository administration, are not effective with the areflexic bowel because of the absence of the sacral reflex arc.

Manual evacuation of stool, in conjunction with techniques used to increase intra-abdominal pressure to move stool into the rectum, are used in management of the areflexic bowel. *Manual evacuation* should be performed with the patient in a sitting position as soon as his or her condition warrants, to increase intra-abdominal pressure and thereby help force stool through the rectum and flaccid anal sphincters. Flexion of the hips and knees, with feet supported on a stool, assists in assuming a squatting position. The Valsalva maneuver, forward bends, sitting push-ups, and abdominal massage also are used. Because lesions of the conus medullaris are usually at or below the T12–L1 vertebral level, some of the abdominal muscles that aid in defecation are intact. As a result, techniques to increase intra-abdominal pressure generally are effective. Upper extremity function is usually good with this level lesion, and the individual can assume responsibility for the procedure.

A gloved and well-lubricated finger is inserted into the rectum in a posterior direction to avoid pressure on the bladder. The rectum is then digitally emptied of stool. The procedure should be performed slowly and cautiously to avoid trauma to the desensitized rectum.

Motor Paralytic Bowel (Anterior Horn Cells or S2, S3, S4 Ventral Root Lesions)

Disease of the anterior horn cells or S2, S3, and S4 ventral roots results in *motor paralytic bowel*. Lesions of this type may be secondary to poliomyelitis, intervertebral disk disease, trauma, or tumor.

☐ Constipation Related to Motor Paralytic Bowel

Sensation is intact, but the bulbocavernous reflex is absent. An areflexic bowel is exhibited with sensory sparing. The major elimination problem the individual faces with this type of lesion is constipation. Fecal incontinence is rare except in widespread disease (Staas & DeNault, 1973).

The *goal* of interventions with motor paralytic areflexic bowel is the prevention of constipation. The individual has sensory awareness of rectal fullness, but does not have the added advantage of the sacral reflex arc to stimulate peristalsis. A sluggish bowel results. Intervention strategies are those that are used with other types of neurogenic bowel dysfunction in which constipation is a problem and include nursing assessment of bowel habits and nutrition as well as physical and functional status. Planning for a scheduled bowel routine takes advantage of the gastrocolic reflex and establishes a habit time for elimination. A diet high in fiber accompanied by adequate fluids will prevent a hard, constipating stool. Physical activity and exercise are encouraged to promote peristalsis. Positioning and techniques to increase intra-abdominal pressure to aid in stool evacuation are employed. The use of medications for routine long-term management is avoided (see section "Principles of Bowel Management").

Sensory Paralytic Bowel (Dorsal Horn Cells, Sacral Dorsal Roots, or Cells of Origin Lesions)

Lesions that involve sacral (S2, S3, S4) dorsal roots, cells of origin, or the dorsal horns of the spinal cord result in sensory paralysis with sparing of the upper and lower motor neurons. Lesions of this type are most commonly seen with diabetes and tabes dorsalis.

☐ **Constipation Related to Sensory Paralytic Bowel**

Defining characteristics of *sensory paralytic* bowel include diminished or absent saddle sensation and normal, decreased, or absent bulbocavernous reflex. Fecal incontinence is rare except in advanced stages (Staas & DeNault, 1973). Sensory paralytic lesions generally result in either a hyporeflexic or an areflexic bowel.

Management of the sensory paralytic bowel is directed toward prevention of constipation that occurs as a result of diminished sensory awareness of distended rectum and slowed colonic motility. Chronic constipation can lead to overdistention of the colon, with further loss of tone. The occurrence of megacolon must be avoided. *Nursing intervention* focuses on strategies used with other types of neurogenic bowel in relation to prevention of constipation. The plan of care is based on assessment of nutrition and bowel habit history. Planning for a consistant habit time for evacuation is important, particularly if awareness of the need to defecate is impaired. A high fiber diet with adequate fluid intake is stressed for prevention of a hard, dry, constipating stool and should preclude the use of medication. Physical activity and exercise aid in improving colonic motility. Positioning and procedures to increase intraabdominal pressure assist in moving stool through the rectum to be evacuated (see section "Principles of Bowel Management"). Table 29–2 summarizes nursing problems and management related to the types of neurogenic bowel.

PRINCIPLES OF BOWEL MANAGEMENT

Goals of Bowel Management

Bowel management is a planned program that uses a comprehensive and individualized approach based on nursing assessment and the specific type of bowel dysfunction present to predetermine the method and timing of evacuation. A well-planned, workable bowel program makes it possible for the individual to regain control over defecation when voluntary control is precluded because of motor or sensory dysfunction. The goals of an effective bowel care program are as follows:

1. The program focuses on establishing a regular, predictable, and reliable time for evacuation to prevent accidental or spontaneous bowel movements.
2. The program must be consistent and maintained, yet flexible enough to meet the needs of the individual's lifestyle. It must be convenient and practical to fit into one's daily activities comfortably.
3. The program should ensure adequate elimination to maintain satisfactory bowel function and prevent complications.

Implementing a Bowel Management Program

In addition to determination of type of bowel dysfunction exhibited and a comprehensive assessment of preexisting conditions affecting bowel elimination, there are other factors that must be considered in the planning and implementation of a bowel management program.

Timing

Planning a consistent schedule for time of evacuation is of the utmost importance in establishing a predictable and reliable bowel routine. In the acute care stages, a morning schedule may be most convenient. As activity and mobility increase, however, a program needs to be developed into which previous bowel habits and the routine the individual will follow after discharge are incorporated. A person's life should not be governed by a

TABLE 29–2. NEUROGENIC BOWEL DYSFUNCTIONS—NURSING MANAGEMENT.

Level of Lesion	Dysfunction Classification	Incontinence Characteristics	Nursing Interventions	Potential Problems
Cortical and subcortical	Uninhibited	Sense of urgency, involuntary defecation that may be infrequent or frequent	Consistent habit time Elimination record Physical exercise High fluid intake High fiber foods Suppository as needed	Constipation
Spinal cord above S2, S3, S4	Reflex Automatic	Infrequent Sudden Unexpected Occurs without warning	Stimulus–response evacuation Suppository use Digital stimulation Consistent habit time with planned evacuation every 2–3 days Elimination record Physical exercise High fluid intake High fiber foods Valsalva maneuver Techniques to increase intra-abdominal pressure at evacuation	Fecal impaction Autonomic dysreflexia
Spinal cord at S2, S3, S4, or cauda equina	Areflexic–flaccid Autonomous	May be frequent if rectum not emptied of stool Induced by physical exertion	Manual evacuation Maintain firm stool Maintain empty rectum Consistent habit time with planned evacuation daily Elimination record Physical exercise High fluid intake	Fecal retention with oozing of stool

Anterior horn cells or S2, S3, S4 ventral roots	Motor paralytic	Infrequent	High fiber foods Valsalva maneuver Techniques to increase intra-abdominal pressure at evacuation Consistent habit time Elimination record Physical exercise High fluid intake	Constipation
S2, S3, S4 dorsal roots, cells of origin, or dorsal horns	Sensory paralytic	Infrequent	High fiber foods Valsalva maneuver Techniques to increase intra-abdominal pressure at evacuation (Same as Motor paralytic)	Constipation Bowel overdistention

Adapted from Martin et al., 1981.

bowel routine. It may be necessary for the individual to change the time of day of bowel evacuation in order to accommodate such factors as a work or school schedule or time of attendant care. Because it may take 1 or 2 weeks or longer to reestablish a bowel routine on a new schedule, frequent changing of time is discouraged. If it is necessary to change the timing of the bowel care, starting a day early at the new time and administering a mild laxative 8 hours previously will get the bowel started on the new schedule.

Evacuation should be scheduled 15 to 30 minutes after a meal, generally in the morning or evening, to take advantage of gastrocolic reflex action. Drinking a warm liquid before defecation also may assist in stimulating peristalsis. Frequency of evacuation is individualized to the type of bowel dysfunction present, the preonset bowel habits, and the present lifestyle. A pattern of soft, formed stools without spontaneous accidental stools between planned bowel care intervals is the goal. Maintaining a bowel record or flow sheet will assist in evaluating the effectiveness of the routine. The longer stool remains in the colon, the drier and harder it becomes, increasing the potential for constipation and fecal impaction. Generally, more than 3 days between evacuations is not advised.

Once a workable elimination schedule has been attained, it should be maintained. If the schedule is upset, it may take weeks to reestablish a reliable new schedule. It is, therefore, critical to encourage active patient participation in the planning stages so that the schedule is tailored to specific needs and lifestyle.

Diet

Frequency and consistency of stool are related to type and amount of food and fluid ingested. In addition to being well balanced, the diet must provide adequate fiber. Fiber increases the bulk of the feces by enhancing water absorption. A diet that has inadequate fiber will result in a hard, dry, constipating stool. High fiber foods include nuts, the bran of whole grain, rather than refined, breads and cereals, and the cellulose of fresh fruits and vegetables with skins and seeds (Table 29–3).

Foods that previously had a constipating effect, caused excessively loose stool, or otherwise upset the bowel regimen probably will have similar effects on the neurogenic bowel. Foods that have a natural laxative effect, such as certain fruits and juices, or alcohol, initially should be ingested cautiously so that their effects can be evaluated.

Exercise

Physical activity and exercise aid in the digestive process, promote peristalsis, and aid in

TABLE 29–3. HIGH FIBER FOODS.

Fruits	
Apples[a]	Grapefruit
Apricots[a]	Peaches
Cherries	Pears
Figs	Plums
Oranges	Prunes
Berries	Dried fruits

Vegetables	
Asparagus	Lima beans
Baked beans	Onions
Broccoli	Peas (all varieties)
Brussel sprouts	Peppers
Cabbage	Potato skins
Carrots	Radishes
Cauliflower	Spinach
Celery	Squash
Corn	Tomatoes
Eggplant	Turnips
Green beans	

Whole Grain Products	
Wheat bran	Rye crisp
Wheat germ	Wheat crisp
Cracked wheat	Brown bread
Whole wheat bread	Cornmeal
Pumpernickel bread	Brown rice

Cereals	Miscellaneous
Oatmeal	Nuts
Bran	Sunflower seeds
Shredded wheat	Popcorn

[a]Should be eaten unpeeled for maximum fiber content.

elimination. Elimination is dependent on the integration of smooth and skeletal muscular activity as well as visceral reflex patterns. Immobility may interfere with these mechanisms, resulting in constipation. The primary muscles involved in defecation, the abdominals, the diaphragm, and the levator ani, work simultaneously to increase intra-abdominal pressure and expel the fecel mass. Immobility contributes to muscular atrophy, loss of tone, and generalized weakness. As a result, the individual is unable to assist with the defecation process, and retention or incomplete evacuation results. As the individual's activity level increases, so does the physiologic response of elimination.

As soon as the individual's condition warrants, encouraging participation in the daily care regimen will increase general conditioning as well as bowel function. Basic daily activities, such as bathing, dressing, and transfer activities, in addition to participating in therapies, will aid in the process. Active exercise, such as pelvic tilting, hiking hips off the bed, range of motion, turning in bed, and wheelchair push-ups, will promote intestinal motility, muscular strengthening, and elimination.

Positioning and Facilitatory Techniques

Bowel care may have to take place in bed immediately after the onset of disability. Bedpans should not be used for people with sensory impairment because of the risk of pressure sores; rather, incontinent pads should be used for bowel care in bed. Positioning can capitalize on the anatomic position of the descending and sigmoid colon. Positioning on the left side promotes absorption and increases the effectiveness of suppositories or enemas by using gravity. After stimulation, positioning on the right side aids in stool expulsion.

As soon as the condition allows, a sitting position should be used for bowel care. The sitting position facilitates the use of gravity and increases intra-abdominal pressure for ease in stool expulsion. A squatting position with the knees higher than the hips is achieved by supporting the feet on a footstool; this position further facilitates increased intra-abdominal pressure. As functional ability permits, bowel care should progress from a commode chair to a raised toilet seat or a standard seat with padding when there is sensory loss. A raised toilet seat or a commode chair with a side opening aids in access to the anal area for suppository insertion, manual stimulation, or evacuation of stool and cleansing. The seat must be in good repair, with adequate padding, to prevent pressure or trauma. As soon as the individual's ability permits, participation in bowel care should be an expectation, with gradual progression to self-care if appropriate.

Defecation is initiated by inhalation followed by exhalation against a closed glottis, with simultaneous tightening of the abdominal muscles. This action increases intra-abdominal pressure, thus forcing stool into the rectum. This procedure called the *Valsalva maneuver* and described as bearing-down requires strength and tone in the abdominal and pelvic muscles and is dependent on intact innervation to the lower thoracic cord (T6–12). Generalized debilitation, atrophy, or a spinal cord lesion above the T12 level results in weakness or paralysis of these accessory muscles and ineffective Valsalva maneuver. The use of various techniques, however, can mimic a Valsalva-type response. Such exercise as forward bends and push-ups from the toilet seat (if balance and ability permit) during elimination assist in the defecation process. Abdominal massage in a clockwise direction, following the anatomic course of the colon, also facilitates evacuation. In the presence of hypertension or cardiovascular disease, the Valsalva maneuver may be contraindicated.

Medications

Bowel stimulants, including laxatives, stool softeners, and bulk-producing agents, frequently are abused and considered as a cure-all for elimination problems. Because the planning and management of a bowel care program is generally a nursing function, nurses must be knowledgeable about the action, effects, and consequences of long-term use of bowel medications for safe and appropriate use. In addition, numerous medications have a systemic effect on bowel function. This necessitates assessment of the individual's total medication profile.

Medications are not used in lieu of other methods, such as diet, fluids, and exercise, for bowel management. Short-term and judicious use of medications may be indicated, however, during establishment of the bowel management routine or if a need exists to reestablish a disrupted routine.

A wide variety of *oral agents*, including bowel stimulants, stool softeners, and bulk producers, is used in establishing a bowel care routine. Discussion of specific drugs and their effects can be found in pharmacology textbooks. General considerations in regard to bowel care planning and maintenance are shown in Table 29–4.

Insertion of a rectal *suppository* initiates reflexes that stimulate peristalsis of the colon and rectum, with resulting relaxation of the anal sphincters for the purpose of facilitating defecation. To be effective, suppositories must be in contact with the mucosa and not placed in the fecal mass. Therefore, stool should be manually removed from the rectum before suppository insertion. The suppository must be inserted above the anal sphincters.

Enemas

Large-volume enemas are not used in a routine bowel care program. Persistent use of enemas can result in diminished bowel tone by overstretching the bowel and causing a loss of the colon's natural elasticity. The end result is a bowel that is more sluggish and prone to further constipation.

During the administration of an enema, the neurogenic bowel can go into spasm and trap fluid in the bowel segment behind the spastic area. If the enema is of large volume, the pressure exerted on the intestinal walls could result in rupture. In the case of a flaccid colon, the enema fluid can flow in without resistance, and the bowel may balloon to accommodate the volume and rupture, since there is no muscle tone or contraction force to express the fluid. Perforation of the rectum can occur as a result of enema tip trauma if the patient has rectal sensory loss.

If a large enema is necessary for cleansing purposes before surgical or diagnostic procedures, it should be administered cautiously and slowly and only by a skilled person (Ireland, 1978). The enema tip should be well lubricated, introduced slowly and carefully, and not inserted more than 6 cm. The patient should be properly positioned and instructed not to move.

COMPLICATIONS ASSOCIATED WITH CONSTIPATION IN PEOPLE WITH NEUROGENIC BOWEL

Constipation is the most common general nursing diagnosis related to neurogenic bowel dysfunction. It is characterized by hard, dry

TABLE 29–4. PRINCIPLES OF MEDICATION USE IN BOWEL MANAGEMENT.

- The effect and action time of drugs may be altered in the presence of neurogenic bowel, which can take 24 hours longer to respond than a normal bowel. Usual suggested dosages may result in cumulative effects that are difficult to control. Beginning with the minimum recommended dose and increasing the dose gradually until effective is recommended.
- Plan bowel evacuation to coincide with peak effectiveness of oral medication.
- The use of bulk-forming medications requires adequate fluid intake to prevent constipation and obstruction.
- Should medications need adjusting, only one element of the bowel program should be changed at a time and sufficient time allowed to evaluate results (at least three days) (Zejdlik, 1983).
- Use of harsh laxatives is avoided.
- Enemas and laxatives ordered in preparation for diagnostic tests may upset an established, workable bowel routine. The routine may take several weeks to reestablish. A modified bowel preparation is generally indicated for the individual with neurogenic bowel.

stool, increased difficulty in passing stool, and inadequate or infrequent results of bowel care. Because of the interrupted neural pathways, bowel motility is decreased and movement of stool through the colon is slowed, resulting in increased reabsorption of fluid from the stool. The longer stool remains in the colon, the drier and harder it becomes. Fecal impaction (a mass of stool that blocks the bowel) may result if stool is allowed to accumulate.

Nursing management of constipation is discussed relative to the various types of neurogenic bowel. Failure to prevent or resolve constipation may result in several serious problems, including megacolon, diarrhea, autonomic dysreflexia, and hemorrhoids.

Megacolon may be described as a hypertrophied and dilated colon that may be associated with prolonged constipation. Alternating episodes of diarrhea and constipation may be present. Megacolon may result from long-term overdistention of the bowel secondary to progressive accumulation of stool and subsequent loss of bowel tone. Long-term laxative abuse or injudicious use of large-volume enemas also can predispose to megacolon. In neurogenic bowel dysfunction, when diminished bowel tone is already present, long-term overdistention leads to further atony and can result in megacolon. Maintaining an effective bowel care regimen that inhibits chronic severe constipation prevents the development of megacolon.

Diarrhea is defined as an increased frequency and fluid consistency of stool. In the presence of neurogenic bowel dysfunction, diarrhea generally is a result of a gastrointestinal disturbance rather than an infectious process. Although an infectious process is infrequently the underlying cause, the possibility must not be ignored. Initial intervention in the treatment of diarrhea is to determine and eliminate its cause. Diarrhea often is related to the ingestion of foods or fluids that may have a laxative effect, such as spicy foods, large amounts of fruit juices, or excessive alcohol intake. It is important to investigate the individual's diet and bowel habit history. Foods that the individual had difficulty tolerating previously will likely have a similar effect after disability. New foods should be introduced one at a time and taken in moderation to evaluate the effect. Certain medications, such as antibiotics, or the excessive use of antacids or laxatives may cause diarrhea. Ingesting buttermilk or yogurt while on antibiotic therapy is often helpful in alleviating diarrhea.

The presence of a *fecal impaction* must be ruled out. Loose stools that occur suddenly and in large amounts are generally characteristic of diarrhea; however, the frequent or continuous oozing of small amounts of liquid stool is usually indicative of inadequate bowel emptying or fecal impaction. The elimination record should be assessed for sufficiency of results at planned elimination times. If elimination has been inadequate, fecal impaction should be suspected.

Autonomic dysreflexia is discussed in the section "Reflex Neurogenic Bowel" in this chapter.

Hemorrhoids are dilated veins under the mucous membranes in the anal and rectal areas. Bleeding may or may not be present. Hemorrhoidal pain and itching experienced by sensory intact individuals may not be present in neurologic dysfunction. Neurogenic bowel dysfunction may predispose the individual to hemorrhoidal development. An altered autonomic nervous system produces a general passive state of vasodilation, hampering venous return from the rectal area. Lack of position change or extended time periods sitting on the toilet can further complicate the picture (Zejdlik, 1983). Excessive straining at defecation, overly vigorous digital stimulation, or rough manual removal of hard stool over time can predispose to hemorrhoids. The individual with a spinal cord lesion at the level of the conus medullaris may be at particular risk because of further compromised venous return as a result of flaccid paralysis.

Nursing focuses on prevention of the occurrence and progression of the problem. Pressure reliefs in the wheelchair and on the toilet, as well as limitation of sitting time on the toilet, will assist in preventing progressive venous stasis in the rectal area. Constipation should be prevented. Digital stimulation and manual evacuation of stool should be gentle, using a glove and plenty of lubricant. Excessive straining must be avoided. External hemorrhoids should be replaced in the anal canal after bowel care. Use of anti-inflammatory suppositories or a topical ointment may be indicated. If bleeding is present, the amount should be noted.

PSYCHOSOCIAL IMPLICATIONS

Elimination is a basic physiologic need that is particularly significant to the person with neurogenic bowel dysfunction. This basic need must be satisfied for realization of the higher needs: security, love and belonging, self-esteem, and self-actualization. Planning, initiating, and maintaining a successful bowel elimination program prevents the occurrence of physical complications. The physical complications in themselves do not have as great a significance for the individual as the psychosocial ramifications of the complications. For example, diarrhea in itself may have little meaning for the individual; however, the fear of an accidental evacuation because of liquid stools has a tremendous impact. Constipation may have little significance until the individual is faced with its complications. If it takes 2 hours three times a week for the individual to perform bowel care, socialization or vocational activities will become secondary. If excessive energies are required to meet the basic needs of elimination, higher level needs cannot be attained. Bowel management must fit the individual's lifestyle. Problems associated with bowel dysfunction should not be accepted as inevitable; they must be anticipated and prevented.

An alteration of bowel function affects the individual and his or her total environment. The individual is part of the environment from which he or she has come, including culture, family, job, and community. The nurse also becomes part of this environment. The nurse must explore and acquire an understanding of the environment from which the individual came to plan future goals effectively. What does bowel dysfunction and its consequences mean to the individual?

The nurse is constantly teaching during patient interactions. As a result, the patient should gain a thorough knowledge of the normal and altered physiology of elimination and the variables affecting elimination. The influence of diet, fluid, and exercise should be understood, as should specific bowel management techniques and complications.

In addition to the responsibility of educating the patient, family, and other care providers, the nurse *also* has a supportive role. Understanding and encouragement are of utmost importance. Impaired bowel function in itself has an emotional impact on the individual. Although optimal independence within functional limitations is encouraged and strived for, total independence is not always possible. If functional limitations necessitate the physical assistance of another person for the performance of bowel care, the problem is amplified. Who will perform bowel care at home? This problem should be explored with the individual and the partner if indicated. It may not be conducive in a sexual relationship for the partner to provide bowel care, and, if possible, alternative arrangements should be planned, such as an attendant or home health aide. The nurse must be sensitive to the myriad of emotions associated with altered bowel function.

REFERENCES

Ireland, P. (1978). *Spinal cord injury care manual for nurses.* New York: Eastern Paralyzed Veterans Association.

Kewalramani, L.S. (1979). Neurogenic gastroduodenal ulceration and bleeding associated with spinal cord injuries. *The Journal of Trauma, 19*(4), 259.

Martin, N., Holt, N., & Hicks, D. (1981). *Comprehensive rehabilitation nursing.* New York: McGraw-Hill.

Perkash, I. (1982). Management of neurogenic dysfunction of the bladder and bowel. In F.J.

Kottke, G.K. Stillwell, & J.F. Lehmann (Eds.), *Krusen's handbook of phsycial medicine and rehabilitation* (3rd ed.). Philadelphia: Saunders.

Rudy, E.B. (1984). *Advanced neurological and neurosurgical nursing.* St. Louis: Mosby.

Staas, W.E. Jr., & DeNault, P.M. (1973). Bowel control. *American Family Physician, 7*(1), 90.

Wurster, R.D., & Randall, W.C. (1975). Cardiovascular responses to bladder distension in patients with spinal transection. *American Journal of Physiology, 228*(4), 1288.

Zejdlik, C.P. (1983). *Management of spinal cord injury.* Belmont, MA: Wadsworth.

SECTION 8. HUMAN SEXUALITY PHENOMENA

30

Human Sexuality: An Overview

Nancy F. Woods

DIMENSIONS OF HUMAN SEXUALITY AND SEXUAL HEALTH

Human sexuality is a complex phenomenon. Our sexuality pervades our biologic being, our sense of ourselves, and the way we relate to other human beings. Human sexuality is a multidimensional construct, with sexual function, sexual self-concept, and sexual roles and relationships constituting important dimensions. *Sexual function* refers to the ability of the individual to give and receive sexual pleasure. *Sexual self-concept* refers to the image one has of oneself as a man or a woman and the evaluation of one's adequacy in that role. Sexual self-concept also includes body image, reflecting the abstract representation of one's body and the evaluation of that image against personal and cultural standards. *Sexual relationships* refer to interpersonal relationships in which our sexuality is expressed. These dimensions have important correlates in expression of sexual health and are mirrored in the World Health Organization definition of sexual health as the "positive integration of the somatic, emotional, intellectual, and social aspects of sexual being in ways that are posi- tively enriching and that enhance personality, communication, and love" (World Health Organization, 1975, p. 6). This chapter examines the complex of biologic function, self-concept, and role relationships as they develop throughout the life span.

HUMAN SEXUALITY AND HUMAN DEVELOPMENT

Beginnings

Humans are sexual beings from the moment of fertilization. Chromosomal sex establishes the first of a series of developmental influences on our sexuality. The male's sperm contributes either an X or a Y chromosome, which combines with the female's X chromosome, resulting in the XX (female) or XY (male) combination (Fig. 30–1).

After fertilization, there are critical points in the evolution of gender identity: the point at which induction of development of internal and external genitalia occurs and the point at which the hypothalamus takes on a male or female pattern. At about 5 to 6 weeks of fetal life, the XX or XY chromosomal com-

Figure 30-1. Fetal sexual development.

Chromosomal sex XX or XY

By 6 weeks of fetal life: Gonad differentiates to testis

By 12 weeks of fetal life:
- Wolffian duct system suppressed, Müllerian duct system develops
- Testis produces fetal androgen and MIS
- Müllerian duct system suppressed, Wolffian duct system develops
- Internal female reproductive system develops
- Internal male reproductive system develops

From 12 weeks of fetal life to birth:
- Androgen liberated
- External female genitals develop
- External male genitals develop
- Female cyclic pattern established in brain
- Male acyclic pattern established in brain

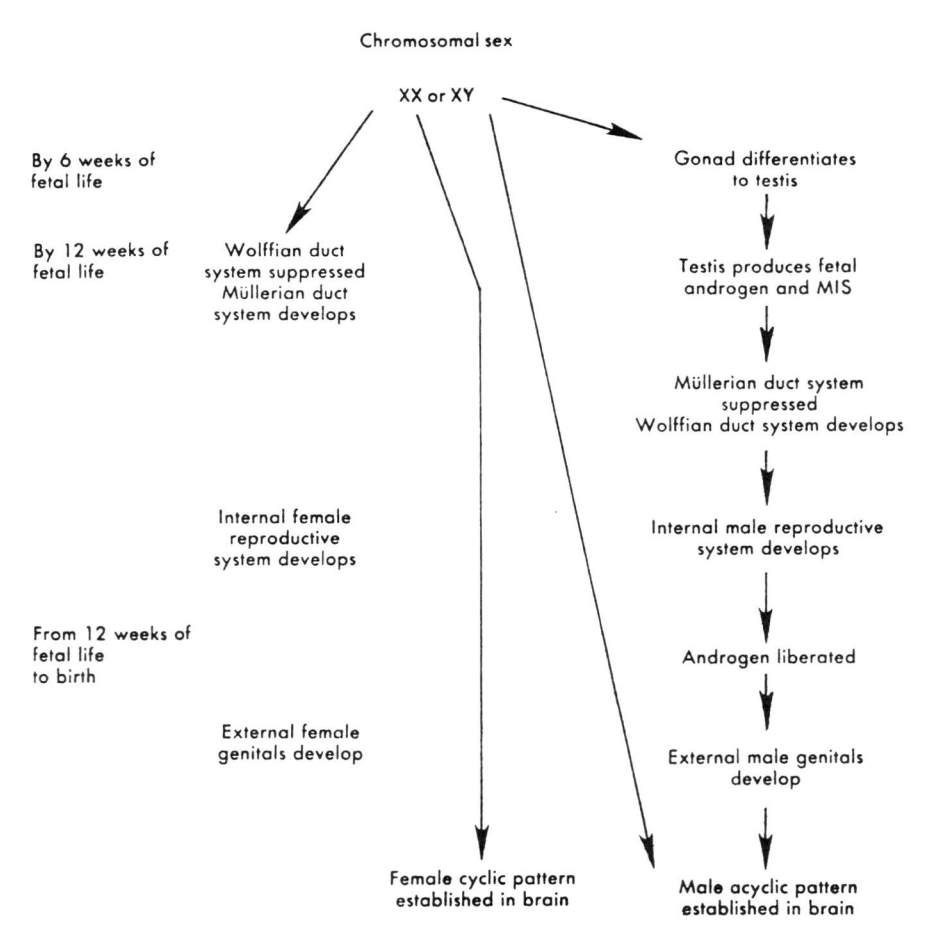

Figure 30–1. Fetal sexual development. *(Reproduced by permission from: N.F. Woods.* Human Sexuality in Health and Illness *[3rd ed.]. St. Louis, 1984, The C.V. Mosby Co.)*

bination determines whether undifferentiated fetal gonads will develop as ovaries or testes. Further differentiation occurs in response to secretion of fetal androgen in the male fetus. If androgens are not present at critical periods and in appropriate amounts, male structures will not develop from the wolffian ducts, and the fetus with XY chromosomes will develop female genitalia. Biologic sex is well established by the 12th week of fetal life. Although there does not appear to be a hormone necessary for induction of the ovarian function in female fetuses, estrogen is necessary for full development of female genitalia (Money & Erhardt, 1972).

Another critical stage occurs around the time of birth, at which point another set of sexual controls is introduced. Testosterone is thought to influence the hypothalamus in such a way that it develops a male acyclic pattern for the release of pituitary gonadotropins. In the female, a cyclic pattern of gonadotropin release is established (Money & Erhardt, 1972).

Although the infant is born with an established chromosomal sex, gender identity and gender role are not yet established. Gender identity is the feeling that one is male, female, or ambivalent. Usually gender identity is solidified in children by the time they are age 3. Caretakers assign gender shortly after birth of the child, and their behavior confirms and reinforces the child's sense of maleness or femaleness. Children also respond to cues from their own bodies. For example, they respond to the appearance of the genitals and to verbal and nonverbal messages from caretakers in relation to their developing sense of self as female, male, or ambivalent. Gender role, the outward expression of one's gender, is learned early in life. Distinctions between appropriate masculine and feminine behavior vary greatly between cultures. In western cultures, these distinctions are becoming much less rigid, with the androgynous person (individuals who possess both female and male characteristics) becoming synonymous with a healthy person.

Sexual development continues throughout the life span, with each component of sexuality being influenced by biologic development as well as sociocultural forces. Some of the significant developmental experiences related to sexual function, sexual self-concept, and sexual relationships are outlined in Table 30–1.

Human Sexual Responses

Human sexual response illustrates the interplay of biology, society, and culture with the individual's thoughts, feelings, and experiences. Masters and Johnson's pioneering work (1966) in the area of human sexual response contributed greatly to our understanding of the physiologic aspects of sexual function. Their studies revealed that the changes that accompany human sexual response result from two physiologic mechanisms: vasocongestion and myotonia. *Vasocongestion* is the primary response to sexual stimulation and refers to the engorgement of blood vessels with blood. Vasocongestion is responsible for swelling of vascular tissues in both women and men and for vaginal lubrication in women. *Myotonia* refers to muscle tension, seen in the contraction of the women's perivaginal muscles and the man's vas deferens and urethra during orgasm. Both vasocongestion and myotonia occur throughout the body with sexual response. Sexual response is thus best thought of as a total body response rather than a genital response.

Masters and Johnson's (1966) original concept of the human sexual response cycle has been revised in the work of Kaplan (1979). Kaplan describes human sexual response as consisting of three phases: desire, excitement, and orgasm. These phases are related components of sexual response but are governed by separate neurophysiologic systems. Her concept of sexual response is useful for understanding the physiology of sexual response, the consequences of pathophysiology, the etiology of sexual dysfunctions, and appropriate therapies.

The *desire phase* of sexual response refers to the experience of sexual appetite or drive produced by the activation of neural systems in the brain. Sexual desire is experienced as sensations that move the person to seek out sexual activity. Although the precise neurons involved in sexual desire are unknown, it is believed to involve the limbic system and the preoptic nuclei of the hypothalamus. It is likely that the brain's sexual centers have either neural of chemical connections with the pleasure centers of the brain. The pleasure centers are stimulated during sexual activity, resulting in the pleasurable quality of sexual behavior. Some suggest that the pleasure centers are stimulated by release of endorphins with sexual behavior. Stimulation of the pain centers can inhibit sexual desire. If an object or situation evokes pain, it will cease to evoke desire.

Testosterone is important in mediating sexual desire in both men and women, and low levels of testosterone are associated with low levels of sexual desire. Luteinizing hormone also may be important in mediating sexual desire. Two neurotransmitters, serotonin (5HT) and dopamine, are believed to be important in mediating sexual desire: serotonin acts as an inhibitor and dopamine as a stimulant to the sexual centers of the brain.

TABLE 30–1. SIGNIFICANT DEVELOPMENTAL EXPERIENCE RELATED TO SEXUAL FUNCTION, SEXUAL SELF-CONCEPT, AND SEXUAL RELATIONSHIPS.

	Sexual Function	Sexual Self-Concept	Sexual Role–Relationship
Infancy	• Orgasmic potential present • Erectile function present	• Gender identity reinforced • Association of sexuality and good–bad • Distinction between self and others	
Childhood	• Genital pleasuring and explanation • Engages in sensual activity (e.g., hugging)	• Core gender identity solidified (by age 3)	• Sex role differences learned • Discrimination between male and female role models • Learns sexual vocabulary
Preschool	• Sex play • Exploration of own body and those of playmates • Self-pleasuring (masturbation)		• Learns about sex roles • Parental attachment and identification
School age		• Curiosity about sex • Sexual fears and fantasies • Interest in aspects of sexual development • Self-awareness as sexual being	• Same-sex friends
Adolescent, prepubertal	• Menarche • Seminal emissions	• Concerns about body image	• Same-sex sexual experiences as part of friendship
Early adolescence	• Awkwardness in first sexual encounter (50% not sexually active) • Masturbation, petting	• Sexual thoughts, fantasies • Anxiety over inadequacy, lack of partner, virginity	• Beginning appropriate sex friendships • Dating • Learning
Late adolescence	• May or may not be sexually active	• Responsibility for sexual activity	• Learning intimacy in relationship • Sex role behaviors, lifestyles explained
Young adult	• Experimentation with sexual positions, expression • Explanation of techniques	• Responsibility for sexual health, e.g., contraception, STD prevention • Development of adult sexual value system, tolerance for others	• Learning to give and receive pleasure • Long-term commitment to relationship
Middle adult	• Adaptation to altered sexual function, e.g., vaginal dryness of menopause, slower erections	• Accept body image changes related to aging	• Adjustment of relationship as roles change

TABLE 30–1. SIGNIFICANT DEVELOPMENTAL EXPERIENCE RELATED TO SEXUAL FUNCTION, SEXUAL SELF-CONCEPT, AND SEXUAL RELATIONSHIPS. *(Continued)*

	Sexual Function	Sexual Self-Concept	Sexual Role–Relationship
Late adult	• Slower sexual function	• Accept slowed sexual response cycle without ending sexual aspects of relationship	• Develop new ways for sharing sexual pleasure and intimacy with aging • Adaptation to loss of partner or illness of partner

After Mims, 1978.

Bonding to another person and love are both powerful stimuli to sexual desire. Many other stimuli are capable of evoking sexual desire, including sight, smell, and other sensory cues. Many of these stimuli are conditioned by the culture. Fear and pain are the most potent inhibitors of sexual desire. Neural connections between the sexual centers and other parts of the brain make it possible for people to turn off sexual desire when other stimuli are more important or when it is not adaptive to the individual to pursue sexual activity. These same connections also make it possible to enhance sexual desire.

During the *excitement phase* of sexual response, the level of sexual tension intensifies. Physiologic changes characteristic of the excitement phase, swelling of the genitalia and vaginal lubrication, are produced by reflex vasodilation of the genital blood vessels. Two centers in the spinal cord (S2–S4 and T11–L2) cause the arterioles to dilate. This vasodilation causes the genitals to swell and changes their shape to adapt to their reproductive function. Vasocongestion is primarily a parasympathetically mediated response. Intense sympathetic response, such as that produced by fear and anxiety, can instantly lead to loss of erection. It is believed that erection is governed by two spinal reflex centers. The thoracolumbar center (psychogenic) appears to respond more to psychic stimuli, whereas the sacral center is stimulated by tactile input to the genitals. It is believed that the spinal reflex centers and the higher neural connections are analogous in males and females.

Orgasm refers to the peak and release of sexual tension. The orgasm phase of sexual response is characterized by a genital reflex governed by spinal neural centers and consists of reflex contractions of certain genital muscles. Sensory influences that trigger orgasm enter the cord via the pudendal nerve at the sacral level: the efferents are T11 and L2. Orgasmic sensations have been described in several ways, but women tend to note one or more of these forms: vulval, uterine, and blended. The vulval orgasm involves involuntary contractions of the orgasmic platform, the vascular tissue at the outer third of the woman's vagina, and the labia minora. The uterine orgasm depends on deep stimulation of the cervix that displaces the uterus, thus stimulating the peritoneum. Blended orgasms combine features of both the vulval and uterine variety.

Even in the presence of complete spinal cord transection, people experience nocturnal emissions and orgasms. Cognitional eroticism persists independent of sensation in the genitalia. The brain seems to be able to function independent of the spinal cord, just as the genitalia of spinal cord injured people work reflexively and independently of the brain.

Variations in Sexual Expression

Sexual pleasure may be experienced in a variety of ways. Culture influences the forms of sexual expression deemed acceptable and one's value system about sexual behavior. Indeed, the culture plays an important role in defining what is normal. The search for a definition of "normal" becomes futile as one observes the variety of forms of sexual expression that is acceptable across various cultures. Instead of becoming obsessed with what is normal, Comfort (1975) suggests that we consider what meaning a behavior has for any individual, whether it impoverishes or enriches the lives of that person and any others with whom the sexual relations are shared, and finally, whether the behavior is tolerable by the society.

Sexual Pleasuring

Each culture provides for a variety of erotic behaviors, but nearly all are concerned with sexual modesty. Incest taboos are common to most societies, although the definition of incest varies from culture to culture. Each society has some form of legal system to regulate sexual behavior; for example, sexual intercourse may be restricted to marriage, or premarital sexual freedom may be encouraged.

Beach (1977) found that the approaches to sexual pleasuring were highly variable between and within cultures. The position used for intercourse was highly variable, including female astride (on top), male astride, side to side, or squatting. In some cultures, women are expected to initiate sexual activity, but in others, only males are to do so. Even the duration of the sex act is regulated by the culture; in some, men are encouraged to ejaculate rapidly, whereas in others, the man's ability to prolong intromission is valued. Sexual stimulation is highly variable. Although kissing is nearly ubiquitous, in some cultures it is regarded as unsanitary. Stimulation of the female breasts either manually or orally is common. Manipulation of the female genitalia by the male is a common prelude to penile intromission. Oral stimulation of the woman's genitals (cunnilingus) is common to many cultures, and somewhat less common is oral stimulation of the male's genitals (fellatio). Painful stimulation is sometimes used to enhance arousal. Although the circumstances surrounding coitus vary from culture to culture, usually privacy is important. Sexual frequency also may be governed by norms; for example, intercourse may be prohibited during menses, lactation, pregnancy, and before hunts or wars.

Although heterosexuality is the most prevalent form of sexual expression in the cultures that have been studied, it is rarely the only type of sexual behavior in which people engage.

Sexual Behavior

There are many variations in sexual behavior that involve variation in partners or aim. For example, heterosexuals choose partners of the opposite six, whereas homosexuals seek partners of the same sex. Bisexuals choose both same-sex and opposite-sex partners at various times.

Homosexuality

Because homosexuality is a very prevalent and poorly understood sexual variation, it is discussed here in more detail than other variations. Two recent investigations have made a significant contribution to our knowledge of homosexuality. The Institute for Sex Research conducted a large study of homosexuals in the San Francisco Bay area (Bell & Weinberg, 1978), and Masters and Johnson (1979) have published the results of their research.

Bell and Weinberg (1978) studied 979 homosexual men and women and a comparison group of 477 heterosexuals from the San Francisco area. Through extensive interviews, these investigators determined that homosexuality involved much more than just sexual practices. Men and women in the homosexual sample varied in the degree to which they were involved in homosexual and heterosexual experiences, ranging along a continuum from those with exclusively homosexual feelings and behaviors to those with more heterosexual than homosexual feelings and behaviors. Homosexuals were predominantly covert about their homosexuality, although frequently their families were aware of their sexual preferences. Many common assumptions about homosexuality were not supported by this study. For example, homosexuals could not be typified as sexually hyperactive or hypoactive. The investigation made clear the uniqueness of homosexual lifestyles and the differences in lifestyles for men and women. "Cruising" (purposefully searching for a partner), for example, was common among men but less common among women. Men tended to have more partners than women, but both men and women preferred a relatively steady relationship with a lover.

The homosexual men and women in this study used a variety of sexual techniques. Men most frequently used fellatio, hand–genital contact, and anal intercourse, and women most frequently participated in masturbation and cunnilingus with their partners. Sexual problems were more commonly reported by men than by women and included difficulty meeting a partner and meeting the partner's sexual request. Although sexually transmitted disease was a common health problem for homosexual men, this was not the case for lesbian women.

Bell and Weinberg found that the homosexuals they interviewed were involved in a variety of relationships, ranging from a quasimarriage to having multiple short-term contacts. Some were not involved in a relationship, had little sexual interest, and regretted their homosexuality.

When psychologic adjustment of the homosexual sample was compared with that of the heterosexual group, it was apparent that the homosexuals who were in dysfunctional sexual relationships and who were asexual were less well adjusted than heterosexuals. However, when the comparison was restricted to those who were functional (had little regret about homosexuality) or were in a coupled relationship, homosexuals were no more distressed than the heterosexuals.

Masters and Johnson (1979) compared the physiology of sexual response in homosexuals and heterosexuals in the laboratory setting. They found no significant difference in the homosexual and heterosexual subjects' facility for orgasm in response to masturbation, partner manipulation, fellatio, or cunnilingus. There were no demonstrable physiologic differences in the sexual response cycles of homosexuals and heterosexuals. Instead, homosexual women responded in the same manner as heterosexual women, and similar results were obtained for men.

Aging and Human Sexuality

Research on sexuality and aging disconfirms the stereotypes of the elderly as either disinterested in sex or abnormally obsessed with it. For many aging persons, sexuality is an important dimension of living.

Although there is a decline in reports of sexual interest and activity with aging, there is no single point in the life cycle at which sexual activity ceases for all. Many investigators have demonstrated that both sexual interest and activity persist well into the seventh, eighth, and ninth decades of life (Kinsey et al., 1948, 1954; Pfeiffer et al., 1969, 1972). Studies suggest that sexual activity is part of life for people in their 60's, with 40% to 65% being sexually active; 10% to 20% of those over 75 report sexual activity, and some older people report increased patterns of sexual activity and increased interest with age.

Changes in sexual function occur gradually throughout the life span, and some may pass unnoticed. Processes essential for sexual response tend to occur more slowly with age, and the phase-specific changes may appear somewhat less intense. Nevertheless, the capacity for sexual pleasure persists among the elderly who are in reasonably good health.

As women age, there are gradual changes in their genitalia and breasts reflecting the change in estrogen levels. Delay in the production of vaginal lubrication may occur in some women, and others notice that the vagina becomes smaller in both diameter and length. In general, vasocongestive responses are less pronounced. Some women may experience painful intercourse because of slow or absent vaginal lubrication and thinning of the vaginal walls. Use of a water-soluble lubricant and having a sensitive, informed sexual partner are both helpful (Masters & Johnson, 1966).

Age-related changes in men parallel those seen in women. As men age, the time necessary to experience an erection increases, and the erection is likely to be less full than earlier in life. As with women, vasocongestive responses are less pronounced, and muscular contraction is less intense (Masters & Johnson, 1966).

For many older people, absence of a sexual partner through death or illness means lack of sexual opportunity. Some find this frustrating, and others inhibit their sexual desire. Still others find new opportunities for sexual pleasure and explore alternative means of obtaining sexual pleasure, such as masturbation or partner stimulation. Usually the most common reason given by both men and women for discontinuing sexual activity is the inability of the male partner to have an erection (Pfeiffer & Davis, 1972).

ASSESSING SEXUAL HEALTH

Assessment of sexual health begins with a sexual history and is supplemented by data about the person's general health, such as that obtained from the physical examination or general health history.

A brief sexual assessment can be based on a few short questions that are integrated into the health history (Table 30–2). The approach described here deals with the person's role and relationship: sexual self-concept and sexual function. Often, it is necessary to ask only the first or second item and the client will volunteer data related to the latter items. When a specific problem is identified that requires a referral to another clinician or when more data are needed for planning an approach to a specific problem, a sexual problem history can be obtained.

Sexual Problem History

The sexual problem history may be used in conjunction with the brief history described

TABLE 30–2. BRIEF SEXUAL ASSESSMENT QUESTIONS.

- Has being ill[a] interfered with your being a: mother, father, wife, husband?
- Has your surgery[a] changed the way you see yourself as a: man, woman?
- Has your disability[a] affected your sexual function?

[a]These items were adapted from McPhetridge (1968). The appropriate situation could be substituted for illness, surgery, or disability.

or alone in the context of sexual counseling or therapy. Although the parameters explored in a sexual problem history vary with the theoretical framework guiding the nurses' practice, there are commonalities to be explored regardless of the approach to therapy. The approach described here was suggested by Annon (1974).

The first component of the sexual problem history is a *description*, in the client's terms, of the current problem or concerns. Next, the *onset and course* of the problem are explored. The practitioner may wish to inquire about the client's age when the problem began, whether it had an insidious onset or occurred suddenly, whether the client can identify any precipitating events, and whether there are other life events associated with the sexual problem. The course of the sexual problem can be described in terms of its fluctuations over time, such as with the changing intensity of a disease process, and if the problem has any functional relationships to such phenomena as medication or alcohol use.

Of great importance is the client's *conception of the cause and persistence of the problem*. These data will enable the nurse to respond directly to the client's concerns rather than dealing with them directly.

Past attempts at treatment and their results may be explored, including evaluations by other health practitioners, such as physicians, the use of other professional help, such as professional counselors, and the attempts that the client has made to cope with the problem.

The last component of the sexual problem history includes an examination of the *client's current expectations and the goals* identified for treatment. A woman complaining of the inability to have orgasm may have the expectation of having orgasm with intercourse rather than by self-stimulation. If her expectations are not stated precisely, the practitioner may inappropriately treat her with the latter goal in mind or refer her to a practitioner whose approach to therapy would not be congruent with her goals.

Diagnosing sexual problems frequently is difficult. Often sexual problems are entangled in problems with relationships or with intrapersonal problems. As a consequence, the sexual problem may be a symptom of another problem, such as a power struggle in a relationship or of depression. Eliciting a careful description of the problem is, therefore, essential.

Disorders at any level of the nervous system have the potential to influence some or all of the phases of sexual response. Cerebral lesions or strong emotion may inhibit the desire phase or the reflex responses of the excitement phase. Lesions of the brainstem and spinal cord may interrupt partially or completely the connections between cognitively mediated desire and the effector systems necessary to achieve intercourse. Neuropathies and spinal cord lesions that affect sensation in large parts of the body, particularly erotic areas, may decrease the sensory components of desire. Autonomic neuropathies, lesions of the sacral cord and cauda equina, and peripheral neuropathies may prevent any reflex activity in the excitement and orgasmic phases, while leaving desire intact.

Preservation of reflex activity in the genital area makes physical intercourse potenitally achievable for the person with spinal cord damage. Loss of such reflexes prevents intercourse but does not prevent sexual expression and is not necessarily damaging to sexual health. People with dysfunction of physical sexual response do not lose their sexuality and can achieve intimacy and affection with alternative forms of expression.

Physical Examination

Although most dimensions of sexual health are best assessed by means of a sexual history, physical assessment techniques provide useful data about potential changes in sexual function, particularly when the client has a health problem involving the nervous system. Examination of sexual response is not necessary if there is no history of a problem with sexual function or evidence of functional loss of lower extremity function. Sensation, volitional control, and reflex tone each provide important data about potential capacity for sexual response. Aspects of the neurologic examination of both men and women are directed toward determining the segmental level of injury (or peripheral level of injury, as in cauda equina lesions), as well as completeness or incompleteness of spinal cord transections. Comarr and Vigue (1978) recommend that the sexual assessment be similar to that made for neurogenic bladder and bowel (see Chapter 27).

Rectal examination evaluates reflex motor function of the sacral cord segments S2, S3, and S4, important in reflex erection in men and sexual lubrication and swelling in women. Reflex control is assessed by inserting a gloved, lubricated finger into the rectum and noting the presence or absence of pressure from the contracting sphincter and then asking the client to voluntarily contract the sphincter and note the presence or absence of pressure on the gloved finger (Fig. 30–2). The bulbocavernous reflex is another way to elicit the anal reflex. Squeezing the glans penis in the male, or the glans clitoris in the female produces contraction of the anal sphincter if the reflex is present. Alternatively, one may elicit the anal reflex by stimulating the perianal skin lightly and observing for contraction of the sphincter. This response is often termed the "anal wink."

If sensation is abnormal in the lower extremities and trunk or if there is a history of injury involving the spinal cord, the sensory examination should include response to touch and pin over the genital and rectal areas (Fig. 30–3.), as well as careful mapping of sensation

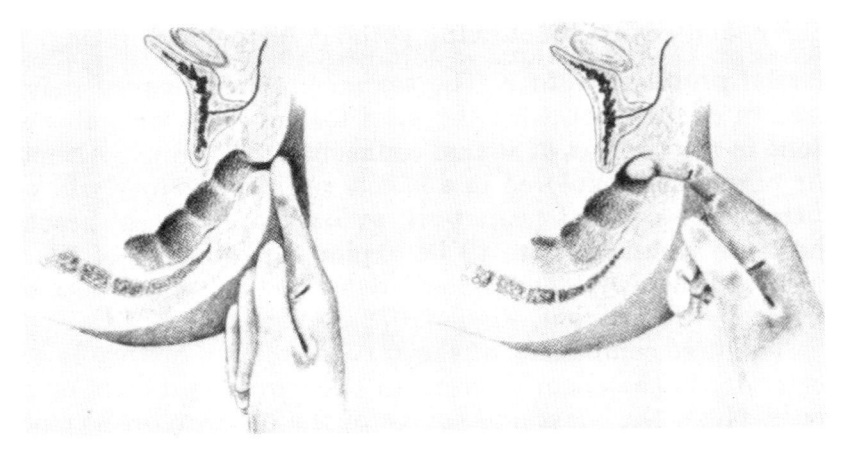

Figure 30–2. Examining the anal sphincter reflex. *(From Mitchell et al. [1984]. Neurological assessment for nursing practice.)*

over the trunk and lower extremities. Such findings help determine the potential for residual sexual response, as discussed in Chapter 31. Finally, reflex penile erection in men should be noted in response to sensory stimuli.

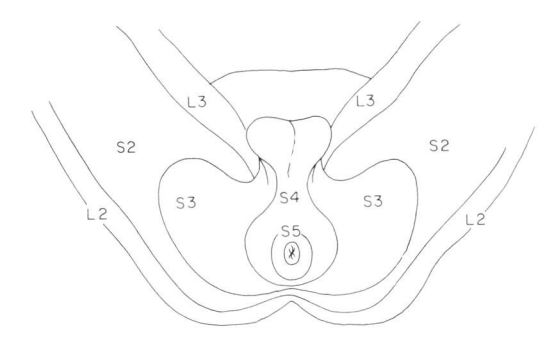

Figure 30–3. Sensory mapping of genital and rectal areas. L2, L3 indicates areas innervated by sensory roots entering the spinal column at lumbar vertebrae. S2–5 are areas sending sensory fibers to enter the spinal column at sacral levels. *(From Mitchell et al. [1984]. Neurological assessment for nursing practice.)*

REFERENCES

Annon, J. (1974). *The behavioral treatment of sexual problems.* Honolulu: Enabling Systems.

Beach, F. (Ed.). (1977). *Human sexuality in four perspectives.* Baltimore: Johns Hopkins University Press.

Bell, A., & Weinberg, M. (1978) *Homosexualities.* New York: Simon & Schuster.

Comarr, A., & Vigue, M. (1978). Sexual counseling among male and female patients with spinal cord and/or cauda equina injury. *American Journal of Physical Medicine, 57,* 107, 215.

Comfort, A. (1975). The normal in sexual behavior: An ethological view. *Journal of Sex Education and Therapy, 2,* 1.

Kinsey, A.C., Pomeroy, W., Martin, C., & Bebhard, P. (1948). *Sexual behavior in the human male.* Philadelphia: Saunders.

Kinsey, A. C., Pomeroy, W., Martin, C., & Bebhard, P. (1954). *Sexual behavior in the human female.* Philadelphia: Saunders.

McPhetridge, L.M. (1968). Nursing history: One means to personalize care. *American Journal of Nursing, 68,* 68.

Masters, W., & Johnson, V. (1966). *Human sexual response.* Boston: Little, Brown.

Masters, W., & Johnson, V. (1979). *Homosexuality in perspective.* Boston: Little, Brown.

Mims, F. (1978). A model to promote sexual health care. *Nursing Outlook, 26* (2), 121.

Money, J., & Erhardt, A. (1972). *Man and woman, boy and girl.* Baltimore: Johns Hopkins University Press.
Pfeiffer, E., & Davis, G.C. (1972). Determinants of sexual behavior in middle and old age. *Journal of the American Geriatric Society, 20,* 151.
Pfeiffer, E., Verwoerdt, A., & Davis, G.C. (1972). Sexual behavior in middle life. *American Journal of Psychiatry, 128,* 1262.
Pfeiffer, E., Verwoerdt, A., & Wang, H.S. (1969). The natural history of sexual behavior in a biologically advantaged group of aged individuals. *Journal of Gerontology, 23,* 193.
World Health Organization. (1975). Education and treatment in human sexuality: The training of health professionals. Report of a WHO meeting. *Technical Report Series,* no. 572, Geneva: WHO.

BIBLIOGRAPHY

Frank, E., Anderson, C., & Rubenstein, D. (1978). Frequency of sexual dysfunction in "normal couples." *New England Journal of Medicine, 299,* 111.
Kaplan, H.S. (1974). *The new sex therapy.* New York: Brunner/Mazel.
Kaplan, H.S. (1979). *Disorders of sexual desire and other new concepts and techniques in sex therapy.* New York: Brunner/Mazel.
Masters, W., & Johnson, V. (1970). *Human sexual adequacy.* Boston: Little, Brown.
Whitley, M., & Willingham, D. (1978). Adding a sexual assessment to the health interview. *Journal of Psychiatric Nursing and Mental Health Services, 16* (4), 17.

31

Alterations in Human Sexuality

Nancy F. Woods

Alterations in several aspects of human sexuality occur throughout the life span, frequently in response to illness. In general, these may be categorized as sexual dysfunctions, alterations in sexual self-concept, and alterations in sexual relationships. This chapter explores nursing diagnoses and management of each of these, with special emphasis on problems that clients with nervous system problems are likely to experience.

HUMAN RESPONSES IN SEXUAL DYSFUNCTIONS

Contemporary systems for the classification of sexual dysfunction include five major categories: desire phase, arousal phase, and orgasm phase dysfunctions, coital pain, and dissatisfaction with sexual frequency (Kaplan, 1974, 1979; Schover et al., 1982). Each broad category of dysfunction includes several specific types of problem. Moreover, each problem can be described as lifelong or not lifelong and global or situational. Qualifying information can be included in the diagnostic statement. The conventions used by Schover et al. (1982) are used in this discussion.

Alterations in Sexual Desire

Alterations in sexual desire include low sexual desire and sexual aversion. Low desire is defined on the basis of frequency of masturbation and partner activity as well as self-reports of desire for a partner and incidence of fantasy, erotic dreams, or seeking out erotic stimuli. Aversion to sex is defined as a clearly negative reaction to sex. Low sexual desire and sexual aversion form a continuum. Aversion is characterized by a clearly negative reaction to sex.

Alterations in sexual desire, including low sexual desire and aversion, can be attributed to both physiologic and psychosocial factors. Depression, severe stress states, certain pharmacologic agents, low androgen levels, and certain illnesses can interfere with sexual desire. Low sexual desire is a frequent concomitant of depression and may reflect severe stress. Many pharmacologic agents, including narcotics, sedatives, alcohol, centrally acting antihypertensives (such as reserpine and methyldopa) and testosterene antagonists, are associated with low sexual desire. Illnesses producing discomfort or malaise are linked to low sexual desire.

Desire phase dysfunctions may occur in response to conscious or unconscious thought processes (Kaplan, 1979). Sexual desire can be turned off by turning on physiologic inhibiting mechanisms associated with anger or fear. Fear and anger can occur as a result of personal conflicts about success and intimacy, complex intrapsychic problems, or severe relationship problems. Anger may be directed at the partner. Anxieties linked to childhood experiences, such as sexual abuse, pressure to have sexual relations, repeated unpleasurable experiences, and guilt, also may interfere with sexual desire.

Diagnosis of alterations in sexual desire is based on the individual's description of frequency of sexual activity and desire for erotic stimuli. Sexual aversion reflects a clearly negative reaction to sex, not just lack of interest. These diagnoses are based on data obtained from a sexual problem history similar to that described in Chapter 30. An important aspect of diagnosis is determining what, if any, qualifying information is pertinent. The diagnosis might be low sexual desire related to malaise from a chronic illness, low sexual desire related to effects of medication, or low sexual desire related to resentment toward a partner. Each of these diagnoses would imply different therapeutic strategies. Several nursing diagnoses related to sexual desire are presented as follows:

Nursing diagnoses of low sexual desire in clients with nervous system problems
Low sexual desire related to:
    Low energy level
    Medication regimen
    Severe stress
    Chronic pain
    Partner's poor health
    Partner's lack of acceptance of illness

Nursing interventions for low sexual desire and sexual aversion are directed to the underlying causes when they can be identified. When the diagnosis is low sexual desire related to low energy levels in a person with chronic illness, therapeutic strategies might include counseling the person to identify times when energy levels are high and attempting sexual activity then. Another strategy might be resting before sexual activity is anticipated. When low sexual desire is related to pharmacologic agents, it is sometimes possible to consult with the client's physician to alter the therapeutic regimen to enchance sexual desire (Table 31-1). When the diagnosis is low sexual desire related to anger directed toward a partner, referral for couple's counseling may be the optimum therapeutic alternative. Sexual aversion is most appropriately treated in the context of sex therapy or intensive psychotherapy.

> Ms. Barbara Thomas, 35 years old, has recently been diagnosed with multiple sclerosis. Her symptoms include transient numbness in her lower extremities, occasional urinary incontinence, and fatigue. She notes a decrease in sexual desire over the past 6 months, which she attributes to her fatigue and anxiety about being incontinent during sexual activity. Her partner of the last 6 years has been sensitive to her altered sexual desire and attributes it to her illness. Ms. Thomas has been able to give pleasure to her partner by having intercourse but says she just does not feel any motivation to initiate sexual activity with her partner or to stimulate herself sexually. She is "too tired."

A diagnosis of recent low sexual desire related to fatigue and anxiety about potential incontinence suggested the following therapeutic strategies:

1. Enhance sexual desire by planning rest periods before opportunities for sexual activity.
2. Reduce anxiety about incontinence by emptying bladder before sexual activity, discussing the possibility of incontinence with the partner, and using a protective sheet on the bed.

TABLE 31-1. DRUG EFFECTS ON HUMAN SEXUAL BEHAVIOR.

Drug or Drug Category	Effect	Probable Mechanism of Action
Oral contraceptives	Positive	Permits separation of sexual activity from concern about conception

Antihypertensives
  Clonidine (Catapres)
  Guanethidine (Ismelin)
  Methyldopa (Aldomet)
  Propranolol (Inderal)
  Reserpine (Serpasil)
  Trimethaphan (Arfonad)
	Negative	Peripheral blockade of nervous innervation of sex glands

Antidepressants
  Amitriptyline (Elavil)
  Desipramine (Norpramin, Pertofrane)
  Imipramine (Tofranil)
  Nortriptyline (Aventyl)
  Pargyline (Eutonyl)
  Phenelzine sulfate (Nardil)
  Protriptyline (Vivactil)
  Tranylcypromine (Parnate)
	Negative	Central depression; peripheral blockade of nervous innervation of sex glands

Antihistamines
  Chlorpheniramine (Chlor-Trimeton)
  Diphenhydramine (Benadryl)
  Promethazine (Phenergan)
	Negative	Blockade of parasympathetic nervous innervation of sex glands

Antispasmodics
  Glycopyrrolate methobromide (Robinul)
  Hexocyclium (Tral)
  Methantheline (Banthine)
  Poldine (Nacton)
	Negative	Ganglionic blockade of nervous innervation of sex glands

Sedatives and tranquilizers
  Benperidol
  Chlordiazepoxide (Librium)
  Chlorpromazine (Thorazine, Megaphen)
  Chlorprothixene (Taractan)
	Negative	Central sedation; blockade of autonomic innervation of sex glands; suppression of hypothalamic and pituitary function

Diazepam (Valium)
  Mesoridazine (Serentil)
  Methaqualone (Quaalude)
  Phenoxybenzamine (Dibenzyline)
  Prochlorperazine (Compazine)
  Thioridazine (Mellaril)
	Positive	Tranquilization and relaxation

Ethyl alcohol	Negative	Central depression; suppression of motor activity; diuresis
	Transiently positive	Release of inhibitions; relaxation
Barbiturates	Negative	Central depression; suppression of motor activity; hypnosis

Diuretics
  Bendroflumethiazide (Naturetin)
  Chlorthiazide (Diuril)
  Spironolactone (Aldactone)
	Negative	Diuresis

Sex hormone preparations
  Cyproterone acetate
  Methandrostenolone (Dianabol)
  Nandrolane phenpropionate (Durabolin)
  Norethandrolone (Nilevar)
	Negative	Antiandrogenic effects on sexual function; loss of libido; decreased potency

Methadone	Negative	Suppresses secondary sex organ function in men

TABLE 31-1. DRUG EFFECTS ON HUMAN SEXUAL BEHAVIOR. *(Continued)*

Drug or Drug Category	Effect	Probable Mechanism of Action
Potassium nitrate (saltpeter)	Questionable	Diuresis
Cantharis (Spanish fly)	Negative	Irritation and inflammation of genitourinary tract; systemic poisoning
Yohimbine	Questionable	Stimulation of lower spinal nerve centers
Strychnine	Questionable	Stimulation of neuraxis; priapism

Narcotics and psychoactive drugs
  Amphetamines
  Cocaine
	Negative	Central depression; decreased libido and impaired potency

Heroin
  LSD
  Marijuana
  Methadone
  Morphine
	Transiently positive	Release of inhibitions; increased suggestibility; relaxation

L-Dopa and p-chlorophenylalanine (PCPA)	Questionable	Improvement of well-being
Amyl nitrite	Questionable	Vasodilation of genitourinary tract; smooth muscle relaxation
Caffeine	Questionable	Central nervous system stimulant
Vitamin E	Questionable	Supports fertility in laboratory animals
Selenium	Questionable	Supports fertility in laboratory animals
Lithium carbonate	Questionable	Produces broad endocrine changes; diuresis
Clomiphene citrate (Clomid)	Questionable	Stimulates gonadotropic hormones; enhances expectations of achieving pregnancy
Bromocriptine (Parlodel)	Questionable	Stimulates gonadotropic hormones
Cimetidine (Tagamet)	Negative	Unknown
Clofibrate (Atromid S)	Questionable	Unknown
Disulfiram (Antabuse)	None by itself; negative with alcohol	Blocks alcohol metabolism; produces aldehyde syndrome

Reproduced by permission from N.F. Woods. Human sexuality in health and illness (3rd ed.). St. Louis, 1984, The C.V. Mosby Co.

Outcomes of these strategies include improvement in sexual desire, and Ms. Thomas and her partner's understanding of reasons for low sexual desire and concerns about incontinence.

Another example of altered sexual desire is that related to aversion in the partner. Often the sequelae of nervous system dysfunction produce bodily changes in the client and demands on the partner to participate in caretaking situations. Both of these situations may alter the partner's sexual desire.

Alterations in Sexual Arousal

There are several varieties of alteration in sexual arousal (sometimes referred to as excitement phase dysfunctions), including:

- Decreased subjective arousal
- Difficulty attaining an erection
- Difficulty maintaining an erection
- Difficulty in both attaining and maintaining an erection
- Decreased subjective arousal coupled with difficulty in attaining an erection or difficulty maintaining an erection or both
- Decreased physiologic arousal in women
- Decreased physiologic and subjective arousal in women.

Schover et al. (1982) distinguished between feelings of subjective arousal and physiologic arousal. They state that some clients report diminished vasocongestion without a loss of erotic sensation. It is possible for both men and women to experience a problem in physiologic aspects of arousal without a problem of subjective feelings of arousal, or vice versa. This diagnostic system offers precision in diagnosis of problems related to erection, since some men have problems attaining an erection, some with maintaining an erection, and some with both aspects.

Problems related to sexual arousal have their origins in body–mind interaction. It should be noted that transient episodes of difficulty in attaining or maintaining erection are common, with 50% of men experiencing them. Pharmacologic agents, such as those shown in Table 31–1, can interfere with physiologic correlates of sexual arousal in men and women. Disorders that affect vascular function, such as diabetes or Leriche syndrome, can impair erection in men and vasocongestion in women.

The aging process is associated with less intense vasocongestive response to sexual stimuli. Problems with vaginal lubrication and swelling are associated with menopausal changes in estrogen levels in some women.

Performance anxiety and fear of failure are commonly associated with arousal phase dysfunctions. In some instances, anxiety is produced by complex causes.

Diagnosis of arousal phase sexual dysfunction is usually based on *defining characteristics* obtained from a sexual problem history and physical examination. The physical examination may or may not provide evidence of arousal phase dysfunction. There may be reflex erection or swelling present with a pelvic or rectal examination, but their absence does not indicate dysfunction. Absence of sensation or alterations of sensation also may be evident in the physical examination (see Chapter 30). As with desire phase dysfunctions, diagnoses can be modified to indicate whether or not the problem is lifelong and situation specific; for example, it is possible to have a lifelong diagnosis of difficulty attaining an erection or decreased subjective arousal that is situational, that is, linked to an illness.

For people with nervous system problems, it is important to reflect on underlying neurophysiologic mechanisms involved in sexual arousal. The area of the parasympathetic outflow (S2, S3, S4) is important in both reflex erection in men and lubrication and swelling in women. Although sexual function is largely an autonomic function, the neurologic assessment is primarily a somatic examination, and the conclusions about autonomic function are made by inference from somatic findings. The distinction can be made between suprasegmental (upper motor neuron) and segmental (lower motor neuron) types of sexual function by means of data obtained from rectal examination. When reflex tone is present in the external sphincter, suprasegmental (upper motor neuron) disruption to sexual function exists. When reflex tone is not present in the external rectal sphincter, segmental dysfunction exists. The likelihood of experiencing erections is much greater for men with suprasegmental lesions.

Sensation and volitional control are important in assessing sexual function. When all sensation (pinprick, light touch) is absent from the genital area (penile, scrotal, perianal, vulval skin) *bilaterally* and when volitional control of the external rectal sphincter is absent, it can be inferred that the spinal cord has been functionally transected. The typical consequences are that sexual sensations are not perceived. There are, however, indications that spinal cord injured women with complete lesions perceive sensations associated with deep vaginal penetration. It is possible that pressure on the cervix causes stimuli to ascend to cortical levels via the autonomic nervous system. When any sensation or volitional control of the rectal sphincter is present, it can be inferred that the spinal cord is only partially transected, and the lesion is termed imcomplete. Both the completeness of the lesion and the segmental level have an important effect on prognosis for sexual function (Comarr & Vigue, 1978). Table 31–2 summarizes the effects of spinal cord injury on sexual functioning.

Inhibition of autonomic outflow can interfere with the vasocongestive aspects of

TABLE 31–2. SEXUAL RESPONSE OF PEOPLE WITH COMPLETE LESIONS OF THE SPINAL CORD.

Location of Cord Lesion	Sexual Function
C1–C3	• Male: Reflex erection from stimulation of genital region or thighs likely. Psychogenic erection from sexual thoughts not possible. Erogenous areas may develop above line of injury. No change in libido. • Female: Little study done. If lubrication analogous to erection, expect reflex lubrication similar to reflexogenic erection. As in male, will not feel sensations or be aware of lubrication unless it is pointed out. No change in libidinal drive. Fertility retained.
C4–C5	• Male: Reflex erection likely. Psychogenic erection impossible. Extragenital erogenous zones above level of injury likely. Nongenital orgasm reported. No ejaculation. Oral sex with partner possible. No change in libido. • Female: Reflex lubrication likely. Psychogenic lubrication unlikely. Extragenital erogenous zones above level of injury likely. Nongenital orgasm reported. Oral sex with partner possible. No change in libido. Fertility retained.
C6	• Male: As for C4–C5 level of injury. Holding and caressing now possible due to ability to use deltoids and biceps. • Female: As for C4–C5, with holding and caressing possible. Fertility retained.
C7–C8	• Male and female: Increased potential for use of hands to give pleasure to self and partner.
T1	• Male and female: As for C7–C8 level of injury, but with increased fine motor hand dexterity.
T2–T5	• Male and female: Commonly reported orgasmic experiences from nipple stimulation. Reflex erection and lubrication not seen.
T6–T12	• Male: Still generally unable to have psychogenic erection. Also unlikely to have reflex erection. • Female: Water-soluble lubricant needed for intercourse because of decreased reflex lubrication. Libidinal drive remains same. Fertility retained.
L1–L2	• Male: Psychogenic stimulation and erection possible between T12 and L2 level of injury. Reflex erections possible but unlikely below L1 and L2. • Female: Psychogenic erection of clitoris, lubrication, labial swelling, and skin flush possible but unlikely. Fertility retained.
L3–L4	• Male and female: No reflexogenic erection or lubrication. Psychogenic genital sexual reactions unlikely.
L5–S1	• Male and female: Extragenital sexual potential great. Erection and lubrication unlikely either through reflexogenic or psychogenic means.
S2–S4	• Male: Reflex erection possible. Ejaculation possible (may be retrograde).

Modified from Weinberg, 1982.

sexual arousal, although not with subjective components of sexual arousal. Although swelling and lubrication may be altered, sensations associated with sexual arousal may be experienced in areas of the body not affected by neurologic description.

Some diagnoses of desire phase dysfunction include:

• Decreased vasocongestion related to spinal cord injury

• Decreased subjective arousal related to fear of failure
• Difficulty maintaining an erection related to neuropathy

Nursing interventions for arousal phase dysfunctions usually are directed at reducing anxiety (performance anxiety or fear of failure) and collaborating with the physician in correcting or transcending physiologic problems if possible. Reduction of anxiety usually is accomplished through desensitization exercises in which women and men are instructed to use erotic imagery to approximate the sexual situations that evoke anxiety. Gradually, the erotic images approach the actual situation. Another therapeutic strategy involves structuring sexual encounters so they are not demanding. Exercises in which emphasis is placed on pleasure versus performance are suggested. These exercises emphasize sensual aspects of touch; often genital touching is prohibited. A special form of nondemanding encounter is called "sensate focus" and involves sequential pleasuring by oneself or a partner, gradually approximating the type of sexual activity (masturbation or intercourse) the individual desires. Fantasy or forms of stimulation other than by a partner can be used in conjunction with sensate focus exercises.

Arousal phase dysfunctions attributable to disrupted neurophysiologic functioning are common among people with nervous system problems. Therapeutic strategies can be directed toward altering or transcending the physiologic problem, which sometimes can be altered; for example, medication regimens that interfere with vasocongestion can be modified to restore sexual function. Sometimes therapeutic agents used to treat underlying medical problems may have positive effects on sexual dysfunction, as is sometimes noted with the use of steroids. Therapeutic strategies directed toward transcending arousal phase problems include techniques that amplify erotic sensations in parts of the body unaffected by pathology. For example, a woman with a sacral and compression injury may learn to amplify the erotic sensations she perceives in her breasts to the point of experiencing orgasm with breast stimulation.

> Mr. Michael Williams, 63 years old, experienced a ruptured cerebral aneurysm 6 months previously during sexual activity with his wife of 40 years. His aneurysm was successfully corrected surgically. He currently desires sexual activity and feels aroused but says he loses his erection too quickly to have intercourse. He is aware that he thinks about the experience of the cerebral hemorrhage and is fearful of its recurrence. Mr. Williams is currently taking propranolol. Mrs. William also is concerned about her husband's welfare and worries that her sexual interest may have been responsible for the initial hemorrhage and fears a recurrence.

A diagnosis of difficulty maintaining an erection, not lifelong, related to fear of a recurrence of cerebral hemorrhage and to medication suggests the following therapeutic strategies:

1. Reduce anxiety about sexual encounters through desensitization exercises using imagery to approximate feeling aroused, feeling an erection, and having intercourse.
2. Monitor response to desensitization exercises, progressing to sensate focus exercises with partner.
3. Monitor response to sensate focus exercises, progressing to intercourse with partner.
4. Monitor medication regimen; if counseling related to anxiety is not effective, discuss alteration of medication regimen.

Outcomes of these strategies include improvement in sexual arousal, being able to maintain an erection, and reduction of anxiety about sexual activity for Mr. Williams.

A diagnosis of anxiety related to her husband's well-being and fear of dangerous outcomes of sexual activity for Mrs. Williams suggests the following therapeutic strategies:

1. Counsel Mrs. Williams about the likelihood of recurrence of cerebral hemorrhage.
2. Involve Mrs. Williams in discussions of densensitization and sensate focus exercises.

Outcomes for Mrs. Williams should include an improved understanding of her husband's risk of untoward outcomes of sexual activity and reduced anxiety during sexual activity.

Alterations in Orgasm

Orgasm phase dysfunctions include problems with ejaculatory function and orgasm and with perception of pleasure associated with orgasm. Ejaculatory dysfunctions include premature ejaculation and inhibited ejaculation. Premature ejaculation occurs when men ejaculate too rapidly. Usually the definition is based on the individual's or the couple's definition of what is too rapid rather than some universally accepted standard. Premature ejaculation may occur before intromission or shortly after intromission. Men who experience premature ejaculation often do not perceive erotic sensations before orgasm and, instead, progress rapidly from low to very high levels of arousal. Often, an underlying problem is anxiety related to the experience of erotic sensations, and a variety of mechanisms has been suggested, including a learned behavior of rapid ejaculation, fear, anger, and anxiety.

Inhibited ejaculation, sometimes termed "retarded ejaculation," implies on inability to ejaculate at all during sexual activity or the requirement for an extended period of time to ejaculate, even in the presence of adequate stimulation. Some men have never ejaculated, even with masturbation; others have not ejaculated intravaginally. Inhibited ejaculation is often associated with lack of trust or anger in a relationship. Neurophysiologic and other medical conditions, as well as medications, can interfere with ejaculation and stimulation and may be responsible for inhibited ejaculation (Table 31-1).

Other problems men experience that are related to orgasm include anhedonic orgasm, which occurs when the client ejaculates with normal force but experiences no sensation, or inhibition of ejaculation, in which emission occurs resulting in seepage of semen rather than forceful ejaculation, and lack of pleasurable sensation is experienced. Ejaculation sometimes occurs with a flaccid penis and, in other instances, anhedonic orgasms may occur without penile flaccidity. Rapid ejaculation with a flaccid penis may occur, with or without sensation of pleasure (Schover et al., 1982).

Orgasmic dysfunctions in women include anorgasmia, a global incapacity to reach orgasm. A woman may be situationally inorgasmic, having orgasms with masturbation or partner manipulation. Anorgasmia with intercourse is a common dysfunction. Diagnoses include:

- Inorgasmic except with masturbation
- Inorgasmic except with partner manipulation
- Inorgasmic except with masturbation and partner manipulation
- Infrequent coital orgasms
- Inorgasmic except for vibrator or mechanical stimulation

Mechanisms responsible for orgasmic phase dysfunctions include inadequate stimulation or obsessive self-observation. More remote mechanisms include fear or loss of control over sexual or aggressive impulses.

Diagnosis of orgasm phase dysfunctions is based on a sexual history and physical examination. Particular emphasis is placed on differentiating the type of dysfunction and if the problem is lifelong or situationally related or global in nature.

It is important to assume that both physiologic and psychosocial mechanisms may be involved in orgasm phase dysfunctions among people who have nervous system problems. For example, a man who has a spinal cord injury affecting ejaculation may experience retrograde ejaculation—ejaculation of semen into the bladder—or may experience orgasm with a flaccid penis, common outcomes of spinal cord injury. The dysfunction may be premature ejaculation, not simply a consequence of the nervous system damage but also a consequence of the anxiety surrounding sexual activity. In short, a clinician cannot safely assume that because nervous system damage is present, it is the sole explanation for the dysfunction.

Nursing interventions for anorgasmia include structuring the situations for sexual activity to achieve stimulation under the most tranquil conditions possible. Some options include distraction from self-observation through the use of fantasy and the use of fantasy or imagery along with self-pleasuring exercises. In some instances, immobility interferes with pleasuring, and in others, lack of sensation or altered sensation interferes with orgasmic experience.

Strategies for premature ejaculation include use of the start–stop technique, in which stimulation is withdrawn intermittently to increase awareness of erotic sensations and to increase tolerance of the pleasure associated with sexual arousal.

Strategies for retarded ejaculation include the use of manual stimulation, gradually approximating vaginal intercourse. Relaxation and stimulation can be paired, or stimulation, along with distraction by fantasy, can be attempted.

> Ms. Linda McCarthy, 28 years old, fell from a horse, sustaining a complete spinal cord transection at L3–L4. Before her accident, she had been orgasmic with intercourse. Since she completed her rehabilitation program, she has had intercourse several times with her husband, has noted vaginal lubrication, has some sensation with deep penile penetration, but does not experience orgasm with intercourse.

A diagnosis of anorgasmia related to decreased sensory perception implies, as therapeutic strategies, enhancing erotic sensations through:

1. Sensate focus exercises to identify areas of maximum pleasure
2. Use of imagery to enhance sensations of sexual arousal
3. Rehearsal of communication regarding sexual pleasuring with her husband

Outcomes of these strategies include enhancement of erotic sensation, with improved understanding by both Ms. McCarthy and her husband of how to enhance pleasure, and experience of orgasm with intercourse for Ms. McCarthy.

> Ms. Debby Fox, a 23-year-old woman with cerebral palsy, has never been orgasmic, although she experiences sexual desire and feels aroused, that is, she perceives vaginal wetness. She does not have a sexual partner. Because of spasticity she is unable to pleasure herself manually.

A diagnosis of anorgasmia, lifelong, related to limited mobility suggests the following therapeutic strategies:

1. Use of vibrator and hand splint to provide sexual stimulation
2. Use of imagery to enhance sexual pleasure

Outcomes of these strategies include enhanced ability to attain sexual stimulation and orgasm.

Alterations in Sexual Self-Concept

An individual's sexual self-concept can be altered dramatically as a consequence of illness. Sexual self-concept includes the notion we have of ourselves as men or women, masculine or feminine. Sexual self-concept reflects body image and evaluation of one's adequacy as a man or a woman.

Surgery or injuries may cause changes in body image that may affect sexual self-concept. Sometimes a person who is ill takes on the identity of the illness, making it difficult to integrate sexuality with the role changes that accompany being sick. Embarrassment and shame associated with changes in one's body due to muscle wasting, spasticity appliances, and other bodily changes may produce intense anxiety about sexual activity and a pervasive sense of inadequacy.

Some of the nursing diagnoses associated with altered sexual self-concept include:

- Anxiety about sexual encounters related to altered body image
- Altered sexual self-concept related to sick role experiences
- Altered sexual self-concept related to partner's response

Diagnoses are based on the sexual history as outlined in Chapter 30. Often the concerns about sexual self-concept exist independent of experiences of sexual dysfunction.

Nursing interventions for enhancing sexual self-concept include those directed at acceptance and transcendence of altered body image:

1. Transcendence of the sick role
2. Enhanced support from a partner

Particular emphasis is focused on helping the client experience validation of himself or herself in a relationship. Reducing anxiety about sexual encounters because of changed body image involves acceptance and transcendence of a changed body. Often support from others who have coped with a similar health problem is invaluable. Rehearsing explanations of the health problem with the client also may be helpful. Exchanging information between clients about how to cope in sexual situations contributes to a broader array of coping strategies. Validation of the person's sexual self-image, that is, comments about the image he or she projects, are helpful.

Transcendence of the sick role is fostered by care environments that encourage client-involvement decision making and emphasize client efficacy. Attributions by others about the illness can either reinforce the client's self-image as sick or encourage the view of self as well and living with a challenge. The client can be encouraged to adopt a self-image consistent with remaining a healthy person in spite of pathology.

Obtaining support from a partner can enhance sexual self-concept. Some clients need assistance in building the social skills necessary to obtain support. These skills include the ability to communicate clearly and comfortably in sexual contexts.

> Olav Anderson, a 22-year-old logger, sustained a crushing cauda equina injury in a logging accident. He has regained some mobility in his lower extremities but does not have bowel control or erections. He has been severely depressed since the injury, referring to the loss of his "manhood" and his occupation as a logger. He refers to himself as "a crip" in front of his male friends and says they pity him.

A diagnosis of altered sexual self-concept related to loss of erections and his occupation implies the following therapeutic strategies:

1. Introduce the client to another spinal cord injured client who has adapted successfully to the injury and has a positive self-concept.
2. Invite the client to rehabilitation unit group meetings that include discussions of sexual adaptation.
3. Rehearse explanations to potential partners about his injury and its effects.
4. Provide anticipatory guidance regarding sexual challenges he may experience.
5. Discuss alternative strategies for sexual pleasuring that he may find satisfying for himself or a partner.
6. Refer the client for occupational counseling and retraining.

Outcomes of these strategies should include improved sexual self-concept as evidenced by a decrease in negative references to himself and by an increase in positive self-statements. Long-term goals are a positive sense of his sexuality and ability to be involved in a sexual relationship.

Alterations in Sexual Relationships

Sexual relationships are altered, sometimes profoundly, by illness. Value conflicts about sexual activity, difficulty communicating about sexual issues, dissatisfaction with sexual frequency, partner's inability to provide stimulation, inability to please a partner, and conflicts over the timing of sexual activity are a few of the difficulties couples can experience in their relationships.

In many instances, the partner has no acceptable outlet for sexual activity other than the ill person. When the client is ill, the partner may be forced to inhibit his or her sexual desire. Sometimes, partners who are also caretakers experience fatigue related to caretaking, which lowers sexual desire. In other instances, the partner may experience role confusion when required to care for the client *and* be a lover; for example, performing catheter care or a bowel regimen may be inconsistent with expressing physical love with the same person. In some couples, the partner may feel guilty or abnormal about initiating sexual activity with the person who is ill.

Alterations in sexual relationships as a result of illness are diagnosed through interview, optimally with both partners individually and together. Some nursing diagnoses related to altered sexual relationships include:

- Value conflicts related to alternative forms of sexual expression
- Dissatisfaction with lowered sexual frequency
- Dissatisfaction with partner stimulation
- Conflicts over timing of sexual activity

Nursing interventions are directed toward facilitating satisfactory involvement in a sexual relationship and emphasize sexual desires and dissatisfactions. Primary interventions include helping clients and partners communicate clearly and comfortably about their concerns and problems. Groups of clients and partners dealing with the same concerns are particularly helpful in this regard. Strategies include:

1. Modeling effective communcation
2. Providing information about the health problem and its effects on sexuality
3. Rehearsing communication about difficulties

> Sandra Miller, partner of a 30-year-old male involved in an automobile accident with resultant S2–S4 injury, is concerned about lack of vaginal stimulation. Her partner is able to have partial erections, but she has difficulty experiencing orgasm because of resultant decreased vaginal stimulation.

A diagnosis of dissatisfaction with stimulation consequent to partner's erectile dysfunction implies the following therapeutic strategies:

1. Provision of information about the effects of S2–S4 injury and partial erection
2. Provision of information about alternative stimulation, for example, use of technique for insertion of penis, use of vibrator or manual stimulation as a complement
3. Rehearsal of communication about sexually satisfying stimuli and providing feedback

REFERENCES

Comarr, A. & Vigue, M. (1978). Sexual counseling among male and female patients with spinal cord and/or cauda equina injury. *American Journal or Physical Medicine 57*, 107, 215.

Kaplan, H.S. (1974). *The new sex therapy.* New York: Brunner/Mazel.

Kaplan, H.S. (1979). *Disorders of sexual desire and other new concepts and techniques in sex therapy.* New York: Brunner/Mazel.

Schover, L., Friedman, M., Weiler, S., Heiman, J., & LoPiccolo, J. (1982). Multiaxial problem-oriented system for sexual dysfunctions. *Archives of General Psychiatry, 39,* 614.

BIBLIOGRAPHY

Anderson F., & Bardach, J.L. (1983). Sexuality and neuromuscular disease: A pilot study. *International Rehabilitation Medicine, 5,* 21.

Besterman, E.M. (1983). How disturbing are side effects of beta blockers? *European Heart Journal, 4[suppl],* D 143.

Bors, E., & Comarr, A.E. (1960). Neurological disturbances of sexual function, with special reference to 529 patients with spinal cord injury. *Urological Survey, 10,* 191.

Boyer, G., & Boyer, J. (1982). Sexuality and aging. *Nursing Clinics of North America, 17,* 421.

Bullard, D.G., & Knight, S.E. (1981). *Sexuality and physical disability: Personal perspectives.* St. Louis: Mosby.

Bush, P. (1980). *Drugs, alcohol and sex.* New York: Richard Marek.

Comarr, A.E. (1970). Sexual function among patients with spinal cord injury. *Urologia Internationalis, 25,* 134.

Fletcher, S. (1982). Learning needs related to sexual functioning of the neurologially impaired individual. In M.J. Van Meter (Ed.), *Neurological care: A guide to patient education* (p. 23). New York, Appleton-Century-Crofts.

Florian, V., & Shurka, E. (1983). Non-disabled opinions on sexual activities and family roles for disabled persons, and disabled persons' view of these opinions. *International Rehabilitation Medicine, 5,* 17.

Gatens, C. (1984). Sexuality and disability. In N.F. Woods (Ed.), *Human sexuality in health and illness* (3d ed.) (p. 341). St. Louis: Mosby.

Hale, J., Norman, A.D., Bogle, J., & Shaul, S. (1978). *Within reach: Providing family planning services to physically disabled women.* New York: Human Sciences Press.

Heslinga, K. (1974). *Not made of stone.* Springfield, IL: Thomas.

Humphrey, M., & Kinsella, G. (1980). Sexual life after stroke. *Sexuality and Disability, 3,* 150.

Lilius, H.G., Valtenen, E.J., & Wikstron, J. (1976). Sexual problems in patients suffering from multiple sclerosis. *Journal of Chronic Disease, 29,* 643.

Mooney, T.O., Cole, T.M., & Chilgren, R.A. (1975). *Sexual options for paraplegics and quadriplegics.* Boston: Little, Brown.

Phelps, G., Brown, M., Chen, J., Dunn, M., Lloyd, E., Stafanick, M.L., Davidson, J.M., & Perkash, I. (1983). Sexual experience and plasma testosterone levels in male veterans after spinal cord injury. *Archives of Physical Medicine and Rehabilitation, 64,* 47.

Robinault, I.P. (1978). *Sex, society and the disabled.* New York: Harper & Row.

Shaul, S., Bogle, J., Hale, J., & Norman, A.D. (1978). *Toward intimacy.* New York: Human Sciences Press.

Sjogren, K. (1983). Sexuality after stroke with hemiplegia. II: With special regard to partnership adjustment and to fulfillment. *Scandinavian Journal of Rehabilitation Medicine, 15,* 63.

Sjogren, K., Damber, J.E., & Liliequist, B. (1983). Sexuality after stroke with hemiplegia. I: Aspects of sexual function. *Scandinavian Journal of Rehabilitation Medicine, 15,* 55.

Steiger, J.C., & Brockway, J.A. (1980). Sexual enhancement in spinal cord injured patients. *Sexuality and Disability, 3,* 84.

Weinberg, J.S. (1982). Human sexuality and spinal cord injury. *Nursing Clinics of North America, 17,* 407.

Whitley, M., & Berke, P. (1984). Sexuality and diabetes. In N.F. Woods (Ed.), *Human sexuality in health and illness* (3d ed.) (p. 328). St. Louis: Mosby.

SECTION 9. SELF-CARE PHENOMENA

32

Self-Care: An Overview

Margaret Auld Bruya

SELF-CARE AND ITS RELATION TO NURSING PRACTICE

The basic role and importance of self-evaluation and self-care in health and during health deviations is of widespread concern to nurses. This chapter identifies self-care as a range of learned individual behaviors, health maintenance lifestyles, use of preventive health services, and symptom evaluation. The focus is on the developmental aspects of self-care practices, the role of family, and cultural practices. Alterations in self-care practices in relation to illness, particularly neurologic, are viewed as a deviation from the expected or developmental norm.

Developmental Aspects
A growing body of literature is available on self-care and self-care practices. Most authors agree that self-care is the basic level of health care in all societies. As such, self-care is considered a deliberate action of which the outcome is foreseen. It is not considered random or erratic behavior but behavior that is the result of thoughtful and deliberate choices. Common wisdom, the behavior and set of rules and logic, is a pattern many of us learn through acculturation. The patterns of normal self-care practice for each society reflect the extent to which scientific data and knowledge application are developed and available to the public. Some behaviors are enduring and culturally prescribed; others are current fashion and may be more transient (e.g., aerobic exercise).

Achievement of self-care ability in general is an anticipated outcome for humans. In pregnancy, it is normal for the mother to fantasize about the outcome of her pregnancy as a normal being. Being normal presumes the ability to experience sensation (e.g., taste, touch), to move at will (e.g., first one crawls, then walks, then runs), to have cognition, consciousness, and affect.

During the course of normal growth and development, the nervous system enables the individual to respond in an integrated fashion to the external and internal environments. Integrating the function of all body systems allows maximal use of the communication network among all body systems and facilitates learning and retention. When the integration function of the human nervous system is impaired, the ability to develop self-care and self-care health practices may be altered. The nurse's essential role in assessing potential for self-care is to evaluate the extent of neurologic dysfunction, including neuroendocrine function or dysfunction, to examine the stage of physical, psychologic, and psychosocial development of the individual, and to consider the sociocultural aspects.

Role of the Family and Social Group

The degree of attainment of self-care and self-care health practices is influenced primarily by the family group. In many cultures, it is the wife–mother who assumes this important role. The practices of self-care espoused by the family are affected by the position of the individual in that family as well as the roles assumed in that family. Litman (1971), however, found that the primary caretaker's knowledge about health and disease as well as knowledge about health care practices may be limited or erroneous. Other researchers have focused on the various family structures and functions in relation to sociocultural differences, looking for explanations for the findings of poorer health, health practices, and health outcomes among people in lower social class groups. One research study reported that 70% of the symptoms documented in a family health calendar were taken care of by the family or maternal involvement (Pratt, 1976).

Within a family group, people who can produce effective self-care must have essential health care knowledge of themselves as well as knowledge of environmental conditions (Orem, 1980). In order to effectively care for self or family, the individual making such decisions needs to have the requisite knowledge as well as be rational and reasonable in judgments. Disadvantages could occur in family-influenced self-care practices when a considerable lack of knowledge limits the ability to perform home care techniques, even those as simple as temperature determination.

Other disadvantages of family-influenced self-care health practices could be related to the level of the previous life experiences of the members. Orem (1980) claims, without research substantiation, that the essential elements to meet specific self-care demands are predicated on the ability to initiate and persevere in self-care to achieve desired results. She claims an ability to achieve this results from:

1. Having knowledge and skills
2. Being motivated to initiate and continue effects
3. Being committed to meeting particular demands for care
4. Being able to execute the movements required
5. Having energy and a sense of well-being sufficient to initiate and sustain self-care

The dominant beliefs and practices of the culture may determine the relationship of the family's role in self-care and the use of professional health care services.

Cultural Factors

In every culture, self-care is learned through human interaction within the context of the sociocultural group. Leininger (1978) suggests that culturally variant groups view illness in two ways. One group perceives illness to be largely a personal body experience. The other group categorizes illness as extrapersonal, or outside the body. For this group, illness might be viewed as resulting from angered spirits. Such difference may account for the manner in which self-care practices are learned. The group who believe that illness is a personal and internal body experience tend to use more technical and physical self-care, whereas those who view illness as an extrapersonal experience would not consider self-care as relevant to health.

Birenbaum's views (1981) confirm this culturally acquired viewpoint. One's group membership and social ties may establish barriers or promote access to seeking professional health care. Working with multiethnic migrants, Byerly (1980) found that there was a great deal of moving in and out of lay and traditional systems and subsystems as the circumstances dictated.

Early cultural conditioning determines a person's attitudes and reactions to healing beliefs and practices, including self-care practices. When immigration and migration occur, blurring and partial assimilation of one's early and newly acquired health and self-care beliefs may occur. Typically, assimilation into a dominant culture influences an individual, but rather than fully embracing the dominant culture, the individual, and subsequently family members for whom he or she shares responsibility, develops bicultural values. The family choices reflect this bicultural use of alternate health beliefs and practices (Orque et al., 1983).

The Orque et al. (1983) text, is an excellent resource for a full description of cultural variation of health and self-care practices. The emphasis on personal or situational control of self-care practices and health care actions for a number of culturally diverse populations is explored. The belief that culturally prescribed healing remedies may help a person psychologically is subscribed to by many blacks; however when such practices fail, a medical person is sought (Orque et al., 1983). Trust in God and in Curanderos (folk healers) characterizes Latinos, whereas Filipinos and Chinese gravitate toward bicultural health practices when assimilated into the more dominant western culture (Orque et al, 1983).

Nurses need knowledge of the variety of cultural influences that have an impact on self-care and health practices. A repertory of cognitive, perceptual, manipulative, communication, and interpersonal skills is essential to exercise self-care practices, and each is influenced by cultural values and beliefs. Viewing a client in the context of his or her cultural orientation and heritage should assist the nurse to facilitate the deliberate performance of health behaviors designed to assist the best outcome. Societal values and influences and individual hierarchies of values in seeking and using the predominant health services of the society all influence health outcomes.

Economic Factors

Economic detriments, such as market supply, demand, and distribution of professional health personnel and services influence one's self-care. Abundant lay literature is available to the literate public. The self-treatment component of self-care is thought to represent growing discomfort and disgruntlement with the perceived dysfunctional aspects and effects of contemporary health service systems. Self-treatment in response to this disgruntlement is not universal but may reflect the historical reliance on one's own emotional and physical resources (Dean, 1981).

Third-party payment, Medicare, and Medicaid programs have made professional care available to more people. This pattern is changing rapidly from the many options available to eligible subscribers in the 1960s to severely curtailed funded professional services available today. In professional health services, the result has been drastic cuts in lengths of hospital stay, more acutely ill persons being discharged from agencies sooner, and the necessity for greater home nursing skills to treat such people. The need to learn self-care skills in managing chronic illness is increased by these factors.

Either as a supplement to or as a substitute for professional services, self-care practices vary among and between individuals. Developmental, social, cultural, economic, religious, and health factors and values have an impact on one's ability to integrate self-care into the living pattern. Nurses must recall that, in order to exercise self-care, one must have knowledge of one's abilities and limitations. It is said that nursing and the provision of nursing services begin when an individual or groups of individuals do not or cannot meet self-care action requirements for health (Orem, 1980).

COMPONENTS AND ASSESSMENT OF SELF-CARE

The ability to self-care is conceptually automatic after one has learned how to do so. Beginning with childhood, one learns to perfect attainment of a comfortable level of self-care. Given a broad range of physical, biologic, and social conditions, individuals who have successfully mastered previous learning can adapt their repertory of abilities and limitations accordingly and are able to estimate their measure of self-care. The power to exercise self-care includes vigilance to the goal; attention to the task; available, usable physical energy; motivation to perform necessary tasks; appropriate technical knowledge; and ability to reason, make reasoned decisions, and conceptualize the plan as an action (Orem, 1980). Support systems, in the form of family, traditions, societal norms, religious and spiritual values, also affect self-care.

The equilibrium achieved in the prototypical model of an individual able to care for self can be contrasted to the disequilibrium of one whose skills are no longer operative. Acute or chronic illness, accidents, or extremes in neuroendocrine balance can bring chaos to the individual or to the support systems for that individual. Neurologic or orthopedic damage from an accident may render an individual unable to move, to experience sensations sufficiently to protect vital functions, or to think clearly enough to make decisions. Similarly, a mildly injured or head-injured person whose forte in the past was a strong memory may experience extreme frustrations in coping with the day-to-day short-term memory needed to read the daily newspapers. A person with hypersecretion of a hormone may experience alterations in affect. Habituated self-care practices are severely affected in each of these examples.

The manner in which deviation from usual self-care practices affects an individual relates back to his or her developmental stage. A young child is not expected to perform extensive self-care practices or to exert extensive personal control over health and health actions. Rather, a responsible adult typically does this. The nurse's role is to respect the client's (including the adult) perceived needs rather than impose the nurse's perceived need. A parallel exists in an adult whom we anticipate to be developmentally mature but whose role may be altered or deviated from the norm.

Assessment of the impact of a neurologic disorder on self-care would then be expected to include: (1) the extent to which the deviation has an impact on mobility, sensation, cognition, coping, consciousness, affect, and support system(s), (2) level of development, (3) prior self-care practices, (4) economic and human resources, and (5) cultural beliefs and norms regarding self-care.

When deviations from self-care occur, the effect is not solely on the individual. The nurse must evaluate that person's role in the family, the age, sex, cultural, and social preferences, the health care situation (e.g., temporary or chronic), the knowledge, and the pathology involved.

The assessment of self-care usually follows a hierarchical model, from being able to perform basic activities of daily living (ADL) to the exercise of a degree of perfection in self-care management. When a client appears to have intact neurologic systems necessary for the exercise of self-care and has the cognitive abilities to do so, yet does not exercise self-care options to the extent the nurse thinks optimal, conflict may occur. In such situations, it may be necessary for the nurse to look beyond the physiologic and psychosocial parameters and investigate cultural patterning.

SUMMARY

The concept of self-care is viewed from developmental, sociocultural, and humanistic dimensions. This view serves as a basis to understand and to learn to view the ability for self-care and self-care practices from a broader perspective than simply providing for one's own activities of daily living. Nursing's role to assess abilities and limitations for self-care are needed when caring for human beings who cannot care for themselves.

REFERENCES

Birenbaum, A. (Ed.). (1981). *Health care and society*. Montclair, NJ: Allenheld, Osmun & Co.

Byerly, E.L. (1980). *Health care alternatives of multiethnic migrants*. A Report to the Division of Nursing, Nursing Research Branch, Public

Health Service, Dept. of Health and Human Services. Grant NU00592.
Dean, K. (1981). Self-care responses to illness: a selected review. *Social Science in Medicine, 15A*, 673.
Leininger, M. (1978). *Transcultural nursing: Concepts, theories and practices.* New York: Wiley.
Litman, T. (1971). Health care and the family: A three-generation analysis. *Medical Care, 9(3)*, 67.
Orem, D.E. (1980). *Nursing: Concepts of practice* (2nd ed.). New York: McGraw-Hill.
Orque, M.S., Block, B., & Monroy, L.A. (1983). *Ethnic nursing care.* St. Louis: Mosby.
Pratt, T. (1976). *Family structure and effective health behavior.* Boston: Houghton-Mifflin.

BIBLIOGRAPHY

Aamodt, A.A. (1978). The care component in a health and healing system. In Bauwens, E.E. (Ed.), *The anthropology of health.* St. Louis: Mosby.
Antrobus, M. (1981). Self-care in sickness and in health. *Nursing Times, 10*(342), 347.
Brownlee, A.J. (1978). *Community culture and care.* St. Louis: Mosby.
Cammermeyer, M. (1983). A growth model of self-care for neurologically impaired people. *Journal of Neorosurgical Nursing, 15*(5), 299.
Caporael-Katz, B. (1983). Health, self-care and power: Shifting the balance. *Topics in Clinical Nursing, 5*(3), 31.
Cousins, N. (1976). The anatomy of an illness as perceived by the patient. *New England Journal of Medicine, 295*(26), 1458.
Cousins, N. (1979). *Anatomy of an illness as perceived by the patient.* New York: Bantam Books.
Damant, M. (1981). The meaning of self-care. *Community Outlook,* 11, 373.
Decker, S.D., & Kinzel, S. (1985). Learned helplessness and decreased social interaction in elderly disabled persons. *Rehabilitation Nursing, 10*(2), 31.
Dickson, G.L., & Lee-Villasenor, H. (1982). Nursing theory and practice: A self-care approach. *Advances in Nursing Science, 5*(1), 29.

Goodin, B. (1984). Self-care in health. *Lamp, 41*(5), 24.
Harper, D.C. (1984). Application of Orem's theoretical constructs to self-care medication behaviors in the elderly. *Advances in Nursing Science, 6*(3), 29.
Hyde, A. (1975). The phenomenon of caring: Part I. *Nursing Research Report, 10*(1), 1, 10.
Hyde, A. (1976). The phenomenon of caring: Parts II, III. *Nursing Research Report,* 11, 2, 15.
Hyde, A. (1977). The phenomenon of caring: Part IV. *Nursing Research Report,* 12, 2.
Johns, J.L. (1985). Self-care today in search of an identity. *Nursing and Health Care, 6*(3), 153.
Katz, S., Branch, L.G., Branson, M.H., Papsidero, J.A., Beck, J.C., & Greer, D.S. (1983). Active life expectancy. *New England Journal of Medicine, 309*(20), 1218.
Kearney, B.Y., & Fleischer, B.J. (1979). Development of an instrument to measure exercise of self-care agency. *Research in Nursing & Health, 2*(1), 25.
Kerr, J.A. (1985). Adharance and self-care. *Heart and Lung, 14*(1), 24.
Leininger, M. (1977). The essence and central focus of nursing: The phenomenon of caring, Part V. *Nursing Research Report, 12*(1), 2, 14.
Levin, L.S., Katz, A.H., & Halst, E. (1979). *Self-care: Lay initiatives in health.* New York: Prodist.
Nelson, D. (1984). Nurse managed rehabilitation. *Nursing Management, 15*(3), 30.
Orem, D.E. (Ed.). (1979). The Nursing Development Conference Group. *Concept formalization in nursing.* Boston: Little, Brown.
Pattulo, A.W., & Barnard, K.E. (1968). Teaching menstrual hygiene to the mentally retarded. *American Journal of Nursing, 68*(12), 2572.
Schlotfeldt, R.M. (1976). Accountability: A critical dimension in health care. In M. Leininger (Ed.), *Transcultural health care issues and conditions.* Philadelphia: Davis.
Winegrad, C.H. (1984). Mental status tests and the capacity for self-care. *Journal of the American Geriatric Society, 32*(1), 49.

33

Alterations in Self-Care

Christina Mumma

Many individuals focused on their independence when asked what they miss most about their lives before having a stroke compared to life after the stroke. (Mumma, 1986). Common statements were:

> I miss being able to go where I want, when I want.
> I'm helpless now; have to depend on others for everything.
> Everything I enjoyed is gone since the stroke; I'm of no use to anyone now.

People who acquire neurologic dysfunction as a result of cerebrovascular accident (CVA) or other diseases or injuries are likely to experience a variety of alterations in self-care. These self-care deficits vary in both quality, or type of deficit, and quantity, or severity of deficit.

CONTINUUM OF SELF-CARE

The type of self-care discussed most often in the nursing literature can be categorized as activities of daily living (ADL). Hickey (1986) defined ADLs as "self-care activities that must be independently accomplished each day in order for the patient to assume responsibility for his own needs and to actively participate in society (p. 183). The self-care activities usually included are self-feeding, bathing, dressing, grooming, toileting, and home care skills (Orem, 1971; Snyder, 1983; Rehabilitation Core Curriculum, 1981). Whether a person must be totally independent in the performance of basic self-care tasks to be an active participant in society is debatable. There are many people with disabilities who depend on others for assistance with such personal self-care activities as bathing, dressing, and toileting but maintain full-time jobs and display considerable productivity and creativity. They are certainly active participants in society. The self is considerably more than the body that is fed, bathed, dressed, toileted, and provided a home. Thus, as discussed in Chapter 32, self-care can be thought of in much broader terms.

Orem (1980) built her model of nursing around the concept of self-care. She states that nursing is the assistance of individuals in the provision and management of self-care in order to sustain life and health, recover from

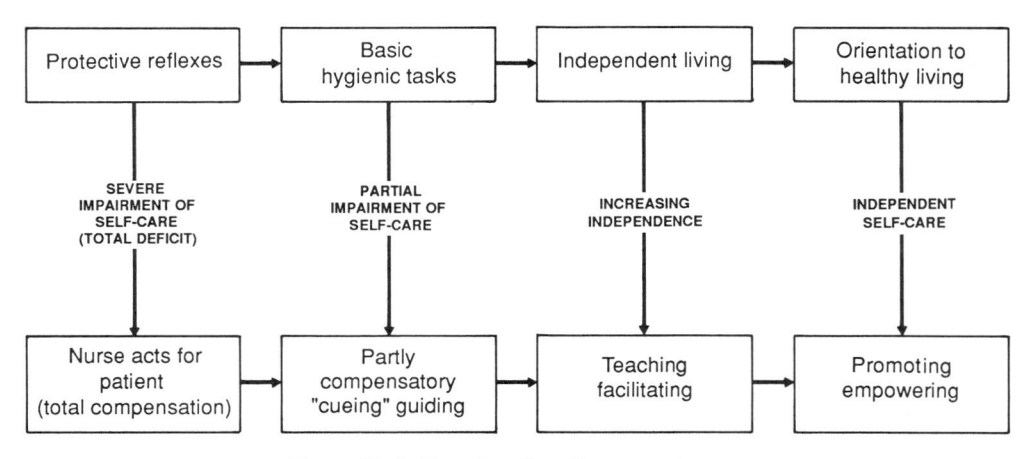

```
┌─────────────────┐    ┌─────────────────┐    ┌─────────────────┐    ┌─────────────────┐
│ Protective      │───▶│ Basic           │───▶│ Independent     │───▶│ Orientation to  │
│ reflexes        │    │ hygienic tasks  │    │ living          │    │ healthy living  │
└─────────────────┘    └─────────────────┘    └─────────────────┘    └─────────────────┘
         │                      │                      │                      │
   SEVERE                 PARTIAL                 INCREASING            INDEPENDENT
   IMPAIRMENT OF          IMPAIRMENT OF           INDEPENDENCE          SELF-CARE
   SELF-CARE              SELF-CARE
   (TOTAL DEFICIT)
         ▼                      ▼                      ▼                      ▼
┌─────────────────┐    ┌─────────────────┐    ┌─────────────────┐    ┌─────────────────┐
│ Nurse acts for  │───▶│ Partly          │───▶│ Teaching        │───▶│ Promoting       │
│ patient         │    │ compensatory    │    │ facilitating    │    │ empowering      │
│ (total          │    │ "cueing" guiding│    │                 │    │                 │
│ compensation)   │    │                 │    │                 │    │                 │
└─────────────────┘    └─────────────────┘    └─────────────────┘    └─────────────────┘
```

Figure 33-1. Alterations in self-care continuum.

disease or injury, and cope with the effects of disease or injury. Methods and amounts of nursing care required depend on the type and severity of alterations in self-care. Self-care ability can be considered as a continuum from inability to perform any self-care activities (total self-care deficit) to ability to perform all self-care activities independently. The broadest interpretation of alterations in self-care would allow for growth and expansion of self, not just self-care deficits. Obviously, people are more likely to come to the attention of nurses and the health care system for "too little" self-care rather than for "too much" self-care. Figure 33-1 illustrates the continuum of alterations in self-care, with examples of nursing interventions at various points along the continuum.

The purpose of this chapter is to examine alterations in self-care typically experienced by individuals with nervous system dysfunction. Illustrative case examples are provided in relation to the following areas of the self-care continuum depicted in Figure 33-1: protective reflexes, basic hygienic tasks, independent living, and orientation to healthy living. The discussion of each type of self-care alteration includes manifestations and human responses. Manifestations involve the relationship of the alteration in self-care to neuroanatomy and neurophysiology. Each self-care alteration is viewed as a human response to multiple phenomena. The neurologic dysfunction resulting from nervous system injury or disease is usually the most important phenomenon to which the individual is responding. Other influencing phenomena include intrapersonal factors (e.g., beliefs, values, self-esteem), interpersonal factors (e.g., relationships with loved ones and caregivers), and environmental factors (e.g., the treatment environment, health care system). Since the phenomena listed are in continuous, dynamic interaction, alterations in self-care are highly complex human responses.

ALTERATIONS IN SELF-CARE

Alterations in Self-Care: Protective Reflexes

The manifestations, or neuroanatomic evidence, within the nervous system of an individual functioning at the level of protective reflexes have left that person dependent on others to meet all self-care needs. Nervous system dysfunction severe enough to cause coma is the result of cortical damage leading to indirect interruption of the ascending reticular activating system (ARAS) or a direct lesion of the ARAS, for example, a brainstem injury (Alcorn, 1983).

Case Study 1

Joshua J is a 21-year-old male with a medical diagnosis of closed head injury and coma secondary to a motor vehicle accident. He is being cared for in a neurologic–neurosurgical intensive care unit. One week ago, on his 21st birthday, he was struck by a speeding car while driving the new car his parents had given him as a birthday present. Paramedics found Joshua unconscious at the scene of the accident. He was transported to a nearby hospital, where an emergency computerized tomography (CT) scan indicated bilateral intracerebral hemorrhage and contusion but no bleeding into the subdural or epidural spaces. After admission to the intensive care unit, Joshua remained comatose with withdrawal response to painful stimuli only. Joshua's parents were called by the police shortly after the accident and have remained with their son almost constantly since his admission to the hospital. They have been kept informed of Joshua's condition and treatment and have been told that his prognosis for functional recovery is guarded.

Assessment and Goals for the Individual. When an individual has severely impaired level of consciousness, a detailed assessment of self-care abilities is not appropriate and is not possible. Participation in self-care activities requires an individual to be awake and alert. A comatose person would thus be diagnosed as having a *total self-care deficit.* The ongoing evaluation of the comatose individual's level of neurologic functioning with regard to protective reflexes would be performed by adding brainstem reflex assessment to a coma scale (Chapters 5 and 6).

Examples of *goals* that might be established for the individual functioning at the level of protective reflexes are:

- Short-term goal: basic self-care activities will be done for the patient by nurses and family members.

- Long-term goal: Return to maximum level of independence possible in performance of self-care activities.

Nursing Interventions for the Individual. The comatose patient will require what Orem (1980) referred to as a totally compensatory nursing system. To the extent that an individual cannot independently perform needed self-care functions, others will perform those activities. One important consideration is the environment within which care is provided. During the critical care phase, it would be most appropriate to provide care within a specialty unit (neurologic or neurosurgical intensive care unit) if available. Care should be provided by nurses with knowledge, skill, and experience in providing totally compensatory care to comatose patients and their families. It would be advantageous to have clinical nurse specialists (critical care, neurology or neurosurgery) available as resources to the nurses providing direct patient care on a daily basis. The specialist nurses would work in the clinical area with the generalist (staff) nurses, participating in the care of the patient to effect facilitating, guiding, teaching, and role modeling. The specialist thus indirectly delivers care to the patient by influencing the care given by the direct caregiving nurses.

Assessment and Interventions for the Family and Significant Others. When an individual sustains a brain injury that results in coma, the extent of that person's awareness of the situation is unknown. However, the impaired individual's family and significant others are acutely aware of the impact of the profound disability. Their coping capacities are severely tested by having a loved one changed from normally functioning to comatose. Nursing assessment of the family related to the individual's total self-care deficit begins with an evaluation of their understanding of the comatose individual's neurologic condition, prognosis, and inability to manage any aspect of personal self-care. The assessment also should include the extent to which family members are able and willing to be involved in meeting the patient's self-care needs. This ability and willingness to participate in caregiving activities depends to a considerable extent on family members' own grief experience and coping abilities. Such participation may actually facilitate family coping and resolution of grief (Werner-Beland, 1980). Another area of family assessment is the family members' own self-care activities and availability and use of support systems. Examples of possible family-focused goals related to self-care, protective reflexes are:

- Family participation in patient's self-care activities (e.g., bathing, grooming)
- Family member effectively meeting their own self-care needs

Nursing interventions provided by nurse generalists and nurse specialists would be based on this assessment and would be specific to the needs of particular families. The staff nurses would assess family understanding of the patient's condition and involve family members in the day-to-day care of the patient to the extent that individual family members chose to participate. The neurologic nurse specialist would be consulted as needed to promote family participation and teach family members particular skills. The specialist's expertise in the area of family adaptation to disability is particularly helpful in the assessment and interventions related to family members' efforts at meeting their own self-care needs. The specialist would also be a teacher and role model to the staff nurses, thereby promoting and facilitating excellent patient and family care.

Assessment and Interventions for the Community. Community assessment related to profound neurologic impairment primarily involves attempts to gauge the knowledge and understanding of people in the community about catastrophic neurologic events, especially those associated with motor vehicle accidents. Other important areas of assessment include availability of motor vehicle accident prevention and safety promotion programs and legislative requirements for safety promotion (e.g., child restraint and seatbelt use) (Lipe, 1985).

Community-focused interventions by both nurse generalists and nurse specialists are based on a systematic community assessment. Nursing interventions toward advocacy, public education, and political action on behalf of persons with profound neurologic impairments and their families should be coordinated with the ongoing efforts of organizations such as the National Head Injury Foundation.

Alterations in Self-Care: Basic Hygienic Tasks

For many individuals with nervous system dysfunction, alterations in self-care occur in relation to the performance of basic hygienic tasks, such as bathing, dressing, and toileting. The neuroanatomic manifestations of impairment in performance of basic hygienic tasks are primarily in the areas of movement, sensation, and cognitive function. The types of cognitive impairment underlying self-care deficits include memory loss, impaired abstract thinking, easy distractibility, short attention span, impaired judgment, and difficulty transferring learning from one situation to another. Cognitive deficits can often be more impeding of self-care performance and more difficult for family and friends to cope with than other manifestations of neurologic dysfunction, for example, paralysis or communication impairment.

Case Study 2

Jack R is a 66-year-old man who is 5 days post-right cortical CVA (infarction). His stroke resulted in left hemiparesis, left hemisensory deficit, left neglect, and impulsiveness. He has a 20-year history of hypertension and was under treatment with antihypertensive medication. He did not take the medication consistently because he "felt fine" without it. Jack and his wife have been married for over 30 years and have five grown children. He retired last year from his job as a mail carrier for the U.S. Postal Service. His wife is in her middle 50s and works part-time as a dental office receptionist. She enjoys her job and does not want to retire for a least 5 more years. Both Jack and his wife describe him as an active, outgoing person who kept busy all the time and could not tolerate sitting around with nothing to do. Jack frequently asks his nurses when his left arm and leg will return to normal so he can be a "whole man" again.

Assessment for the Individual. There are a number of possible approaches to the assessment of an individual's ability to perform basic hygienic tasks of self-care. One approach is to evaluate specific aspects of nervous system functioning, such as motor ability, sensation, and perceptual ability, and then make prognostic statements about the individual's basic hygienic task performance. A more direct approach is to evaluate the individual's actual performance of such self-care tasks as bathing, toileting, dressing, and self-feeding. A complete neurologic nursing assessment would include the evaluation of basic hygienic task performance, often categorized as ADLs.

One frequently used approach to the assessment of ADLs involves the use of scales that yield functional ability–disability scores. The scales most often referred to in the literature include the PULSES Profile and the Barthel Index (Dudas, 1986; Granger, Gresham 1984; Rehabilitation Core Curriculum, 1981). A scale that is more relevant to a nursing assessment of ADLs is the Enforced Social Dependency scale (ESD) The ESD is a measure of the reliance of the individual on others for the performance of tasks previously accomplished without assistance (Benoliel et al., 1980). The ESD scale was originally developed within research studies of people with cancer and heart disease but has been used recently to measure enforced social dependency within a sample of people poststroke (Mumma, 1984).

The ESD scale is composed of two subscales, Personal Competence and Social Competence (Benoliel et al., 1980). The performance of basic hygienic tasks is measured within the Personal Competence subscale. Assessment of an individual's basic hygienic task performance could lead to the following specific nursing diagnoses (American Nurses' Association & American Association of Neuroscience Nurses, 1985, p. 10):

- Self-care deficit: Impaired ability to feed self
- Self-care deficit: Impaired ability to bathe self
- Self-care deficit: Impaired ability to dress self
- Self-care deficit: Impaired ability to use toilet

Examples of possible individual goals related to the performance of basic hygienic tasks are:

- Short-term goal: Participation in self-feeding with set-up, cueing, and supervision by nursing staff.
- Long-term goal: Demonstration of maximum level of independence possible in performance of basic hygienic tasks (consistent with physical and cognitive limitations).

Nursing Interventions for the Individual. The generalist nurses caring for an individual with impaired ability to perform basic hygienic tasks would use a partly compensatory nursing system for the delivery of nursing care (Orem, 1980). A potentially effective approach to the care of people with impaired ability to perform basic self-care tasks is based on rehabilitation nursing principles. Major principles include (Rehabilitation Core Curriculum, 1981, p. 5):

1. Promotion of health and optimum human potential
2. Focus on individual wholeness and uniqueness
3. Active partnership with clients and their families
4. Provision of supportive environment in which to facilitate independence
5. Emphasis on teaching and preparing individual to return to functional role within family and community
6. Continuity of care for clients and families

Facilitating attainment of the goal of independent performance of basic hygienic tasks requires such nursing interventions as teaching, guiding, cueing, and supporting. The nurse collaborates with other members of the health care team to ensure goal attainment. If the patient is transferred to a rehabilitation setting, the involvement of the multidisciplinary rehabilitation team is explicit. In such settings, goal establishment and care planning are usually team endeavors. Specialist nurses would be available as resources to the generalist nurses.

Assessment and Interventions for the Family and Significant Others. When an individual acquires a neurologic disability that impairs the ability to meet self-care needs, the person's adaptive ability is severely challenged. Adaptive challenges are faced also by the individual's loved ones. Family assessment related to basic hygienic self-care tasks has a number of components. It is important to assess family members' knowledge and skills related to self-care activities as a basis for involving family members in the patient's care and rehabilitation program. It is also essential to assess how the family is coping with a suddenly disabled loved one. Spouses, in particular, will often describe feeling as if they had lost the person they knew before the disabling event (Mumma, 1984). Other aspects of the family assessment include (1) an examination of how family members are caring for themselves and (2) assessment of availability and use of support systems.

Family-focused interventions are based on the nurse's sensitivity to the profound stresses experienced by family members coping with the patient's sudden disability. Nursing interventions designed to provide support to family members can be delivered both individually and in a group setting. Support groups provide participants with the opportunity to discuss their experiences with others in a similar situation—as family members of a newly disabled individual. Additional family interventions are similar to those used with the patient, with the added dimension of interaction among family members. Potentially useful interventions include teaching, guiding, modeling, and active listening. These interventions are discussed in Chapter 17. Most interventions could be provided by nurse generalists, with guidance and assistance as needed by nurse specialists.

Assessment and Interventions for the Community. Community assessment related to self-care—basic hygienic tasks can be organized around the questions: (1) How accessible and receptive is the community to individuals who have impaired self-care ability? (2) Where are the barriers, both architectural and attitudinal, to community involvement of individuals with impaired self-care ability? According to Albrecht (1976), attitudinal barriers can be even more of an impediment than architectural barriers. (3) Are there educational programs available related to disability? (4) How are individuals with disability represented in the media (newspapers and television)? (5) What is occurring in the political and legislative arenas related to advocacy for persons with disability?

Nurse generalists and nurse specialists have a reponsibilty to be involved in community-focused interventions based on systematic community assessment. Interventions include teaching, advocating, and modeling with individuals, groups, and organizations. There are opportunities for nurses to participate in the ongoing work of national and local organizations whose purpose is to provide public education about disabling neurologic conditions.

Alterations in Self-Care: Independent Living

Cognitive functioning would be relatively intact for an individual to have impairment in self-care and yet be capable of independent living. Cortical brain damage to the extent that an individual must rely on others to make decisions and solve problems related to daily living would not be consistent with most definitions of independence. Independence is often a matter of degree and sometimes of definition. No one is totally independent of others, but living independently generally means reliance primarily on oneself to meet the demands of daily living for both personal and social activities (Benoliel et al., 1980).

Neuroanatomic areas in which damage could result in altered performance of self-care with retained ability for independent living include the motor cortex, primary sensory cortex, visual system, subcortical motor systems, motor and sensory tracts in the brainstem and spinal cord, autonomic nervous system, and peripheral nervous system (motor and sensory) (Mitchell et al., 1984).

An example of a nervous system disease that can lead to impaired self-care with retained independent living is multiple sclerosis (MS). The demyelination and plaque formation that occurs with MS can result in interruption of nervous system functioning in any of the areas listed above (Hickey, 1986). The interrupted functioning results in impaired ability to perform self-care activities.

Case Study 3

Nancy L is a 42-year-old woman who was diagnosed with multiple sclerosis (MS) at the age of 30. She had had subtle symptoms, including transient blurring of vision in her right eye and numbness and tingling of both legs for several years before the diagnosis. She said she was actually relieved when told that her symptoms were due to MS because she was worried that they were "just in her head" and that she might be "losing touch with reality." She is divorced and lives alone. She had been married at age 19 and thinks she and her husband would have been divorced "with or without the MS" because they had changed and drifted apart over the years. She has two grown children whom she describes as close to her and concerned but busy with their own lives.

Nancy's current neurologic deficits are primarily due to spinal cord damage from the MS. She has spastic paraparesis, with more strength in the right leg than the left leg. She has been unable to walk for the past 5 years but is independent with the use of her wheelchair. Her home is completely accessible to her wheelchair. She has continuous numbness and tingling in both legs and for the past year has had intermittent numbness in her left arm, especially when very tired. She has been working full-time in a secretarial job but is considering decreasing her work hours because of problems with fatigue. She is active in the local chapter of the National Multiple Sclerosis Society and is knowledgeable about theories of possible causes of MS and currently available treatments. She considers herself fortunate that she is not more disabled than she is. She is determined to remain as independent as possible for as long as possible.

Assessment for the Individual. Comprehensive assessment of an individual's capacity for independent living is generally a collaborative effort by various members of the health care team, for example, nurses, physicians, therapists, and psychologists. Nursing assessment of self-care ability may be aided by tools such as the PULSES profile, Barthel Index, or ESD. It is important to assess the individual's ability to perform self-care skills in the broadest sense, beyond basic hygienic tasks. The ESD scale includes assessment of such activities as work and recreation (Benoliel et al., 1980). A key aspect of the assessment is an evaluation of the individual's ability to solve problems and make decisions related to daily living. Examples of possible goals for an individual at this level of functioning are:

- Maintain as much independence as possible in performance of self-care activities (specify activities)
- Use support system and community resources as needed to enhance independence in self-care

Nursing Interventions for the Individual. As individuals move along the self-care continuum from dependence on others to greater and greater independence, they require less physical nursing assistance. People striving to maintain an independent living situation need less of nurses' doing for them and much more of nurses' teaching, guiding and facilitating. Not all nurses are comfortable with nursing interventions that empower the patient to make decisions and actively manage self-care. For those who are, it is helpful to have nurse specialists available as resources to guide and promote independence on the part of both staff nurses and patients.

Nursing interventions related to independent living involve collaboration with other members of the health care team to ensure that the chosen living situation is resident-friendly, that is, with as few barriers as possible.

Assessment and Interventions for the Family and Significant Others. There are several important aspects of family assessment in relation to independent living. It is important to assess family members' knowledge about independent living and about how the patient can maintain as much independence as possible. Family ability and willingness to be supportive of the patient's independent living is a major factor in the success of any independent living situation. It is worthwhile to examine other stresses and problems within the family occurring concurrently. It is rare that a family is faced with one isolated stressor.

Family-focused interventions are based on this assessment and on the family's specific goals. Interventions primarily involve teaching, supporting, and facilitating. Nurse generalists and nurse specialists work toward assisting the family to promote the patient's independence.

Assessment and Interventions for the Community. Community assessment related to independent living could be based on the questions suggested in the section "Basic Hygienic Tasks" of this chapter. Primary attention should be given to factors within the community that promote independent living and factors that inhibit independent living.

Community-focused interventions by both generalist nurses and nurses specialists should be aimed at strengthening those factors that positively influence independent living and working toward removal of those factors that impede independent living for people with neurologic dysfunction.

Alteration of Self-Care: Orientation to Healthy Living

Can people who are independent in meeting their own self-care needs benefit from nursing intervention? Is it within the nursing domain to work toward health promotion, to help relatively healthy people become healthier? Several authors argue for more involvement of nurses in health education and self-care promotion with people who are not ill or disabled (Caporael-Katz, 1983; Moll, 1982). A large group of people who might benefit from the guidance and teaching provided by nurses focused on orientation to healthy living are those with stress-related or stress-aggravated headaches (migraine, vascular tension, muscle contraction).

The neuroanatomic manifestations of orientation to healthy living encompass the whole brain and, in fact, the whole person. An individual's approach to life and to maintaining or enhancing health and well-being is an integrated, complex response. Specific areas of the brain that play important parts in orientation to life are the frontal lobe and association areas of the cortex, the limbic system, and the autonomic nervous system (Mitchell et al., 1984).

Case Study 4

Linda B is a 34-year-old woman who has had headaches since she was a teenager. She was evaluated recently by a neurologist, who diagnosed her headaches as mixed vascular and muscle tension headaches and recommended that she get counseling in stress management. Linda is married, and her husband is a graduate student in biochemistry. Linda is the primary wage-earner while her husband is in school. They have three healthy, active children, aged 9 years, 7 years, and 18 months. Linda is a Registered Nurse and works full-time in a busy family practice clinic. She acknowledges that there are many stressors in her life right now and that her headaches are much worse during and immediately after particularly stressful times. The major stressors identified by Linda are (1) financial worries, (2) husband too busy with school to have much time for Linda and the children, (3) she would like to be at home with her toddler more—to work 3 days per week instead of full-time, and (4) she never has time for herself—to do what she wants to do or just to be alone.

Linda has a headache at least 2 or 3 days each week. The headaches range in intensity from mild (3 on a scale of 10) to fairly severe (7 on a scale of 10). When her headache is at its worst, her head throbs, she feels irritable and nauseated, and only wants to get away from everything and go to sleep. She eats a fairly balanced diet, drinks too much caffeine (in her opinion), does not smoke, and drinks alcohol (wine with dinner) about once a week. She sleeps about 7 hours per night but does not feel rested in the morning and feels tired by midafternoon. She would like to exercise regularly but does not know where she would fit it in. She misses work about 1 day per month with a headache; most of the time she just keeps working even though her head hurts. She occasionally cancels or postpones activities because she has a headache. She expresses high motivation to do something to relieve her headaches and manage stress more effectively.

Assessment for the Individual. Nursing assessment of an individual who is functioning at the highest level of the self-care continuum (Fig. 33–1) differs from the assessments previously described in this chapter. A person like Linda has no difficulty meeting her own basic hygienic needs and is living independently. She, in fact, has several people dependent on her to varying degrees. The primary focus of the assessment of someone's orientation to healthy living is an evaluation of lifestyle and health habits, including sleep patterns, diet, exercise, smoking, and consumption of alchohol and caffeine. Special emphasis should be given to exploring identified stressors in the individual's life and current and past coping strategies. Based on systematic assessment of an individual's situation, possible *goals* might be:

- Short-term goal: Consistent practice of a relaxation technique three times per day for about 5 minutes, each time resulting in subjective feeling of calmness and relaxation.
- Long-term goal: Decreased frequency and intensity of headaches.

Nursing Interventions for the Individual. A person with very little difficulty performing personal self-care tasks and living independently may not have much opportunity for interaction with nurses in health care settings. There are nurse specialists in outpatient settings and in the community who provide stress management and health promotion services. In order for health-promoting and self-care-enhancing nursing interventions to be used, they must be available and highly visible in the community. It is the responsibility of nurse providers of such interventions to make themselves known.

Appropriate nursing interventions for individuals at the most independent levels of the self-care continuum (Fig. 33–1) include teaching, facilitating, validating, and role-modeling. According to Tomlin (1983) "as nurses engage increasingly in more effective caring for themselves as whole persons, they provide a powerful model for clients to reach ever healthier levels of self-caring" (p. 59). This does not mean that nurses are expected to be perfect in the performance of their own self-caring activities but that they are actively moving toward health in their own lives. Nurses have the opportunity and the responsibility to teach the value of healthy living by their own self-caring behaviors.

Assessment and Interventions for the Family and Significant Others. Human beings are individuals and at the same time members of families and other interacting, reciprocally influencing systems. Thus, a complete assessment of an individual's orientation to healthy living includes aspects of the individual's key influencing relationships. The assessment focuses on the self-care practices of family members and others indentified by the individual as significant. Relationships should be examined in relation to various types of support (emotional, instrumental) received and provided. Another key aspect of relationships is the extent to which they are a source of stress for the people involved.

Family-focused interventions related to healthy living should be similar to those used in the care of the individual. Appropriate interventions with relatively healthy families include teaching, facilitating, supporting, and promoting self-care. In addition to working with family members as individuals, it is important to conduct teaching and support sessions with significant family members and the client as a group. Family sessions provide the opportunity for all involved to hear the same information. The nurses facilitating the sessions should model health-promoting interactions with the client while being observed by family members. These interventions are generally enacted by nurse specialists or nurse generalists who have developed skills in family assessment and intervention.

Assessment and Interventions for the Community. Community assessment related to orientation to healthy living could be centered on several broad questions. Is the community healthy—environmentally, attitudinally, interactionally? What is the community doing to promote healthy living? Who are the key people in the community who are working toward a healthy community? What are the major barriers or impediments to healthy living within the community? What is the local community doing to promote health in the larger community—the nation? the world?

Interventions toward the goal of community health can be implemented by both nurse generalists and nurse specialists. Nursing as a profession and nurses as individuals have the responsibility to promote an orientation to healthy living within the community.

SUMMARY

This chapter discusses alterations in self-care that result from nervous system dysfunction. The levels of self-care alteration explored are (1) protective reflexes, (2) basic hygienic tasks, (3) independent living, and (4) orientation to healthy living. Self-care can be thought of as a continuum, from maximum dependence in performance of self-care activities to maximum independence. As such, self-care encompasses more than the frequently referred to ADLs: bathing, feeding, dressing, toileting.

Alterations in self-care are complex human responses to multiple phenomena. Nurse generalists and nurse specialists in various care settings have special opportunities to participate with patients and their loved ones in confronting the effects and challenges of altered self-care performance.

REFERENCES

Albrecht, G.L. (Ed.). (1976). *The sociology of physical disability and rehabilitation*. Pittsburgh: University of Pittsburgh Press.

Alcorn, M.H. (1983). Altered levels of responsiveness: Decreased response. In M. Snyder (Ed.), *A guide to neurological and neurosurgical nursing*. New York: Wiley.

American Nurses' Association Council on Medical-Surgical Nursing Practice and American Association of Neuroscience Nurses. (1985). *Neuroscience nursing practice: Process and outcome criteria for selected diagnoses*. Kansas City, MO: American Nurses' Association.

Benoliel, J.Q., McCorkle, R., & Young, K. (1980). Development of a social dependency scale. *Research in Nursing and Health, 3*, 3.

Caporael-Katz, B. (1983). Health, self-care and power: shifting the balance. *Topics in Clinical Nursing, 5*(3), 31.

Dudas, S. (1986). Nursing diagnoses and interventions for the rehabilitation of the stroke patient. *Nursing Clinics of North America, 21*(2), 345.

Granger, C.V. & Gresham, G. E. (Eds.). (1984). *Functional assessment in rehabilitation medicine*. Baltimore: Williams & Wilkins.

Hickey, J.V. (1986). *The clinical practice of neurological and neurosurgical nursing.* Philadelphia: Lippincott.

Lipe, H.P. (1985). Prevention of nervous system trauma from travel in motor vehicles. *Journal of Neurosurgical Nursing, 17*(2), 77.

Mitchell, P.H., Ozuna, J., Cammermeyer, M., & Woods, N.F. (1984). *Neurological assessment for nursing practice.* Reston, VA: Reston.

Moll, J.A. (1982). High-level wellness and the nurse. *Topics in Clinical Nursing, 4*(1), 61.

Mumma, C. (1984). The effects of disability following a cerebrovascular accident on older individuals and on their marital relationships. Unpublished doctoral dissertation, University of Washington, Seattle.

Mumma, C. (1986). Perceived losses following stroke. *Rehabilitation Nursing, 11*(3), 19.

Orem, D.E. (1980). *Nursing: Concepts of practice.* 2d ed. New York: McGraw-Hill.

Rehabilitation Nursing: Concepts and practice, A core curriculum. (1981). Evanston, Il,: Rehabilitation Nursing Institute.

Snyder M. (1983). *A guide to neurological and neurosurgical nursing.* New York: Wiley.

Tomlin, E. (1983). Self-care. In J. Lindberg, M. Hunter, & A. Kruszewski (Eds.), *Introduction to person-centered nursing* (p. 51). Philadelphia: Lippincott.

Werner-Beland, J.A. (1980). *Grief responses to long-term illness and disability.* Reston, VA: Reston.

BIBLIOGRAPHY

Cammermeyer, M. (1983). A growth model of self-care for neurologically impaired people. *Journal of Neurosurgical Nursing, 15*(5), 299.

Kearney, B.Y., & Fleisher, B.J. (1979). Development of an instrument to measure exercise of self-care agency. *Research in Nursing and Health, 2*(1), 25.

APPENDIX

Neuroscience Nursing Practice: Process and Outcome Standards for Selected Diagnoses*

INTRODUCTION

As the professional society for nursing in the United States, the American Nurses' Association is responsible for defining nursing, establishing the scope of nursing practice, and setting standards for professional nursing practice. During the past 15 years, the association has published a number of documents that have delineated generic standards for nursing practice and standards for specific areas of nursing practice.

In 1973, ANA published *Standards of Nursing Practice*.[1] These standards remain the generic standards for the profession; they provide direction for determining the quality of nursing care a client receives. In 1974, the ANA Division on Medical-Surgical Nursing Practice developed *Standards of Medical-Surgical Nursing Practice*. This document was intended to provide a "basic model by which the quality of medical-surgical nursing practice may be measured."[2] In response to the identified need to address the quality of nursing care within the area of neurological and neurosurgical nursing practice, a joint committee of the American Nurses' Association and the American Association of Neurosurgical Nurses (now the American Association of Neuroscience Nurses) was convened. This committee developed *Standards of Neurological and Neurosurgical Nursing Practice*, published in 1977.[3] The joint committee reviewed this publication in 1981 and decided that further development was necessary to reflect the current state of knowledge in this field.

The most recent definition of nursing as "the diagnosis and treatment of human responses to actual or potential health problems," stated in the ANA publication *Nursing: A Social Policy Statement*, has guided the preparation of this document.[4] A conceptual framework was developed and published, early in the developmental process, by the American Association of Neuroscience Nurses (AANN) to order the approach to revising the standards and to begin delineating the scope of neuroscience nursing practice.[5] As a part of the development of this conceptual framework, nurse members of AANN were surveyed and expressed agreement on the phenomena of particular concern in their current practice. The phenomena of concern are the human responses that are the focus of nursing intervention.

Because this document, *Neuroscience Nursing Practice: Process and Outcome Criteria for Selected Diagnoses*, is intended for national use, those involved in its development have made a concerted

---

*Reprinted by permission of the American Nurses' Association and American Association of Neuroscience Nurses. Kansas City, MO: American Nurses' Association, 1985.

attempt to incorporate the values reflected within the generic *Standards of Nursing Practice*. These values include a deliberate use of the nursing process in providing care, the inclusion of the client in decision making regarding care, an emphasis on health, and the recognition of the necessity for collaboration in providing nursing care.

This document represents a pioneering effort to guide the implementation of the generic *Standards of Nursing Practice* within the field of neuroscience nursing. The intent of this document is to provide a general framework by which the quality (or outcomes) of care in neuroscience nursing practice may be evaluated. It is significant that the development of this framework required reaching consensus on the current level of knowledge in this field. In order to represent areas of consensus accurately, the work of the joint committee has evolved through several critical periods of modification.

First, in the absence of an agreed-upon classification system or taxonomy of nursing diagnoses for the profession, the joint committee selected broad classifications, that is, diagnostic categories for the field of neuroscience nursing. These were derived from the phenomena of particular concern to neuroscience nursing practice, as identified through the survey of AANN members. The second phase involved the identification of common nursing diagnoses (or subclassifications) in this field for each diagnostic category. Finally, implementation (process and outcome) criteria were identified for each nursing diagnosis. Together these nursing diagnoses and related implementation criteria constitute the contemporary focus in the neuroscience practice area and serve as broad guidelines for the nurse generalists providing care to individuals with nervous system dysfunction. The draft document received extensive field review; this document includes revisions made following the field review.

Document Overview

The six broad diagnostic categories presented in this publication are consciousness and cognition, communication, mobility, sensation, rest and sleep, and sexuality. General assessment parameters for each of the six diagnostic categories are suggested in the Appendix. The Bibliography will lead the reader to additional sources pertinent to this document, including readings that address specific parameters, scales, and tools for obtaining objective and subjective data.

Nursing Diagnoses

Specific nursing diagnoses have been identified within the broad diagnostic categories. The committee began its identification of nursing diagnoses using the list of nursing diagnoses accepted for clinical testing by the North American Nursing Diagnosis Association (NANDA). Since it is recognized that NANDA's list is a beginning list and not by any means a complete list, the committee modified some nursing diagnoses and identified new diagnoses to reflect the uniqueness of neuroscience nursing practice. The determination of diagnoses is not intended to be exhaustive within each category. Rather, these nursing diagnoses are those agreed upon as having "high incidence" and a unique application in the current practice of neuroscience nursing.

Defining Characteristics

A central focus in the development of this document was the identification of defining characteristics for each nursing diagnosis. The defining characteristics listed in this document represent factors that should be considered in determining a valid nursing diagnosis. Not all of the defining characteristics, however, need to be present in making the given nursing diagnosis. Many of the lists of defining characteristics are extensive, so critical assessment factors will not be overlooked by the nurse.

The joint committee acknowledges the absence of etiologies and/or risk factors for each nursing diagnosis. While recognizing the value and implications of causality or etiology as critical to the development of nursing's scientific base for practice, the state of knowledge within the field of neuroscience nursing is not yet sufficient to allow consensus on etiology. The evolution of a more complete conceptual system will necessitate the identification of the phenomena of concern in neuroscience nursing—including defining characteristics and causal factors. This document represents a developmental step toward a more complete conceptual system and offers further impetus for rigorous scientific investigation. The identification of etiology should constitute a focal activity for the enhancement and subsequent revision of this document.

Process Criteria

Process criteria have been developed for each nursing diagnosis. These criteria indicate broad areas of nursing intervention (care) that are expected to accomplish the stated outcomes for the given nursing diagnosis. These nursing interventions are not intended to be exhaustive or prescriptive in nature. Instead, these criteria (which focus on the delivery of nursing care) identify broad areas to guide or suggest relevant nursing interventions. These process criteria provide a range of alternatives for selection, ordering, and prioritization based upon the nursing assessment.

Outcome Criteria

One or more outcomes have been identified for each nursing diagnosis. These outcomes are the expected changes in the health status of the client following nursing intervention. The outcome criteria reflect either the biological response to nursing intervention or the acquisition and assimilation of knowledge, attitudes, or skills by the client, family, and significant others. A concerted attempt has been made to identify realistic, measurable, and attainable outcomes.

Where "knowledge deficit in the individual, family, and significant others" is the nursing diagnosis, the outcome is stated relative to the behavior of the family and significant others. The joint committee took the position that knowledge deficit, as a nursing diagnosis, must have a specific focus so that appropriate nursing interventions can be taken. For the purpose of this document, the general defining characteristics for "knowledge deficit in the individual, family, and significant others" are that these persons have no knowledge of or no prior experience with the client's condition.

Use of this Document

This document is intended for use by the nurse generalist practicing in any setting with individuals experiencing actual or potential nervous system dysfunction. The use and evaluation of the diagnostically related implementation criteria as a general framework for improving the quality of nursing care to this client population are of primary importance.

However, as previously mentioned, this document reflects the current state of knowledge in this field. As such, this work is provisional, dynamic, and subject to testing and subsequent change. It follows, then, that a secondary purpose of this document is to promote the validation of these nursing diagnoses and related criteria in order to evaluate more effectively the processes and outcomes of professional nursing practice in the field of neuroscience nursing.

This continuing development depends upon the document's use and its critical evaluation by clinical specialists and nurse scientists committed to the delineation of the nature and scope of neuroscience nursing practice and to this field's contributions to the profession's scientific base for practice. The authors submit this challenge to nurses practicing in the field of neuroscience.

PROCESS AND OUTCOME STANDARDS FOR SELECTED NURSING DIAGNOSES

Diagnostic Category: Consciousness and Cognition

Defining Characteristics	Process Criteria	Outcome Criteria

High Risk of Secondary Brain Injury

One or more of the following:
• Decreased responsiveness
• Generalized motor response to stimuli
• Abnormal flexion or extension posture upon stimulation
• Decreased pupillary reaction
• Unequal pupils
• Decreased or absent brainstem reflexes
• Altered respiratory rate and/or rhythm
• Confusion
• Disorientation
• Altered behavior (restless, combative)
	• The nurse identifies the individual's baseline level of brain function, including responsiveness, pupillary size and reaction, brainstem reflexes, respiratory rate and rhythm, and behavior.
	• The nurse institutes measures to promote cerebral perfusion, including as needed:
	  • Avoiding or minimizing hypoxia through measures such as maintenance of airway, ventilation, circulation, and administration of oxygen and other prescribed therapy.
	  • Avoiding or minimizing hypercapnia through measures such as maintenance of airway, ventilation, circulation, and positioning.
	  • Avoiding or minimizing hypotension or hypertension through measures such as administering prescribed medication, controlling untoward effects of medication, and positioning.
	  • Avoiding or minimizing increased intracranial pressure through measures such as positioning and controlling the environmental stimuli, intrathoracic pressure, body temperature, and fluid volume.
	• The nurse monitors clinical and physiologicl parameters, modifying treatment as indicated according to preestablished protocols.
	• The nurse promptly collaborates with others as determined by mutual protocols if changes indicate deterioration, and administers prescribed therapy.
		• The risk of secondary brain injury is minimized, as reflected by the stabilization of documented clinical indicators at or above the baseline.
		• The risk of secondary brain injury is minimized, as reflected by stabilization of documented physiological indicators (such as oxygen and carbon dioxide levels, blood pressure, and intracranial pressure) within predetermined parameters.

(continued)

Defining Characteristics	Process Criteria	Outcome Criteria

Altered Level of Responsiveness: Decreased

One or more of the following:
- No response to stimuli
- Generalized motor response to stimuli
- Localized motor or verbal response to stimuli

- The nurse monitors behavioral responsiveness.
- The nurse coordinates a program that includes tactile, gustatory, olfactory, visual, and auditory stimuli.

- The individual progresses to a higher level of responsiveness.

Altered Level of Responsiveness: Heightened

One or more of the following:
- Confused and agitated response to stimuli
- Misperception
- Delusion
- Hallucination
- Anxiety
- Aggression
- Combativeness

- The nurse protects the individual from harming others or himself or herself by measures such as:
  - Maximizing perception of relevant stimuli.
  - Structuring the environment to reduce overall stimulation and distraction.
  - Correcting misperceptions, delusions, and hallucinations in a calm, factual manner.
  - Involving the individual in simple motor activities to decrease agitation.
  - Using physical and/or chemical restraints appropriately.

- The individual does not harm others or himself or herself.
- The individual progresses to a higher level of responsiveness.

Altered Level of Responsiveness: Inappropriate Behaviors and Moods

One or more of the following:
- Confused, nonagitated, and inappropriate response to stimuli
- Emotional lability
- Emotional and/or behavioral outbursts
- Incontinence
- Sexual advances
- Sexual self-pleasuring in public
- Failure to recognize behavior as inappropriate
- Apathy
- Flat affect

- The nurse uses and serves as a role model in using measures to control inappropriate behavior, such as:
  - Acknowledging behavior in a calm, factual manner.
  - Distracting or redirecting.
  - Physically or chemically controlling behavior as necessary.
- Teaching the family and significant others measures to control inappropriate behavior.
- The nurse institutes a behavior modification program if the individual has decreased ability to monitor or control behavior.
- The nurse collaborates with the behavioral management professional.

- The individual's episodes and/or duration of inappropriate behavior and inappropriate mood changes decrease.
- The family and significant others demonstrate effective intervention during episodes of inappropriate behaviors and/or inappropriate mood changes.

(continued)

Diagnostic Category: Consciousness and Cognition *(continued)*

Defining Characteristics	Process Criteria	Outcome Criteria

Uncompensated Cognitive Deficit (specify type of deficit)

One or more of the following:
- Confused but appropriate response to stimuli
- Automatic but appropriate response to stimuli
- Disorientation, which may include disorientation to time, person, and/or place
- Memory deficit
- Impaired judgment
- Lack of insight
- Lack of awareness of impairment or physical limitations
- Impaired ability to recognize body parts, objects, and persons
- Inability to follow left-right commands
- Acalculia
- Impaired problem solving

- The nurse acknowledges the individual's disability and coordinates daily activities as necessary.
- The nurse uses compensation techniques, such as:
  - Structuring the environment to ensure safety, consistency, and minimal distractions.
  - Avoiding left-right directions.
  - Utilizing repetition, verbal cues, and memory aids.
  - Providing reinforcement by ensuring success.
  - Encouraging the individual to touch and look at the affected body parts.
- The nurse teaches safety awareness and compensation techniques to the individual, family, and significant others.
- The nurse institutes measures to minimize episodes of perseveration, such as the use of verbal cues, teaching, and intervention.

- The individual sustains no injury caused by cognitive deficit.
- The individual, family, and significant others use compensation techniques.
- The family and significant others adopt methods to promote the individual's use of compensation techniques.

Total Health Management Deficit: Irreversible

One or more of the following:
- Irreversible inability to perceive self-care needs
- Irreversible inability to plan, organize, and/or sequence self-care
- Irreversible inability to manage health needs

- The nurse provides for feeding, bathing, dressing, and toileting.
- The nurse institutes measures to maintain fluid balance, elimination, and rest and sleep.
- The nurse institutes measures to maintain skin integrity and joint mobility.
- The nurse provides appropriate assistance.
- The nurse institutes measures to ensure safety.

- The individual's hygiene, nutrition, and elimination needs are met.
- The individual sustains no complications of immobility.

Self-Care Deficit (specify feeding, bathing, dressing, toileting)

One or more of the following:
- Partial ability to recognize self-care needs
- Partial ability to plan, organize, and/or sequence self-care
- Partial ability to recognize limitations when performing self-care
- Partial ability to recognize and use assistive devices

- The nurse provides opportunities for the individual to engage in self-care through measures such as:
  - Using cognitive compensation techniques.
  - Performing self-care in an appropriate environment.
  - Separating activities into individual steps.

- The individual engages in self-care activities consistent with physical and cognitive limitations.
- The family and significant others demonstrate measures to promote the individual's self-care abilities.
- The individual, family, and significant others demonstrate safety awareness when engaging in self-care activities.

Defining Characteristics	Process Criteria	Outcome Criteria

Self-Care Deficit (specify feeding, bathing, dressing, toileting) (continued)

- The nurse teaches family and significant others measures to promote individual's self-care.
- The nurse teaches and/or reinforces safe, appropriate use and maintenance of assistive devices.
- The nurse collaborates with occupational and physical therapists.
- The nurse institutes measures to ensure safety.

Knowledge Deficit in the Family and Significant Others (regarding behavioral responses)

- The nurse teaches the meaning of behavioral responses.
- The nurse provides information about the individual's condition, treatment plan, and prognosis.
- The nurse teaches methods of effective interaction.
- The nurse teaches methods of environmental manipulation.

- The family and significant others interpret and explain behavioral responses in terms of brain dysfunction.
- The family and significant others verbalize realistic expectations of the individual.
- The family and significant others state and/or demonstrate effective interaction and methods to manipulate the environment.

Anticipatory or Actual Grieving of the Family and Significant Others

One or more of the following:
- Verbal report of actual or perceived loss
- Anticipation of loss imposed by disease or therapy

- The nurse provides opportunities for the family and significant others to verbalize thoughts and feelings.
- The nurse provides support to the family and significant others throughout the grief process.
- The nurse provides information about community resources such as self-help groups, financial aid, and transportation.
- The nurse institutes measures to promote the ability of the family and significant others to make decisions such as identification of strengths and resources.
- The nurse collaborates with other professionals such as the clinical nurse specialist, social worker, psychiatrist, and clergy as appropriate.
- The nurse collaborates with other professionals to offer the family and significant others the opportunity to consider organ donation in the event of actual or inevitable brain death.

- The family and significant others express grief to members of the health care team.
- The family and significant others participate in decision making related to treatment.
- The family and significant others plan realistically for the future.

Diagnostic Category: Communication

Defining Characteristics	Process Criteria	Outcome Criteria

Impaired Communication

One or more of the following:
• Impaired verbal language
• Impaired written language
• Impaired speech programming
• Impaired writing programming
• Impaired articulation
• Impaired modulation
• Impaired ability to write
• Impaired ability to make gestures
	• The nurse anticipates the individual's needs until an effective method of communication is developed.
	• The nurse provides an alternative method of communication when possible.
	• The nurse collaborates with the speech therapist.
	• The nurse teaches measures to promote communication, such as:
	  Using assistive devices.
	  Controlling environmental distraction.
	  Reducing anxiety.
	  Decreasing the speed of communication.
		• The individual communicates that needs are being met.
		• The individual begins to establish a defined method of communication.
		• The individual uses assistive devices appropriately.
		• The individual demonstrates ways to maximize his or her ability to communicate.

Knowledge Deficit in the Family and Significant Others[a]

	• The nurse teaches the nature of the communication disability.
	• The nurse teaches and serves as a role model in taking measures to promote the individual's ability to communicate, such as:
	  • Removing and reducing environmental distractions.
	  • Allotting time for the practice of communication and the use of assistive devices.
	  • Adjusting the length of the session to complement the individual's attention span.
	  • Planning successful experiences for each practice session.
		• The family and significant others state the nature of the individual's communication disability.
		• The family and significant others demonstrate measures to maximize the individual's ability to communicate.

[a]Regarding the nature of the communication disability and/or measures to promote the individual's ability to communicate.

Diagnostic Category: Mobility

Defining Characteristics	Process Criteria	Outcome Criteria

Impaired Physical Mobility

One or more of the following:
- Inability to move purposefully within the physical environment, including mobility in bed, transfer, ambulation, and locomotion
- Vasomotor instability
- Imposed restriction of movement, including mechanical constraints and medical protocols
- Reluctance to move

- The nurse provides for the individual both active and passive range of motion exercises and active and passive weightbearing.
- The nurse positions the individual in correct functional alignment.
- The nurse provides support for the individual's extremities during sitting, standing, and ambulation.
- The nurse uses assistive devices as appropriate.
- The nurse institutes a schedule for turning and repositioning.
- The nurse collaborates with physical and occupational therapists in developing and using safe and effective techniques for transfer, ambulation, and locomotion.
- The nurse institutes measures to promote vasomotor adaptability.
- The nurse monitors blood pressure and pulse before, during, and after activity.
- The nurse plans a daily routine to provide pain relief and rest before and after activity.
- The nurse teaches measures to conserve energy and reduce fatigue.
- The nurse uses assistive cough techniques, suctioning, and other pulmonary hygiene measures.
- The nurse collaborates with occupational and speech therapists in developing and using techniques for chewing and swallowing.

- The individual achieves safe mobility and vasomotor stability within the limits imposed by his or her physical status.
- The individual's pulse and blood pressure remain within safe parameters during activity.
- The individual moves, transfers, and ambulates with or without assistance and/or devices or propels his or her wheelchair.
- The individual sustains no complications of immobility.

High Risk of Ventilatory Insufficiency or Atelectasis

One or more of the following:
- Airway obstruction
- Reduced vital capacity (hypoventilation)
- Weak or paralyzed respiratory muscles

- The nurse recognizes risk and monitors respiratory status.
- The nurse positions the individual to prevent obstruction and promote increased ventilation.
- The nurse uses devices to promote lung expansion.
- The nurse provides ventilatory support when indicated.

- The individual's risk of atelectasis is minimized.
- The individual is adequately ventilated.

(continued)

Diagnostic Category: Mobility *(continued)*

Defining Characteristics	Process Criteria	Outcome Criteria

Total Self-Care Deficit

Inability to:
- Feed, bathe, dress, and toilet
- Move about in bed
- Transfer
- Ambulate
- Initiate, sustain, or terminate movement
- Grasp and/or grip
- Voluntarily perform skilled motor activities
- Manipulate tools and utensils

- The nurse provides for the feeding, bathing, dressing, and toileting of the individual.

- The individual's hygiene, nutrition, and elimination needs are met.

Partial Self-Care Deficit

Partial ability to:
- Feed, bathe, dress, and toilet
- Move about in bed
- Transfer
- Ambulate
- Propel a wheelchair
- Initiate, sustain, and terminate movement
- Grasp and/or grip
- Voluntarily perform skilled motor activities
- Manipulate tools and utensils

- The nurse provides the individual with opportunities to assist with self-care.
- The nurse provides equipment, devices, and/or assistance as appropriate.
- The nurse intervenes before the individual becomes excessively fatigued or frustrated.
- The nurse institutes safety measures.
- The nurse structures the environment to provide accessibility.
- The nurse collaborates with physical and occupational therapists to promote self-care.

- The individual participates in self-care at a level consistent with his or her limitations, with or without assistance and/or devices.
- The individual sustains no injury while performing self-care.

High Risk of Aspiration

One or more of the following:
- Inability to move the body or change the position of the head
- Inability to control the muscles of the tongue, mouth, or pharynx
- Difficulty chewing or swallowing
- Difficulty supporting the head in an upright position.

- The nurse recognizes risk and monitors respiratory sounds and vital signs.
- The nurse positions the individual to facilitate drainage of secretions and vomitus.
- The nurse initiates measures to reduce or prevent vomiting.
- The nurse selects foods of appropriate consistency.

- The individual's risk of aspiration is minimized.

Defining Characteristics	Process Criteria	Outcome Criteria
	High Risk of Aspiration (continued)	

• Impaired ability to clear the upper or lower airway
• Pooling of secretions in the upper airway
	• The nurse allows adequate time for chewing and swallowing.
	• The nurse raises the head of the bed when the individual eats unless there are contraindications for that position.
	• The nurse uses appropriate feeding devices and techniques.
	• The nurse institutes safety measures when administering nasogastric and/or gastric feedings, such as:
	  • Supporting the head in an upright position.
	  • Checking for the presence of residual in the stomach prior to feeding.
	  • Checking tube placement prior to feeding.	

	High Risk of Corneal Ulceration	
One or more of the following: • Reduced or absent blink • Reduced frequency of blink • Impaired ability to close eye(s)	• The nurse recognizes risk and monitors for corneal alteration. • The nurse initiates protocols to protect the cornea, such as eyedrops, other lubrication, and protective patching.	• The individual's corneas are intact and free from abrasion or ulceration.
	Knowledge Deficit in the Family and Significant Others[a]	
	• The nurse instructs the family and significant others about the nature of the deficit. • The nurse demonstrates the skills and techniques needed to provide care and assistance to the individual.	• The family and significant others verbalize an understanding of the mobility deficit. • The family and significant others demonstrate skill in carrying out care techniques. • The family and significant others demonstrate appropriate techniques to improve the individual's mobility.

[a]Regarding the nature of mobility deficits and skills to provide care and assistance to the individual.

Diagnostic Category: Sensation

Defining Characteristics	Process Criteria	Outcome Criteria
	Uncompensated Sensory Deficit	

One or more of the following:
• Impaired vision
• Impaired hearing
• Impaired proprioception
• Impaired smell
• Impaired taste
• Impaired tactile sensation
• Impaired ability to sense sources of potential injury
	• The nurse orients the individual to the environment, utilizing intact senses.
	• The nurse modifies the environment and daily routines in such ways as:
	  • Permanent placement of furniture and articles.
	  • Adaptation of the telephone, door bells, and warning devices.
	• The nurse provides detailed information and instruction related to the disability and compensatory techniques and devices.
	• The nurse plans care and routines to allow for slower response and adaptation.
	• The nurse uses aids and assistive devices as appropriate in care activities.
	• The nurse institutes appropriate safety precautions, such as:
	  • Providing assistance and supervision.
	  • Eliminating or reducing environmental hazards.
		• The individual communicates a sense of comfort and security within the environment.
		• The individual uses assistive devices and compensatory techniques correctly.
		• The individual sustains no burns, falls, wounds, or pressure injuries.

	Pain: Chronic	

One or more of the following:
• Communication of pain or discomfort
• Exhibition of such behaviors as:
  • Restlessness or agitation
  • Avoidance of activity
  • Altered muscle tone
  • Preoccupation with or guarding of the painful part
  • Irritability
  • Fatigue
  • Emotional lability
  • Withdrawal
  • Disruption of cycle of sleeping and waking
  • Disruption of eating pattern
	The nurse promotes adaptation to pain by instituting such measures as:
	• Acknowledging the existence of pain.
	• Assisting the individual to identify the situations and factors that precipitate or intensify pain.
	• Assisting the individual to adjust his or her lifestyle to reduce pain-producing situations and factors.
	• Assisting the individual to use the prescribed pain regimes for maximum benefit.
	• Collaborating with pain management specialists to develop appropriate cutaneous, affective, and cognitive treatment modalities.
	• Collaborating with other care providers to establish a management plan.
		• The individual participates in developing, carrying out, and evaluating the management plan.
		• The individual reports an improved sense of well-being and/or increased satisfaction with relationships, lifestyle, and with himself or herself.
		• The individual reports engaging in positive social interaction with others.
		• The family and significant others support the management plan.

Defining Characteristics	Process Criteria	Outcome Criteria

Pain: Chronic (continued)

- Teaching the individual, family, and significant others about the nature of the pain.
- Providing guidance regarding anticipated lifestyle changes.
- Providing opportunities for the individual to verbalize feelings related to the chronicity of the pain.
- Providing positive reinforcement for health-promoting behaviors and encouraging appropriate use of caregivers and support systems.

Self-Care Deficit (specify type of deficit)

One or more of the following:
- Impaired visual ability to direct one's own movement and locate and/or use self-care articles
- Impaired ability to distinguish environmental temperatures
- Impaired ability to recognize articles by touch
- Impaired ability to perceive physical injury
- Impaired ability to perceive the position of body parts

- The nurse provides the individual with opportunities to participate in self-care using intact senses, compensatory techniques, and devices.
- The nurse structures the environment and daily routine to maximize the individual's self-care ability.
- The nurse collaborates with physical and occupational therapists to develop techniques for self-care.
- The nurse teaches and reinforces the use of compensatory echniques, such as:
  - Memorizing the placement of furniture and articles.
  - Coding clothing to distinguish front and back and colors.
  - Using thermometers or unimpaired body parts to measure environmental temperatures.
  - Monitoring and protecting the body.
  - Strengthening eye-hand coordination.

- The individual performs self-care using compensatory techniques and devices, with or without assistance from others.

Knowledge Deficit in the Family and Significant Others[a]

- The nurse teaches the family and significant others the nature of the sensory deficit(s).
- The nurse teaches and demonstrates safety precautions.
- The nurse teaches assistive techniques.

- The family and significant others verbalize an understanding of the sensory deficit(s).
- The family and significant others demonstrate safety precautions and assistive techniques.

[a]Regarding both the nature of the sensory deficit and the safety precautions and techniques that may assist the individual.

Diagnostic Category: Rest and Sleep

Defining Characteristics	Process Criteria	Outcome Criteria
	Activity Intolerance: Easily Fatigued	
One or more of the following: • Exertional discomfort • Difficulty completing activities • Verbal report of fatigue	• The nurse assists the individual to prioritize activities. • The nurse teaches measures to establish a rest–activity pattern that conserves energy and avoids fatigue.	• The individual establishes a rest–activity pattern that allows the individual to accomplish prioritized activities.
	Sleep Pattern Disturbance	

One or more of the following:
• Less sleep than normal
• Continuous environmental stimuli
• Interrupted sleep
• Altered behavior or mood in the presence of any of the above
• Report or observation of difficulty initiating sleep, restlessness during sleep, or daytime somnolence
• Verbal report of not feeling well rested
• Verbal report of altered sleep pattern
• Verbal report of distraction by environmental stimuli
• Verbal report of anxiety or pain at night
	• The nurse institutes measures to promote adequate sleep periods, such as:
	  • Maintaining a cycle of light and darkness.
	  • Minimizing nighttime noise and treatments.
	  • Using monitoring techniques and equipment that minimize the need to awaken the individual.
	• The nurse identifies the nature of the sleep pattern disturbance.
	• The nurse institutes and teaches measures to promote sleep, such as:
	  • Managing dietary and chemical substance intake.
	  • Maintaining consistent times to go to bed and arise.
	  • Manipulating the environment.
	  • Positioning.
	  • Managing activity, exercise, and work factors.
	  • Limiting the frequency and length of naps.
	  • Collaborating with the physician regarding the medication regime.
	• The nurse institutes measures to promote the management of anxiety, such as:
	  • Encouraging the verbalization of fears and concerns.
	  • Teaching relaxation techniques.
	• The nurse institutes measures to promote the management of pain (see the process criteria for the diagnosis of "pain: chronic," within the diagnostic category of sensation).
	• The nurse collaborates with the appropriate specialist.
	• The nurse provides information about available resources.
		• The individual describes the nature of the sleep pattern disturbance.
		• The individual carries out measures to promote sleep.
		• The individual has undisturbed periods for sleep.
		• The individual reports feeling rested upon awakening.

Diagnostic Category: Sexuality

Defining Characteristics	Process Criteria	Outcome Criteria
	Alteration in Sexual Identity	

One or more of the following:
• Verbalization of a problem with sexual identity
• Report of an alteration in a perceived sex role
• Report of an alteration in a relationship with a significant other
• Seeking of confirmation of desirability
	• The nurse institutes measures to promote the individual's awareness of his or her sexual identity, such as:
	  • Conveying recognition and acceptance of the individual's sexuality.
	  • Manipulating the environment to prevent embarrassment.
	  • Assisting the individual with physical appearance.
	• The nurse assists the individual to resume sexual roles.
		• The individual verbalizes the perception of himself or herself as a sexual being possessing sexual characteristics and needs.
		• The individual demonstrates interest in maintaining his or her physical appearance.

	Sexual Dysfunction	

One or more of the following:
• Actual or perceived limitation imposed by the disease and/or therapy
• Report of inability to achieve the desired sexual satisfaction
• Report of an alteration in achieving the desired sexual satisfaction
	• The nurse institutes measures to promote the individual's sexual functioning, such as:
	  • Teaching the nature of the sexual dysfunction.
	  • Manipulating the environment to facilitate the desired physical intimacy.
	  • Providing resource information.
	  • Encouraging the individual to seek sexual counseling.
	  • Collaborating with the sex counselor.
	• The nurse teaches measures to promote sexual expression and satisfaction, such as:
	  • Pain management regimes.
	  • Methods of bowel and bladder control.
	  • Alternate positions and time of day.
	  • Exploration of different sexual behaviors.
		• The individual describes the nature of the sexual dysfunction.
		• The individual performs measures to promote sexual expression and satisfaction.
		• The individual reports satisfaction with the achievable level of sexual functioning.

	Knowledge Deficit in the Partner[a]	

	• The nurse teaches the partner the nature of the sexual dysfunction.
	• The nurse teaches measures to promote sexual expression and satisfaction, such as:
	  • Alternate positions and time of day.
	  • Exploration of different sexual behaviors.
	• The nurse provides resource information.
	• The nurse encourages the partner to seek sexual counseling.
	• The nurse collaborates with the sex counselor.
		• The partner describes the nature of the sexual dysfunction.
		• The partner uses appropriate resources to begin establishing a satisfying pattern of sexual behavior.

[a] Regarding the nature of the sexual dysfunction and measures to promote sexual expression and satisfaction.

SUGGESTED ASSESSMENT PARAMETERS FOR DIAGNOSTIC CATEGORIES

Assessment Parameters for Consciousness and Cognition

Behavioral response (e.g., eye opening, motor movement, and speech) to stimuli
Pupillary size, shape, and reaction to light (direct and consensual)
Eye movements at rest
Brainstem reflexes—swallowing, gag, corneal, cough, and oculocephalic reflexes
Breathing pattern
Blood pressure
Rate, rhythm, and volume of arterial pulses
Temperature
Percussion notes and breath sounds
Orientation to self, person, place, and time
Immediate, recent, and remote memory
General fund of knowledge
Ability to calculate
Abstraction (abstract reasoning)
Problem-solving skills and ability to form judgments
Overall mood
General behavior
Presence of illusion, delusions, and/or hallucinations
Nutritional status and patterns
Ability to carry out self-care patterns
The family's and significant others' perceptions of the individual's consciousness, coma, cognition

Assessment Parameters for Communication

Recognition and interpretation of spoken language
Recognition and interpretation of written language
Production of spontaneous speech
Repetition
Identification of familiar objects
Mass, tone, and strength of musculature of the face and the arms and hands
Motor coordination of speech structures and the arms and hands
Function of cranial nerves, except olfactory
Current method(s) of communication, including use of body language
The individual's, family's, and significant others' knowledge deficits and learning abilities
The individual's, family's, and significant others' readiness to learn
The individual's, family's, and significant others' preferences for teaching–learning strategies

Assessment Parameters for Mobility

Reflex function of cranial nerve V (trigeminal nerve)
Reflex and motor function of cranial nerve VII (facial nerve)
Reflex function of cranial nerves IX and X (glossopharyngeal and vagus nerves)
Function of cranial nerve XI (spinal accessory nerve)
Mass, tone, and strength of musculature
Degree and distribution of abnormal and/or involuntary movement
Deep tendon and pathological reflexes
Degree and distribution of disturbances in cutaneous sensations
Degree and distribution of disturbances in deep sensations
Cerebellar function (coordination)
Posture and/or station
Gait
Joint appearance and size, mobility, and function
Skeletal changes
Changes in mobility
Ability to carry out self-care patterns
Changes in nutritional patterns
Changes in elimination patterns
Ability to maintain patterns of sexual expression
Blood pressure lying, sitting, and standing
Respiratory movement, frequency, depth, chest expansion, and pattern
Vital capacity or tidal volume
Voice sounds, percussion notes, and breath sounds
The individual's, family's, and significant others' knowledge deficits and learning abilities
The individual's, family's, and significant others' readiness to learn
The individual's, family's, and significant others' preferences for teaching–learning strategies

Assessment Parameters for Sensation

Function of cranial nerve I (olfactory nerve)
Function of cranial nerve II (optic nerve)
Sensory and reflex function of cranial nerve V (trigeminal nerve)
Taste function of cranial nerve VII (facial nerve)
Function of cranial nerve VIII (vestibulocochlear nerve)
Sensory and reflex function of cranial nerves IX and X (glossopharyngeal and vagus nerves)
Degree and distribution of disturbance in cutaneous sensations, including pain
Degree and distribution of disturbance in deep sensations, including proprioception and pain

Degree, distribution, and extent of cortical sensation disturbance
Mass, tone, and strength of musculature in area(s) of sensory disturbance
Reflexes in the area(s) of sensory disturbance, station, and/or gait
Cerebellar function of body part(s) involved in sensory disturbance
Ability to carry out self-care patterns and patterns of sexual expression
General appearance
Skin appearance, color, and texture in affected body part(s)
Sweating function of involved cutaneous tissues
Joint appearance, mobility, and function in affected body part(s)
Changes in sleep patterns, elimination patterns, and nutrition patterns
Ability to carry out self-care patterns
Changes in psychosocial patterns with pain: assess involved anatomical structures and physiological systems
The individual's, family's, and significant others' knowledge deficits and learning abilities
The individual's, family's, and significant others' readiness to learn
The individual's, family's, and significant others' preferences for teaching–learning strategies

Assessment Parameters for Rest and Sleep

Past sleep history, including sleep environment, bedtime routines, and sleep aids from the individual, family, and significant others
Current sleep pattern
Past sleep pattern
Current rest and activity pattern
Past rest and activity pattern
Drug history, including alcohol
History of seizure disorder
Mental status
Pain: assess involved anatomical structures and physiological systems
Muscle strength and tone
Presence of abnormal motor movement
Respiratory status
Cardiovascular status
Blood pressure
Weight
Neck appearance

Assessment Parameters for Sexuality

General appearance
Degree and distribution of disturbance in cutaneous sensation
Degree and distribution of disturbance in deep sensation
Mass, tone, and strength of musculature
Degree and distribution of involuntary muscle movement
Superficial and deep tendon reflexes
Changes in psychosocial patterns
Changes in roles
Changes in elimination patterns
Drug history, including alcohol
The individual's and the partner's knowledge and attitudes about sexuality and sexual function
The individual's and the partner's concepts of self and others as sexual beings
Changes in sexual expression patterns and function
Satisfaction with sexual expression
The individual's and the partner's willingness to explore alternative methods of sexual expression

REFERENCES

1. American Nurses' Association. (1973). *Standards of nursing practice*. Kansas City, MO: The Association.
2. American Nurses' Association. (1974). *Standards of medical-surgical nursing practice*. Kansas City, MO: The Association, 3.
3. American Nurses' Association's Division on Medical-Surgical Nursing Practice and the American Association of Neurosurgical Nurses. (1977). *Standards of neurological and neurosurgical nursing practice*. Kansas City, MO: The Association.
4. American Nurses' Association. (1980). *Nursing: A social policy statement*. Kansas City, MO: The Association, 9.
5. American Association of Neuroscience Nurses. (April 1984). The AANN Conceptual Framework. *Journal of Neurosurgical Nursing 16*(2), 117.

BIBLIOGRAPHY

Adams, R. D., & Victor, M. (1981). *Principles of neurology* (2nd ed.). New York: McGraw-Hill.
American Nurses' Association. (1980). *Nursing: A social policy statement*. Kansas City, MO: The Association.

American Nurses' Association. (1974). *Standards of medical-surgical nursing practice.* Kansas City, MO: The Association.

American Nurses' Association. (1977). *Standards of neurological and neurosurgical nursing practice.* Kansas City, MO: The Association.

American Nurses' Association. (1973). *Standards of nursing practice.* Kansas City, MO: The Association.

American Association of Neuroscience Nurses. (1984). The AANN Conceptual Framework. *Journal of Neurosurgical Nursing, 16*(2), 117.

American Association of Neuroscience Nursing. (1974, 1983). *Core curriculum.* Chicago: The Association.

Armstrong, M. E., (1980). Current concepts in pain. *AORN Journal, 80*(9), 383.

Boss, B. J. (1984). Dysphasias versus dysarthrias versus dyspraxias: Distinguishing features, 2 parts. *Journal or Neurosurgical Nursing, 16*(3), 151; *16*(4), 211.

Brody, H. (1982). The lie that heals: The ethics of giving placebos. *Annals of Internal Medicine, 97*(1), 112.

Carpenito, L. J. (1983). *Nursing diagnosis: Application to clinical practice.* Philadelphia: Lippincott.

Diagnostic classification of sleep and arousal disorders. (1979). *Sleep, 2*(1), 1.

Goodwin, J. S., Goodwin, J. M., & Vogel, A. V. (1982). Placebo misuse. *Nursing, 12*(2), 82.

Gordon, M. (1982, 1985). *Manual of nursing diagnosis.* New York: McGraw-Hill.

Hauri, P. (1982) *The sleep disorders: Current Concepts.* Kalamazoo, MI: Upjohn.

Hayter, J. (1980). The rhythm of sleep. *American Journal of Nursing, 80*(3), 457.

Hickey, J. (1981). *The clinical practice of neurological and neurosurgical nursing.* Philadelphia: Lippincott.

Johnson, J. H., & Cryan, M. (1979). Homonymous hemianopsia: Assessment and nursing management. *American Journal of Nursing, 79*(12), 2131.

Kim, M. J., McFarland, G. K., McLane, A. M. (Eds.). (1984). *Pocket guide to nursing diagnosis.* St. Louis: Mosby.

Livingston, R. B. (1984) Neural integration. In E. D. Frohlick (Ed.), *Pathophysiology: Altered regulatory mechanisms in disease.* Philadelphia: Lippincott.

Luce, J. M., Thompson, T. L., Getto, C. J., et al. (1979). New concepts of chronic pain and their implications. *Hospital Practice, 14*(4), 113.

Mahney, E. K. (1980). Alterations in cognitive functioning in brain-damaged patients. *Nursing Clinics of North America, 15*(2), 283.

Mancall, E. I., (1978). *Alper and Mancall's essentials of the neurological examination.* Philadelphia: Davis.

McCaffery, M. (1979). *Nursing management of the patient with pain* (2nd ed). Philadelphia: Lippincott.

Mitchell, P. H., Cammermeyer, M., Ozuna, J., & Woods, N.F. (1984). *Neurological Assessment for nursing practice.* Reston, VA: Reston.

Norman, S. (1979). Diagnostic Categories for the patient with a right hemisphere lesion. *American Journal of Nursing, 79*(12), 2126.

Norman, S. & Bratz, R. (1979). Understanding Aphasia. *American Journal of Nursing, 79*(12), 2135.

Plum, F. & Posner, J. (1980). *The diagnosis of stupor and coma* (2nd ed.) Philadelphia: Davis.

O'Brien, M. T., & Pallett, P.J. (1978). *Total care of the stroke patient.* Boston: Little, Brown.

Snyder, M. (Ed.). (1983). *A guide to neurological and neurosurgical nursing.* New York: Wiley.

Taylor, J. W. & Ballenger, S. (1980). *Neurological dysfunctions and nursing interventions.* New York: McGraw-Hill.

Wachter-Shikora (Powers), N. (1981). Pain theories and their relevance to the pediatrics population. *Issues in Comprehensive Pediatric Nursing, 5*(5–6), 321.

Wallhagen, M. I. (1979). The split brain: Implications for care and rehabilitation. *American Journal of Nursing, 79*(12), 2118.

Walseben, J. (1982). Sleep disorders. *American Journal of Nursing, 82*(6), 936.

Wells, C. R. (1977). *Dementia* (2nd ed.). Philadelphia: Davis.

Index

AANN. *See* American Association of Neuroscience Nurses.
Abdomen, assessment of, 426–427
Absence spell, generalized, 100
Abstraction, 204–205
Acalculia, 206
Accountability, 6
Acetylcholine, 62, 272–273
Acetylcholinesterase, 272–273
Achromatopsia, 196, 198
Acoustic neurinomas, 30
Acromegaly, 30
ACTH, 118
Actin, 270–271
Active range of motion exercises, 313
Activities of daily living (ADL)
    assessment chart, 286t–288t
    assessment in mobility disfunction, 298
    scales for, 284
    self-care and, 489, 493
Adaptive capacity, intracranial, 76–77
Adenomas, pituitary, 30
Adenosine triphosphate (ATP), 271
ADL. *See* Activities of Daily Living.
Adrenocorticotrophic hormone (ACTH), 118
Advocacy, 6, 51–52
Affiliative relationships
    altered, 259–266
        case study, 261
        human responses in, 260–266
    assessment of, 252, 255–257
        framework for, 256t
    forms of, 248–250
    goals of, 250–252
    human needs met through, 251–252
    impact of neurologic disorders on, 259–260
    nature of, 247–248
    overview, 247–257t
    theoretical frameworks
        communication, 255
        developmental, 254–255
        institutional, 252–253
        interactional, 254
        psychoanalytic, 253
        situational, 254
        structural-functional, 253
Age(ing)
    brain changes and, 151–152
    changes in sensory components of nervous system, 374, 375t
    cognition and, 151–152
    communication ability and, 214–215
    motor function and, 277–278
    peripheral nerve changes, 386

Italicized letters following page numbers indicate tables (*t*) and figures (*f*).

INDEX

Age(ing) *(cont.)*
 "premature social," 335
 sexual arousal and, 475
 sexuality and, 465–466
 sleep disturbances and, 121–122
 sleep patterns and, 118
Ageusia, 376
Aggression
 case study, 88–89
 definitions of, 85–86
 potential for violence, 93–94
Agnosia, 196–197, 203
Airway clearance, insufficient, 350
Akinesia, 276
Alcohol
 sleep and, 130–131
 withdrawal delirium, case study, 89–90
Aldosterone, circadian rhythmn and, 118
Alertness
 deficits in, 194
 problems of, 192–194
Alexia, 197
Alzheimer's bodies, 151
Alzheimer's disease
 dementias of, 24, 227
 neurologic involvement, 25
Ambient sleep temperature, 130
Amenorrhea, 30
American Association of Neuroscience Nurses (AANN)
 phenomena identified by, 12
American Association of Neurosurgical Nurses (AANN)
 founding of, 5
 Scope of Practice Statement, 6–8
American Nurses' Association (ANA)
 Neuroscience Nursing Practice: Process and Outcome Criteria for Selected Diagnoses, 501–502
 Nursing: A Social Policy Statement, 3–4, 9, 11–12, 501
 Standards of Nursing Practice, 501–502
Amnesia
 anterograde, 145, 147, 173
 in physiologic disturbances, 171
 posttraumatic, 173
 in psychologic disturbances, 171
 retrograde, 145, 173
Amnesic aphasia, 224–225
Amusia, 197
Amygdala, hyperarousal and, 87*f*, 88
Amyotrophic lateral sclerosis, 26–27, 221
Analgesia, 385
Analgesics, 406–407

Anal reflex, 426, 467
Anal sphincter, 419
Anal wink, 426, 467
Androgens, 139
Anesthesia, 385
Anger, 265
Anhedonic orgasm, 478
Anomic aphasia, 224–225
Anorgasmia, 478–479
Anosmia, 376
Anosodiaphoria, 197
Anosognosia, 197
Anterior chamber, 368
Anterior horn of spinal cord, 362
Anterograde amnesia, 145, 147, 173
Anterolateral sensory system, 363
Antiepilepsy drugs
 noncompliance, 105–107
 overdose, 109
Anxiety
 acute pain responses and, 399–400
 from diagnosis, 261–262
 from painful procedures, 408–409
 reduction, 262
Aphasia
 anomic, 224–225
 Broca's, 223*t*
 case study, 235–236
 conduction (central), 225
 description of, 222–225
 interventions for, 236
 sensory, acoustic or receptive (Wernicke's), 223*t*, 224
 transcortical motor, 225
 transcortical sensory, 225
 verbal communication alteration and, 380–381
Apnea
 central, 125
 mixed, 125–126
 obstructive or upper airway, 125
Apraxia
 definition of, 209
 of speech, 221–222
Aqueous (of the eye), 368
Architectural barriers, 279–280
Argyll-Robertson pupils, 368
Arousal
 assessment, 63–65*t*
 classification of disorders, 63*f*
 decreased, 63, 188–194*t*
  case study, 70–73
  in CNS impairments, 75–76

Italicized letters following page numbers indicate tables (*t*) and figures (*f*).

diagnoses from reduced environmental interaction, 79–82
diagnoses related to pathophysiologic state, 74–79
etiology, 67–70
inadequate resources for, 82–83
responses to auditory and somatic sensory stimuli, 81–82
sudden-onset coma case study, 73–74t
definition, 58
disorders
    alertness problems, 192–194
    speed of processing, 192
disorders of, 68f
increased, 63, 85. *See also* Hyperarousal.
    anatomic basis of, 86–88f
    case studies, 88–90
    human responses, 90–96
    manifestations, 85–86
intermittent loss of, 99–112
    human responses to, 100–112
    injury potential, 102–103
    nursing roles in management, 112
    sources, 99–100
manifesting behaviors, 58
neuroanatomic basis, 59–61f
neurochemical basis, 61–62
normal alterations in, 62–63
sleep disorders. *See* Sleep-wake pattern disorders.
Arteriosclerosis, 306
Arteriovenous malformation, case study, 73–74
Artificial larynx, 243–244
Ascending reticular activating system, 120, 490–491
Aseptic meningitis, 35
Assessment. *See* under specific phenomena or condition.
Assistive devices
    for communication disorders, 241–245
    for mobility, 278, 300
    for self-feeding, 329f, 349, 354
Association and naming deficits, 198–199
Astereognosis, 150–151
Asterognosia, 197
Astrocytomas, 29, 30
Asymbolia for pain, 197
Ataxic dysarthria, 219
Atelectasis, 307
ATP, 271
Attention
    deficits, 188–194t
        alertness problems, 192–194
        speed of processing, 192
    directed, neural network for, 191–192f
    pain perception and, 401
Audiologic evaluation, 234

Auditory agnosia, 197
Auditory cortex, disorders of, 149–150
Auditory-spatial analysis disorders, 199–200
Auditory stimuli, psychophysiologic alarm response and, 81–82
Auditory verbal agnosia, 222
Augmentative communication systems
    goals of, 241–242
    types of devices, 242–245
Aura, 34–35
Automatic processing, 191
Autonomic dysreflexia
    case study, 435
    description of, 446–448
Autonomic nervous system responses, in decreased arousal, 81–82
Autonomous bladder, 436
Autotopagnosia, 197
Awareness, intermittent loss of, 112
Axis I of the nervous system
    altered responses
        with CVA, 20–21
        with vascular headaches, 23
    degenerative disorders, 23–25
    infectious disorders, 35–36
    tumors
        human responses, 30–31
        symptoms, 28
Axis II of the nervous system
    altered responses with CVA, 21–22
    degenerative disorders, 25–27
    infectious disorders, 35–36
    tumors, human responses, 30–31
Axis III of the nervous system
    altered responses with CVA, 22
    degenerative disorders, 25–27
    infectious disorders of, 36–37
    neoplasms, 30–31
Axis IV of the nervous system
    degenerative disorders, 25–27, 27–28
    neuromuscular disorders, 31–33

Bacterial meningitis, 35
Balance, conditions affecting, 375–376
Balint's syndrome, 199
Barium enema, 428
Barriers, to mobility, 340–341
Barthel Index, 284, 288–289, 290t, 493, 495
Basal ganglia, 276–277
Basilar artery, occlusion or hemorrhage, 21–22
Beds
    for pressure sore prevention, 314
    for respiratory care during immobility, 312

Behavior
  acute pain responses, 398–399
  factors influencing sleep, 131–132
  goal-oriented, 147
  indicators of ineffective coping, 95
  in memory deficit, observations of, 177–178
  responses to chronic pain, 400
  sexual, 464
Behavioral output, 67–68
Behavior modification, 94
Bell's palsy, 369
Biofeedback, 48–49
Bitemporal hemianopsia, 368
Bladder
  anatomy, 419, 420
  elimination, 419–422
    alterations in, 431–439
    alternate management methods, 439
  neurogenic, 422
Bladder neck, 41
Blood gases, abnormalities, with impaired mobility, 329–330
Body image disturbance, 391–392
Body temperature, circadian rhythmn and, 118–119
Bonding, 463
Botulism, 32
Bowel
  areflexic or flaccid, 447–448
  elimination, 422–424
    immobility and, 314
    management, positioning, and facilitatory techniques, 453
    psychosocial implications of alterations, 456
  history, 428
  incontinence, related to neurogenic bowel, 443–444
  management
    implementation of program, 449–454t
    principles of, 449–454
  motor paralytic, 448
  neurogenic
    human responses to, 441–449
    neuraxial levels of, 442t
  retraining, 445–446
  stimulation techniques, 446
  uninhibited, 441, 443
Bowel stimulants, 453–454
Bradykinesia, 24, 27
Brain
  age-related changes, 151–152
  anatomy
    cognition and, 138–139
  dominant and nondominant hemispheres, 146f
  functional organization, 155–156, 186–187, 200–201
  herniation, potential after neurosurgery, 71–72
  holistic formulations of cerebral function, 186–187
  left hemisphere, 139
  regions of specific memory alteration, 174t
  right hemisphere, 139
  tissue
    degeneration, memory loss from, 173
    surgical loss, memory loss from, 174
Brain abscess, 36
Brain edema. See Cerebral edema.
Brain injury, high risk of, 504
Brain swelling, 71
Brain tissue, infarction of, 306
Brain tumors. See Central nervous system, tumors.
Brainstem
  altered responses with CVA, 21–22
  axis II. See Axis II of the nervous system.
  neoplasms, 30
  reticular activating system, 363
Brainstem lesions, 303–304
Brainstem nuclei, 276
Breathing, ineffective patterns, 312
Broca's area, 217
Brodman's area, 369
Brown-Séquard syndrome, 364–365
Bulbocavernous reflex, 426

Calcium, muscle contraction and, 271
Calculation process, 205–206
  disorders of, 206
Cardiac arrhythmias, 75
Cardiac output, immobility and, 307
Cardiovascular system, effects of immobility, 307
Carotid artery, internal, CVA and, 21
Cataplexy, 126
Catecholamines, circadian rhythmn and, 118
Cauda equina, 362
Causalgia, 366, 385
Central apnea, 125
Central cord syndrome, 365
Central hearing loss, 367
Central nervous system
  decreased arousal with impairments, 75–76
  defecation and, 424
  impaired processing, 68–69
  micturation regulation and, 421
  taste pathway, 369
  trauma, 33–34

Italicized letters following page numbers indicate tables (t) and figures (f).

tumors
  classification by neural structures, 30–31
  classification by type of tissue involved, 28–30
  of coverings, 29
  of supportive tissue, 29
Central somesthetic sensory system, 363–366
Cerebellar artery
  disorders of, 22
  thrombosis of, 22
Cerebellar astrocytoma, 30
Cerebellar dyssynergy, ipsilateral, 22
Cerebellopontine angle tumors, 30
Cerebellum
  axis II. See Axis II of the nervous system.
  dysfunction of, 277
  hemorrhage into, 22
  ischemia, 22
  movement and, 277
  neoplasms, 30
Cerebral artery, cerebrovascular accident and, 21
Cerebral cortex
  deficits, anatomic correlates for, 146f
  organization of, 146f
Cerebral edema, 71
Cerebral embolism, 20
Cerebral hemispheres
  axis I. See Axis I of the nervous system.
  neoplasms, 30
Cerebral hemorrhage, 20
Cerebral infarct, 69
Cerebral ischemia, 69
Cerebral thrombosis, 20
Cerebrovascular accident
  altered responses
    in axis I, 20–21
    in axis II, 21–22
    of axis III, 22
  case study
    alteration of special senses and, 377–381
    basic hygienic tasks and, 492–494
    immobility and, 310–311
  cerebral arterial distribution and, 21
  communication and, 235–236
  community implications, 316
  decreased arousal in, 69
  incidence, 20
  pathophysiology, 306
Cerebrovascular disorders. See also Cerebrovascular accident.
  vascular headache, 22–23
Cervical cord injury, case study, 309–310
C fibers, 361
Cholesteatomas, 29
Chondrosarcomas, 29

Chordomas, 29
Choroid, 367
Choroid plexus papillomas, 29
Chosen families, 249
Chromosomal sex, 459–460f
Ciliary body, 36
Circadian sleep-wake cycle, 118–119
Clasp-knife phenomenon, 304
Clostridium botulinium toxin, 32
Clostridium tetani, 36
Cluster headaches, 22
Coding
  deficit in, 201
  definition of, 200–201
Cognition
  age-related changes, normal, 151–152
  aggregate field view, 138
  alterations in processing, 185–209. See also Cognitive processing.
  assessment, 155–168, 517
    case study, 162–164f
    in clinical setting, 155
    evaluation of functions, 157t
    integration of nursing and neuropsychologic assessment, 160–164f
    neurobehavioral cognitive status examination text booklet, 166–169f
    types of, 156–160
  brain anatomy and, 138–139
  central processing, impaired function of, 200–206t
  deficits
    irreversible, 506
    in sensation and perception, 194–196
    uncompensated, 506
  definitions, concepts, and theories, 137–138
  disorders of pattern recognition, 196–200
  functions
    comparison of mental status examinations, 161t
    impairment of output processing, 206–209
    specific tests of, 160
  input processes, deficits of, 188–196t
  localization view, 138–139
  neuroanatomy for, 143–152f
  neurophysiology of primary abilities, 143–151f
  normal development, 139–142t
Cognitive–linguistic disorders
  description of, 225–226
  generalized intellectual impairment, 226–227
Cognitive processing
  altered, human responses to, 188–209
  domains of, 187–188
    central processing, 187–188
    input stage, 187–188
    output stage, 187–188

Cognitive processing (cont.)
  input function, impaired, 188–196t
  models of, 185–187
  nursing model, 187, 188f
Cohabitation, 249
Cold application, 411–412
Colloid cysts, 29
Colon, 422
Color association disorders, 199
Color-naming defects, 198–199
Column tract, dorsal or posterior, 362–363
Coma
  assessment of, 63–64t
  case study, 73–74t
  decreased arousal, 67
  etiology
    head injury, 69
    nontraumatic, 79
    structural and metabolic disorders, 67–68
  prognosis, family knowledge deficit and, 78–79
Comfort, alteration in. See Discomfort.
Communication
  ability, evaluation in elimination, 427
  assessment parameters, 516
  augmentative systems of, 241–245
  of consciousness, impairment of, 69–70
  disorders, 217–227t, 508
    acute and long-term implications, 227–228
    alterations from dysarthria and dysphonia, 333
    expressive and cognitive–linguistic deficits, 237–241
    expressive aphasia, case study, 240–241
    neurogenic, management of, 231–245
    neuroscience nursing role, 231–232
    overview, 213–229
    sensory–perceptual alterations from sensory overload, 236–237
    verbal, alterations from hearing impairment and aphasia, 380–381
  human responses to alterations, 232–241
  language, mechanism of, 217
Communication chart, 242–243
Community
  consequences
    of acute pain, 409
    of chronic pain, 416
    of sensory alteration, 382
  diagnoses
    for ineffective family coping, 266
    peripheral sensation alteration, 393–394
  effects of communication disorders on, 227
  knowledge deficit
    epilepsy stigma and, 111–112
    head injury prevention, 79
    on immobility, 340–341
    on increased behavioral arousal, 96
  resources
    for immobility, 316–317, 341
Community-focused interventions
  advocacy, 51–52
  public education, 51
  for self-care deficits, 494, 496, 497–498
Complex cognitive operations, 138
Complex partial seizure, 100, 103
Computers, as communication assistive devices, 243
Concept
  definition, 10
  formation of, 201, 203–206
  historical development of nursing and, 10–11
  vs. phenomenon, 10
Conceptual concreteness, 205
Conceptualizations, 204
Conduction aphasia, 225
Conductive hearing loss, 367, 375
Cones, of the eye, 367
Congenital tumors, 29
Consciousness
  altered level of, 201
  arousal. See Arousal.
  assessment parameters, 516
  concept of, 10
  content of, 156
  decreased, associated human responses, 70–83
  defining characteristics, 504–507
  definition, 57–58
  impaired, total self-care deficit, 491–492
  outcome criteria, 504–507
  overview, 57–65
  process criteria, 504–507
  rhythmic alterations in, 115–132. See also Sleep.
Constipation
  with autonomous neurogenic bowel, 447–448
  decreased activity and, 332–333
  motor paralytic bowel and, 448
  with neurogenic bowel, complications of, 454–456
  sensory paralytic bowel and, 449
Contractures, 313, 320
Controlled processing, 191
Coordination assessment, 294
Coping
  ineffective, by family and/or significant others
    in abnormally increased arousal cases, 95–96

Italicized letters following page numbers indicate tables (t) and figures (f).

in brain injury cases, 82
in chronic immobility cases, 339
in chronic pain cases, 414–415
in epilepsy and syncope, 109–110
in hyperarousal cases, 95–96
in peripheral sensation alteration cases, 392–393
related to limited situational support, 262–265
use of denial, 103–104
ineffective, family and/or significant others
in acute pain cases, 406–408
ineffective, individual
with abrupt alteration of mobility, 314–315
with chronic immobility, 334–335
with chronic pain, 410
patterns, 299*t*
skills instruction for, 408
Cornea, 367
Cortical defects, anatomic correlates, 147, 148*t*
Corticosteroid therapy, for myasthenia gravis, 31–32
Corticotropin, 118
Cortisol, 118
Counseling, for families and significant others, 50–51
Counterirritation, 412
Cover-uncover test, 291–292
Cranial nerves, functional assessement of, 292–294
Craniopharyngiomas, 29, 30
Craniotomy
decreased arousal after, case study, 73–74
postoperative period
potential for brain herniation, 71–72
potential for intracranial hypertension, 72–73
potential for brain swelling, 37
Creatinine clearance, 425
Credé maneuver, 436
Crisis theory, chronic illness and, 319–320
Cultural factors
influences in pain expression, 401
self-care and, 484–485
Cushing's syndrome, 30
CVA. *See* Cerebrovascular accident.

Daily Activity Diary, 413
Dance therapy, 44
DC potential theory, 143
Decisional control, 46
Decision-making patterns, 261
Deconditioning effects, 320
Decubitus ulcers, 309
Deep breathing exercises, 408–409
Deep tendon reflexes, 294–297*t*
Deep venous thrombosis, immobility and, 307
Defecation
neurogenic control of, 423–424*f*
reflexes, 419, 423
system, anatomy of, 422
Defining characteristics, 502. *See also* under specific diagnoses.
Degenerative disorders. *See also* specific disorders.
of axes II, III and IV, 25–27
of axis I, 23–25
of axis IV, 27–28
characteristics, 23
Delirium
from alcohol withdrawal, case study, 89–90
characteristics of, 86
Delta sleep, 116
Delta sleep-inducing peptide, 121
Dementias
of Alzheimer's disease, 24, 227
clinical course, 25
etiology, 227
incidence, 24–25
symptoms, 25
Denial
of epilepsy, 103–104, 110
interventions for, 265
Depression, chronic pain and, 400–401
Dermatomes, 361
Dermatomyositis, 33
Detrusor sphincter dyssynergia, 438–439
Development, human
self-care abilities and, 483–484
sexuality and, 459–466*t*
Developmental remnants, tumors of, 29
Diabetes insipidus, hyperosmolar state of, 75
Diabetes mellitus
case study, 386–388, 437–438
peripheral neuropathy and, 386–388
Diadochokinesis, 238
Diarrhea, 455
Diazepam, for sleep terrors, 129
Diencephalon
axis I. *See* Axis I of the nervous system.
lesions, 60
neoplasms, 30
Diet. *See also* Nutrition.
bowel elimination and, 424
high fiber foods, 452*t*
neurogenic bowel dysfunction management and, 452
Digestion
neurogenic control of, 423
process of, 422
Digital stimulation techniques, for defecation, 446
Diplopia, 333
Disability, meanings for, 284
Discomfort
with chronic immobility, 334

Discomfort (cont.)
  interventions for, 404–405
  with peripheral sensation alteration, 389
Discrimination, two-point, 371
Disuse syndrome, 80
Divided attention deficits, 191
  assessment, 193–194
L-Dopa, 206
Dopamine, 62, 461
Dorsal column system, 363
Dorsal horn, 362
Dream anxiety attacks, 129
Dreaming, 118
Drugs. *See also* specific drugs.
  for aggression, 94
  for bowel management, 454*t*
  consciousness altering, 69
  effects on sexual behavior, 473*t*–474*t*
  history, in elimination assessment, 428
  for stimulation of bowel elimination, 453–454
Duchenne muscular dystrophy, 32–33
Dysarthrias
  altered communication and, 333
  description of, 218–221
Dysesthesias, 334, 385
Dysgraphia, 222
Dyskinesia, 276
Dyslexia, 222
Dysphagia
  inadequate nutrition and, 332
  interventions, 354
  radiographic assessment, 353*f*
  treatment guidelines, 353–354
Dysphonia, altered communication and, 333
Dyspraxia
  definition of, 209
  of speech, 221–222

Eating, motor component assessment, 292
Economic factor, self-care and, 485
Education, public. *See* Public education.
Ejaculatory dysfunctions, 478
Electroencephalogram (EEG)
  of alertness disorders, 193
  during non-REM, 116
  during wakefulness, 115–116
Electromyogram (EMG)
  during non-REM, 116
  during REM, 117

Elimination
  alteration, immobility and, 313–314
  assessment of, 424–428
  bowel, alterations in, 441–456
  effects of immobility, 308
  gastrointestinal assessment, 426–428
  neurourologic assessment, 424–426
  overview, 419–428
Emotional deprivation, 265–266
Encephalitis, 35–36
Enemas, 454
Enforced Social Dependency scale (ESD), 493
Environment
  barrier-free, 279–280
  factors influencing sleep, 130–131
  impact on mobility, 299–301*t*
  mobility and, 279–280
  nervous system development impairment and, 142
  pressure sore developmental and, 80–81
Enzymatic cofactors, 61, 62
Ependymoma, 29–30
Epidermoid cysts, 29
Epidural hematoma, 69
Epilepsy
  alteration in family process, 110–111
  community diagnoses, 111–112
  denial of, 103–104
  fear and, 101–102
  knowledge deficit, 107–108*t*, 111–112
  memory deficit, 109
  noncompliance, 105–107
  role disturbance, 105
  seizure classification, 34–35, 100
  sense of smell and, 369–370
  social isolation in, 104–105
    assessment of, 104
    goals for nursing management, 104–105
  stigma related to knowledge deficit, 111–112
Equilibrium, 256
Excessive daytime sleepiness, assessment of, 125
Excitation–contraction coupling, 271
Exercise
  bowel elimination and, 452–453
  classifications of, 43–44
  sleep and, 131
Experimental or predictive studies, 17
Expressive transmission disorders, 228–229
Extraocular muscle
  anatomy, 368
  assessment of function, 290, 292*f*

Italicized letters following page numbers indicate tables (*t*) and figures (*f*).

Eye, anatomy, 367–368

Facial nerve assessment, 293
Factor S, 121
Fainting, 99
Falls, potential for, in Parkinson's disease, 324
Family
  achieved, nonbiologic, 249
  acute immobility and, 315–316
  assessment, 260–261
  consequences
    of acute pain, 409
    of chronic pain, 415–416
    of sensory alteration, 381–382
  coping ability of, 261. *See also* under Coping.
  crisis potential, 315–316
  effects of communication disorders on, 227
  extended, 248–249
  healthy biologic or achieved, characteristics of, 249–250
  influence of neuroscience nurse, 228
  knowledge deficit. *See* Knowledge deficit, family and significant others.
  legal and biologic, 248–249
  married childbearing or traditional, 248
  models of pain experience, 401
  new definition of, 248
  process alterations
    assessment of, 111
    in epilepsy, 110–111
  roles
    changes, ineffective coping and, 392–393
    disruption of, 265
    self-care attainment and, 484
    single parent, 248
  support groups for, 263–264
Family-focused interventions, for self-care deficits, 494, 496, 497–498
Family of origin, 249
Fatigue
  etiology, 320
  low sexual desire from, 472, 474
Fear
  of addiction, 406
  assessment of, 101
  intermittent loss of arousal and, 100–102
    etiologies, 100–101
Fecal impaction
  diagnosis of, 455
  potential with reflex neurogenic bowel, 444–446
Feedback, 257
Feeding
  interventions for swallowing dysfunction, 356
  self-feeding with motor impairment, 329
Feet, pressure distribution, 387, 388*f*
Fertilization, 459
Fetal sexual development, 459–460*f*
Fiber, dietary, 452*t*
Fibers, nerve, 361
Fictive kin, 249
Fifth nerve tumors, 30
Final common pathway, 270
Flaccid dysarthria, 218
Flexibility, deficit of, 205
Floor bed, 90–91*f*
Focused attention deficits, 191, 193
Food(s)
  high fiber, 452*t*
  intake, sleep and, 130–131
Fractionated recognition, 204
Friedreich's ataxia, 219
Friends. *See also* Significant others.
  as family, 249
Frontal lobe, selective damage, 208
Functional assessment, relationship to impairment, disability, and handicap model, 285*f*
Functional Life Scale (FLS), 284
Functional profiles, 284

Galveston Orientation and Amnesia Test (GOAT), 160, 175, 178, 179*f*
Gamma-aminobutyric acid (GABA), 62
Gastrocolic reflex, 419, 423
Gastrointestinal system, assessment of elimination, 426–428
Gate control theory, 397, 399*f*
Gender identity, 461
Gender role, 461
General interaction chemical theory of sleep, 120–121
General interpretive area, dysfunction of, 150–151
Generalized seizures, 35
General systems theory, 255–256
Glandular tumors, 30
Glasgow Coma Scale, 10, 63–64*t*
Glial cells, 62
Glioblastoma multiforme, 29
Gliomas, 29, 30
Global instruments, for functional assessment of mobility, 283–284
Glossopharyngeal nerve, 293
Goal-oriented behavior, 147
Goals for nursing management. *See* under specific conditions.
Golgi tendon organs, 274–275
Graphesthesia, 371
Gray matter, 362

Grieving, anticipatory or actual, 507
Grounded theory, 16
Group interventions, 50
Growth hormone, secretion, sleep-dependent nature of, 116
Guillain-Barré syndrome
 diminished behavioral output in, 69
 incidence, 27
 motor paralytic bladder, 436–437
Guilt, 265

Hallucinations, 93
Halstead-Reitan Battery, 158
Haustra, 422
Headaches, orientation to healthy living, 496–498
Head injury
 case study, 88–89, 174–175, 492–493
 coma from, 69
 incidence, 33–34
 prognosis, 78–79
 Rancho Los Amigos Levels of Cognitive Functioning Scale, 89t
Health Belief Model, 106, 108t
Health care market, impact on neuroscience nursing, 8
Health maintenance, with chronic immobility, 338–339
Health practices, self-care
 cultural factors, 484–485
 developmental aspects, 483–484
 economic factors, 485
 social and family aspects, 484
Health promotion, in peripheral sensation alteration, 393–394
Hearing
 assessment of, 371
 and balance, conditions affecting, 375–376
 central auditory system, 366
 loss, 222
  central, 367
  conductive, 367
  injury potential and, 379–380
  sensorineural, nongenetic causes, 367
 mechanism, 217
 peripheral components, 366
 physiology of, 366–367
Hearing aids, 244–245
Heart rate, immobility and, 307
Heat application, 411
Helplessness, 262
Hemiplegia, 303–304
Hemophilus influenza, bacterial meningitis, 35

Hemorrhage
 intracerebral, 69
 intracranial, 306
Hemorrhoids, 455–456
Hemotomas, 34
Herpes simplex, encephalitis from, 35–36
Herpes zoster, somatic sensation and, 365–366
Heschl's gyrus, 217
Hesitancy, related to uninhibited neurogenic bladder, 432–433
Hippocampus
 hyperarousal and, 87f, 88
 long-term memory and, 145
Home maintenance management deficit, with chronic immobility, 337–338
Homosexuality, 464–465
Honorary kin, 249
Hope, 49–50
Horner's syndrome, 22, 368
Humor, as intervention, 49
Huntington's disease
 chorea, 227
 etiology, 24
 impaired respiratory function, 329–333
 incidence and prevalence, 24
 motor signs, 24
 movement problems in, 320
 symptoms, 25
 vision alteration, 333
17-Hydroxycorticosteroid excretion, circadian rhythmn and, 118
Hygiene
 in hyperarousal, 92
 performance with neurologic impairment, 492–494
Hypalgesia, 385
Hyperalgesia, 385
Hyperalimentation, 77
Hyperammonemia, 67
Hyperarousal
 case studies, 88–90
 etiologies, 86t
 goals for nursing management, 91, 92, 94
 manifestations, anatomic basis, 86–88
 nutrition alterations, 91–92
 patient diagnosis, 90–94
 potential for violence, 93–94
 sensory-perceptual alterations, 93
 sleep pattern alterations, 93
 sources of, 63
 thought processes alterations in, 93
  goals for nursing management, 93

Italicized letters following page numbers indicate tables (*t*) and figures (*f*).

Hyperemia, 71
Hyperesthesia, 385
Hyperkinesia, 220, 276
Hyperkinetic dysarthria, 220–221f
Hypermetabolism, nutritional deficit from, 77–78
Hyperosmolar state, 75
Hyperreflexia
  case study, 435
  description of, 446–448
Hypesthesia, 385
Hypnagogic hallucinations, 127
Hypoarousal, 63
Hypogeusia, 376
Hypoglycemia, 67
Hypokinesia, 220, 276
Hypokinetic dysarthria, 220
Hypoosmolar state, 75
Hyposmia, 376
Hypothalamus
  functions of, 364
  hyperarousal and, 86, 87f
  testosterone and, 460
Hypoxia, 67

Ia afferent fibers, 273–274
Imagery, 45, 404, 407–408
Immobility, acute
  human responses to, 307–309
    cardiovascular effects, 307
    elimination effects, 308
    integumentary effects, 309
    metabolic effects, 308
    musculoskeletal effects, 308–309
    respiratory effects, 307–308
  impact of, 269–270
  nursing diagnoses
    for community, 316–317
    for family and significant others, 315–316
Immobility, chronic
  flow sheet for monitoring, 322f
  human responses to, 321–341
  impact of, 269–270
  with muscular dystrophy, 327–328
  myasthenia gravis case studies, 325
  from neurosurgical procedure, 37
  nursing diagnoses for family and significant others, 339–340
  nursing diagnoses for individual, 321–322
  Parkinson's disease case studies, 322–323
  pathophysiology, 319
Infants, sleep cycle in, 117–118
Infection
  assessment, 78
  potential, related to invasive monitoring devices, 78
  types of disorders, 35–37
Infectious neuropathies, 386
Inflammatory myopathies, 33
Information processing system
  automatic, 191
  central processing, 187t
  controlled, 191
  input, 187t
    definition, 257
    diminished, 68
    impaired, 188–196t
    speed of processing deficits, 192
  models of, 185–187
  output, 187t
    diminished, 69–70
Infratentorial craniotomy, 37
Injury potential
  assessment, 102
    in hyperarousal, 90
  from diminished or absent sensation, 389–390
  hearing impairment and, 379–380
  for hyperarousal, 90–92
  immobility and, 315
  with intermittent loss of arousal, 102–103
  from loss of proprioception or vibration, 390
  Parkinson's disease, 323–325
  peripheral sensation alteration and, 389–390
  vision impairment and, 379–380
Input. See Information processing system, input.
Insight, definition of, 138
Intake and output monitoring, in CNS impaired patients, 76
Integration disorders of language, 229
Integumentary system, immobility effects, 309
Intellectual impairment, generalized, 226–227
Intentional movement, deficits of, 209
Intermediolateral cell column, 362
Internal memory aids, 181
Interventions, nursing. See under specific phenomena or conditions.
Intracerebral hemorrhage, 69
Intracranial adaptive capacity, decreased, 76–77
Intracranial hemorrhage, 306
Intracranial hypertension
  with decreased intracranial adaptive capacity, 76–77
  postoperative potential, 72–73
Intramural plexus of intestine, 423
Invasive monitoring devices, infection potential and, 78
Iris, 367
Isokinetic exercise, 43
Isometric exercise, 43
Isotonic exercise, 43

Jakob-Creutzfeldt disease, 227
Jebsen Test for Hand Function, 284
Journal intervention, 51
Judgment
  definition of, 138
  impaired, 207–208

Katz Index of ADL, 284
Kidneys, 419, 420
Kinetic bed, 312
Knowledge, nursing
  clinical, sources and development of, 12–14
  current status of, 14–15
  developing science in nursing and, 15–17
Knowledge deficit
  of community
    about resources for affiliative relationships, 266
    epilepsy stigma and, 111–112
    on increased arousal, 96
    on mobility resources, 340–341
  of family and significant others
    on chronic immobility, 339–340
    on coma, 78–79
    on communication impairment, 508
    on consciousness and cognition disorders, 507
    on hyperarousal, 95
    on increased arousal, 95
    on neurologic dysfunction, 266
    on peripheral sensation alteration, 393
  of individual
    on chronic immobility, 336–337
    on epilepsy, 107–108t
Korsakoff's psychosis (syndrome), 145, 147, 173

Laminae, 362
Laminectomy, 37
Language
  acquisition, 214–215
  definition of, 213–214
  integration disorders, 222–225t
    characteristics of, 224t
  mechanism, 217
Larynx, 215
  artificial, 243–244
Lateral geniculate body, 368
Lateral horn, 362
Lateral spinothalamic tract, 362
Learning
  definition of, 137
  research method and, 15–17f
Lens, 368
Leptomeninges, tumors of, 29
Lhermitte's sign, 366
Limbic system, hyperarousal and, 86–88f
Lipid, content of brain, 152
Lipofuscin, 151
Localization view, 138
Locked-in syndrome, 21–22, 69–70
Lou Gehrig's disease (amyotrophic lateral sclerosis), 26–27, 221

Magnetic resonance imaging, of multiple sclerosis, 26
Manual evacuation of stool, 448
Marriage, childless dyadic, 248
Massage, 48, 404
Mass movements, 423
McGill Pain Questionnaire (MPQ), 402–403
Means-end analysis, impaired, 207
Mechanoreceptors, 360t
Medication. *See* Drugs; specific medication.
Medullary syndromes, from vascular disorders, 22
Medulloblastomas, 28, 30
Megacolon, 455
Memory
  alterations in, 171–182
  deficit, manifestations of, 177–180
  definition of, 137
  long-term
    episodic, 172
    secondary or remote, 172
    semantic, 172
    visual and verbal, 172
  loss, 152–153
    behavioral observations, 177–178
    brain regions of specific alterations, 174t
    case studies, 174–177
    defining characteristics of, 109
    in epilepsy, 109
    formal assessment tools, 178–180t
    goals of nursing management, 181
    human responses to, 177–181
    interventions for, 180–181
    "islands" of, 173
    nursing diagnoses for individual, 180
    pathophysiology of, 173–177
    types of, 173–174
  REM sleep and, 117
  sensory, 172–173
  short-term or primary, 172

Italicized letters following page numbers indicate tables (t) and figures (f).

systems
  goal-oriented behavior and, 147
  long-term, 143–147f
  short-term, 143, 144f, 147f
  theories of, 171–173
  working, 172
Memory trace, 200–201
Meningiomas, 29, 30
Meningitis, 35
Mental status examinations
  comparisons, 161t
  for memory loss, 178
Meperidine, 405f, 406, 407f
Metabolic disorders, causing coma, 67
Metabolic waste products, consciousness altering, 69
Metabolism, effects of immobility, 308
Metastatic tumors, 30
Micturition
  neural regulation of, 420–422f
  process of, 419–422
Midazolam, 128
Migraine headache
  medical therapy, 23
  prevalence, 22
  symptoms, 22–23
Milieu therapy, 413
Mini-Mental State (MMS), 159
Minnesota Multiphasic Personality Inventory (MMPI), 157–158, 400
Mixed dysarthrias, 221
Mobility. *See also* Immobility, acute; Immobility, chronic.
  abrupt alteration of, 303–317
    associated diagnoses, 313–315
    case studies, 309–312
    neuroanatomic correlates of, 303–306
    nursing diagnosis related to individual, 312–313
    pathophysiology of common conditions, 306–307
  altered
    swallowing dysfunction with, 345–356
  assessment, 283–301f
    functional, 283–289f
  assessment parameters, 517–518
  chronic illness and, 319–321
  environment and, 279–280
  essential elements, 283f
  impaired, 509
    aspiration risk, 510–511
    assessment of, 312–313
    associated nursing diagnoses, 332–339
    corneal ulceration risk, 511
    with decreased behavioral arousal, 80
    knowledge deficit of family and significant other, 512

respiratory function impairments, 329–332
    self-care deficit, 328–329
      partial, 511
      total, 511
    ventilatory insufficiency risk, 510
  individual strengths and weaknesses, 298–299
  motivation, role of, 278–279
  overview, 269–280
  physical dimension of, 289–297t
  psychosocial dimension, 297–299
Monitoring, skin, for pressure sores, 81
Monoamines, 62
Monoamine theory of sleep, 120–121
Mononeuropathies, 27–28
Motivation, in mobility, 278–279
Motor cortex, 217, 275–276
Motor function, aging and, 277–278
Motor neurons
  description, 273–275
  diseases, 26–27
  suprasegmental and segmental, 270
Motor output, disorders, 69–70
Motor paralytic bowel, 448
Motor paralytic neurogenic bladder, 432t, 436–437
Motor response, 208–209
Motor-speech mechanism, 217
Motor strip, 217
Motor systems, relationship of components, 271f
Motor unit, 273, 321
Movement
  assessment, 289t
    history data, 291t
    screening examination of neurologic function, 291t
  compensated, 278
  definition, 283
  neuroanatomy of, 270–278
  neurophysiology of, 270–278
  patient interventions, 41–44f
  problems, in chronic neurologic conditions, 320–321
Movement therapy, 44
Multiple sclerosis
  case study
    of bladder elimination, 433–435
    of self-care aspects, 495–496
  cost per individual, 25
  description, 221
  etiology, 25–26
  risk, 25
  self-care deficit interventions, 328–329
  signs and symptoms, 26
  somatic sensation and, 366
  syndrome classification, 26
  treatment, 26
  vision disorders, 368

Multiple Sleep Latency Test, 125
Munich Coma Scale, 64, 65*t*
Muscle
   contraction, 270–272, 274
   relationship of receptors and spinal cord, 274*f*
   relaxation, progressive, 42–43*f*
   strength, 294, 313
   tension, altered in lumbar area, 411–412
   tone, 294, 313
Muscle mass, 294
Muscle spindles, 273–275
Muscular dystrophy
   case study, 327–328
   description, 32–33
   impaired respiratory function, 329–333
Musculoskeletal system, immobility effects, 308–309
Music intervention, 47
Myasthenia gravis
   activity intolerance, 325–327
   case study, 325
   impaired respiratory function, 329–333
   incidence and prevalence, 31
   medical therapy, 31–32
   neuromuscular junction and, 273
   self-care deficit interventions, 328–329
   symptoms, 31
Myofibrils, 270
Myopathies, chronic, 32–33
Myosin, 270–271
Myotonia, 461
Myotonic muscular dystrophy, 33

Naming and association deficits, 198–199
Narcolepsy, 126–127
Narcolepsy-cataplexy, case study, 127–128
Narcotics, adverse effects, 406, 407*t*
Needs, basic human, hierarchy of, 298–299
Negative pressure ventilators, 331
Neisseria meningitidis, bacterial meningitis, 35
Neoplasms. *See* Tumors.
Nerve sheath tumors, 30
Nervous system
   development, macroscopic and microscopic changes, 140*t*–142*t*
   dysfunction, relevant phenomena in, 9–10. *See also* specific phenomena.
   structural and functional changes with age, 374, 375*t*
Neuralgia, 385
Neuraxis. *See also* Axis I, Axis II, Axis III, Axis IV, of the nervous system.
   classifications, 20
Neuritic plaques, 151
Neuroastrocytomas, 28
Neurobehavioral batteries, 157–158
Neurobehavioral Cognitive Status Examination (NCSE), 160, 166–169*f*, 178
Neurobehavioral Mental Status Examination (NMSE), 178
Neurobehavioral Rating Scale (NRS), 175, 178
Neurogenic bladder
   definition of, 422
   human responses to, 431–439
   motor paralytic, 436–437
   pathophysiology and management techniques, 432*t*
   psychosocial concerns, 438
   reflex, 432*t*, 435–436
   sensory paralytic, 437–438
   uninhibited, 432–435*t*
   urinary complications, 438–439
Neurogenic bowel
   constipation and, complications of, 454–456
   human responses to, 441–449
   nursing management, 450*t*–451*t*
   patterns with spinal cord lesions, 444–448
   psychosocial implications, 456
Neurologic disorders. *See also* specific disorders.
   diagnosis and treatment, 19–20
   impact on affiliative relationships, 259–260
Neuromuscular disorders, 31–33
Neuromuscular junction, 272–273*f*
Neuromuscular transmission, 272–273*f*
Neuronal elements, primitive, tumors of, 28
Neurons
   metabolic substrates, 61–62
   tumors of, 28
Neuropathy, 27–28, 386. *See also* specific neuropathy.
Neuropsychologic assessments, indications to formalize, 161*t*
Neuropsychologic screening tests, 158–160
Neuropsychologist, referral to, 234
Neuroscience nurse, role and influence, in communication disorders, 227–228
Neuroscience nurse specialist
   functions of, 4–5
   role in peripheral sensation alteration, 394
Neuroscience nursing
   clinical knowledge
     from authority, 13–14
     current status, 14–15
     from experience, 13
     from science, 14

Italicized letters following page numbers indicate tables (*t*) and figures (*f*).

sources and development of, 12–17
  from tradition, 13
conceptual framework, 5–6
fundamental concerns, 9–10
practice, definition of, 5–8
relationship to nursing profession, 3–4
scope of practice, 6–8
specialization, 4–5
Neurosurgery
  decreased arousal after, case study, 70–73
  patient care, generally, 37
Neurosyphilis, 368
Neurotransmitters. *See also* specific neurotransmitters.
  central, 62
  consciousness and, 61, 62
  sleep and, 120, 121
Neurotrauma, 33–34
Nociceptors, 360
Noise, nighttime, effect on sleep, 130
Noncompliance
  with altered sensation, 390–391
  with antiepilepsy drugs, 105–107
  assessment of, 105–106
Non-rapid eye movement sleep (non-REM), 116, 119–120
Nonspecific alerting, 58
Norepinephrine, 62
Nosocomial infection, 78
Number writing, in sensory function discrimination, 371
Nurse generalist, care of, peripheral sensation alteration, 394
Nursing diagnoses. *See also* under specific conditions.
  definition of, 502
  process and outcome criteria for, 504–517
Nursing intervention. *See* under specific condition or phenomena.
Nursing management strategies. *See also* under specific conditions.
  interventions for patients, 41–50f
Nursing profession
  historical development, 10–11
  neuroscience nursing and, 3–4
  scientific methods, 15–17
  specialization, 4–5
Nutrition. *See also* Diet.
  alterations
    in hyperarousal, 91–92
    in swallowing dysfunctions, 350, 355–356
  altered taste and smell and, 382–383
  assessment
    of deficit, 77
    in hyperarousal, 91
  history, in elimination assessment, 427

inadequate, dysphagia and, 332
  for swallowing dysfunction, 348–349

Occlusive disease, 306
Occlusive plastic film, 314
Occupation, mobility and, 269
Off periods, 323
Olfactory tract, trauma, 369
Oligodendrogliomas, 29
Operants, 400
Optic nerve, 368
Optic neuritis, 368
Oral peripheral examination, 238
Orgasm
  alterations in, 477–479
  definition of, 463
Osteomas, 29
Outcome criteria, 503
Output. *See* Information processing system, output.

Paced Auditory Serial Addition Task (PASAT), 192
Pain
  acute
    case study, 403–404
    consequences of, 409
    etiology and medical management, 404t
    human responses in, 402–409
    nursing diagnoses, 404–409f
    responses, types of, 398–400
    vs. chronic, 398–402
  assessment, 370, 402–403t, 410
  chronic
    benign, 400
    case study, 410–415
    consequences of, 415–416
    human responses to, 410–415
    multidisciplinary management of, 414t
    nursing diagnoses and interventions, 415t
    responses, types of, 400–401
    vs. acute, 398–402
  gate control theory, 397, 399f
  influencing factors, 401–402
  neurophysiology of, 397–398
  with peripheral sensation alteration, 389
  preoccupation related to narrowed focus of attention, 413–414
Pain behavior, 400
Pain Rating Scale (PRS), 402–403
Palatopharyngeal sphincter, 215–216
Papillomas, choroid plexus, 29
Paradoxical sleep. *See* Rapid eye movement sleep.
Paralytic ileus, 308, 445

Paraplegia, 305
Parasomnias, 129
Parasympathetic nervous system
  defecation and, 423–424
  micturation regulation and, 421–422
Paresthesia, 385
Parietal lobe, 364
Parietal lobe lesions, somatic sensation and, 365
Parkinson's disease
  basal ganglia dysfunction, 277
  case study, 322–323f
  with dementia, 25
  description of, 23–24
  etiology, 23
  falls, potential for, 324
  human responses, 24
  hypokinesia of, 220, 276
  impaired respiratory function, 329–333
  incidence, 23
  injury potential, 323–325
  medical therapy, 24
  movement problems in, 320
  self-care deficit interventions, 328–329
  skin breakdown potential, 325
  surgical treatment, 24
  symptoms, 23–24
  vision alteration, 333
Partial seizures, 34–35
Passive movement, 370
Passive range of motion exercises, 313
Patient diagnoses, abnormally increased arousal, 90–94
Patient interventions. *See also* under specific condition.
  cognitive, 44–46
  hope, 49–50
  humor, 49
  movement and proprioception, 41–44
  presence, 50
  sensory, 46–49
  timing, 49
Pattern recognition deficits, assessment of, 197
Perception, 173, 373
Peripheral nerves. *See* Axis IV of the nervous system.
Peripheral neuropathy, case study, 311–312, 386–388
Peripheral pathway, for taste, 369
Peripheral sensation alterations, 385–394
  human responses to, 389–394
  nursing roles, 394
Peripheral somesthetic sensory system
  dermatomes, 361
  fibers, 360–361
  receptors, 359–360

  spinal cord, 361–363
Personality characteristics, influence on pain responses, 402
Phenomena
  in ANA Social Policy Statement, 11–12
  historical development of nursing and, 10–11
  identified by AANN, 12
  relevant to nervous system dysfunction, 9–10. *See also* specific phenomena.
  vs. concept, 10
Phenomenology, 15–16
Phonation, 215
Physical examination, for sexual problem assessment, 467–468f
Physiologic responses, to acute pain, 398
Pick's disease, 227
Pinealomas, 30
Pituitary adenomas, 30
Pituitary gland, dysfunction, 30
Pituitary tumors, 368
Planning, 207–208
Pleasuring, sexual, 464
Pneumobelt, 331
Poisons, consciousness depression and, 69
Poliomyelitis, 36
Polymositis, 33
Polyneuropathies. *See* specific polyneuropathies.
Portable Short Mental Status Questionnaire (PSMSQ), 159
Position sense assessment, 370
Positive pressure devices, 331
Posterior fossa tumors, 29, 30. *See also* Astrocytomas.
Posttetanic potential theory, 143
Posttraumatic amnesia, 173
Postural drainage, 331, 332f
Posture, 294
Potassium, urinary, circadian rhythmn and, 118
Powerlessness, 262
PPQRST, 402, 403t
Prefrontal area
  hyperarousal and, 87f, 88
  unilateral lesions, 208
Premature ejaculation, 478, 479
Presence intervention, 50
Pressure sores
  developmental factors, 309
    environment related, 80–81
    patient related, 80
  prevention, 314
  risk patients, goals for nursing management, 81
  types, 80

Italicized letters following page numbers indicate tables (*t*) and figures (*f*).

Primary image, 204–205
Problem solving, impaired, 207
Process criteria, 502–503
Processing, central nervous system, impaired, 68–69
Processing of sensory input, 67
Proctosigmoidoscopy, 428
Progressive muscle relaxation, 42–43f
Prolactin, circadian rhythmn and, 118
Proprioception
 loss, injury potential and, 390
 patient interventions, 41–44f
Prosopagnosia, 196, 197
Protein
 development and, 139
 synthesis, REM sleep and, 117
 total brain, aging and, 152
Psychosocial implications
 of altered bowel elimination, 456
 of mobility, 297–299
Public education, 51
 for epilepsy, 111–112
 for stroke prevention, 316
Pulmonary embolism, immobility and, 307
PULSES, 284, 493, 495
Pupillary abnormalities, 368
Purposeful touch, 47–48

Quadriplegia
 case study, 435–436
 segmental disruption and, 304–305

Radiology, diagnostic assessment of elimination, 425–426
Rancho Los Amigos Levels of Cognitive Functioning Scale, 64, 89t
Rapid eye movement sleep
 rebound phenomenon, 117, 120
 sleep deprivation and, 119–120
Rathke's pouch, 29
Rational empiric studies, 16–17
Raynaud's disease, 412
Reasoning, definition of, 138
Receptive communicative and cognitive–linguistic deficits, 232–235
 assessment, 233–234
Receptive transmission disorders, 228
Receptors, sensory, 359–360, 361t
Rectal examination, 467, 468f
Referrals, 238
Reflexes, assessment of, 294–297t
Reflex neurogenic bowel, 444–446
Registration, 201

Reitan-Indiana Aphasia Screen, 158–159, 159–160
Relaxation techniques, 412
Reminiscence, 46
Remorse, 265
REM-triggering protein substance R, 121
Renin, 118
Research, descriptive phase, 15–17f
Resistive exercises, 313
Resources, inadequate, for long-term decreased arousal patients, 82–83
Respiration, speech production and, 215
Respiratory system
 assessment, 330
 depression, from narcotics, 406
 effects of immobility, 307–308
 interventions, for immobile patients, 312
 sleep-induced impairment, 125–126
Responsiveness
 altered levels, inappropriate behaviors and moods, 505
 decreased level of, 505
 heightened level of, 505
Rest and sleep
 activity intolerance, 514
 assessment parameters, 517
 sleep pattern disturbance, 514
Retarded ejaculation, 478, 479
Reticular activating system, 59–60f, 363
Reticular formation, 144f
Reticuloendothelial system, tumors, 29
Retina, 367–368
Retrograde amnesia, 145, 173
Reverberating circuit theory, 143
Rinne test, 371
Rocking bed, 312
Rods, 367
Role disturbance
 assessment, 105
 in epilepsy and syncope, 105
Role modeling, by nurse, 95
Roy Adaptation Model of Nursing, 187

Saddle sensation, 426
Safety measures, for hyperarousal, 90–93f
Scientific methods, in nursing, 15–17
Sclera, 367
Seeing. See Vision.
Segmental disorders, 321
Segmental neurons, disruption, 304–306
Segmental spinal cord organization, 275
Seizures
 definition of, 34–35
 fear of, during pregnancy, 102

Seizures (cont.)
    injury potential from, 102–103
    nursing roles in management, 112
    pathophysiology, 99–100
Self-actualization needs, 299
Self-care
    alterations, 489–498
        basic hygienic tasks, 492–494
        case study, 492–493
        independent living, 494–496
        orientation to healthy living, 496–498
        protective reflexes, 490–492
    assessment, 486
        in hyperarousal, 92
    components and assessment of, 485–486
    continuum of, 489–490f
    deficit, 506–507
        with decreased behavioral arousal, 79–80
        in hyperarousal, 92
        immobility and, 313
        interventions, in muscular dystrophy, 328–329
        in muscular dystrophy, 328–329
        scale, 92t
        total, 491–492
        with vision loss, 378–379
    relationship to nursing practice, 483–485
Self-concept
    mobility and, 297–298
    sexual, 459
        alterations in, 479–480
Self-perception, mobility and, 297–298
Senile plaques, 151
Sensate focus, 477
Sensation
    alteration, consequences of, 381–382
    assessment
        parameters, 516–517
        of somatic and special senses, 370–371
    central somesthetic sensory system, 363–366
    of chronic pain, 512–513
    deficits in, 194–196
    of genital and anal areas, 467–468f
    knowledge deficit in family and significant others, 514
    overview, 359–371
    peripheral, alteration in, 385–394
        causes of, 385–386
        pathologic causes, 386
    peripheral somesthetic sensory system, 359–363
    self-care deficit, 513
    somatic, altering conditions, 364–366

special senses. *See also* specific senses.
    alteration of, 373–383
    uncompensated sensory deficit, 512
Senses, human responses to alteration, 377–381
Sensorineural hearing loss, 367, 375
Sensory deprivation, 68
Sensory function
    age-related changes, 375t
    discrimination of, 370–371
Sensory information
    analysis of, 147–151
    definition of, 44–45, 408
    input, 59
    output, 60–61
    processing, 59–60f, 156
Sensory input, 67
    afferent, 362
Sensory interventions, 46–49
Sensory memory, 172–173
Sensory paralytic bowel, 449
Sensory–perceptual alterations
    assessment, 93
    goals for nursing management, 93
    in hyperarousal, 93
Septal complex, hyperarousal and, 87f, 88
Sequencing disorder, 209
Serotonin, 62, 461
Sexual behavior, drugs affecting, 473t–474t
Sexual desire
    alterations in, 471–472, 474
    aversion to sex, 471
    low, 471
Sexual dysfunctions
    altered sexual arousal, 474–477
    with chronic immobility, 334
    classification of, 471
    defining characteristics, 515
    human responses in, 471–481
    immobility and, 314
    orgasm alterations, 477–479
    outcome criteria, 515
    process criteria, 515
    self-concept alterations, 479–480
    sexual relationship alteration, 480–481
Sexual expression, movement and, 269
Sexual function, 459
Sexual health assessment, 466–468t
Sexuality
    aging and, 465–466
    alteration in sexual identity, 515
    assessing sexual health, 466–468t

Italicized letters following page numbers indicate tables (*t*) and figures (*f*).

assessment parameters, 517
dimensions and sexual health, 459
human development and, 459–466t
human sexual responses, 461, 463
knowledge deficit in partner, 515
variations in sexual expression, 463–465
Sexual problem, history, 466
Sexual relationships, 459
Sexual response
  desire phase, 461
  excitement phase, 463
Sexual self-concept
  alterations in, 479–480
  definition of, 459
Significant others. *See* Family; Friends.
Skeletal muscle, neurophysiology and neuroanatomy of movement, 270–272
Skin
  immobility, impairments with, 314
  impairment potential
    in nutritional and self-care deficits, 80–81
    in Parkinson's disease, 325
    in peripheral sensation alteration, 392
Sleep
  anatomic and biochemical correlates, 120–121
  arousal, normal alteration of, 62–63
  deprivation, 119–120
  duration, 119
  non-rapid eye movement, 116
  patterns, 117–120
    circadian sleep-wake cycle, 118–119
    physiologic and psychologic correlates, 115–117
    rapid eye movement (REM), 117
    slow wave or delta, 116
    wakefulness and, 115–116
Sleep apnea syndromes, 125–126
Sleep cycle, 117–118
Sleep disturbances, age and, 121–122
Sleep history, 124
Sleep hygiene, 129–132
Sleep-inducing factors, 121
Sleep log, 124
Sleep paralysis, 126–127
Sleep terrors, 129
Sleep–wake pattern disorders
  diagnostic classification, 123t
  excessive somnolence, 124–127
  human responses to, 121–132
  of initiating and maintaining sleep, 122, 124
  parasomnias, 129
  of sleep–wake schedule, 128–129
Sleep–wake pattern disturbances
  in hyperarousal, 93
  with peripheral sensation alteration, 392

Sleepwalking, 129
Slow wave sleep, 116
Smell, sense of
  altered, nutrition and, 382–383
  assessment of, 371
  description of, 369–370
  dysfunction, etiologies of, 376
Snellen eye chart, 371
Social group, self-care attainment and, 484
Social isolation
  with chronic immobility, 335–336
  in epilepsy, 104–105
Socialization, assessment of, 336
Social network intervention, 264–265
Social rejection, fear of, 101–102
Socioeconomic factors, 402
Somatic sensation, assessment, 370–371
Somatic stimuli, responses to, with decreased arousal, 81–82
Somatosensory agnosia, 197
Somesthetic cortex, 147–149
Somnabulism, 129
Sound stimuli, 366–367
Spastic dysarthria, 218
Spatial analysis, 199
Specialization in nursing, 4–5
Speech, mechanism, 215–216f
Speed of processing, 194
Spinal cord
  anterior, thrombosis of, 22
  axis III. *See* Axis III of the nervous system.
  posterior, ischemia or thrombosis of, 22
  segmental organization, 275
  tracts, 275
  tumors, 30–31
    extramedullary and intramedullary, 30
Spinal cord lesions
  incomplete, 364–365
  injury types, 34
  neurogenic bowel dysfunction
    autonomous neurogenic bowel, 446–448
    reflex neurogenic bowel, 444–446
  pathophysiology of, 306–307
  sexual response with, 475, 476t
  somatic sensation alteration and, 364
Spinal muscular atrophies, 27
Spinal nerves, 362
Spinal shock, 305–306
Spinocerebellar tract, 363
Spinothalamic tract, anterior or lateral, 362
Stercognosis, 371
Stigma, peripheral sensation alteration and, 393
Stimuli
  external, 59

Stimuli *(cont.)*
  internal, 59
  responsiveness to, 67. *See also* Arousal.
Stool
  content of, 422
  manual evacuation of, 448
Streptococcus pneumoniae, bacterial meningitis, 35
Stress
  progressive muscle relaxation for, 42–43*f*
  sleep and, 132
Stress ulceration, 445
Striate area, 368
Stroke. *See* Cerebrovascular accident.
Stroke volume, immobility and, 307
Subarachnoid hemorrhage, 20, 82
Subdural hematoma, 69
Superficial reflexes, 295*t*
Support groups, 95
Suppository, rectal, 454
Supramarginal gyrus dysfunction, 150–151
Suprasegmental disorders, 321
Suprasegmental neurons, disruption, 303–304
Swallowing
  assessment, 347–353*f*
    speech-communication disorders program, 352–357
  difficult
    behavioral manifestations of, 346–354*f*
    case study, 354–355
    nursing diagnoses, 355–356
  dysfunction
    with altered mobility, 345–356
    case study, 349
    ineffective airway clearance, 350
    nursing diagnoses, 350
    treatment guidelines, 348–349
  normal phases, 345–346
Sympathetic nervous system
  defecation and, 424
  micturation and, 422
Symptom Checklist-90, Revised (SCL-90-R), 157–158
Syncope
  causes of, 99
  injury potential from, 102–103
  role disturbance and, 105
Syndrome of inappropriate antidiuretic hormone (SIADH), 75
Syringomyelia, 365

Taste, sense of
  altered, nutrition and, 382–383
  assessment of, 371
  description of, 369
  dysfunction, etiology of, 376
Taylor Number Series, 159
Temperature
  ambient sleep, 130
  perception, assessment of, 370
Temporal information, 408
Temporal lobe, hyperarousal and, 87*f*, 88
Tendon receptors, 273–275
Teniae coli, 422
Tennessee Self-Concept Scale, 269
TENS, 411, 412
Tension, 257
Teratomas, 29
Testosterone, 460, 461
Tetanus, 36–37
Thalamic lesions, somatic sensation and, 365
Thalamotomy, 24
Thalamus, 364
Therapeutic touch, 46–47
Thermoreceptors, 360, 361*t*
Thinking, definition of, 137
Third-party payment, 485
Thought
  definition of, 137–138
  elaboration of, 151
Thought processes, alterations, in hyperarousal, 93
Throughput, 256
Thyroid hormone, development and, 139
Thyrotropin, circadian rhythmn and, 118
Tic douloureux (trigeminal neuralgia), 365
Timing, patient intervention and, 49
Tonic alertness deficit, 194
Tonic–clonic seizure, 100–103
Topographic disorientation, 197
Touch, sense of
  deficits, 376
  light, assessment of, 370
  purposeful, 47–48
  uncompensated deficits, 378*t*
Touch deprivation, 265–266
Toxic neuropathies, 386
Trail Making Test, 159
Transcortical sensory aphasia, 225
Transient ischemic attacks (TIA), 20
Transmission
  definition of, 218, 228
  disorders of, 219*t*
    characteristics, 220*t*
    expressive, 218–222

Italicized letters following page numbers indicate tables (*t*) and figures (*f*).

receptive, 222
Transportation, motorized scooter, 327f
Transportation, public, 317
Trauma, memory loss from, 173
Trendelenburg position, 331, 332f
Trigeminal nerve, 292–293
Trigeminal neuralgia, 365
Tropomyosin, 270
Troponin, 270
L-Tryptophan, 121
T-tubules, 271
Tumors
    classification of, 28–31
    incidence in central nervous system, 28
    olfactory, 369
Two-point discrimination, 371

Unilateral neglect, 191–192, 194
Ureters, 420
Urethra, 419, 420
Urgency
    from uninhibited neurogenic bladder, 432–433
    from uninhibited neurogenic bowel, 443
        case study, 443–444
Urinalysis, 425
Urinary elimination, immobility and, 313–314
Urinary frequency, 432–433
Urinary infection, clinical signs of, 438
Urinary retention
    with autonomous neurogenic bladder, 435–436
    with motor paralytic bladder, 436–437
    with sensory paralytic bladder, 437–438
Urinary system, anatomy, 420
Urine cultures, 425
Urodynamic evaluation, 426

Vagus nerve, 293
Valsalva maneuver, 436, 453
Vascular headache, 22–23
Vasocongestion
    alteration, 475–476
    in normal sexual response, 461, 463
Vegetative state, persistent, 82–83
Ventilation, monitoring, in CNS impaired patients, 76
Ventilatory support, 331
Verger-DeJerine syndrome, 365
Vibration, sense of

assessment of, 370
    loss, injury potential and, 390
Vigilance, 58, 63. *See also* Arousal.
Violence, potential, in hyperarousal, 93–94
Vision
    alteration, from ocular muscle weakness, 333–334
    anatomy and physiology, 367–368
    assessment, 333
    disorders of, 368
    impairment, neurologic disorders causing, 374–375
    loss, case study, 377–381
    motor component assessment, 290–292
    testing, 371
Visual acuity
    assessment, 371
    decreased, 378
Visual agnosia, 196
Visual cortex, disorders of, 149
Visual disturbances, 199–200
Visual field
    assessment, 371
    defects, 378
    definition of, 368
Visualization, 45
Visual pathway, 368
Vitreous body, 368
Vocal tract, points of articulation, 215–216f
Vocational rehabilitation programs, 316
Voiding, 419–422
Voiding history, 424

Wakefulness, 115–116
Walking, motor functioning assessment, 294–297t
Wallenberg syndrome, 22
Weakness, 320
Weber's test, 371
Wechsler Adult Intelligence Scale (WAIS), 158
Wechsler Memory Scale, 178
Werdnig-Hoffmann disease, 27
Wernicke's aphasia, 150, 223–224
Wernicke's area, 217
Wheelchairs, 278
White matter, 362–363
Wilson's disease, 221
Word blindness, 197
Workplace family, 249
Work schedules, sleep disturbed by, 128–129